METHODS IN MOLECULAR BIOLOGY

For further volumes:
http://www.springer.com/series/7651

Veterinary Infection Biology: Molecular Diagnostics and High-Throughput Strategies

Edited by

Mónica V. Cunha

Instituto Nacional de Investigação Agrária e Veterinária, Lisbon, Portugal

Centro de Biologia Ambiental, Faculdade de Ciências, Universidade de Lisbon, Lisbon, Portugal

João Inácio

Instituto Nacional de Investigação Agrária e Veterinária, Lisbon, Portugal

School of Pharmacy and Biomolecular Sciences, University of Brighton, United Kingdom

Humana Press

Editors
Mónica V. Cunha
Instituto Nacional de Investigação
Agrária e Veterinária
Lisbon, Portugal

Centro de Biologia Ambiental
Faculdade de Ciências, Universidade de Lisbon
Lisbon, Portugal

João Inácio
Instituto Nacional de Investigação
Agrária e Veterinária
Lisbon, Portugal

School of Pharmacy and Biomolecular Sciences
University of Brighton
United Kingdom

ISSN 1064-3745 ISSN 1940-6029 (electronic)
ISBN 978-1-4939-2003-7 ISBN 978-1-4939-2004-4 (eBook)
DOI 10.1007/978-1-4939-2004-4
Springer New York Heidelberg Dordrecht London

Library of Congress Control Number: 2014953901

Printed on acid-free paper

Humana Press is a brand of Springer
Springer is part of Springer Science+Business Media (www.springer.com)

Foreword

Infectious diseases of domestic and wild animals have a tremendous impact on the economy and public health worldwide. Sixty percent of the pathogens that cause diseases in humans have their source in animals (whether domestic or wild), as do 75 % of emerging human diseases and 80 % of the pathogens that potentially could be used in bioterrorism. Animal diseases that are transmissible to humans (collectively known as zoonoses), such as avian influenza, rabies, bovine tuberculosis, and brucellosis, represent a very relevant public health threat worldwide, being imperative to prevent and/or control them. Likewise, pathogens that are not zoonotic but have a negative impact on livestock production, and the associated financial income, should not be overlooked. Some estimates suggest that world production of food animals is reduced by more than 20 % due to disease, which may be particularly important in developing countries where the unavailability of animal protein is socially impacting and inevitably exacerbates infectious diseases risk.

The World Organization for Animal Health (OIE) was created in 1924 with the aim of controlling the international spread of infectious animal diseases, but currently, over and above this original mission, the new mandate is "*to improve animal health worldwide.*" The OIE builds its expertise on a global network of Reference Laboratories and Collaborating Centers that play an essential role in prevention, detection, surveillance, and control of animal diseases worldwide. Reference Laboratories serve as centers of scientific and technical expertise for official listed diseases and have particular responsibility for carrying out confirmatory diagnostic tests for these diseases. Collaborating Centers are centers of expertise in key competences related to the management of a particular animal health issue, such as epidemiology, diagnosis, risk analysis, welfare, or veterinary training. This global network of excellence enables OIE to remain at the forefront of world veterinary scientific expertise and successfully carry out its activities, providing authoritative scientific opinions and advice on key topics, such as animal health and welfare and diagnostic techniques. Moreover, the OIE is involved in the preparation of standards on diagnostic assays and their official validation which are published in the *OIE Terrestrial Manual* and *Aquatic Manual* and updated annually by the World Assembly of the Delegates of the OIE (available from www.oie.int).

The achievements of biotechnology are significantly contributing to the development of novel, rapid, and powerful diagnostic assays for animal diseases, namely based on molecular approaches, such as standard and real-time polymerase chain reaction and isothermal nucleic acid amplification methods. The recent advent of high-throughput sequencing technologies is also boosting the prompt detection of all microbes in a sample, uncovering novel pathogens and significantly advancing veterinary diagnostic microbiology. Furthermore, the analysis of single nucleotide and large sequence polymorphisms in the genome of pathogens provides novel information on their traits, such as virulence and antimicrobial resistance determinants, and supports epidemiological studies. Outstandingly, biotechnology is enabling the development of diagnostic kits that can ultimately be used in point-of-decision settings, away from centralized laboratories to assist in local decision-making, for instance during an outbreak. OIE is aware of the opportunities and challenges that these novel molecular-based approaches bring to veterinary diagnosis and several OIE Reference

Laboratories and Collaborating Centers are also dedicated to *Research and Development* activities on these fields. In this context, the present Springer's book on the use of molecular biology strategies in veterinary laboratory practice showcases the versatility of the veterinarian profession in meeting the challenges posed by the continuous advance of science, namely in the biotechnology field. The editors have succeeded in bringing together an impressive group of renowned collaborating authors, primarily veterinary doctors and researchers of veterinary science, from institutions with established and prized expertise in the fields of molecular biology and veterinary diagnostics, including several OIE Reference Laboratories and Collaborating Centers. This book provides therefore an excellent and authoritative overview of molecular biology strategies for pathogen detection and characterization, along with the most recent technological innovations and their potential to reconstruct transmission chains and to disclose pathogen biology, evolution, and interaction with the host. Beyond the techniques, the book also discusses the integration of these new molecular approaches in the framework of veterinary practice and animal health management. In recognition of the challenge faced by the public and private components of Veterinary Services and all veterinarians to improve the animal health status worldwide, this book may aid veterinary laboratories in setting up molecular diagnosis valences and is a valuable resource to veterinary doctors and laboratory technicians, researchers, and students of veterinary medicine and science interested in knowing more about these challenging, but promising molecular strategies to unravel animal infectious diseases.

Bernard Vallat

Director General
World Organization for Animal Health (OIE)

Preface

Infectious diseases of animals represent a significant economic burden to economies worldwide and may raise relevant Public Health concerns. Molecular diagnostics has emerged as the fastest growing and trending segment of the in vitro diagnostics industry and seems also promising in the veterinary sector, providing novel and powerful tools that enable the fast and accurate diagnosis of animal diseases.

In this book, we provide an overview of molecular biology tools for pathogen detection and characterization, along with potential applications to disclose pathogen biology and interaction with the host. In Part I, biobanking, biosafety and good laboratory practices, biological specimen collection and processing, quality assurance and control, and validation of molecular diagnostic assays for veterinary use are concisely introduced as a basis for the molecular strategies enclosed in protocol sections. The significance and integration of molecular biology methods in the framework of veterinary practice are discussed, along with a SWOT analysis presenting our view on the advantages, limitations, opportunities and weaknesses, or challenges, of these approaches. The rationale is on the techniques and applications rather than the pathogen or disease models. Part II is dedicated to the molecular detection and identification of animal pathogens using a wide range of established techniques and covering, also, emerging diagnosis approaches. A brief overview of the advances on nanoscience and microfluidics is provided, including a discussion on how the recent developments in these research fields may be translated into field deployable biosensors. Part III addresses genotyping tools for assessing the genetic landscape and epidemiology of pathogens. Part IV introduces integrative omics and high-throughput technologies as powerful research tools, yielding massive amounts of information that may ultimately improve the control and management of infectious diseases. We strived to span a broad range of molecular approaches, from simple and affordable to emerging and sophisticated, which we anticipate will be useful for veterinary doctors and laboratory technicians, researchers, and students of veterinary medicine and science.

Lisbon, Portugal

Mónica V. Cunha
João Inácio

Acknowledgements

The editors were supported by Fundacão para a Ciência e Tecnologia (FCT, Portugal) through projects PTDC/CVT/111634/2009 (JI) and PTDC/CVT/117794/2010 and in the framework of Projecto 3599—Promover a Produção Científica e Desenvolvimento Tecnológico e a Constituição de Redes Temáticas (MVC). Alice Santos (INIAV IP, Lisbon, Portugal) is acknowledged for the cover image artwork. The authors of Chap. 17 are acknowledged for providing the fluorescence microscopy image used in the artwork.

Contents

Contributors

AHMED AHMED • *WHO/FAO/OIE and National Collaborating Centre for Reference and Research on Leptospirosis, Department of Biomedical Research, Royal Tropical Institute (KIT), Amsterdam, The Netherlands*

SANDRA ANTUNES • *Instituto de Higiene e Medicina Tropical, Universidade Nova de Lisboa, Lisbon, Portugal*

ALICIA ARANAZ • *Departamento de Sanidad Animal, Facultad de Veterinaria, Universidad Complutense de Madrid, Madrid, Spain*

MARIA BALLESTER • *Centre de Recerca en Sanitat Animal (CReSA), UAB-IRTA, Campus de la Universitat Autònoma de Barcelona, Bellaterra (Cerdanyola del Vallès), Spain; Centre de Recerca en Agrigenòmica (CRAG), Consorci CSIC-IRTA-UAB-UB, Bellaterra, Spain; Departament de Ciència Animal i dels Aliments, Facultat de Veterinària, Universitat Autònoma de Barcelona, Bellaterra, Spain*

KRISTIANE BARINGTON • *Department of Veterinary Disease Biology, Faculty of Health and Medical Sciences, University of Copenhagen, Frederiksberg C, Denmark*

CARRIE BATTEN • *The Pirbright Institute, Surrey, UK*

SÁNDOR BELÁK • *OIE Collaborating Centre for the Biotechnology-based Diagnosis of Infectious Diseases in Veterinary Medicine, Swedish University of Agricultural Sciences (SLU), Uppsala, Sweden; Department of Biomedical Sciences and Veterinary Public Health (BVF), Swedish University of Agricultural Sciences (SLU), Uppsala, Sweden; The National Veterinary Institute (SVA), Uppsala, Sweden*

THOMAS BJARNSHOLT • *Department of International Health, Immunology and Microbiology, Costerton Biofilm Center, Faculty of Health and Medical Sciences, University of Copenhagen, Frederiksberg C, Denmark; Department of Clinical Microbiology, Copenhagen University Hospital, Copenhagen, Denmark*

STEVEN VAN BORM • *Veterinary and Agrochemical Research Center, Brussels, Belgium*

ANA BOTELHO • *Instituto Nacional de Investigação Agrária e Veterinária IP, Lisbon, Portugal*

METTE BOYE • *National Veterinary Institute, Technical University of Denmark, Kongens Lyngby, Denmark*

BRONWYN E. CAMPBELL • *Department of Veterinary Science, The University of Melbourne, Parkville, VIC, Australia*

CINZIA CANTACESSI • *Department of Veterinary Science, The University of Melbourne, Parkville, VIC, Australia*

ANA CANTO • *Instituto Nacional de Investigação Agrária e Veterinária IP, Lisbon, Portugal*

ANA CLÁUDIA CARREIRA • *iMed.UL—Research Institute for Medicines and Pharmaceutical Sciences, Nanomedicine & Drug Delivery Systems Group, Faculdade de Farmácia, Universidade de Lisboa, Lisbon, Portugal; Instituto Nacional de Investigação Agrária e Veterinária, I.P. (INIAV, I.P.), Lisbon, Portugal*

LÉLIA CHAMBEL • *Centro de Biodiversidade, Genómica Integrativa e Funcional, Faculdade de Ciências, Universidade de Lisboa, Lisbon, Portugal*

STEFANO CINOTTI • *Cell Culture CentreA, Istituto Zooprofilattico Sperimentale della Lombardia e dell'Emilia Romagna (IZSLER), Brescia, Italy*

PEDRO COSTA • *Instituto Nacional de Investigação Agrária e Veterinária IP, Lisbon, Portugal; Instituto de Higiene e Medicina Tropical, Universidade Nova de Lisboa, Lisbon, Portugal*

ISABEL COUTO • *Instituto de Higiene e Medicina Tropical, Universidade Nova de Lisboa, Lisbon, Portugal*

MÓNICA V. CUNHA • *Instituto Nacional de Investigação Agrária e Veterinária IP, Lisbon, Portugal; Centro de Biologia Ambiental, Faculdade de Ciências, Universidade de Lisbon, Lisbon, Portugal*

SYLVIANE DERZELLE • *Bacterial Zoonosis Unit, Animal Health Laboratory, University Paris-Est, Anses, Maisons-Alfort, France*

ANA DOMINGOS • *Centro de Malária e Outras Doenças Tropicais; Instituto de Higiene e Medicina Tropical, Universidade Nova de Lisboa, Lisbon, Portugal*

SILVIA DOTTI • *Cell Culture Centre, Istituto Zooprofilattico Sperimentale della Lombardia e dell'Emilia Romagna (IZSLER), Brescia, Italy*

MANSOUR EL-MATBOULI • *Clinical Division of Fish Medicine, University of Veterinary Medicine, Vienna, Austria*

MAURA FERRARI • *Cell Culture Centre, Istituto Zooprofilattico Sperimentale della Lombardia e dell'Emilia Romagna (IZSLER), Brescia, Italy*

ANA S. FERREIRA • *Instituto Nacional de Investigação Agrária e Veterinária IP, Lisbon, Portugal*

LUÍS FONSECA • *Department of Bioengineering, Instituto Superior Técnico (IST), Institute for Biotechnology and Bioengineering (IBB), Centre for Biological and Chemical Engineering, Lisbon, Portugal*

GRAHAM FREIMANIS • *The Pirbright Institute, Pirbright, UK*

JOACHIM FREY • *Institute of Veterinary Bacteriology, Vetsuisse Faculty, University of Bern, Bern, Switzerland*

LORRAINE FROST • *The Pirbright Institute, Surrey, UK*

JOSÉ DE LA FUENTE • *SaBio, Instituto de Investigación en Recursos Cinegéticos IREC, UCLM-JCCM, Ciudad Real, Spain; Department of Veterinary Pathobiology, Center for Veterinary Health Sciences, Oklahoma State University, Stillwater, OK, USA*

ALICE FUSARO • *Istituto Zooprofilattico Sperimentale delle Venezie, Padova, Italy*

GIULIANO GAROFOLO • *Istituto Zooprofilattico Sperimentale dell'Abruzzo e del Molise "G. Caporale"—National and OIE Reference Laboratory for Brucellosis, Teramo, Italy*

ROBIN B. GASSER • *Department of Veterinary and Agricultural Sciences, The University of Melbourne, Parkville, VIC, Australia; Institute of Parasitology and Tropical Veterinary Medicine, Berlin, Germany*

JACINTO GOMES • *Instituto Nacional de Investigação Agrária e Veterinária IP, Lisbon, Portugal*

FREDRIK GRANBERG • *OIE Collaborating Centre for the Biotechnology-based Diagnosis of Infectious Diseases in Veterinary Medicine, Swedish University of Agricultural Sciences (SLU), Uppsala, Sweden; Department of Biomedical Sciences and Veterinary*

Public Health (BVF), Swedish University of Agricultural Sciences (SLU), Uppsala, Sweden

IRENE R. GRANT • *Institute for Global Food Security, School of Biological Sciences, Queen's University Belfast, Northern Ireland, UK*

RUDY A. HARTSKEERL • *WHO/FAO/OIE and National Collaborating Centre for Reference and Research on Leptospirosis, Department of Biomedical Research, Royal Tropical Institute (KIT), Amsterdam, The Netherlands*

ANDREAS HOFMANN • *Structural Chemistry Program, Eskitis Institute, Griffith University, Brisbane, QLD, Australia*

DIRK HÖPER • *Friedrich Loeffler Institut—Federal Research Institute for Animal Health, Riems (Greifswald), Germany*

ANA HURTADO • *Department of Animal Health, NEIKER—Instituto Vasco de Investigación y Desarrollo Agrario, Bizkaia, Spain*

JOÃO INÁCIO • *Instituto Nacional de Investigação Agrária e Veterinária IP, Lisbon, Portugal; School of Pharmacy and Biomolecular Sciences, University of Brighton, Brighton, UK*

HENRIK ELVANG JENSEN • *Department of Veterinary Disease Biology, Faculty of Health and Medical Sciences, University of Copenhagen, Frederiksberg C, Denmark*

LOUISE KRUSE JENSEN • *Department of Veterinary Disease Biology, Faculty of Health and Medical Sciences, University of Copenhagen, Frederiksberg C, Denmark*

AARON R. JEX • *Faculty of Veterinary and Agricultural Sciences, The University of Melbourne, Parkville, VIC, Australia*

OSKAR E. KARLSSON • *OIE Collaborating Centre for the Biotechnology-based Diagnosis of Infectious Diseases in Veterinary Medicine, Swedish University of Agricultural Sciences (SLU), Uppsala, Sweden; Department of Biomedical Sciences and Veterinary Public Health (BVF), Swedish University of Agricultural Sciences (SLU), Uppsala, Sweden*

DONALD P. KING • *The Pirbright Institute, Pirbright, UK*

JOSEPH KOZLOVAC • *United States Department of Agriculture (USDA), Agricultural Research Service (ARS), Office of National Programs, Beltsville, MD, USA*

PETER KUHNERT • *Institute of Veterinary Bacteriology, Vetsuisse Faculty, University of Bern, Bern, Switzerland*

CÉLIA LEÃO • *Instituto Nacional de Investigação Agrária e Veterinária IP, Lisbon, Portugal*

MIKAEL LEIJON • *OIE Collaborating Centre for the Biotechnology-based Diagnosis of Infectious Diseases in Veterinary Medicine, Uppsala, Sweden; The National Veterinary Institute (SVA), Uppsala, Sweden*

LIHONG LIU • *OIE Collaborating Centre for the Biotechnology-based Diagnosis of Infectious Diseases in Veterinary Medicine, Uppsala, Sweden; The National Veterinary Institute (SVA), Uppsala, Sweden*

TINA LOMBARDO • *Cell Culture Centre, Istituto Zooprofilattico Sperimentale della Lombardia e dell'Emilia Romagna (IZSLER), Brescia, Italy*

PETRA MOEBIUS • *Institute of Molecular Pathogenesis at Friedrich-Loeffler-Institut (Federal Research Institute for Animal Health), Jena, Germany*

ISABELLA MONNE • *Istituto Zooprofilattico Sperimentale delle Venezie, Padova, Italy*

RICHARD ORTON • *Institute of Biodiversity, Animal Health and Comparative Medicine, University of Glasgow, Glasgow, UK*

Chris Oura • *School of Veterinary Medicine, University of the West Indies, St. Augustine, Trinidad and Tobago*

Marina Popara • *SaBio, Instituto de Investigación en Recursos Cinegéticos IREC, UCLM-JCCM, Ciudad Real, Spain*

Susanne Elisabeth Pors • *Department of Veterinary Disease Biology, Faculty of Health and Medical Sciences, University of Copenhagen, Frederiksberg C, Denmark*

Fernando Rodriguez • *Centre de Recerca en Sanitat Animal (CReSA), UAB-IRTA, Campus de la Universitat Autònoma de Barcelona, Bellaterra (Cerdanyola del Vallès), Spain*

Florian Roeber • *Faculty of Veterinary and Agricultural Sciences, The University of Melbourne, Parkville, VIC, Australia; AusDiagnostics Pty. Ltd., Beaconsfield, NSW, Australia*

Toon Rosseel • *Veterinary and Agrochemical Research Center, Brussels, Belgium*

Anke Ruettger • *Institute of Molecular Pathogenesis at Friedrich-Loeffler-Institut (Federal Research Institute for Animal Health), Jena, Germany*

Konrad Sachse • *Institute of Molecular Pathogenesis at Friedrich-Loeffler-Institut (Federal Research Institute for Animal Health), Jena, Germany*

Mona Saleh • *Clinical Division of Fish Medicine, University of Veterinary Medicine, Vienna, Austria*

Susan Sanchez • *Athens Veterinary Diagnostic Laboratory, College of Veterinary Medicine, The University of Georgia, Athens, GA, USA*

Ilda Santos-Sanches • *Centro de Recursos Microbiológicos, Departamento de Ciências da Vida, Faculdade de Ciências e Tecnologia, Universidade Nova de Lisboa, Lisbon, Portugal*

Nick Saunders • *Public Health England (PHE), Microbiology Services Colindale, London, UK*

Beverly Schmitt • *United States Department of Agriculture (USDA), Animal and Plant Health Inspection Service, National Veterinary Services Laboratories, Ames, Iowa, USA*

Christiane Schnee • *Institute of Molecular Pathogenesis at Friedrich-Loeffler-Institut (Federal Research Institute for Animal Health), Jena, Germany*

Holly Sellers • *Poultry Diagnostic and Research Center, College of Veterinary Medicine, The University of Georgia, Athens, GA, USA*

Ian Sharp • *Public Health England (PHE), Microbiology Services Colindale, London, UK*

Hatem Soliman • *Clinical Division of Fish Medicine, University of Veterinary Medicine, Vienna, Austria; Fish Medicine and Managements, Department of Animal Medicine, Faculty of Veterinary Medicine, Assiut University, Assiut, Egypt*

Linda D. Stewart • *Institute for Global Food Security, School of Biological Sciences, Queen's University Belfast, Northern Ireland, UK*

Fernando Teles • *Laboratory of Mycology/Microbiology Unit and Centre for Malaria and Tropical Diseases (CMDT), Institute of Hygiene and Tropical Medicine (IHMT), Universidade Nova de Lisboa (UNL), Lisbon, Portugal*

Rogério Tenreiro • *Centro de Biodiversidade, Genómica Integrativa e Funcional, Faculdade de Ciências, Universidade de Lisboa, Lisbon, Portugal*

SIMON THIERRY • *Bacterial Zoonosis Unit, Animal Health Laboratory, University Paris-Est, Anses, Maisons-Alfort, France*
BERNARD VALLAT • *World Organization for Animal Health (OIE), Paris, France*
RICCARDO VILLA • *Cell Culture Centre, Istituto Zooprofilattico Sperimentale della Lombardia e dell'Emilia Romagna (IZSLER), Brescia, Italy*
MARGARITA VILLAR • *SaBio, Instituto de Investigación en Recursos Cinegéticos IREC, UCLM-JCCM, Ciudad Real, Spain*
MIGUEL VIVEIROS • *Instituto de Higiene e Medicina Tropical, Universidade Nova de Lisboa, Lisbon, Portugal*

Part I

Introducing Nucleic Acid Testing in the Veterinary Laboratory

Chapter 1

Overview and Challenges of Molecular Technologies in the Veterinary Microbiology Laboratory

Mónica V. Cunha and João Inácio

Abstract

Terrestrial, aquatic, and aerial animals, either domestic or wild, humans, and plants all face similar health threats caused by infectious agents. Multifaceted anthropic pressure caused by an increasingly growing and resource-demanding human population has affected biodiversity at all scales, from the DNA molecule to the pathogen, to the ecosystem level, leading to species declines and extinctions and, also, to host-pathogen coevolution processes.

Technological developments over the last century have also led to quantic jumps in laboratorial testing that have highly impacted animal health and welfare, ameliorated animal management and animal trade, safeguarded public health, and ultimately helped to "secure" biodiversity. In particular, the field of molecular diagnostics experienced tremendous technical progresses over the last two decades that significantly have contributed to our ability to study microbial pathogens in the clinical and research laboratories. This chapter highlights the strengths, weaknesses, opportunities, and threats (or challenges) of molecular technologies in the framework of a veterinary microbiology laboratory, in view of the latest advances.

Key words Molecular diagnostics, Veterinary microbiology, Nucleic acid testing, Animal health, Animal welfare, Public health, Biodiversity, Validation, In-house, Molecular assays, Quality assurance, Quality control

1 Introduction

Active and passive surveillance of infectious diseases in farmed and wild animals enable the detection of (re)emergent pathogens and the monitoring of endemic and/or zoonotic diseases and, ultimately, back up stakeholders, supporting national and international policies aimed at the protection of animal health and welfare, food security and public health, and the trade of animals and animal products. During recent years, the world has witnessed the emergence or reemergence of a number of major animal diseases such as foot-and-mouth disease (FMD), bluetongue, classical swine fever (CSF), and avian influenza, which are emblematic examples of the overwhelming economic, social, and public health impacts that animal diseases may cause. Effective surveillance and control of animal

Mónica V. Cunha and João Inácio (eds.), *Veterinary Infection Biology: Molecular Diagnostics and High-Throughput Strategies*, Methods in Molecular Biology, vol. 1247, DOI 10.1007/978-1-4939-2004-4_1, © Springer Science+Business Media New York 2015

diseases require a rapid and accurate detection of the etiological agent by the use of effective diagnostic tests. Veterinary microbiology laboratories play a fundamental role in this context, the main purposes being the detection, identification, and characterization of any pathogenic organisms present in a diverse range of biological samples, such as tissues, blood, urine, and other fluids collected from suspect animals. The characterization of the microorganisms may include drug susceptibility testing and genotyping of the isolates for epidemiological purposes, which is essential to track sources and routes of infection, as well as for pathogen population studies. The direct observation by optical microscopy of biological samples, usually stained by different processes, may give a first indication of the presence of a microorganism. Histopathological examination of hematoxylin-eosin-stained paraffin-embedded tissues may also give indications on the infectious disease and the putative agent, thus potentially complementing the diagnostic algorithm. However, the confirmation of an infection usually involves the isolation of the causative agent(s), followed by identification through additional phenotypic tests. Also widely used are immunological-based diagnostic methods relying on the specific binding between antigens and antibodies. These methods allow detecting the presence of antibodies produced in response to an antigen, or the presence of an antigen, through various experimental formats, such as agglutination tests, immunofluorescence, and ELISA. All these laboratory diagnostic approaches are based on the analyses of phenotypic characteristics of the microorganisms and can be designated as traditional, classical, or conventional methods. In contrast, the so-called molecular diagnostics methods detect or analyze, in the majority of the cases, genotypic characteristics of the microorganisms, such as the presence of certain genes or their respective polymorphisms. In this context, it is possible to identify the microorganisms at different taxonomic levels, from domain to species, and even down to intraspecific levels, through the analysis of genes or other genome regions. Moreover, relevant information can be obtained about pathogenic microorganisms by the analysis of molecular determinants encoding virulence factors (e.g., toxins) or conferring antimicrobial resistance. Importantly, in this field are the availability, appropriateness, and accuracy of diagnostic and phenotypic characterization tests to avoid selective pressure from unnecessary or erroneous antimicrobial use during therapy.

The field of molecular diagnostics experienced tremendous technological developments in the last two decades that have contributed significantly to our ability to study microbial pathogens in the clinical laboratory. Molecular methods have thus been taking an increasingly important role, supporting, complementing, and, in some cases, even replacing the conventional methods. This chapter highlights some of the strengths, weaknesses, opportunities, and threats (or challenges) of molecular technologies designed for the diagnosis of infectious diseases in animals.

2 Molecular Diagnostics Market

Molecular diagnostics appears as one of the highest growth segments within the overall in vitro diagnostics (IVD) market, which is currently estimated at approximately € 36,000 million, and is fourth in terms of sales behind the segments of immunology, blood glucose tests, and clinical chemistry [1]. The market for molecular diagnostics thus passed from a nonexistent dimension in 1990 to over € 3,000 million in 2011, with a forecast of € 4,980 million for 2016 [1], corresponding to a compound annual growth rate (CAGR) of almost 11 %. In this segment, nearly two thirds of the market value corresponds to the use of molecular tests for the diagnosis of infectious diseases and to the study of their agents (approximately € 1,950 million in 2011), including sales of reagents, equipments, services, products for extraction of nucleic acids, and other consumables. Of this amount, approximately € 1,155 million (59 %) is dedicated to the diagnosis of viral diseases, with a particular emphasis on real-time PCR-based tests. The remaining amount corresponds mainly to the diagnosis of bacterial infections, with particular emphasis for microorganisms such as *Chlamydia trachomatis*, *Neisseria gonorrhoeae*, methicillin-resistant *Staphylococcus aureus* (MRSA), and *Clostridium difficile*. The market for molecular diagnostics of fungal agents and other eukaryotic parasites is still very small.

The overall veterinary IVD market is a fraction of that of the human market and was recently estimated at € 2,064 million (in 2013), with a forecast of € 3,030 million in 2018, representing a CAGR of about 8 % [2]. The market is mainly driven by the growing incidences of disease outbreaks and of zoonotic diseases, the increasing companion animal market (backed up by the rise in the adoption of pets), the increase in the disposable incomes in developing countries, and a rising demand for clinical diagnostic tests specifically designed for food-producing animals (in order to meet the demand for safe meat and dairy products and the increasing number of livestock) [2]. The majority of sales occur in the United States (45 %) and Europe (30 %), but the demand for veterinary diagnostic tests is steadily growing in the Asia-Pacific and Latin American countries. The main segments of the veterinary IVD market are clinical chemistry, immunodiagnosis, and hematology, with the fourth position corresponding to the molecular diagnostics, with a total market value estimated at around € 292 million. This last figure should increase to approximately € 500 million in 2018 [2].

3 Brief Overview of Molecular Technologies in the Veterinary Microbiology Laboratory

Molecular methods have two main applications in the veterinary microbiology laboratories. Firstly, and probably the most common, these methods are used as tools to identify, characterize, and genotype the microorganisms following their culture and isolation from samples. Secondly, these methods can be used to detect pathogen nucleic acids directly in the biological samples, allowing working with inactivated materials, thereby reducing the risk of environmental contamination and occupational infection when the pathogens are also zoonotic. The molecular diagnostics technologies comprise basically two main strategies: the hybridization and the amplification of nucleic acids, although many systems based on the amplification include additional steps of hybridization to identify the amplified products.

The direct hybridization with labeled DNA probes allows the identification of microorganisms cultured from biological samples and, in some cases, the direct detection of their presence in those samples. Among the firstly described applications of nucleic acid hybridization methods in the veterinary context, we find, for example, the detection of bovine herpesvirus type 1 in bovine exudates [3] and of *Trypanosoma evansi* in infected blood samples [4]. In a more recent example, the hybridization with specific complementary DNA probes has allowed the discrimination between *Streptococcus* species associated with mastitis in cattle [5]. Despite their high specificity, the applications based on the direct hybridization of nucleic acids were never really adopted for the clinical routine diagnosis, since they are very labor-intensive, costly, and slow. Additionally, these applications usually have a reduced sensitivity since a high number of target DNA copies must be present in the sample. To circumvent this difficulty, in vitro cultivation may yield a high number of the target microorganisms, bringing an additional limitation in cases where the handling of large quantities of viable pathogens is not recommended.

The most used nucleic acid amplification technology in veterinary microbiology laboratories is, undoubtedly, the polymerase chain reaction (PCR), introduced in the mid-1980s [6]. Reverse transcriptase PCR was also introduced at that time, allowing producing copies of DNA from RNA templates [7]. Among the first applications of PCR in the veterinary field, we find examples for the detection of porcine herpesvirus type I (causing Aujeszky disease) [8]; of *Neorickettsia risticii* (formerly, *Ehrlichia risticii*) [9], implicated in the Potomac horse fever; of the equine herpesvirus type 1 [10], responsible for respiratory, neurological, and abortion problems in horses; of *Toxoplasma gondii* in sheep [11]; and of *Babesia* and *Theileria* parasites in cattle [12], among others. There are currently thousands of published works describing the use of PCR-based methods to detect, identify, and characterize pathogenic microorganisms of veterinary relevance, these methods being particularly useful for the study of fastidious organisms that are difficult or impossible to cultivate in artificial media, such as viruses and bacteria of the genera *Brucella*, *Mycobacterium*, *Rickettsia*, and *Chlamydia*, among many others. An important landmark that greatly contributed to the accumulation and popularity of molecular technologies in diagnostic laboratories, including the veterinary context, was the introduction of the real-time PCR in the mid-1990s [13, 14], enabling the detection of amplified nucleic acids as they are being synthesized. This technology also allows quantifying the number of copies of template nucleic acids present in a sample, useful, for example, to estimate viral loads, to monitor the success of antimicrobial therapies, and to potentially discriminate infection, colonization, or contamination of the samples. The technology of real-time PCR has been widely exploited to support the diagnosis of viral diseases, of which many are notifiable to the World Organisation for Animal Health (OIE), such as FMD, CSF, and bluetongue [15]. Many other applications have also been developed to detect veterinary-relevant bacteria, such as particular ecotypes within the *Mycobacterium tuberculosis* complex species [16] and eukaryotic parasites, such as *Theileria annulata* [17].

Among the strategies for nucleic acid amplification are also worthy of note those based on isothermal processes. For example, the technology of nucleic acid sequence-based amplification (NASBA) has been used to develop diagnostic tests for several viruses with single-stranded RNA genomes, such as the FMD virus [18]. In another example, the technology of loop-mediated isothermal amplification (LAMP) has gained increasing interest in recent years for the use in molecular diagnostics tests, and there are also several references within a veterinary context, for example, for the detection of the CSF virus [19], the FMD virus [20], and species of *Brucella* [21].

The DNA fragments amplified by PCR or by other technology of nucleic acid amplification can also be analyzed by hybridization with DNA probes immobilized on solid supports (reverse hybridization), such as nylon or nitrocellulose membranes, glass, or other materials. The reverse hybridization technology on nylon or nitrocellulose membranes has been used, for example, to detect and identify species of *Babesia* and *Theileria* directly from blood samples of cattle [22, 23], and to genotype *Mycobacterium bovis* and other veterinary-relevant tuberculous mycobacteria by spoligotyping [24, 25]. Several systems are currently commercialized that may enable a differential diagnosis result within hours. High-density systems for reverse hybridization have been also developed, commonly known as microarrays, allowing the simultaneous analysis of hundreds to thousands of different genomic targets in the same assay. Microarrays are particularly useful for studies of gene expression, and, although still very expensive, some applications have also been described for the detection and identification of veterinary-relevant pathogens such as *Mycoplasma* spp. [26].

Nucleic acid sequencing has also become common for microbiological diagnostic laboratories due to the rapid technological developments in this field and the consequent reduction of associated costs. The sequencing of certain genes or other genomic regions amplified by PCR enables to easily identify and genotype the microorganisms, by using, for example, multilocus sequence typing (MLST) approaches [27]. The more recent introduction of the next-generation sequencing and metagenomics technologies has, among other applications, allowed the discovery and characterization of newly emerging or unknown pathogens, independently from culture, excellent examples being the identification of the Schmallenberg virus [28] that recently affected cattle in Europe, or the recognition of viruses that affect bees [29].

4 SWOT Analysis of Molecular Diagnostics Technologies

The available information in the literature on the development and application of molecular diagnostics methods is profuse, including the description of methods for the detection and identification of veterinary-relevant pathogens causing diseases listed by the OIE. However, relatively few molecular methods in the form of widespread tests or diagnostic services have been successfully arriving to the IVD market and seldom have been adopted officially by national and international veterinary authorities as reference methods for a particular animal infection or disease. The use of molecular tests turns out to be optional in most laboratories, being used only when the classical diagnostic methods do not allow a satisfactory response [30]. Despite the great advantages normally associated with molecular diagnostics technologies, for example, in terms of specificity and sensitivity, accuracy, and speed of response, laboratories face several challenges in the implementation and use of these methods and, sometimes, in the interpretation of the clinical relevance of the results. In Table 1, we detail our view on the most relevant strengths, current weaknesses, opportunities, and threats, or challenges, associated with molecular diagnostics technologies, possibly contributing to a better comprehension of the current state of the art of the IVD segment in the context of veterinary diagnosis and to outline some clues regarding the future.

The implementation and use of molecular methods is usually more expensive when compared to the classic microbiological diagnostic tests, since they usually require a relatively sophisticated laboratory infrastructure and equipments, and reagents and consumables are also typically more costly. In addition, the procedures may be more demanding and/or have increased complexity, in particular to prevent the occurrence of cross-contamination that may lead to false-positive results, which in turn require more specialized technical personnel. However, the simplification and increasing automation of various procedures have been contributing to a greater integration of molecular diagnostics methods in

Table 1
SWOT analysis of molecular diagnostics technologies in the veterinary microbiology laboratory

Strengths	Weaknesses
• Overall higher analytical and diagnostic sensitivities and specificities, higher accuracy, and shorter time-to-result • Suitable for the analysis of a large number of samples (e.g., *high sample throughput in automated systems*) • Suitable for the detection of a wide range of pathogens, at different taxonomic levels (e.g., *virus, bacteria, fungi, protozoa, and other eukaryotic parasites; detects fastidious microorganisms and those that cannot be cultured*) • Allow the discovery and characterization of newly emerging or unknown pathogens (e.g., *broad-range PCR assays or metagenomics*) • Can be also used after the starting of antimicrobial therapy (*results not affected by the presence of antimicrobials in samples*) • Eventual delays in sample collection, transport, and storage have less effects on the final result (*DNA is a very stable molecule*) • Suitable for identifying antimicrobial resistance and highly virulent strains (*by targeting the respective trait-associated genes*) • Possibility to detect several pathogens or respective genetic traits simultaneously (*multiplexing capability, allowing to obtain more information per single test, at a lower cost*) • Suitable for the direct analysis of a wide range of biological samples (e.g., *tissues, blood, and other fluids; nucleic acids of the pathogens can be detected directly in the samples, allowing to work with inactivated materials*) • Possibility of quantification of target nucleic acids in samples (e.g., *to assess viral load in the blood, to discriminate between infection, colonization, and contamination, to guide treatments, and to monitor progress of disease*) • High discriminatory power for microorganisms typing (e.g., *to track sources of infection, assess transmission chains and epidemiology studies*) • Molecular data is easily shared using public databases online, and a wide range of bioinformatics tools for analysis is available	• Higher costs for establishing a molecular biology laboratory (*including facilities, equipments, and skilled technicians*) • Comparatively more expensive reagents and consumables (*also usually requiring more costly transportation and storage conditions, such as a cold chain*) • Usually requires technically complex procedures (*with meticulous following of effective standard operating procedures and quality control; accuracy, reproducibility, and reliability of some assays may depend on the expertise of the technician and of other factors such as instruments calibration and batch-to-batch variation of reagents*) • Higher potential for the occurrence of false-positive results (e.g., *due to specimen contamination by target nucleic acids*) • Higher potential for the occurrence of false-negative results (e.g., *related to the difficulty of extracting pathogens nucleic acids from some specimens or to the presence of inhibitors of amplification reactions*) • Nucleic acid detection may not always prove involvement in infectious processes (e.g., *in active* vs. *latent infections, asymptomatic animal carriers, and opportunistic pathogens members of the normal microbial flora*) • Nucleic acid detection cannot usually differentiate between viable and nonviable microorganisms (*unless the molecular target is, for example, messenger RNA, which is more technically demanding*) • Single use of molecular techniques does not allow archiving of samples for future study (e.g., *microorganisms are not normally isolated in pure culture, which can limit epidemiological surveillance*)

(continued)

Table 1 (continued)

Opportunities	Threats
• molecular diagnostics is one of the highest growth segments within the IVD market • Rising demand for clinical diagnostic tests for food-producing and companion animals • Less strict regulations in the veterinary IVD sector can promote a more rapid adoption of new technologies (*when compared with the human IVD sector*) • Professional guidelines and educational efforts to disseminate molecular diagnostics and data interpretation • Increasing automation of molecular diagnostic assays (*contributing to a greater integration in diagnostic laboratories, making also possible the remote analysis, and lowering the cost per test*) • Demand for diagnostic tests for use in the point of decision (e.g., *directly at farms, slaughterhouses, or local veterinary clinics and laboratories*) • Demand for the development of simple, efficient, and fast nucleic acid extraction and purification assays • Novel technologies becoming more mature for the development of alternative molecular diagnostic tests (e.g., *microfluidics and nanotechnology; biosensors*) • Novel applications and increasing affordability of next-generation sequencing approaches (e.g., *metagenomics*) • Increased amounts of gene and genome sequences information in publicly available databases • Some expertise in classical diagnostic methods is disappearing (e.g., *expertise in virus culture and electronic microscopy*)	• Pressure to keep a low cost per analysis in the veterinary field (*which is more pronounced in the livestock segment than in the companion animal segment, including pets and horses; may limit a more widespread adoption of molecular diagnostics technologies*) • Lack of harmonization between the molecular tests used among different laboratories (*which may yield contradicting results, also related with different levels of exigency in the implementation of these tests*) • Clear algorithms for the use and interpretation of the medical relevance of molecular results may be difficult to establish (*standards for reporting molecular data and respective interpretative criteria need to be established for most infectious diseases*) • Conservatism of the medical personnel in the adoption and prescription of new diagnostics technologies (*also associated with the usually little importance given to molecular diagnostics technologies in veterinary medical curricula*) • Difficulty in assessing reference materials and good gold standard methods to validate molecular tests

clinical laboratories. With the currently available technology, it is now possible to process and extract nucleic acids from hundreds of samples and proceed to analysis for defined genetic markers in less than a working day. Thus, the ability of molecular-based methods to analyze hundreds or thousands of samples in a short time, and a greater speed to reach the final results (also potentially contributing to limit the use of unnecessary empirical antimicrobial therapies), may generate substantial savings, making these technologies more competitive in terms of cost per analysis. An earlier detection of the infectious agents in diseased or carrier animals may also limit the spread of these pathogens to neighbor animals (and even to humans) and improve the overall quality of the veterinary service.

Another important aspect is related to the sensitivity of molecular methods. It is widely recognized that the analytical sensitivity of these methods is extremely high, particularly in those based on the amplification of nucleic acids, often being possible to detect the presence of a single copy of the target nucleic acid in the reaction mixture. In contrast, the performance of molecular methods may become unsatisfactory for the detection of nucleic acids directly from samples, yielding false-negative results. A problem still largely unsolved concerns the processes of extraction and purification of nucleic acids from biological samples (e.g., blood or tissues). The extraction and purification of microbial nucleic acids from some biological matrices prove to be complicated, due to the intrinsic characteristics of the agents (e.g., difficulty to lyse cell walls, such as in bacteria from the *Mycobacterium tuberculosis* complex), due to the presence of a much higher proportion of nucleic acids from host animals, or related to the presence of inhibitory compounds in the nucleic acid extracts that may affect the success of the amplification reactions [16]. Protocols for the extraction of nucleic acids, including several steps of mechanical, chemical, or enzymatic lysis, and several purification steps can be efficiently used in research, but are not practical or are too expensive for routine use. Thus, the availability of efficient, consistent, and reproducible nucleic acid extraction processes adapted for difficult biological matrices, yet affordable and simple to use, is still an unmet need that has hindered the widespread routine use of molecular methods in the veterinary microbiology laboratory. The consistency of the extraction process becomes even more critical if the aim involves the quantification of the pathogenic agents in the samples.

Another major challenge of molecular diagnostics lies in the lack of harmonization of the operational procedures used among different laboratories, which contrasts greatly with the situation of conventional diagnostic methods, whose use is very standardized. In veterinary medicine, molecular tests are largely designed in-house and implemented locally in different laboratories, as there are fewer commercial diagnostic kits available (also due to the smaller IVD market). Thus, to detect the same agent in the same type of sample, laboratories may use different methods for the extraction of nucleic acids and/or discrepant primer sequences and/or diverse amplification conditions. Consequently, the comparison of results among different laboratories is complicated and may even be contradictory, an illustrative example being the discrepant results for the PCR-based diagnosis of feline immunodeficiency virus (FIV) infection in cats by different laboratories using parallel samples [31]. The level of optimization and exigency in the implementation of molecular diagnostics methods varies greatly from laboratory to laboratory, from those that simply reproduce a particular system that has been described elsewhere in the literature, offering little quality control to those who effectively conduct a technical validation and quality control of the methods, assessing their specificity, sensitivity, and positive and negative predictive values, among other features.

Important in this context is the availability of reference materials and adequate gold standard diagnostic methods to validate and assess the performance of molecular tests. International agencies, such as the OIE, are making efforts to alert for the need for international standardization and validation of molecular tests for the use in veterinary microbiology laboratories and are making available relevant guidelines and procedures toward that aim. Nevertheless, since there is currently no major regulatory validation hurdles for the marketing of veterinary molecular diagnostic tests for infectious diseases, veterinarians and technicians must keep themselves informed and be smart buyers of these tests or services [32].

Perhaps one of the major challenges with regard to the molecular diagnostics technologies is precisely the interpretation of the clinical relevance of a positive or negative test. A negative result, which may indicate the absence of the agent, should always be interpreted considering the limitations of the specificity and sensitivity of the molecular test since, as mentioned above, false-negative results may occur, for example, due to the inefficiency of the nucleic acid extraction methods. With respect to the positive tests, the interpretation could be considered straightforward, for example, in cases where the presence of a particular pathogenic agent implies the occurrence of disease. However, a positive amplification result does not always mean that the agent is present in the sample in a viable state. The agent may be dead or nonviable, or there may be only remnants of nucleic acids (e.g., in animals that began therapy or when the agents have been successfully eliminated by the immune system) [33]. An interesting but yet unanswered question for different infectious diseases is how long the nucleic acid of causal agent may remain detectable in the samples after treatment and/or recovery of the animals. In other cases, nucleic acid detection may not mean that the animal is effectively ill, for example, in cases of latent infections, in asymptomatic carrier animals, in hosts in equilibrium with the agent, and when dealing with ubiquitous microorganisms. The vaccination of animals may also interfere with the performance or interpretation of molecular diagnostics assays, the detection of FIV in vaccinated cats being a good illustrative example of this limitation [31]. Moreover, when the disease is caused by opportunistic pathogens belonging to the normal microbial flora of animals, the interpretation of a positive molecular test also becomes more difficult, being necessary to differentiate between colonization and active infection. Veterinary doctors and technicians should be aware of the enhanced accuracy and speed of molecular tests for the diagnosis of infections but also to understand their limitations. Thus, clear algorithms for the use of molecular tests must be settled for each disease (and eventually for each animal species), establishing the appropriate specimen to collect, the suitable timing for collection, and the proper test to use, namely, regarding qualitative versus quantitative response, and whether it is fit for purpose (i.e., fulfills the needs of the situation). The clinician should be aware of the pathogenesis of each pathogen and collect the most adequate sample for its detection since the analysis of the wrong sample type is a common mistake leading to false-negative results [34]. A clear reporting of molecular data by diagnostic laboratories, an effective communication between the laboratory and the clinical settings, and clear interpretative criteria for the results have also to be established, requiring well-designed clinical studies. Molecular results should be analyzed considering the limitations of the techniques, the epidemiological context, and, preferably, where appropriate, in complement to the classical methods in a search for various relevant phenotypic and genotypic characteristics of the agents. Ultimately, the veterinarian should bring together all these results within the context of the set of clinical signs and symptoms exhibited by the suspect animal(s), to reach a final diagnosis.

Very few studies attempted to investigate the need for education in the field of molecular diagnostics technologies among veterinary practitioners. As an example, a recent survey assessed the knowledge and clinical use of PCR-based diagnostics in equine practice by diplomates of the American College of Veterinary Internal Medicine [34]. Noteworthy, the results of this study mostly express our own perception on the level of existing knowledge about these technologies and its applications in the general veterinary community. Although the majority of the surveyed veterinarians reported being familiar with the principles of nucleic acid amplification, just over half of respondents knew the difference between standard and real-time PCR. Most of these professionals also reported to regularly submit samples to specialized laboratories for the PCR detection of pathogens. However, this study found surprising that blood was the most commonly submitted sample, given that the majority of respiratory, enteric, and neurologic equine pathogens are not detectable in the peripheral blood [34]. Particularly relevant, this survey found that specialized information about molecular diagnostics is not routinely accessible to practicing veterinarians, and most of these professionals emphasized the need for an improved and continuing education on these technologies. Professional guidelines and educational efforts should be therefore increasingly developed to disseminate the best practices in molecular diagnostics and data interpretation and directed to all the people in the diagnostic chain, from the owner, farmer, or professional that collects the sample to the person that reports the result and the veterinarian that has to make an enlighten evidence-based decision.

During easily transmitted and economically impacting disease outbreaks, such as FMD, the early detection of infection is particularly important but is often impractical to test all the samples in centralized reference laboratories. Moreover, in many regions of the globe, even the veterinary reference laboratories may not be adequately equipped to face these threats. In this context, the availability of diagnostic methods for use in the point of decision (e.g., directly at farms, slaughterhouses, or local veterinary clinics or laboratories) is particularly relevant and is forecasted to represent a major opportunity for the IVD market. Molecular diagnostics methods generally are not applicable in these circumstances, requiring the use of sophisticated and expensive equipments operated by skilled technicians. The increasing availability of portable thermal cyclers may be potentially useful for a wider use of molecular technologies, allowing their implementation closest to the regions where outbreaks occur (e.g., in regional laboratories or in the field) [15]. The use of isothermal technologies for the amplification of nucleic acids, such as LAMP, may also prove useful in this context because of its lesser requirement for sophisticated equipments. The detection of amplified products by electrophoresis is not practical outside the laboratory, but disposable strips for lateral flow detection of nucleic acids are also already commercially available [19]. Other fields experiencing great developments are microfluidics and nanotechnology. The procedures normally required for the molecular detection of pathogens in biological samples, including cell lysis, extraction of nucleic acids, amplification of specific genomic targets, and their detection, can all potentially be integrated into autonomous miniaturized microfluidic systems, enabling the development of molecular diagnostics devices (commonly referred to as lab-on-a-chip), which can be used in the point of decision [35–40]. Nanotechnologies have also sparked interest in the development of new diagnostic tests, including molecular tests, taking advantage of the unique properties that many materials exhibit at the nanoscale [41, 42]. Biosensors based on these technologies are likely to eliminate the need for any steps of extraction and amplification of nucleic acids from samples [42], and several prototypes were recently described in the literature for the detection of viruses and bacteria.

5 Conclusion

The unprecedented growth of human population, increasingly demanding for more food supplies and animal protein, changes in land use, globalization, industrialization, deforestation, and climate change, among others, have cumulatively and irreversibly affected biodiversity at all scales, from the DNA molecule to the ecosystem level. All animals, either domestic or wild, and humans face similar health challenges imposed by pathogenic agents. Over the last century, laboratorial tests had a tremendous impact on animal health and welfare, contributing to ameliorate animal management and animal trade, helping to protect public health, and ultimately helping to minimize biodiversity loss. The growing technological innovations in molecularly based tests have contributed to more rapid pathogen detection results and to the certification of the sanitary status of animal or animal groups, to increase our understanding of the epidemiology of pathogens, to support their control and eradication, and to provide guidance to policy makers. On a more fundamental perspective, molecular technologies have also been crucial to increase our understanding on pathogen biology, including interaction and coevolution with the host and, also, on xenobiotic (including antimicrobial drugs) resistance.

Unquestionably, molecular technologies have broadened up the scope of veterinary diagnostics and will be increasingly used for the rapid diagnosis and study of the pathogenesis and epidemiology of infectious diseases. It is likely that in the near future, as has happened in recent years, molecular methods will replace some currently used classical diagnostic tests, providing significant improvements in specificity, sensitivity, and speed of responses. However, the pathogenicity of a microorganism is a complex phenomenon resulting from mechanisms and interactions at the genomic, regulatory, and expression levels. Thus, a complete picture of the characteristics of a microorganism, especially those relevant for their pathogenicity and interaction with their hosts, can hardly be achieved only on the basis of the analysis of their genome. The real added value of molecular technologies will be their complementarily use with conventional microbiological tests, properly integrated in a laboratorial diagnostic and research algorithm, allowing the collection and analysis of multivariate phenotypic and genotypic characteristics of pathogenic microorganisms.

Acknowledgments

This work was supported by Fundacão para a Ciência e Tecnologia (FCT) through projects PTDC/CVT/111634/2009 and PTDC/CVT/117794/2010 and in the framework of Projecto 3599—Promover a Produção Científica e Desenvolvimento Tecnológico e a Constituição de Redes Temáticas.

References

1. Hughes MD (2013) Molecular diagnostics, market trends and outlook. Enterprise Analysis Corporation (www.eacorp.com), Stamford, United States
2. Anonymous (2014) Veterinary diagnostics market by products (clinical chemistry, hematology analyzers, molecular diagnostics, immunodiagnostics, diagnostics imaging), by animals (companion, food-producing, dog, livestock, poultry, swine): global forecast to 2018. Markets and Markets, Dallas, United States (*Executive Summary*)
3. Dorman MA, Blair CD, Collins JK et al (1985) Detection of bovine herpesvirus 1 DNA immobilized on nitrocellulose by hybridization with biotinylated DNA probes. J Clin Microbiol 22:990–995
4. Viseshakul N, Panyim S (1990) Specific DNA probe for the sensitive detection of *Trypanosoma evansi*. Southeast Asian J Trop Med Public Health 21:21–27
5. Almeida A, Albuquerque P, Araújo R, Ribeiro N, Tavares F (2013) Detection and discrimination of common bovine mastitis-causing streptococci. Vet Microbiol 164:370–377
6. Saiki RK, Scharf S, Faloona F et al (1985) Enzymatic amplification of beta-globin genomic sequences and restriction site analysis for diagnosis of sickle cell anemia. Science 230:1350–1354
7. Kawasaki ES, Clark SS, Coyne MY et al (1988) Diagnosis of chronic myeloid and acute lymphocytic leukemias by detection of leukemia-specific mRNA sequences amplified in vitro. Proc Natl Acad Sci U S A 85:5698–5702
8. Belák S, Ballagi-Pordány A, Flensburg J et al (1989) Detection of pseudorabies virus DNA sequences by the polymerase chain reaction. Arch Virol 108:279–286
9. Biswas B, Mukherjee D, Mattingly-Napier BL et al (1991) Diagnostic application of polymerase chain reaction for detection of *Ehrlichia risticii* in equine monocytic ehrlichiosis (Potomac horse fever). J Clin Microbiol 29:2228–2233
10. Ballagi-Pordány A, Klingeborn B, Flensburg J et al (1990) Equine herpesvirus type 1: detection of viral DNA sequences in aborted fetuses with the polymerase chain reaction. Vet Microbiol 22:373–381
11. Wheeler R, Wilmore H, Savva D et al (1990) Diagnosis of ovine toxoplasmosis using PCR. Vet Rec 126:249
12. Figueroa JV, Chieves LP, Johnson GS et al (1992) Detection of *Babesia bigemina*-infected carriers by polymerase chain reaction amplification. J Clin Microbiol 30:2576–2582
13. Heid CA, Stevens J, Livak KJ et al (1996) Real time quantitative PCR. Genome Res 6: 986–994
14. Williams PM (2009) The beginnings of real-time PCR. Clin Chem 55:833–834
15. Hoffmann B, Beer M, Reid SM et al (2009) A review of RT-PCR technologies used in veterinary virology and disease control: sensitive and specific diagnosis of five livestock diseases notifiable to the World Organisation for Animal Health. Vet Microbiol 139:1–23
16. Costa P, Ferreira AS, Amaro A et al (2013) Enhanced detection of tuberculous mycobacteria in animal tissues using a semi-nested probe-based real-time PCR. PLoS One 8:e81337
17. Santos M, Soares R, Costa P et al (2013) Revisiting the Tams1-encoding gene as a species-specific target for the molecular detection of *Theileria annulata* in bovine blood samples. Ticks Tick Borne Dis 4:72–77
18. Lau LT, Reid SM, King DP et al (2008) Detection of foot-and-mouth disease virus by nucleic acid sequence-based amplification (NASBA). Vet Microbiol 126:101–110
19. Chowdry VK, Luo Y, Widén F et al (2014) Development of a loop-mediated isothermal amplification assay combined with a lateral flow dipstick for rapid and simple detection of classical swine fever virus in the field. J Virol Methods 197:14–18
20. Yamazaki W, Mioulet V, Murray L et al (2013) Development and evaluation of multiplex RT-LAMP assays for rapid and sensitive detection of foot-and-mouth disease virus. J Virol Methods 192:18–24
21. Pérez-Sancho M, García-Seco T, Arrogante L et al (2013) Development and evaluation of an IS711-based loop mediated isothermal amplification method (LAMP) for detection of *Brucella* spp. on clinical samples. Res Vet Sci 95:489–494
22. Gubbels JM, de Vos AP, van der Weide et al (1999) Simultaneous detection of bovine *Theileria* and *Babesia* species by reverse line blot hybridization. J Clin Microbiol 37: 1782–1789
23. Gomes J, Soares R, Santos M et al (2013) Detection of *Theileria* and *Babesia* infections amongst asymptomatic cattle in Portugal. Ticks Tick Borne Dis 4:148–151
24. Kamerbeek J, Schouls L, Kolk A et al (1997) Simultaneous detection and strain differentiation of *Mycobacterium tuberculosis* for diagnosis and epidemiology. J Clin Microbiol 35: 907–914

25. Matos F, Cunha MV, Canto A, Albuquerque T, Amado A, Botelho A (2010) Snapshot of *Mycobacterium bovis* and *Mycobacterium caprae* infections in livestock in an area with a low incidence of bovine tuberculosis. J Clin Microbiol 48:4337–4339
26. Schnee C, Schulsse S, Hotzel H et al (2012) A novel rapid DNA microarray assay enables identification of 37 *Mycoplasma* species and highlights multiple *Mycoplasma* infections. PLoS One 7:e33237
27. Boonsilp S, Thaipadungpanit J, Amornchai P et al (2013) A single multilocus sequence typing (MLST) scheme for seven pathogenic *Leptospira* species. PLoS Negl Trop Dis 7:e1954
28. Hoffmann B, Scheuch M, Höper D et al (2012) Novel orthobunyavirus in Cattle, Europe, 2011. Emerg Infect Dis 18:469–472
29. Granberg F, Vicente-Rubiano M, Rubio-Guerri C et al (2013) Metagenomic detection of viral pathogens in spanish honeybees: co-infection by Aphid Lethal Paralysis, Israel Acute Paralysis and Lake Sinai Viruses. PLoS One 8:e57459
30. Hunt PW (2011) Molecular diagnosis of infections and resistance in veterinary and human parasites. Vet Parasitol 180:12–46
31. Crawford PC, Slater MR, Levy JK (2005) Accuracy of polymerase chain reaction assays for diagnosis of feline immunodeficiency virus infection in cats. J Am Vet Med Assoc 226:1503–1507
32. Daniels JB (2013) Molecular diagnostics for infectious disease in small animal medicine: an overview from the laboratory. Vet Clin North Am Small Anim Pract 43:1373–1384
33. Duarte MD, Henriques AM, Santos-Barros S et al (2013) Snapshot of viral infections in wild carnivores reveals ubiquity of Parvovirus and susceptibility of Egyptian mongoose to Feline Panleukopenia Virus. PLoS One 8:e59399
34. Pusterla N, Mapes S, Leutenegger CM (2006) Survey of the large-animal diplomates of the American College of Veterinary Internal Medicine regarding knowledge and clinical use of polymerase chain reaction: implications for veterinary education. J Vet Med Educ 33: 605–611
35. Bearinger JP, Dugan LC, Baker BR et al (2011) Development and initial results of a low cost, disposable, point-of-care testing device for pathogen detection. IEEE Trans Biomed Eng 58:805–808
36. Beyor N, Seo TS, Liu P et al (2008) Immunomagnetic bead-based cell concentration microdevice for dilute pathogen detection. Biomed Microdevices 10:909–917
37. Kim J, Johnson M, Hill P et al (2009) Microfluidic sample preparation: cell lysis and nucleic acid purification. Integr Biol (Camb) 1:574–586
38. Wen J, Legendre LA, Bienvenue JM et al (2008) Purification of nucleic acids in microfluidic devices. Anal Chem 80:6472–6479
39. Heo J, Hua SZ (2009) An overview of recent strategies in pathogen sensing. Sensors (Basel) 9:4483–4502
40. Ahmad F, Hashsham SA (2012) Miniaturized nucleic acid amplification systems for rapid and point-of-care diagnostics: a review. Anal Chim Acta 733:1–15
41. Jain KK (2003) Nanodiagnostics: application of nanotechnology in molecular diagnostics. Expert Rev Mol Diagn 3:153–161
42. Kaittanis C, Santra S, Perez JM (2010) Emerging nanotechnology-based strategies for the identification of microbial pathogenesis. Adv Drug Deliv Rev 62:408–423

Chapter 2

Significance and Integration of Molecular Diagnostics in the Framework of Veterinary Practice

Alicia Aranaz

Abstract

The field of molecular diagnostics in veterinary practice is rapidly evolving. An array of molecular techniques of different complexity is available to facilitate the fast and specific diagnosis of animal diseases. The choice for the adequate technique is dependent on the mission and attributions of the laboratory and requires both a knowledge of the molecular biology basis and of its limitations.

The ability to quickly detect pathogens and their characteristics would allow for precise decision-making and target measures such as prophylaxis, appropriate therapy, and biosafety plans to control disease outbreaks. In practice, taking benefit of the huge amount of data that can be obtained using molecular techniques highlights the need of collaboration between veterinarians in the laboratory and practitioners.

Key words Molecular diagnostics, PCR, RT-PCR, Veterinary clinical microbiology, Pathogens

1 Introduction

Molecular techniques, fueled by polymerase chain reaction (PCR), have revolutionized the diagnostics in veterinary practice. Molecular approaches are now widely accepted for identification of etiological agents and in many cases have replaced traditional systems based on the more cumbersome phenotypic identification. Several assays are currently described for the detection and identification of many pathogens of the *OIE-listed diseases* and other *diseases of importance to international trade*. However, compared to serological techniques, molecular assays are still officially recommended as prescribed tests only for a limited number of diseases, when concerning the international trade and movement of animals and animal products (http://www.oie.int/en/international-standard-setting/terrestrial-manual).

The development of molecular methods has provided new tools for enhanced surveillance and outbreak detection, and this may result in better implementation of infection control programs. Benefits of using molecular diagnostics are clear in terms of time to

Mónica V. Cunha and João Inácio (eds.), *Veterinary Infection Biology: Molecular Diagnostics and High-Throughput Strategies*, Methods in Molecular Biology, vol. 1247, DOI 10.1007/978-1-4939-2004-4_2, © Springer Science+Business Media New York 2015

result and accuracy; however, laboratories also face several challenges when implementing molecular diagnostic assays, related with throughput, quality control, direct use on clinical samples, or difficulties for the definition of gold standards to assess the techniques. The aim of this chapter is to give an overview of the general uses of molecular techniques in routine work of veterinary diagnostics and to discuss some of their limitations.

2 Basic Approaches in the Laboratory

In the past 20 years, international research efforts have provided an exponential knowledge on pathogen genomic sequences and the availability of molecular technologies of different complexity. This knowledge has resulted in powerful tools that enable the rapid and specific diagnosis of animal diseases [1, 2]. The practical relevance of these techniques is directly related to the problems that the pathogens pose in the laboratory; the more fastidious the pathogen, or noncultivable, the more useful will be the molecular technique. However, for some fast-growing pathogens, biochemical characterization using commercial automated systems is still a valuable tool. Accordingly, molecular techniques are of paramount importance for diagnosis of viral diseases and for some serious bacterial pathogens, such as brucellae, mycobacteria, and rickettsiae, which take considerable time to grow in vitro and/or require specific culture media or cell culture systems, and are not adequate for wide-scale culture-based diagnosis. Moreover, additional time is required for the biochemical or serological identification of the isolates. It is also known that false-negative culture results may occur. To overcome these limitations, efforts have focus on the PCR amplification of nucleic acids directly extracted from clinical specimens or environmental samples. Extensive research and use of these techniques have increased our knowledge of pathogens and epidemiology of the diseases.

Molecular diagnosis of diseases caused by main pathogens of veterinary interest can be applied following two main approaches:

1. Coupled to conventional microbiological culture to identify bacterial or fungal isolates, or cell culture in the case of viruses, replacing the more cumbersome biochemical or serological identification. This requires only a step to inactivate the pathogen and to prepare the nucleic acids that will work as template for the amplification reactions. In many instances, the suspension of the colonies in distilled sterile water and simple boiling is enough for DNA extraction, being suited for laboratories even with minimum resources.
2. Direct detection of the pathogen's nucleic acids in clinical specimens (e.g., tissues, feces, body fluids, and swabs). In this case, the direct detection presents the advantage of rapidity

(which can mean saving up to several months) and the possibility to work with inactivated material, so reducing the risk of laboratory hazards (important when pathogens are also zoonotic). However, the direct detection of pathogen's nucleic acids in clinical samples requires the use of improved DNA/RNA extraction methods. Although amplification-based assays are extremely sensitive when used on microbial cultures, its sensitivity may drop when directly applied to samples eventually containing inhibitors. Protocols requiring many steps involving mechanical, chemical, and enzymatic disruption of microbial cells, or involving commercially available DNA/RNA extraction and purification kits, may be useful and efficient for research activities but may not be adequate or be cost-prohibitive when handling a large number of samples with routine diagnostic purposes, as during disease outbreaks (high pressure to analyze many samples in the minimum period of time) or surveillance (high number of samples during an extended period of time). Furthermore, the use of automated work stations that handle several samples at a time may not be available in resource-limited laboratories. The effectiveness of every nucleic acid extraction protocol depends on the matrix (i.e., type of clinical sample) and the pathogen and needs to be adjusted for each specific combination.

3 Level of Information

Most molecular diagnosis approaches currently used in the routine veterinary laboratory rely in the PCR and its variants, such as nested-PCR and real-time PCR. The performance of these assays mainly depends upon the primers used, which are usually a pair of short oligonucleotide fragments complementary to flanking regions of the target sequence and that will specifically anneal to the microbial genetic material present in the sample. The laboratory can design *in-house* PCRs based on previously well-characterized and validated genomic targets and primers sequences available in scientific publications and online databases. Otherwise, the laboratory staff would need to select novel targets and to design appropriate primers (free software can be downloaded and used for this purpose). Ideally, the primers should be 100 % specific and, at the same time, should detect all variants that are being "hunted"; this may require a balance between the use of conserved and of highly variable genetic regions as complementary targets for those primers. Depending on the primer design strategy, molecular tests can allow the identification of the etiological agents further than the species level, such as distinct groups (lineages) with a characteristic geographic spread, for instance, the *Mycobacterium bovis* clonal complexes [3] or the *Brucella melitensis* groups [4]. The possibility of designing own primers allows to focus diagnosis on local needs and priorities but will require further experimental optimization of the PCR-based reactions in every laboratory. Nevertheless, an increasing number of commercial kits to detect pathogens have become available; some diagnostic kits are certified by the OIE as fit for purpose.

Regarding the number of distinct sequence targets that are detected per amplification reaction, there are two strategies: the use of a single target (singleplex) or of several targets (multiplex). The latter strategy involves the use of multiple different pairs of primers in the same PCR, usually yielding amplification products with distinct lengths. Multiplexing allows for an increased workflow and reduced cost and has been used mainly with the two following objectives:

1. To identify pathogens to the species, or even to the strain level using, e.g., specific genes, genetic regions, or insertion sequences, or specific nucleotide polymorphisms, as complementary targets. Examples are the tests to distinguish the classical *Brucella* species and vaccine strains [5] and to identify the biovars of *B. suis* [6], using standard gel electrophoresis to assess the amplification results, or the test for ruminant *Mycoplasma* spp. using a bead-based liquid suspension array [7].
2. To allow the simultaneous detection of multiple pathogens in a same specimen. This option may be used in a syndromic approach, i.e., to identify the etiology of diseases caused by different pathogens but with similar clinical signs or pathological findings, such as the simultaneous detection of *Chlamydia* spp., *Coxiella burnetii*, and *Neospora caninum* in abortion material from ruminants [8]; the detection of *C. burnetii* and *N. caninum* in equine-aborted fetuses and neonates [9]; and the diagnosis of *Brucella ovis*, *Actinobacillus seminis*, and *Histophilus somni* infection in ram semen [10, 11], among many other examples. In combination with reverse transcription PCR (RT-PCR), this multiplex strategy is being used to detect endemic and different transboundary porcine viruses [12–14]. There is a trend to multiplexing, aiming to develop syndrome-specific assays targeting multiple candidate agents, but the design of the assays needs to be evaluated experimentally in order to check that test sensitivities do not significantly decrease when compared to singleplex testing.

Molecular techniques can be also applied to identify "clones." PCR-based techniques such as multilocus variable-number tandem repeat analysis (MLVA) are less demanding and less time-consuming than other previously used methods, such as the analysis of restriction fragment length polymorphisms (RFLP) or pulse-field gel electrophoresis (PFGE), and provide results that can easily be compared between laboratories. Results obtained with the implementation of these techniques (called molecular epidemiology) may be combined with classical epidemiology to understand the dynamics of an infection and to design control measures.

These results can be worked out with phylogenetic purposes as well. A variety of PCR-based methods have been used, involving, e.g., the study of the presence or absence of large pieces of DNA, called regions of difference (RD) or large sequence polymorphisms (LSPs), which are expected to represent unidirectional evolution events, and of single nucleotide polymorphisms (SNPs), which are fast to test and less prone to homoplasy. As an example, these genomic targets have been used to delineate the phylogeny of the members of the *Mycobacterium tuberculosis* complex [15, 16].

Whole-genome sequencing is becoming affordable and applied to accumulate information on the biology of known pathogens or to disclose novel emerging pathogens. Analysis of complete genomes, or representative parts of the genome, can reveal the probable chain of transmission events and demonstrate the value of such techniques in providing information useful to control programs, as it has been done with the genetic analysis of the complete genome of the foot-and-mouth virus in the last outbreak in the UK [17]. In a near future, application of whole-genome sequencing analysis will offer definitive information about each pathogen.

The detection of unknown pathogens has been possible using broad-based primers with degenerate sequences. A most recent approach consists of a combination of nonspecific amplification and extensive sequencing. This approach requires a sound knowledge of taxonomy and genomics [18]. Furthermore, these new technological trends provide with an enormous amount of data that must be mined by bioinformatics. As an example, the use of a metagenomics approach allowed to identify the Schmallenberg virus, a novel orthobunyavirus that affected cattle in Europe in 2011 [19].

4 The Technique That Is Best Suited for the Laboratory

The choices for the most adequate molecular techniques and equipments are dependent on the mission and attributions of the laboratory. Several methods of nucleic acid amplification have been developed, and some of them are now common in veterinary diagnostics. Thermal cyclers to perform basic PCRs have become compact, easy to use, and (relatively) affordable equipments present in almost every diagnostic infrastructure. PCRs are frequently used in combination with an electrophoretic transfer cell to analyze the molecular weight of the amplified products. Additionally, laboratories may have an imaging system and software for gel documentation.

The success of PCR-based assays relies on its performance and versatility but also in the ease of use and affordability. Standard PCR requires the use of crucial reagents including dNTPs, a thermostable DNA polymerase and the respective buffer, and a pair of well-designed primers to make millions of copies of the deoxyribonucleic acid target in a couple of hours. In theory, the number of copies could reach 2^n, where n is the number of rounds of denaturing-annealing-extension steps. The amplified product (amplicon) can be detected by simple electrophoresis on an agarose gel and staining with a fluorescent dye (e.g., SYBR® Green) that preferentially binds to double-stranded DNA. An internal molecular weight ladder is run at the same time in the gel to estimate the size of the amplicons. The presence of the amplicon of the defined size (in base pairs) indicates the presence of the target DNA and, therefore, of the pathogen. An alternative system of detection consists on reverse hybridization where amplicons are denatured and allowed to hybridize with specific probes (single-stranded DNA) that are immobilized on a membrane strip. Subsequently, bound products may be detected, e.g., using an alkaline phosphatase reaction and a colorimetric detection assay. This system can detect sequences and specific point mutations in a gene and is commonly used to detect genotypes or pathogens (species identification, presence of toxin genes and of other virulence factors), as well as resistances to drugs.

Nested PCR implies the use of two rounds of amplifications with a second set of primers that anneal in a shorter region of the amplicon product from the first round of amplification. This method increases sensitivity and can also increase specificity; the disadvantage is the increased risk of DNA carryover and subsequent potential occurrence of false-positive results.

Detection of ribonucleic acid (RNA) requires a reverse transcription reaction to synthesize a complementary DNA copy which will be subsequently amplified using conventional PCR. Reverse transcription PCR (RT-PCR) is used for gene expression analysis and detection of viral RNA [20].

Real-time PCR enables the amplification and quantification of the amount of specific nucleic acid sequences in the template sample. It has been implemented in many laboratories because the equipment to perform real-time PCR has become reasonably priced, taking into account the array of possibilities it offers. Reactions are carried out in closed tubes, and results are monitored based on fluorescence generated by intercalating dyes or by different fluorophore-labeled probes; fluorescence is proportional to amplification with optimum performance within a defined area of the amplification curve. Readings are detected automatically, and analysis is performed using ad hoc software. Current apparatus can monitor several fluorescence signals (channels) in a single tube. This allows single-tube closed tests, so this format also decreases the problem of contamination. For these reasons, this technique is best suited for routine testing of a large number of samples. Another benefit over conventional endpoint detection is that this technique allows for quantification of target sequences (qPCR); the number of amplification cycles that are required to generate product to cross a threshold cycle (C_t) correlates with the quantity (or copy number) of target sequences in the sample. Real time can be combined with reverse transcription (RT-qPCR or rRT-PCR); a major advantage of this technique is the detection of viral RNA. Several good examples are described for livestock diseases that are notifiable to the OIE, e.g., for foot-and-mouth disease, bluetongue, and classical swine fever, among many others [14, 20]. In humans, this has also been used for monitoring treatment efficacy in some infections.

Microarrays can be used to detect the presence of genes or polymorphisms from the organisms under study or used to detect the presence of pathogens, depending on the design. This technique consists of an array of a large number of specific oligonucleotide probes (complementary to target sequences) spotted on the surface of a solid support ("microchip"); complementary DNA (usually amplified DNA) is hybridized onto it and detected with fluorescent dyes, and then signals are measured and analyzed using specific software. DNA arrays have been exploited to study infectious processes of pathogens, for diagnostics, and to study host-pathogen interactions [21]. This technique is still costly and not affordable for all potential users.

Other techniques, such as fluorescence in situ hybridization (FISH), are restricted to research and are more time-consuming, or under study, and may become popular in the future.

5 Limitations of the Molecular Techniques

The main problems that can affect the performance of PCR-based technologies are the occurrence of false-positive and false-negative results, comparison to gold standards, and interpretation [20, 22]. Awareness of potential problems and control of the underlying causes result in higher confidence and acceptance of the techniques.

Regardless of the type of technique, knowledge of problems associated to amplicon contamination and quality controls should be established since the very beginning. The millions of copies generated by PCRs can act as carryover products and contaminate equipments or reagents and serve as templates that generate false-positive results. To control this pitfall, meticulous good laboratory practices are required, and many laboratories use clearly defined separated areas for the preparation of PCRs ("clean area"), amplification, and post-amplification in order to reduce cross-contamination.

Careful work reduces the need for inactivation of carryover products using enzymatic or chemical treatments. Negative controls are also run in every batch of samples.

False-negative results may arise from the presence of PCR inhibitors in the sample or the presence of foreign DNA (e.g., host eukaryotic DNA) that could interfere with performance of the test, particularly when the amount of nucleic acid from the infectious agent in the sample is low. PCR inhibitors are a heterogeneous class of substances with different properties and mechanisms of action. They are present in a large variety of sample types and may lead to decreased PCR sensitivity or even false-negative PCR results [23]. If this is the case, removal of PCR inhibitors during sample preparation is needed. This problem is relevant when performing direct DNA extraction, in special, when processing complex biological matrices. The amplification of an internal positive control is used to detect inhibitions; these controls can be an endogenous gene (housekeeping genes, such as mammalian beta-actin) that it is present in the specimen or an exogenous control that is added to each sample.

Validation of the tests requires a preliminary assessment involving a comparison to a gold standard reference method. The traditional definitive confirmation of infection has been based on microbiological (in vitro growth on culture media, viral propagation in cell culture) or histopathological diagnosis, but these gold standard techniques may require considerable time, and the sensitivity is not 100 %. Estimates of sensitivity and specificity in comparison with an imperfect gold standard and ancillary tests may provide discrepant results that cause confusion [24]. Interpretation can be specifically problematic when it leads to official or legal consequences in cases when the samples are negative by culture but positive when tested by PCR (since PCR detects nucleic acids from both viable and nonviable organisms).

The use of molecular tests is recommended when the presence of a pathogen implies disease or is a part in the assessment of an eradication program. A negative result, which would indicate the absence of the pathogen, should be interpreted carefully according to the epidemiological context and taking into account the limitations on sensitivity that may be related to the protocol for DNA extraction and the molecular technique itself. On the other hand, in some situations, the identification of pathogen's nucleic acids does not provide a clear etiological answer (e.g., latent, asymptomatic infections, carriers, presence of widespread pathogens), and interpretation of results must be done according to other parameters (epidemiological context) or with the support of additional laboratory diagnostic tools (e.g., serology).

Quality assurance and quality improvement programs need to be developed for increased acceptance of the techniques for routine diagnostic purposes [22, 25]. So far, there has been limited harmonization of techniques. Interlaboratory comparisons, consisting on a same blind-coded panel of samples to be tested simultaneously in several laboratories, are difficult to organize because of logistics and biohazard, but they remain the best system to assess the wide range of diagnostic techniques (commercially available kits and in-house assays) for the specific pathogens. These comparisons allow evaluating the proficiency of the participating laboratories in that precise test. Some good examples are available in the literature [26, 27].

6 Technologies in the Near Future

While it is not possible to foresee the platforms that will become routine in the future, there are two technologies that are standing out in terms of expectancies and reports.

The introduction of inexpensive platforms for massive DNA sequencing has provided culture-independent methods for virus discovery and characterization, surveillance, and outbreak investigation [28]. High-throughput sequencing requires sequence acquisition and complex bioinformatics analysis to assemble the contiguous short reads in order to obtain the correct genomic sequence that can be compared to known microbial sequences. There are several sequencing technologies currently available on the market, each with intrinsic limitations and potential applications [29]. Because of specialized equipment and level of expertise needed, these technologies are still restricted to research on pathogen discovery at highly specialized laboratories. In the future, advancements and simplifications of the associated technology and costs may move sequencing to the forefront position of clinical diagnostics [28].

On the other hand, recent advancements on the use of molecular techniques on-site, at the clinics or at the farm, hold great promise, especially for low-resource scenarios. This option is known as "pen-side testing" of animals, and it is a system analogous to the point-of-care testing or alternate-site testing in human clinics. This consists of tests performed outside the central laboratory using devices that can be easily transported and handled in the field by nonspecialists [30]. Regarding molecular techniques, these employ portable cyclers based on isothermal amplification, for example, nucleic acid sequence-based amplification (NASBA) and loop-mediated isothermal amplification (LAMP). Ideally, analyses are carried out in self-contained sample systems which integrate sample preparation, amplification, and detection steps. This option would be ideal when timely and accurate diagnosis of animals with suspected clinical signs is critical for urgent intervention, such as infections with legal disastrous consequences (e.g., foot-and-mouth disease or avian flu). This pen-site testing can also be a complement to the use of centralized laboratories and a help in geographical areas that do not have easy access to other traditional facilities. Currently, these options are under development; however, other tests, such as the lateral flow devices (immuno-chromatographic strip tests) that can detect antigens or antibodies, seem to be simpler and rapid tools for the use in the field. A good example on the use of these new technologies has been discussed for the diagnosis of food-and-mouth disease in sub-Saharan countries [25]. The definitive chance to replace traditional diagnostic methodologies will depend on cost-effectiveness and practicalities in every situation.

7 Conclusion

The field of molecular diagnostics is rapidly evolving, with an expanding number of techniques and assays. The advisability of each technique depends on the purpose of use and the existing limitations. The ability to quickly detect pathogens and their characteristics (e.g., subtypes, virulence factors, and drug-resistance traits) would allow for precise decision-making and target measures such as prophylaxis, appropriate therapy, and biosafety plans to promptly control disease outbreaks. New tools are needed for diagnosis and surveillance of emergent or reemergent pathogens that may arise from globalization of travels and trade, changes in vector distribution, anthropological pressure on pristine areas, and many other factors. Keeping abreast with this exponentially growing knowledge requires constant dedication. In this sense, to take advantage of these possibilities, future veterinarians must have a global understanding regarding the type of tests that can be applied in the laboratory and the conclusions that can, or cannot, be drawn from the results. In this sense, fundamentals of sequence analysis should become an important item in the teaching program of veterinary medicine, including genes, methods, and databases that should be accessed for sequence comparison [18]. This requirement for long-life learning is extensive to all veterinarians.

In practice, taking benefit of the huge amount of data that can be obtained using molecular techniques highlights the need of collaboration between veterinarians in the laboratory and practitioners. The possibility to detect an extensive number of pathogens in the laboratory does not preclude the need for adequate samples collection and shipment, an adequate anamnesis, and a definition of the objective of the diagnosis from the practitioner. The laboratory must provide an accurate and fast diagnosis and assistance in the interpretation of results. The final diagnosis of the disease and the decision to apply a treatment or a control program must be made by the practitioner according to laboratory results but also to other epidemiological factors.

Currently, the use of molecular techniques is highly variable between countries, with a marked contrast between laboratory facilities in developed and developing countries. Obviously, the concept of "affordable test" depends on the financial availability and cost of imports (equipment, reagents) that are limiting factors in resource-limited countries. Development of diagnostic tests should take into account many epidemiological scenarios, such as endemic and/or zoonotic diseases, and highlights the benefit from exchange of scientific expertise. Appropriate worldwide use of these tools will contribute to the implementation of the "One World, One Health" perspective.

References

1. Schmitt B, Henderson L (2005) Diagnostic tools for animal diseases. Rev Sci Tech 24: 243–250
2. Plummer PJ (2007) Molecular diagnostics for the food animal practitioner. Vet Clin North Am Food Anim Pract 23:481–501
3. Smith NH (2012) The global distribution and phylogeography of *Mycobacterium bovis*. Infect Genet Evol 12:857–865
4. Valdezate S, Navarro A, Villalón P, Carrasco G, Saéz-Nieto JA (2010) Epidemiological and phylogenetic analysis of Spanish human *Brucella melitensis* strains by multiple-locus variable-number tandem-repeat typing, hypervariable octameric oligonucleotide fingerprinting, and *rpoB* typing. J Clin Microbiol 48: 2734–2740
5. López-Goñi I, García-Yoldi D, Marín CM, de Miguel MJ, Muñoz PM, Blasco JM, Jacques I, Grayon M, Cloeckaert A, Ferreira AC, Cardoso R, Corrêa de Sá MI, Walravens K, Albert D, Garin-Bastuji B (2008) Evaluation of a multiplex PCR assay (Bruce-ladder) for molecular typing of all *Brucella* species, including the vaccine strains. J Clin Microbiol 46:3484–3487
6. López-Goñi I, García-Yoldi D, Marín CM, de Miguel MJ, Barquero-Calvo E, Guzmán-Verri C, Albert D, Garin-Bastuji B (2011) New Bruce-ladder multiplex PCR assay for the biovar typing of *Brucella suis* and the discrimination of *Brucella suis* and *Brucella canis*. Vet Microbiol 154:152–155
7. Righter DJ, Rurangirwa FR, Call DR, McElwain TF (2011) Development of a bead-based multiplex PCR assay for the simultaneous detection of multiple *Mycoplasma* species. Vet Microbiol 153:246–256
8. Reisberg K, Selim AM, Gaede W (2013) Simultaneous detection of *Chlamydia* spp., *Coxiella burnetii*, and *Neospora caninum* in abortion material of ruminants by multiplex real-time polymerase chain reaction. J Vet Diagn Invest 25:614–619
9. Leon A, Richard E, Fortier C, Laugier C, Fortier G, Pronost S (2012) Molecular detection of *Coxiella burnetii* and *Neospora caninum* in equine aborted foetuses and neonates. Prev Vet Med 104:179–183
10. Saunders VF, Reddacliff LA, Berg T, Hornitzky M (2007) Multiplex PCR for the detection of *Brucella ovis*, *Actinobacillus seminis*, and *Histophilus somni* in ram semen. Aust Vet J 85: 72–77
11. Moustacas VS, Silva TMA, Costa LF, Xavier MN, Carvalho CA Jr, Costa EA, Paixão TA, Santos RL (2013) Species-specific multiplex PCR for the diagnosis of *Brucella ovis*, *Actinobacillus seminis*, and *Histophilus somni* infection in rams. BMC Vet Res 9:51
12. Giammarioli M, Pellegrini C, Casciari C, De Mia GM (2008) Development of a novel hot-start multiplex PCR for simultaneous detection of classical swine fever virus, African swine fever virus, porcine circovirus type 2, porcine reproductive and respiratory syndrome virus and porcine parvovirus. Vet Res Commun 32: 255–262
13. Xu X-G, Chen G-D, Huang Y, Ding L, Li Z-C, Chang C-D, Wang C-Y, Tong D-W, Liu H-J (2012) Development of multiplex PCR for simultaneous detection of six swine DNA and RNA viruses. J Virol Methods 183:69–74
14. Wernike K, Hoffmann B, Beer M (2013) Single-tube multiplexed molecular detection of endemic porcine viruses in combination with background screening for transboundary diseases. J Clin Microbiol 51:938–944
15. Brosch R, Gordon SV, Marmiesse M, Brodin P, Buchrieser C, Eiglmeier K, Garnier T, Gutiérrez C, Hewinson G, Kremer K, Parsons LM, Pym AS, Samper S, van Soolingen D, Cole ST (2002) A new evolutionary scenario for the

Mycobacterium tuberculosis complex. Proc Natl Acad Sci USA 99:3684–3689

16. Smith NH, Kremer K, Inwald J, Dale J, Driscoll JR, Gordon SV, van Soolingen D, Hewinson RG, Smith JM (2006) Ecotypes of the *Mycobacterium tuberculosis* complex. J Theor Biol 239:220–225
17. Cottam EM, Wadsworth J, Shaw AE, Rowlands RJ, Goatley L, Maan S, Maan NS, Mertens PPC, Ebert K, Li Y, Ryan ED, Juleff N, Ferris NP, Wilesmith JW, Haydon DT, King DP, Paton DJ, Knowles NJ (2008) Transmission pathways of foot-and-mouth disease virus in the United Kingdom in 2007. PLoS Pathog 4:e1000050
18. de Lamballerie X (2009) Essential veterinary education in modern molecular tools for the detection of disease: what veterinarians will need to know about genomics and molecular biology and diagnostics (including bioterrorist weapons) in 2025. Rev Sci Tech 28:657–662
19. Hoffmann B, Scheuch M, Höper D, Jungblut R, Holsteg M, Schirrmeier H, Eschbaumer M, Goller KV, Wernike K, Fischer M, Breithaupt A, Mettenleiter TC, Beer M (2012) Novel orthobunyavirus in cattle, Europe, 2011. Emerg Infect Dis 18:469–472
20. Hoffmann B, Beer M, Reid SM, Mertens P, Oura CA, van Rijn PA, Slomka MJ, Banks J, Brown IH, Alexander DJ, King DP (2009) A review of RT-PCR technologies used in veterinary virology and disease control: sensitive and specific diagnosis of five livestock diseases notifiable to the World Organisation for Animal Health. Vet Microbiol 139:1–23
21. Ojha S, Kostrzynska M (2008) Examination of animal and zoonotic pathogens using microarrays. Vet Res 39:04
22. Yang S, Rothman RE (2004) PCR-based diagnostics for infectious diseases: uses, limitations, and future applications in acute-care settings. Lancet Infect Dis 4:337–348
23. Schrader C, Schielke A, Ellerbroek L, Johne R (2012) PCR inhibitors: occurrence, properties and removal. J Appl Microbiol 113:1014–1026
24. Fulton RW, Confer AW (2012) Laboratory test descriptions for bovine respiratory disease diagnosis and their strengths and weaknesses: gold standards for diagnosis, do they exist? Can Vet J 53:754–761
25. King DP, Madi M, Mioulet V, Wadsworth J, Wright CF, Valdazo-González B, Ferris NP, Knowles NJ, Hammond J (2012) New technologies to diagnose and monitor infectious diseases of livestock: challenges for sub-Saharan Africa. Onderstepoort J Vet Res 79:456
26. Jones RM, Hertwig S, Pitman J, Vipond R, Aspán A, Bölske G, McCaughey C, McKenna JP, van Rotterdam BJ, de Bruin A, Ruuls R, Buijs R, Roest H-J, Sawyer J (2011) Interlaboratory comparison of real-time polymerase chain reaction methods to detect *Coxiella burnetii*, the causative agent of Q fever. J Vet Diagn Invest 23:108–111
27. Wernike K, Bonilauri P, Dauber M, Errington J, LeBlanc N, Revilla-Fernández S, Hjulsager C, Isaksson M, Stadejek T, Beer M, Hoffmann B (2012) Porcine reproductive and respiratory syndrome virus: interlaboratory ring trial to evaluate real-time reverse transcription polymerase chain reaction detection methods. J Vet Diagn Invest 24:855–866
28. Lipkin WI, Firth C (2013) Virus surveillance and discovery. Curr Opin Virol 3:199–204
29. Kircher M, Kelso J (2010) High-throughput DNA sequencing: concepts and limitations. Bioessays 32:524–536
30. Holland CA, Kiechle FL (2005) Point-of-care molecular diagnostic systems: past, present and future. Curr Opin Microbiol 8:504–509

Chapter 3

Biosafety Principles and Practices for the Veterinary Diagnostic Laboratory

Joseph Kozlovac and Beverly Schmitt

Abstract

Good biosafety and biocontainment programs and practices are critical components of the successful operation of any veterinary diagnostic laboratory. In this chapter we provide information and guidance on critical biosafety management program elements, facility requirements, protective equipment, and procedures necessary to ensure that the laboratory worker and the environment are adequately protected in the challenging work environment of the veterinary diagnostic laboratory in general and provide specific guidance for those laboratories employing molecular diagnostic techniques.

Key words Biosafety, Biocontainment, Laboratory biosecurity

1 Introduction

Veterinary diagnostic laboratories play a critical and fundamental role in a country's individual veterinary health and public health systems but also act as a key component to regional and worldwide veterinary health and public health systems. The field of biosafety promotes safe laboratory practices, procedures, and proper use of containment equipment and facilities; promotes responsible activities among laboratory workers; and provides advice on laboratory design. Individuals working in veterinary diagnostic laboratories have occupational exposure to a variety of hazardous materials in the workplace. Diagnostic laboratories are demanding work environments where the pace is hectic, the work load is often heavy, and the pressure to provide rapid, accurate, and reliable results is ever present. Therefore it is of primary importance that institutions have a robust biosafety program in place which ensures that laboratory staffs are well aware of the risks present in the laboratory but more importantly that they understand how to use the protective equipment provided and practice those critical safety behaviors which are based on internationally recognized, scientifically valid best practices.

Mónica V. Cunha and João Inácio (eds.), *Veterinary Infection Biology: Molecular Diagnostics and High-Throughput Strategies*, Methods in Molecular Biology, vol. 1247, DOI 10.1007/978-1-4939-2004-4_3, © Springer Science+Business Media New York 2015

2 Basic Elements of a Biosafety Program

All successful biosafety programs, and indeed any effective safety and health program, will have the following key elements in common: (1) management commitment and leadership, (2) employee participation, (3) hazard identification and assessment, (4) hazard prevention and control, (5) hazard communication and training, and (6) evaluation of program effectiveness [1]. The diagram in Fig. 1 depicts those core elements necessary for an effective biosafety management program, and each will be further discussed below. Biosafety has developed as a distinct and sometimes independent field from industrial safety because of the complexity, unique work environment, and evolving nature of the hazard—biological organisms. Therefore, management commitment must be strong and consistently demonstrable in order for a biosafety program to be developed, implemented, sustained, and continually improved. An organization's leadership sets the tone for the biosafety program, and this begins with the organizational vision and mission statements. A vision statement is the leadership's mental image of the possible and/or desirable future state of the organization (or subcomponent of the organization). In order for the leadership's vision to have impact on employees, it must be communicated in a lasting and dramatic fashion; "Excellent science

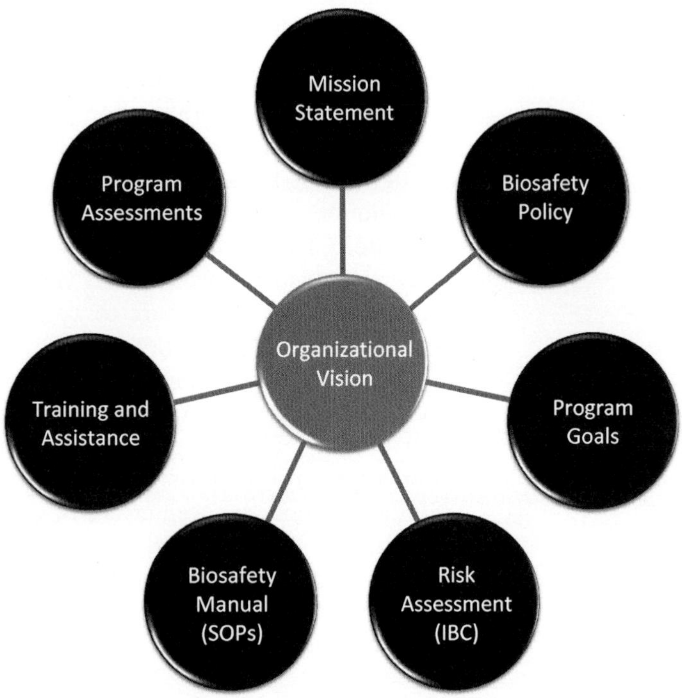

Fig. 1 Biosafety management program core elements

done safely" would be a good example. A mission statement is an organization's vision translated into written form. It should be a short and concise statement of goals and priorities, such as the below example of a mission statement for a biosafety program:

> The purpose of the Biosafety Program is to prevent or minimize employee exposures or the accidental environmental release of hazardous biological agents through the promotion of safe laboratory practices and procedures and proper use of containment equipment and facilities by employees, students, visitors, and contractors.

The biosafety program vision and mission for maximum effectiveness should be able to directly link to the institution's vision and mission statements or goals. An institution's biosafety policy is especially critical in that it defines the roles and responsibilities for the program at all levels, as well as the methodology for defining program goals and how individual accountability at all levels is measured. It is important that the biosafety policy clearly states the intent and direction of institutional leadership, and supporting documentation must identify a chain of responsibility for information on biosafety-related issues. It is important to note that the written biosafety/biocontainment policy is just another mechanism of communicating the policy to the employees. Laboratory supervisors', principal investigators', biosafety and safety professionals', and other institutional leaders' attitude toward biosafety and what they do both as individuals and collectively, or fail to do, is a more powerful expression of the actual biosafety policy and culture than the actual written words of the policy. In other words, a strong biosafety culture will only be created and maintained when all levels of management demonstrate their commitment personally by embodying and rewarding culture-supportive behaviors and conclusively addressing behaviors in others that undermine the culture of safety.

Following clockwise on the diagram of Fig. 1, the fourth through seventh balloon collectively represent universal employee participation through hazard identification and assessment, hazard prevention and control, information and training, and evaluation of program effectiveness. Employee participation is critical to the success of any biosafety program. Employees from all levels within the organization need to be engaged and provided opportunities to actively participate within the biosafety program, such as participating on various safety committees engaged in risk assessment and policy development, participating in active discussions of biosafety topics at regularly scheduled laboratory meetings, inclusion of lab staff on biosafety inspection and audit teams, and, finally, ensuring that employees are involved in determining biosafety-related goals and metrics for their specific work areas. Organizations need to ensure that employees are actively encouraged to report unsafe conditions, accidents, and near misses, as well as making recommendations to improve safety and health within their working environment. The critical components of this encouragement are the creation and enforcement of "whistle-blower"-type protections for those employees that report concerns at a minimum and ideally the creation of a reward structure for reports that encourage safe practices but discourage false or retaliated reporting. As a safety culture is established within an organization and employees adopt those critical safety behaviors as the norm, an environment is created in which risky behaviors are no longer tolerated among peers or management [2]. Of course, any robust biosafety program must include a continuous formal process of hazard identification, risk assessment, hazard prevention, and mitigation, which is conducted by the laboratory supervisor or a committee such as a biosafety committee. We will further discuss these elements in the next section as they are closely related.

3 Risk Assessment for Veterinary Diagnostic Labs

The nature of veterinary diagnostic work, which involves working with samples of unknown status that may contain strict veterinary pathogens or zoonotic pathogens, differs from work conducted in research laboratories where the agent risks are known and can be incorporated into the initial risk assessment. Diagnostic workers who work in (human) public health have a significant and known occupational exposure risk to cultures or tissues containing pathogens that infect humans. However, the risk to those individuals working in veterinary diagnostic laboratories for occupational exposure to pathogens that can infect and cause disease in humans is not negligible. Indeed 65 % of identified infectious diseases in humans are caused by organisms which infect multiple hosts in nature, and 75 % of emerging human infectious diseases over the past three decades have been zoonotic in nature [3]. Accordingly, veterinary health professional and diagnostic workers should be familiar with the principles and practices for preventing transmission of infectious agents (collectively known as "standard precautions"). In 2006, the National Association of State Public Health Veterinarians' (NASPHV) Veterinary Infection Control Committee published a compendium of veterinary standard precautions, *Zoonotic Disease Prevention in Veterinary Personnel* [4], which is an excellent review of the standard precautions one should employ while working with animals in the field, veterinary clinic, and diagnostic labs that handle animal tissues or zoonotic agents. Another excellent reference on standard precautions entitled *Guideline for Isolation Precautions: Preventing Transmission of Infectious Agents in Healthcare Settings* was published in 2007, by the Healthcare Infection Control Practices Advisory Committee (HICPAC) [5]. This guide discusses worker practices and precautions to minimize infectious disease transmission in patient care and diagnostic labs and is another valuable reference for those individuals working in both animal and human diagnostic laboratories.

In addition to occupational risks associated with potentially zoonotic veterinary pathogens, those individuals conducting risk assessment with veterinary pathogens in which humans are not a relevant host must be cognizant of those risk drivers for animal agriculture that are based primarily on the potential economic impact on animal health associated with the release of a veterinary pathogen, as well as the international trade implications of disease [6]. Some agent-specific characteristics that should be evaluated as part of a comprehensive risk assessment involving pathogens of veterinary significance are the following:

- Is the agent endemic or foreign to the region?
- Is the host animal native or exotic to the area?
- What is known regarding the morbidity and mortality caused by the agent, including whether it is exclusively an animal agent or a zoonotic agent?
- Are there effective prophylaxes, treatments, or vaccines available (for animals and/or humans)?
- What are the shedding and transmission patterns of the agent in the relevant host species?
- Will the agent be introduced into species for which there are no data?
- Are there active control or eradication programs for the disease?
- What are the environmental stability, quantity, and concentration of the agent?
- How will the agents be used—in animals (large or small scale), in the field, or in the laboratory?
- What is the host range of the agent and are there ongoing surveillance testing programs?
- Is the agent vector-borne and transmitted, and what is the occurrence of competent vectors? [7].

A risk assessment must also review the operational elements of the proposed work with biological hazards. Diagnostic laboratories need (at a minimum) to conduct risk assessment on the following operational areas:

- Receiving, unpacking, and transfer into the laboratory.
- Initial processing of the sample.
- Preparation of sample for analysis (culture, ELISA, polymerase chain reaction (PCR), etc.) [8].

Although risk assessment methodology can be either quantitative or qualitative, it is recognized that most life science institutions

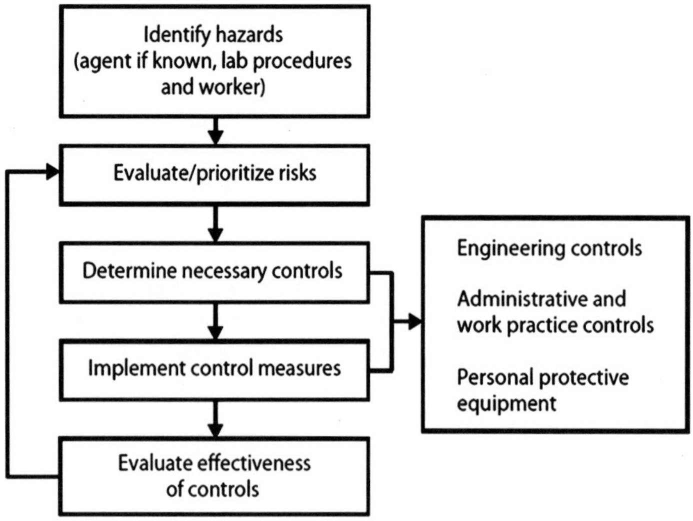

Fig. 2 Risk assessment and management process

favor qualitative methodology such as operational risk management, which is a continuous process that can be broken down into the key steps depicted in the diagram of Fig. 2. For more detailed information on operational risks associated with specific diagnostic activities, the authors recommend that the readers review US Centers for Disease Control and Prevention (CDC): *Guidelines for Safe Work Practices in Human and Animal Medical Diagnostic Laboratories* (www.cdc.gov/mmwr/preview/mmwrhtml/su6101a1.htm) [9]. Finally, a risk assessment must review the training, experience, and competency of the individuals who will be conducting the work with biohazards. The risk for exposures, laboratory-acquired infections, and the unintended release of research, clinical, or diagnostic materials to the environment should ultimately be reduced by ensuring the competency of laboratory workers at all levels. Indeed, many institutions have successfully implemented a formal training and mentoring program for individuals new to the laboratory regardless of previous education and experience elsewhere, and the authors believe this is a practice that should be encouraged at all laboratories. However when working with a new biohazard or a change to work currently performed, the level of risk changes and an evaluation of the risk must be conducted, which includes a review of the experience and competency of the laboratory supervisor and staff as part of this formal risk assessment process. An MMWR supplement *Guidelines for Biosafety Laboratory Competency* was published on behalf of CDC and the Association of Public Health Laboratories (APHL) in 2011 [10]. These competencies outline the essential skills, knowledge, and abilities required for working with biologic agents at the three highest biosafety levels (BSLs) (levels 2, 3, and 4) as defined in the HHS/NIH publication *Biosafety in Microbiological and Biomedical*

Laboratories, 5th edition [11]. This document can be a useful tool in categorizing the level of laboratory competency of staff in a diagnostic laboratory as well as for the development of competency-based biosafety training programs.

Once a valid and complete risk assessment has identified agent hazards, operational hazards, and staff training needs, the individual(s) conducting the risk assessment can minimize those risks through the use of appropriate facility engineering controls, administrative controls, personal protective equipment, and training programs designed to integrate all those factors at the level of individual employee competence.

4 Biocontainment Levels

Many institutions and organizations throughout the world must consider the risks presented by proposed research with agricultural pathogens and make decisions regarding the placement of these pathogens into proper biocontainment and/or biosafety categories [6]. Many countries and international organizations such as the World Organization for Animal Health (OIE) have published guidance to define biocontainment and/or biosafety levels, which provide specific combinations of facility design features, engineering controls, work practices, and personal protective equipment (or alternative barriers) for a range of assigned risks from low to high. The majority of guidance documents recommend that the selection of facility design features, protective equipment, and administrative controls must be informed by a robust, site-specific risk assessment (as earlier described) which takes into consideration agent characteristics, type of work to be conducted, and training and competency of staff conducting the work. The new OIE Manual chapter "Standard for managing biorisk in the veterinary laboratory and animal facilities" was adopted at the May, 2014 OIE General Session. It has not yet been combined with the old Manual chapter on biosafety; that still is a stand-alone chapter although efforts are being made to combine the two in the near future. The new chapter draws heavily from concepts articulated in the CEN Workshop Agreement (CWA) 15793 on Laboratory Biorisk Management which was scheduled to expire in September 2014 but has been transferred to the International Standard Organization (ISO) to be used as the primary source for an ISO deliverable. The new chapter moves away from the traditional approach of describing minimal recommended biocontainment levels to a laboratory-specific risk control measures approach. The authors are supportive of the concepts contained within CWA 15793 and firmly believe that biorisk management programs can be a valuable tool in facilitating good biosafety and laboratory biosecurity practices and applaud OIE for including these concepts as one of the focal points in the new Terrestrial Manual chapter. However, the authors still see value for international organizations in providing minimal biocontainment levels.

5 Minimal Facility Requirements for All Biological Laboratory Work

1. The laboratory should be easy to clean, with surfaces that are impervious to water and resistant to chemicals. There shall be a hand-washing basin near the exit. An emergency shower, including an eye bath, should be present in each laboratory suite appropriate to the risks represented by chemicals and other hazards present.
2. Personnel access to the work area should be restricted; appropriate security measures such as controlled electronic access may be necessary with higher risk agents.
3. The laboratory door should be closed when work is in progress and ventilation should be provided by extracting air from the room (where biosafety cabinets are used, care shall be taken to balance ventilation systems).
4. No infectious materials shall be discarded down laboratory sinks and a method for decontaminating waste materials should be available within the facility (autoclave, etc.).
5. Laboratory windows that open to the outside are not recommended. If a laboratory has operable windows they should be fitted with fly screens [9, 11].

Veterinary diagnostic laboratories routinely receive specimens where a variety of diseases are possible. When the infectious nature of the sample is unknown, it is prudent for initial processing activities to utilize facilities, procedures, and personal protective equipment as described by the World Health Organization (WHO) (www.who.int/csr/resources/publications/biosafety/WHO_CDS_CSR_LYO_2004_11/en) and other internationally recognized guidance as biosafety level 2. Primary containment equipment such as a Class II biological safety cabinet should be used when laboratory manipulations have the potential to generate aerosols or splashes of potentially infectious materials. When the clinical history of the specimen suggests a higher level of containment, that level should be utilized in a similar fashion.

6 Operational Procedures (Emphasis on Molecular Testing)

The use of molecular procedures such as PCR and sequencing does not preempt the need for adequate biosafety and biocontainment procedures to work with diagnostic specimens and/or agents.

Biocontainment and biosafety operating procedures need to be determined and must be based on a risk assessment [12]. Standard operational procedures for handling diagnostic specimens and/or agents are as follows:

1. Access to the laboratory is restricted.
2. Laboratory personnel must wash their hands after handling infectious material and before leaving the laboratory.
3. Eating, drinking, smoking, handling contact lenses, and applying cosmetics or medicinal products are not permitted in areas designated for work with infectious material. Food is stored outside of laboratory work area.
4. Mouth pipetting is prohibited.
5. A policy for handling sharps must be in place.
6. Generation of aerosols must be minimized. Any procedures that are recognized to generate aerosols should be performed in primary containment equipment such as a Class II biological safety cabinet.
7. Work surfaces must be decontaminated before and after manipulation of infectious material.
8. All infectious material must be decontaminated before disposal using a method such as autoclaving.
9. Personnel protective equipment (PPE) must be used based on risk assessment of the infectious material. Examples of PPE are lab coat, gloves (latex, nitrile), and respirator (if a respirator is used that individual should participate in a facility respiratory protection program which includes medical evaluation, training and fit testing).
10. Biosafety cabinets are recommended for work with infectious material as proper use will protect the operator and prevent contamination of the environment [11].

6.1 Special Safety Considerations for Molecular Work

Laboratories performing molecular work may encounter unique safety hazards including electrical shock, ultraviolet light, and caustic, corrosive, carcinogenic, or mutagenic chemicals. High-voltage power sources used in electrophoresis and sequencing equipment should not be used near flammable liquids and gases. Power sources should be serviced only by appropriately trained technicians. Ultraviolet light (UV) is used to visualize nucleic acid bands in gels and to break down DNA and RNA on work surfaces. Special care should be taken to wear eye and skin protection when there is possible exposure to UV light. Chemicals such as phenol, chloroform, ethidium bromide, and guanidine isothiocyanate are commonly used in molecular work such as nucleic acid extraction. Follow the material safety data sheet recommendation when using/disposing of these and other chemicals [9].

6.2 Movement of Extracted DNA/RNA from High to Low Containment Laboratory Areas

A laboratory may have the need to extract RNA/DNA from samples that may be infected with a high-consequence pathogen and subsequently tested at a lower containment level. In these situations, the type of pathogen should be considered with emphasis on whether the extraction method will provide complete inactivation.

Extraction procedures on viruses utilizing protein disruption chemicals such as phenol and guanidine isothiocyanate (GITC) will completely inactivate most viruses [13]. These methods may be less effective for bacterial spores, and the worker may need to introduce a heat treatment step [14]. After extraction, the pellet may be tested at a lower level of biocontainment with a recommended treatment of the tube containing the pellet with a suitable disinfectant. All developed processes should be tested and validated with a robust isolation protocol before implementation.

6.3 Operational Challenges

Molecular techniques such as real-time PCR have demonstrated improved utility in disease outbreaks over conventional techniques such as virus isolation [15]. Real-time PCR performed in a 96-well plate format enables use of high-throughput equipment which can dramatically increase laboratory "surge capacity." Due to the speed and accuracy of the procedure, the total number of samples tested is practically limited primarily by the initial sample processing and reporting steps. While use of PCR in an outbreak can decrease the number of people needed at the bench, it is necessary to adequately staff support positions to handle the initial sample processing and reporting duties.

A great deal of monetary and personnel resources have been dedicated in the last decade to establishing and implementing PCR in low-resource countries, in particular, for avian influenza detection. While PCR is a robust diagnostic tool, this technology has prerequisite infrastructure requirements such as a dependable source of electricity to run specialized equipment (thermo cyclers and analysis software). Lack of resources in low-resource countries will be a continuing challenge to development and sustainment of surveillance programs for animal and zoonotic diseases of concern.

Validation and quality assurance for molecular techniques is very similar to that required by conventional assays—with some special considerations [16]. PCR can lend itself to the use of internal controls that can provide assurance of test performance at several key steps, such as extraction and amplification. It is recommended that validated internal controls be utilized for quality control purposes.

New next-generation sequencing technology is making genomic analysis cheaper and more routinely available to laboratories of any size. From a biosafety perspective, this technology has the same requirements as outlined previously in the chapter.

7 Conclusion

Implementing and maintaining appropriate biosafety measures is one of the most important parts of veterinary diagnostic laboratory operations. Robust and comprehensive risk assessments must be conducted to determine the appropriate protection measures to be utilized in the laboratory. The use of molecular techniques does not preclude the application of adequate biosafety measures to handle the biological risks of pre-extraction diagnostic samples, as well as the general laboratory safety measures needed to address chemical and physical hazards inherent in these procedures.

References

1. Roughton J, Mercurio J (2002) Developing an effective safety culture: a leadership approach. Butterworth-Heinemann, Oxford, UK
2. Gershon R, Karkashian C, Grosch J et al (2000) Hospital safety climate and its relationship with safe work practices and workplace exposure incidents. Am J Infect Control 28:211–221
3. American Veterinary Medical Association (2008) One health: a new professional imperative. http://www.avma.org/onehealth. Accessed 23 Dec 2013
4. National Association of State Public Health Veterinarians (2006) Compendium of veterinary standard precautions: zoonotic disease prevention in veterinary personnel. http://scav.org/Edit/uploads/compendium%20of%20veterinary%20standard%20precautions%202006.pdf. Accessed 23 Dec 2013
5. Siegel JD, Rhinehart E, Jackson M, Chiarello L et al. (2007) Guideline for isolation precautions: preventing transmission of infectious agents in healthcare settings. http://www.cdc.gov/hicpac/pdf/isolation/isolation2007.pdf. Accessed 23 Dec 2013
6. Heckert R, Kozlovac JP (2007) Biosafety levels for animal agriculture pathogens. Appl Biosaf 12:168–174
7. Kozlovac J, Thacker E, Ellis R (2012) Introduction to biocontainment and biosafety concepts as they relate to research with large livestock and wildlife species. In: Richmond JY, Jackman J (eds) Anthology of biosafety XIII. Animal production and protection-challenges, risks and best practices. American Biological Safety Association, Mundelein, IL
8. Pauli U, Griot C, Thür B et al (2012) From the field to the laboratory in an animal disease outbreak situation. In: Richmond JY, Jackman J (eds) Anthology of biosafety XIII. Animal production and protection-challenges, risks and best practices. American Biological Safety Association, Mundelein, IL
9. Centers for Disease Control and Prevention (2012) Guidelines for safe work practices in human and animal medical diagnostic laboratories. MMWR 61(Suppl):1–101
10. Centers for Disease Control and Prevention (2011) Guidelines for biosafety laboratory competency. MMWR 60(02):1–6
11. Centers for Disease Control (2009) Laboratory facilities (secondary barriers). In: U.S. Health and Human Services (ed) Biosafety in microbiological and biomedical laboratories, 5th edn. p 33–35
12. Office des Epizooties (2012) Biosafety and biosecurity in the veterinary microbiology laboratory and animal facilities. In: Manual of diagnostic tests and vaccines for terrestrial animals. 6th edn, Vol 1, Chapter 1.1.2, p 1–11
13. Blow JA, Dohm DJ, Negley DL et al (2004) Virus inactivation by nucleic acid extraction reagents. J Virol Methods 119:195–198
14. Theriault S (2009). Advances in applied research. Public Health Agency of Canada. www.stcu.int/bb2009/download/download.php?id=115. Accessed 23 Dec 2013
15. Crossley B, Hietala S, Shih L et al (2005) High-throughput real-time RT-PCR assay to detect the exotic Newcastle Disease Virus during the California 2002–2003 outbreak. J Vet Diagn Invest 17:124–132
16. Office des Epizooties (2012) Principles and methods of validation of diagnostic assays for infectious diseases. In: Manual of diagnostic tests and vaccines for terrestrial animals. 6th edn, Vol 1, Chapter 1.1.5, p 1–16

Chapter 4

Veterinary Biobank Facility: Development and Management for Diagnostic and Research Purposes

Tina Lombardo, Silvia Dotti, Riccardo Villa, Stefano Cinotti, and Maura Ferrari

Abstract

Biobanking is an essential tool for ensuring easy availability of high-quality biomaterial collections that combine essential samples and epidemiological, clinical, and research data for the scientific community. Specimen collection is an integral part of clinical research. Indeed, every year throughout the world, millions of biological samples are stored for diagnostics and research, but in many fields the lack of biological material and models is a major hindrance for ongoing research. A biobank facility provides suitable samples for large-scale screening studies and database repositories. Software dedicated to biological banks simplify sample registration and identification, the cataloging of sample properties (type of sample/specimen, associated diseases and/or therapeutic protocols, environmental information, etc.), sample tracking, quality assurance, and specimen availability characterized by well-defined features. Biobank facilities must adopt good laboratory practices (GLPs) and a stringent quality control system and also comply with ethical issues, when required.

The creation of a veterinary network can be useful under different aspects: the first one is related to the importance of animal sciences itself to improve research and strategies in the different branches of the veterinary area, and the second aspect is related to the possibility of data management harmonization to improve scientific cooperation.

Key words Biobanking, Biological resources, Quality controls, Cryopreservation, Veterinary medicine

1 Introduction

The word "biobank" is a little over a decade old. It has been used since 1996 [1] to describe collections of various types of biological samples. Biobanks have been defined in a variety of different ways and this has been a major challenge [2]. As reported by Hallmans and Vaught, a biobank may be defined as the long-term storage of biological samples for research or clinical purposes [3]. In addition to storage facilities, a biobank can comprise a complete organization, including biological samples, data, personnel, policies, and procedures, for handling specimens and performing other services, such

Mónica V. Cunha and João Inácio (eds.), *Veterinary Infection Biology: Molecular Diagnostics and High-Throughput Strategies*, Methods in Molecular Biology, vol. 1247, DOI 10.1007/978-1-4939-2004-4_4, © Springer Science+Business Media New York 2015

as database management and scientific studies planning [3]. The Organisation for Economic Co-operation and Development, OECD, defines biobanks as "a collection of biological material, the associated data and information stored in an organized system for a population or a large subset of a population" [4]. Based on this definition, these infrastructures can be seen as components of dedicated research facilities, which enable the linkage of samples, their storage locations, and their "quality assured history since their original time of sampling" with associated, well-documented, clinical data. For managing such a biobank, Yuille et al. [5] have emphasized that an efficient information infrastructure is a critical component in life-science research and have even created the term "biobank informatics" as a discipline, with the purpose of identifying the best coding systems available for storing and retrieving biobank information.

In veterinary medicine, the activity of a biobank should not be limited to the collection of biomaterials, but should involve the processing, cataloging, and distribution of samples to the scientific community for research purposes and therapeutic applications.

The field of "biobanking" has evolved from a simple collection of frozen specimens to a virtual biobank in response to regulation changes, the advances made in biological sciences, and the advent of the computer chip [6].

Biobanks play a pivotal role in research, diagnosis, and production, as they provide high-quality biomaterial that is otherwise difficult or impossible to access for scientists of both human and veterinary medicine; in fact, the availability of high-quality samples is a reported problem and samples stored in improper conditions may lack the expected quality for their use [7]. Human biological specimens have been collected and distributed for many decades and have played a key role in the understanding and treatment of human diseases; in fact, in human medicine, the network of biobanks is advanced, but in veterinary medicine such networking is at a very early stage. Human specimen collections vary widely in biological resources and structure. Furthermore, modern cryopreservation techniques allow the storage of different types of biological samples, ready to be used upon request. The role of biobanks is gradually increasing as they have been identified as a key source of biological tissues to be used in transplantation, tissue engineering, regenerative medicine, pharmaceuticals, and diagnostics. One of the major objectives in Europe is to define concerted actions aimed at developing and sharing best practices and standardizing the procedures [8]. Currently, there is considerable variation in national laws and local practices applied to the processing and storage of biological samples in the various countries throughout the world [2]. This variability complicates the conditions for collaboration among scientists from different countries, reducing the future sharing of research data and samples and the possibility of carrying out collaborative research if regulations are not harmonized [9]. A process to reduce this variability has been initiated, and several sets of standards and best practices, helpful in improving quality of standards for biobank operations and biospecimens, have been published [10].

The Istituto Zooprofilattico Sperimentale della Lombardia e dell'Emilia Romagna (IZSLER) is a veterinarian public institution of the Italian Ministry of Health that includes 16 off-site laboratories and has its headquarters in Brescia. In recent decades, almost all of these laboratories involved in different areas have stored samples of animal origin, resulting from routinely diagnostic procedures and research. This activity has created several biological resources and materials collected according to different quality criteria and without harmonized procedures, depending on the main competence areas of the departments. In order to enhance interoperability and ensure the availability of biological material with well-defined quality features, a centralized infrastructure for storing biological resources in Brescia has been developed. This procedure allows the storage of samples that are controlled by standardized processes. At the same time, within national and international biobank collaborations, studies are performed using a large number of samples from different sources, which could be used for epidemiological researches. For such studies, it is of pivotal importance to establish quality criteria regarding the type of samples, storage conditions, and the availability of specific information. The subsequent paragraphs will describe the experience of IZSLER with the development of a biobank infrastructure, mainly based on biological resources, to be used in the field of diagnosis, research, and microorganism production.

2 Development of a Veterinarian Biobank Infrastructure

The development of a veterinarian biobank infrastructure was based on the following steps: sample census, data recording, quality management system and quality controls, safety and security of the storage area, and personnel.

2.1 Sample Census

The first step consisted in the inventory of the existing resources located in all the different facilities, the purpose of their use and storage, and the amounts of existing aliquots; this approach was necessary to evaluate the space and equipment required for their preservation. In particular, the main aspects were to define the quality standards required and the various biohazard levels, storage conditions, and selection of specific tests to be performed in order to ensure the identity, purity, and suitability of each specific sample. The outcome of this investigation has allowed the detection of 17 different types of biological resources equivalent to 42,683 stored samples. Biological resources from different animal species were subdivided into the following sections: microbiology and parasitology (bacteria, *Chlamydiaceae*, fungi, metazoans, mycoplasmas, *Prototheca* algae, protozoans), virology and prions (viruses, viral pathological materials, prions), biological products (cell cultures, field sera, hybridomas, IgG anti-immunoglobulins, immune sera), and others (chemical compounds, histological materials). On the basis of these findings, it was decided to proceed with the creation of a centralized infrastructure. Biological resources included in the biobank were selected for their suitability, depending on the type of the sample collected and according to specific quality criteria. Due to the presence of unique sample types, for some kind of biological resources (i.e., bacteria, viruses), three different aliquots were considered: the base matrix (master sample) to be used for the preparation of new batches, the working batches originated from the master to be used, and finally the "backup sample" as a deposit rate (usually equal to ¼ of the amount fitted). Storage in a different remote infrastructure is aimed at preserving samples in the event of a technical failure or calamity. This additional "mirror banking" of samples ensures that, if samples are compromised for whatever reason, replicate undamaged aliquots will still be available.

2.2 Data Recording

In order to ensure the traceability of biological samples, a database has been developed with different data recordings, each one specific for a biological resource. All samples are identified by a code and labeled with a bidimensional bar code. Data regarding all individual samples are collected in a software database that allows the number and position of the sample to be traced. In particular, bar codes ensure major reduction of errors in all specimen-handling processes and the possibility of tracking information about manipulation activities according to standard operating procedures (SOPs), quality control results, and loading and unloading order management.

Standard operating procedures mean documented procedures which describe how to perform tests or activities normally not specified in detail in study plans or test guidelines. The database for managing a biobank includes a web-based catalog, which lists the access terms and conditions and the resource characteristics. The catalog is intended to be used as a reference for scientists seeking information about biological samples and data suitable for their research.

2.3 Quality Management System and Quality Controls

Currently, biobanks must follow internationally accepted guidelines and best practices issued by ISBER (International Society for Biological and Environmental Repositories) [11] and BBMRI (Biobanking and Biomedical Resources Research Infrastructure). In particular, BBMRI aims to improve biobanking accessibility and interoperability by harmonizing similar biobanks in different locations and enriching the genotypic and phenotypic data [12]. All biospecimens should be handled according to well-defined protocols, and the whole clinical "biobanking" process should be fully documented, from seeking informed consent from the donor or patient to collecting, transporting, processing, storing, and retrieving the biospecimens [13]. Careful documentation of the methods and conditions used during collection and processing will increase the future value of specimens [14]. Furthermore, quality control programs must be established to check compliance with the standard operating procedures for specimen collection, handling, and analyses [15, 16].

With regard to "animal" biobanks, informed consent is not required; however, all other parameters must be performed according to the same criteria. Biobanking work, including associated laboratory handling specimens, has been performed in a standardized way. It is recommended the use of SOPs with the aim of continuously assessing the methods, materials, and equipment employed. SOPs should consider the specific requirements of analysis platforms and the biological questions to be addressed. However, SOPs can only be applied to prospectively collected samples, whereas for old archived samples, processing has often not been documented in sufficient detail without following specific SOPs, as in the past there was no application of quality management system, and storage of biological materials was performed by scientists with no standardized procedures. In the context of quality management, the scientific use of this material therefore requires special analyses to assess the proper preservation of biomolecules [17]. The recommendations for biobanking activities, quality assurance (QA), and quality control (QC) programs must be followed to ensure the high quality of samples. As described by OECD [18], good laboratory practices (GLPs) are "a quality system concerned with the organizational process and the conditions under which non-clinical health and environmental safety studies are planned, performed, monitored, recorded, archived and reported." The principles of GLPs represent a managerial concept in order to cover the whole organization process, beginning from the planning and arriving to the reporting of the applied procedures. Furthermore, this way of management facilitates the exchange of information and contributes to the protection of human health and the environment. Stability of biological samples depends on the procedures from the time of acquisition to the time of processing and storage; in fact, the use of anticoagulants, stabilizing agents, the time from collection to storage, and the sample handling temperature must all be controlled.

Biological samples can be stored for up to 30 years, but specific protocols are required to reduce the damage induced by preservation techniques [19]. This issue has been widely reported with proposals for rigorous quality controls for each step of the working flow, including collection, processing, and storage [20].

These procedures aimed to assess the preserving conditions depend on the type of biospecimen. Appropriate controls can be applied to cell suspensions (cell viability assays, contamination assays), to DNA and RNA (quantification and purity, function of DNA-modifying enzymes), to tissue morphology, and to viral batches (viral contamination tests, standard microbiological testing methods, and real-time PCR). All strains enrolled in IZSLER collection are submitted to different cultural and molecular biology control tests, in order to evaluate their features, purity, and identity.

However, no appropriate quality controls exist for liquid biosamples (serum, plasma, urine, saliva, cerebrospinal fluid, synovial fluid).

At IZSLER, the activity of the laboratories involved in biobanking is carried out using a quality assurance system in accordance with the requirements of UNI CEI EN ISO/IEC 17025:2005 as well as ISO 9001:2008 quality system for cell cultures. Biological resources are prepared and stored according to internal procedures.

2.4 Personnel

Laboratory activity is based on certain fundamental rules of good microbiological practice for the safe manipulation of biological samples.

Each operator (technician) must follow internal training courses, specific for their activities, positions, and competencies.

The operators should have basic knowledge on various biological topics. First of all, microbiology is one of the main subjects to know, as well as the isolation and cultivation of pathogens. Another important aspect is represented by the information on disinfection of work surfaces, equipment, and environment. Personnel should be aware of the need to minimize the production of aerosols and control other potential risks of contamination between biosamples and workers.

2.5 Control, Safety, and Security of the Storage Area

This is one of the main points that must be monitored and controlled. In fact, it represents a potential risk in the whole storage process. Starting from this point of view, monitoring temperature within mechanical freezers and refrigerators is an important quality assurance measure in addition to general building safety and security to protect against fire, unauthorized entrance, and other usual hazards. Furthermore, all freezers must be protected by a real-time temperature monitoring and alarm system. Alarm systems should be in place to monitor the temperature conditions of mechanical freezers or, for nitrogen freezers, the liquid nitrogen level (Fig. 1). Furthermore, a well-designed biobank software system has been developed to provide the possibility of monitoring the temperature values with an alarm service. Such temperature logging information must be automatically transferred via electronic interface into the biorepository management system and be linked with the

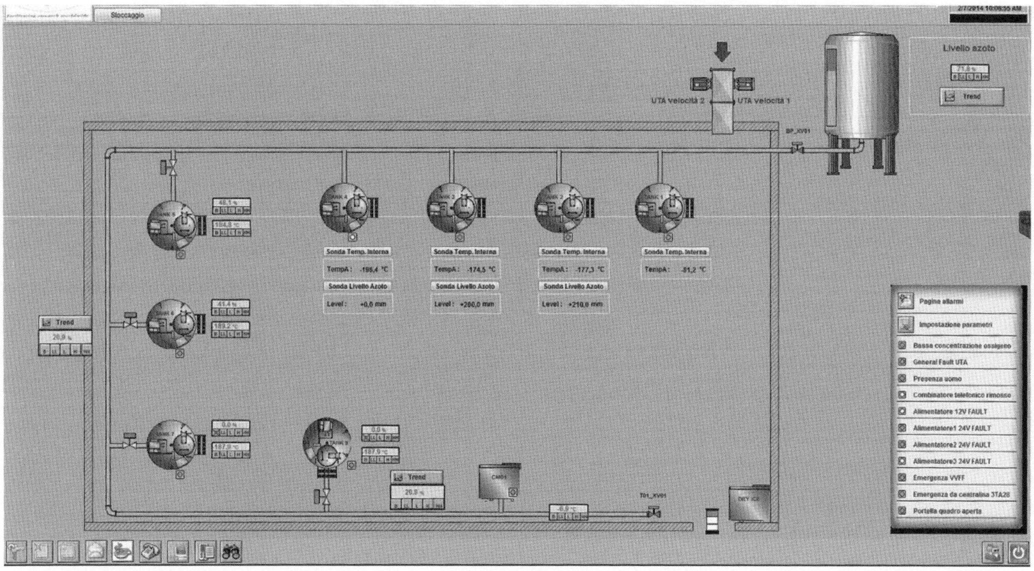

Fig. 1 Illustration of the real-time monitoring and alarm system of the IZSLER Veterinary Biobank facility

samples stored in the corresponding freezer. Any interruption of electrical power should be compensated for within minutes by an independent system, such as a generator with locally controlled production of electrical power. Automatic data logging into a database and the alarm service are very important for quality management of a biobank. If a measured value drifts outside inner or outer thresholds, an alarm is sent to staff members.

3 Sample Types and Preparation

Pre-analytical conditions are a key factor in maintaining the high quality of biospecimens. They are necessary to achieve the highest specificity of the laboratory test used for clinical diagnosis as well as for accurate reproducibility of experiments in the field of biomarker discovery. Inappropriate collection, handling, and storage of samples, as well as errors in data analysis and documentation, may all contribute to the generation of irreproducible and unreliable data. Preservation and optimization of biosample integrity to foster relevant research results and outcomes is a guiding principle of sample management.

The field of veterinarian research is rapidly evolving with new technologies and new standards. Samples are collected and stored also for a long period of time (years) before being used. For this reason, sample handling procedures should be defined and appropriated in order to guarantee a suitable use for the technology of tomorrow.

Biological samples have different storage requirements. For this reason, various approaches can be defined in order to obtain the most correct procedure.

3.1 Blood Samples

The routine use and collection of blood samples for diagnosis has provided general information on optimal methodologies and potential pitfalls.

Although procedures for collecting, processing, storing, and shipping blood components are generally standardized and well documented, several important factors need to be considered.

An important early decision in blood collection is whether to collect anticoagulated blood (consisting of plasma, buffy coat, and red blood cells) or coagulated blood (consisting of serum and red blood cell clot). Hemolysis of the specimen affects the accuracy of laboratory tests, particularly chemical and serological tests; therefore, it should be prevented by employing careful handling techniques according to optimum needle size, proper handling of the tubes, and proper pipetting techniques; however, if hemolysis is observed (pink to red tinge in sample), this information should be recorded [21]. In fact, hemolyzed samples would not be used for proteomics analysis, but destroying them may be unnecessary as any sample is worth saving, unless storage space is constrained. Annotation of all pertinent information about the samples allows the identification of potential factors that could influence outcomes. Serum and plasma specimens are of better quality for analysis if smaller-volume aliquots are initially prepared rather than larger ones that have to be thawed, handled, and refrozen, perhaps several times. Indeed, the ability to provide ready-to-use (RTU) aliquots without additional handling steps facilitates the sharing of samples and provides multiple replicates handled in an identical manner. It is also important to consider new or alternative methods and reagents that may offer longer-term stability or increased efficiency in the collection and preservation of blood [22, 23].

3.2 Cell Cultures

The ability to cryopreserve and successfully recover cell lines has been critical to the conservation of these biological samples, in particular the preservation of stem cells and the preparation of well-characterized cell banks. Indeed, the systematic storage and establishment of cryopreserved banks of cells for the stem cell research community is essential to the promotion of standardization in stem cell research and its use in clinical applications. Despite the significant potential for the use of stem cells in research and therapy, they are challenging to preserve and have been shown to be unstable after prolonged culture, often resulting in permanent alterations in their genetic background, which ultimately alters the phenotype of the culture. The working process related to cell culture isolation, amplification, control, storage, and shipment should be carried out in accordance with a quality management system such as ISO 9001:2008. Preparation and propagation of cell cultures are performed as indicated by international guidelines, and their sensitivity and reproducibility have been evaluated during interlaboratory tests. Each cell culture process provides ideal conditions for the growth of many organisms [24]; for this reason, particular attention must be placed on quality controls that should be performed on all samples with the purpose of assessing their purity and safety. These tests are carried out using microbiology, virology, serology, and molecular biology methods, as reported by the *European Pharmacopoeia* or other international guidelines. These assays are mainly based on in vitro tests. However, in vivo methods are used on laboratory animals, in the absence of validated in vitro systems or as indicated by international guidelines. In particular, the tests usually performed are aimed at detecting contamination from bacteria, fungi, yeasts, and mycoplasmas as well as animal and human viruses for human cell lines. Furthermore, bacterial endotoxin level, tumorigenicity, and cross contamination are investigated. Tests on cell cultures for detecting bacteria, fungi, and yeasts must be performed in an isolation unit, according to the *European Pharmacopoeia*.

3.3 Chlamydiaceae

Serological and molecular screening focused on the identification of chlamydial infections is routinely performed. Isolation of chlamydial species is carried out on cell culture.

Identification of the species belonging to the *Chlamydiaceae* is carried out using molecular tests, i.e., real-time PCR and PCR-RFLP analysis, which amplify specific genome sequences. The identification of new chlamydial species not yet classified is also performed using new real-time PCR and specific gene sequencing.

3.4 Field and Immune Sera

The field sera include samples from different animal species, mainly farmed, pets, and wildlife animals. The samples are collected by blood, sent to IZSLER to be tested in accordance with national or regional control programs or for specific serological tests. All these samples can be used as positive reference due to the presence of antibodies toward a specific pathogen, turning them very useful for retrospective serological surveys and validation of innovative serological tests. All serum samples collected and stored in the biobank are tested toward a panel of pathogens with the aim to know the presence/absence of antibodies.

Different serological techniques can be used and these are reported in specific sheets. Titers of humoral antibodies of serum samples are also registered and values are performed at preestablished intervals. The immune sera consist in polyclonal sera obtained from different animal species (rabbit, goat, mouse, rat, guinea pig) and toward several bacterial and viral antigens. They have been produced with antigens mostly purified and have a specificity panel available at the facility where they have been produced.

3.5 Hybridomas

The hybridomas that produce monoclonal antibodies are selected to be used in in-house diagnostic assays. They were generated to produce monoclonal antibodies against a wide spectrum of viruses, bacteria, and proteins, mainly of veterinary interest, and immunoglobulin isotypes of various animal species that were shown to be strategic tools for both research and diagnostic purposes. Hybridoma cultures are usually collected for freezing during the exponential growth phase and then are submitted to a double series of cloning procedure to assure the stability of the hybridoma and the clonality of the produced antibody. The monoclonal antibodies expressed by each hybridoma are controlled through a series of immunological assays aimed at identifying and characterizing their reactivity profile.

3.6 Microbiological and Parasitological Samples

Bacterial/fungal strains are identified by either phenotypic or genotypic tests. The former consists of microscopic observation and isolation in specific culture media. Identification is made through biochemical tests performed using commercial tests like the "API" or the "Vitek" systems. Genotypic tests, mainly PCR-based, are carried out to detect genes of virulence. Moreover, the 16S rDNA gene sequence analysis can be used to confirm the identity of bacterial species.

Parasites are identified using either phenotypic or genotypic tests. The former consists of microscopic observation and comparison with identification keys. Genotypic tests, mainly PCR-based, are carried out to identify genus or species.

3.7 Prototheca Algae

The identification of *Prototheca* algae (species and eventually subspecies) is currently carried out through microscopic examination, growth in specific culture media, and molecular assays (HMR-PCR, end point PCR, or sequencing).

3.8 Tissue Samples

Tissue samples can be stored in different ways, depending on their intended purpose. Indeed, molecular tools for tissue profiling, such as real-time PCR and expression microarrays, generally require collection of fresh frozen tissues as sources of high-quality RNA. Frozen tissue sections are made from high-quality tissues immediately snap-frozen in liquid nitrogen after being excised and identified by a pathologist. Available tissues include normal, diseased, and tumor animal tissues. The tissues excised are immediately frozen by liquid nitrogen and then stored at −80 °C. Tissue sections of 5–10 μm in thickness are mounted on positively charged glass slides. Furthermore, 0.4–0.7 g samples of standard size could be frozen in blocks into liquid nitrogen for 20–40 min after surgical excision. Otherwise, tissues could be fixed in 10 % neutral formalin for a minimum of 24 h and stored as paraffin blocks of $0.5 \times 1 \times 1$ cm. Formalin fixation and paraffin embedding (FFPE) preserve the morphology and cellular details of tissue samples. Thus, it has become the standard preservation procedure for diagnostic surgical pathology [25]. Historically, the archived FFPE blocks have been successfully used for immunohistochemistry application. However, formalin-fixed archival samples are known to be poor materials for molecular biology applications due to the irreversible modifications caused by formalin fixation on macromolecules. In the last ten years, there has been an exponential increase in the development of molecular assays using FFPE blocks. At present, when sections from FFPE blocks are to be used for molecular extraction, focus is placed on the time of fixation in formalin in order to avoid over-fixation. The advances in the field of molecular biology techniques have attempted to overcome the issue of formalin cross-linking and have successfully extracted DNA, RNA, and proteins, although fragmented.

3.9 Viruses and Viral Pathological Materials

Cell-associated viruses that can be grown in adherent or suspension cell cultures or chorioallantoic membranes of embryonated hen's eggs can be isolated from several types of samples. The main principle of isolating viruses is to choose the most suitable cell line and mechanically lyse infected cells and subsequently carry out several amplification passages to increase the titer in order to produce the master sample and then the working samples. Virus batches are tested for potential microbiological and viral adventitious contaminations; the tests are performed using microbiology, virology, serology, and molecular biology methods. The primary sources of potential viral contamination come from infected animal tissues used to prepare biological reagents and media and during laboratory manipulation. Virus detection and identification can be made by employing several methods, mainly based on serology tests using monoclonal antibodies and standard and real-time PCR. These assays amplify specific viral genome sequences known to be characteristics of a virus with a nucleotide sequence available in database collections. Extraneous viral contaminations can be verified through tests based on molecular biology techniques that allow the detection of viral DNA and RNA of other viruses. Mycoplasma contamination can be detected using real-time PCR methods. Bacterial contamination is determined through inoculation of nonselective culture media. In addition, electron microscopy is available for viral detection and identification using negative staining methods. Such "catchall" methods (able to detect even non-suspected/unknown viruses) benefit from "Airfuge" ultracentrifugation, increasing the sensitivity of the detection level. Indeed, immune electron microscopy methods (IEM and IEM gold) based on the use of hyperimmune sera and/or monoclonal antibodies may help viral identification and classification.

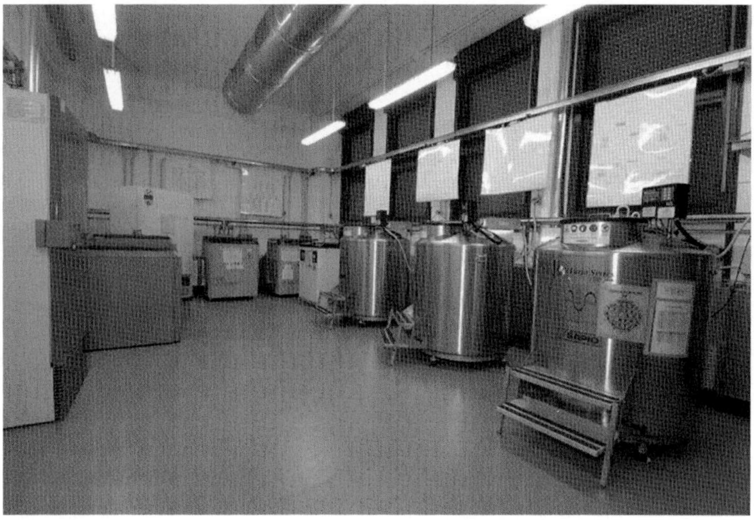

Fig. 2 Cryogenic area for preservation of biological resources

4 Storage of Biological Resources

Proper storage requires the use of cryovials and labeling systems that will withstand the intended storage conditions: vessels, labels, and bar codes or other printing systems are chosen for extended storage periods.

Samples have been deposited in freezers or other appropriate storage containers according to specific storage systems in order to preserve several parameters known to influence the condition of biospecimens.

In accordance with features, intended use and estimated length of storage, specimens may be stored at: room temperature, 4 °C, –20 °C, –80 °C, or –196 °C (vapor phase nitrogen) (Figs. 2 and 3). Temperature is a major variable in specimen management. Moreover microorganisms and viruses can be submitted to lyophilization process that allows preserving viability for a long time. These freeze-dried samples can be stored at 4 °C or at –20 °C, reducing the necessity to have freezers with lower temperature (–80 °C); for these reasons, this is a practical and efficient method for prolonged storage, less expensive, and more available in emerging countries.

5 Application of Biological Resources

Two major formats of biobanks with several subtypes can be distinguished: the population-based biobank and the disease-oriented biobanks, each with distinct and complementary scientific value.

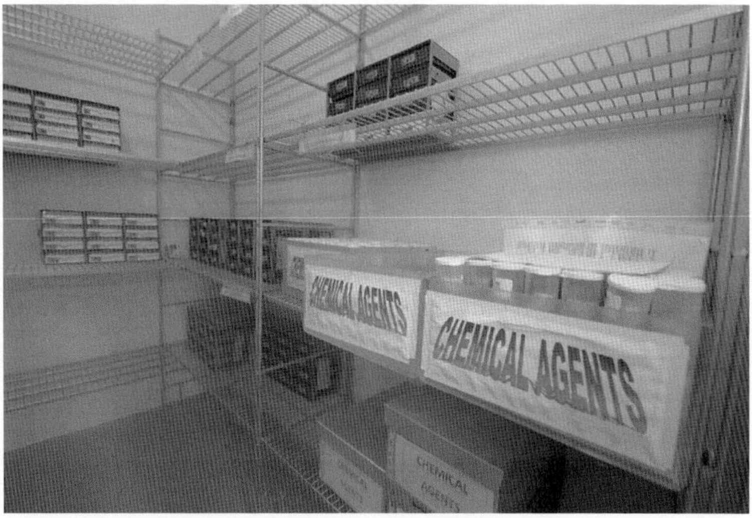

Fig. 3 Freezing area for preservation of biological resources

The most common format is the longitudinal population-based biobank, with biological samples and data from randomly selected individuals of a general population, used as resources for future unspecified research [26–28]. The specific strength of this format is the assessment of the natural frequency of occurrence and progression of common diseases, with special emphasis on predisposing genetic variants and environmental risk factors. In contrast, in disease-oriented biobanks, which may contain tissue, isolated cells, blood, or other body fluids, specimens are collected in the context of medical diagnosis and treatment. These biosamples allow the comparison of different disease stages and/or forms of treatment at a molecular level, in order to evaluate biomarkers for the diagnosis of a disease or assessment of risk/predisposition and prognosis (research purpose), monitoring the recurrence of diseases, prediction of mortality, and response to therapy [29]. The development of precisely defined clinical data elements (CDEs) may help to ensure that clinically relevant data are collected at each time interval [12]. In veterinary medicine, the wide availability of biological samples stored in biobanks provides the basis for research, leading to a better understanding of animal disease biology and the development of new diagnostic tests that require the use of biosamples with well-defined features [13]. The European Technology Platform for Global Animal Health (ETPGAH) has identified the lack of biological material as one of the main gaps in the development of new effective tools for the control and prevention of animal diseases. Biobanks represent an important tool in improving epidemiological research dependent on the availability and quality of the biomaterials but also on the collection of associated data [6]. In particular, for retrospective studies and longitudinal designs for evaluating the course of diseases, the requirements for obtaining time-specific data are even stronger. Furthermore, biological materials are a critical resource for genetic research. Major research in genomics is being pursued to improve the efficiency of selection for healthier animals with disease resistance properties. Molecular genetic tests have been developed to select farm animals with improved traits, for example, removal of the porcine stress syndrome and selection for specific estrogen receptor alleles [30]. The sequencing of the genome to identify new genes and unique regulatory elements holds great promise in providing new information that can be used for livestock production. Currently, in vitro embryo production and embryo transfer are being the preferred means of implementing these new technologies to enhance efficiency of farm animal production. Furthermore, the possibility of developing an integrated approach of genomics and proteomics using bioinformatics is essential for obtaining complete use of the available molecular genetic information. The development of this knowledge will benefit scientists, industry, and breeders considering that the efficiency and accuracy of traditional farm animal selection schemes will be improved by the implementation of molecular data into breeding programs.

6 Role of Biobanks in Veterinary Medicine

A decade ago, biobanks were simply repositories of biospecimens. Clinical data of limited quantity and quality had to be retrieved from hospital information systems retrospectively [31]. Nowadays, biobanks are much more than just collections of biospecimens; in fact, the legal entity "biobank" refers to the management of the samples stored under that label, the huge amount of either clinical or experimental data, and the requirements for their cession [32]. In human medicine the concept of storing biological material represents a consolidated aspect that involved either ethical or scientific tools with a particular regard to both individual and community interests [33]. The recent advances in veterinary medicine have allowed the creation of a biobank for storing animal samples. These resources should be useful for several different aspects. The first is related to the role of veterinary medicine itself, as the biobank allows more detailed information to be obtained regarding all biological resources available, for improving knowledge in several veterinary areas such as food safety, animal health, global climate change, public health emergency, and genetic conservation of biodiversity. The second aspect is related to the possibility of crossing traditional discipline boundaries for future interdisciplinary research, pathogenetic studies on eubacteria and viruses, detection of emerging zoonoses, epidemiological surveys and phylogenetic trees, and genetic evolution studies that play a key role in public health.

The use of biobanks for epidemiological research does not only depend on the availability and quality of the biomaterials, but also on the collection of associated information, such as anamnestic and epidemiological data, purity, and identity of the samples, (testing performed) depending on the biological resource, allowing large-scale screening studies.

Furthermore, experimental investigations and the development of diagnostic tests and vaccines could be transferred to national and international industrial branches.

The BVR (Biobank of Veterinary Resources) of IZSLER infrastructure integrates existing and newly established animal biological samples and data collections, resources, technologies, and expertise to facilitate high-quality medical research, improving standardization and international cooperation. Furthermore, this infrastructure will provide the flexibility needed to facilitate growth of the network with new members and partners. An additional service includes the possibility of storing human and animal biosamples, offering repository services, and ensuring governance systems that provide quality assurance.

7 Remarks and Future Perspectives

The field of biobanks is very complex and diversified, as it deals with the collection, treatment, storage, distribution, and computerization of biological material, not only of human, animal, and plant material, but also that from sources such as fossils and microbes. Biobanks and biospecimens are essential components for several areas of clinical and basic research, and, in fact, public awareness of biospecimens and biobanking has grown significantly [19].

The primary purposes for improving biobank networks are to harmonize and spread quality banking practices to distribute biospecimens with well-defined features and associated data. One of the major obstacles for developing a uniform system of regulation across Europe is the lack of an agreed definition of "biobank" [2].

Biological samples collected at the IZSLER Veterinary Biobank infrastructure could be a key resource for the scientific community. The possibility of creating a veterinary biobanking and biological resource infrastructure in Italy, and then in Europe, will allow the harmonization of standards for sample collection, storage, and techniques of analysis, data management, and preparation of a specific database. One solution to address the issues of standardization of quality and capacity should be the creation of biobank networks [34].

The main challenge of an international biobank network is balancing the need to centralize specimens and resources with the reality of delocalized collection activities, especially in a clinical context. Currently, these networks could be considered as a trade union between human and veterinary medicine, which could significantly develop a multidisciplinary approach for discovering new frontiers within life sciences and patient care.

Interoperability in biobanking represents the key for improving national and international research collaborations [35]. Furthermore, the integration of human and veterinary biobank initiatives should harmonize databank diagnostic and typing methods. There is a considerable variation in national laws and local practices regarding the processing and storage of biological samples, personal information, and data recorded among countries around the world. This variability complicates the conditions for collaboration between scientists from different countries, reducing future sharing of research data and samples. Furthermore, if regulations are not harmonized between nations, the possibility of carrying out collaborative research decreases [29].

Millions of biological samples are stored every year throughout the world for diagnostic and research, but in many fields the lack of biological material and models is a major hindrance for ongoing research. Currently, variability regards the collection, processing, storage, and relative data of the majority of biospecimens available for research and diagnosis. Such heterogeneous practices provide biospecimens of unknown molecular integrity and contribute to irreproducible results, impeding the development of more effective therapeutics and diagnostics [36].

Biobanking plays a crucial role in providing access to high-quality biomaterial, essential not only for human medicine, but also for veterinary medicine. Modern techniques of cryopreservation allow the long-term storage of biological samples for clinical or research purposes comprising a complete organization including biological samples, data, personnel, policies, and procedures for handling specimens and performing other services, such as managing the database and planning scientific studies.

Software dedicated to biological banks facilitate sample registration and identification, the cataloging of sample properties (type of sample/specimen, associated diseases and/or therapeutic protocols, environmental information, etc.), sample tracking, quality assurance, and specimen availability. Biobank facilities must adopt good laboratory practices and a stringent quality control system and comply with ethical issues when required [8].

The necessity for accessing high-quality specimens has increased, along with the necessity for standards to guide the proper collection, processing, storage, and distribution of specimens.

Perhaps more importantly, it is essential to know that the sample used for research and diagnosis is accurately characterized; once the most critical points in a biospecimen processing method have been identified, specific tests or markers to assess the quality of the biospecimen are needed.

If appropriately collected, documented, and stored, biospecimens are a valuable resource that can help answer current and future scientific questions, to meet the needs of emerging technologies [37]. The lack of concerted efforts, together with heterogeneous policy approaches and practices, jeopardizes international collaboration and the sharing of samples and data. A new attitude and strategy for sharing data and promoting cooperation in the field of biobanks may not only have a great impact on public health programs, but also in the development of new biomarkers and drugs.

The importance of biobank networking has been emphasized by many authors, and there are several major biobank networking initiatives worldwide. Currently, international initiatives are emerging in order to find ways to cooperate even in the context of heterogeneous ethical and legal frameworks in which the national biobanks are being established.

Acknowledgments

The authors thank Dr. G. Bontempi, L.R. Scorrano, colleagues of IZSLER, and the personnel of Biobank Infrastructure for practical support and collaboration.

References

1. Loft S, Poulsen HE (1996) Cancer risk in oxidative DNA damage in man. J Mol Med 74: 297–312
2. Kaye J (2006) Do we need a uniform regulatory system for biobanks across Europe? Eur J Hum Genet 14:245–248
3. Hallmans G, Vaught JB (2011) Best practices for establishing a biobank. Methods Mol Biol 675:241–260
4. OECD (2006) Creation and governance of human genetic research databases. OECD Publishing, 25 October 2006. ISBN-92-64-02852-8
5. Yuille M, Van Ommen GJ, Bréchot C et al (2008) Biobanking for Europe. Brief Bioinform 9:14–24
6. Prokosch HU, Beck A, Ganslandt T et al (2010) IT infrastructure components for biobanking. Appl Clin Inf 1:419–429
7. Carter A, Betsou F (2011) Quality assurance in cancer biobanking. Biopreserv Biobank 9: 157–163
8. Végvari A, Welinder C, Lindberg H et al (2011) Biobank resources for future patient care: developments, principles and concepts. J Clin Bioinforma 1:24
9. Zika E, Paci D, Schulte T et al (2010) Biobanks in Europe: prospects for harmonisation and networking. Seville: European Joint Research Commission and Institute for Prospective Technological Studies. http://ftp.jrc.es/EURdoc/JRC57831.pdf. Publications Office of the European Union, Luxembourg
10. Vaught JB, Caboux E, Hainaut P (2010) International efforts to develop biospecimen best practices. Cancer Epidemiol Biomarkers Prev 19:912–915
11. International Society for Biological and Environmental Repositories (ISBER) (2012) Best practices for biorepositories: collection, storage, retrieval, and distribution of biological materials for research. Biopreserv Biobank 10: 79–161
12. Zielhuis GA (2012) Biobanking for epidemiology. Public Health 126:214–216
13. Simeon-Dubach D, Burt AD, Hall PA (2012) Quality really matters: the need to improve specimen quality in biomedical research. J Pathol 228:431–433
14. Huppler Hullsieka K, Georgea M, Brownb SK (2010) Designing and managing a flexible and dynamic biorepository system: a 15 year per-

spective from the CPCRA, ESPRIT, and INSIGHT clinical trial networks. Curr Opin HIV AIDS 5:538–544
15. Betsou F, Barnes R, Burke T et al (2009) Human biospecimen research: experimental protocol and quality control tools. Cancer Epidemiol Biomarkers Prev 18:1017–1025
16. Patiel L, Aarem J, Baekken S et al (2012) Biospecimen quality program in the biobank of the Norwegian Institute of Public Health. Nor Epidemiol 21:225–229
17. Asslaber M, Zatloukal K (2007) Biobanks: transnational, European and global networks. Brief Funct Genomic Proteomic 6:193–201
18. OECD Series on Principles of Good Laboratory Practice and Compliance Monitoring. ENV/JM/MONO(2002)9. The OECD's World Wide Web site. http://www.oecd.org/ehs
19. Vaught J, Lockhart CN (2012) The evolution of biobanking best practices. Clin Chim Acta 413:1569–1575
20. Moore HM, Kelly A, Jewell SD et al (2011) Biospecimen reporting for improved study quality. Biopreserv Biobank 9:57–70
21. Micke P, Ohshima M, Tahmasebpoor S et al (2006) Biobanking of fresh frozen tissue: RNA is stable in nonfixed surgical specimens. Lab Invest 86:202–211
22. Vaught JB (2006) Blood collection, shipment, processing, and storage. Cancer Epidemiol Biomarkers Prev 15:1582–1584
23. Tuck MK, Chan DW, Chia D et al (2009) Standard operating procedures for serum and plasma collection: early detection research network consensus statement standard operating procedure integration working group. J Proteome Res 8:113–117
24. Cobo F, Stacey GN, Hunt C et al (2005) Microbiological control in stem cell banks: approaches to standardization. Appl Microbiol Biotechnol 68:456–466
25. Kokkat TJ, Patel MS, McGarvey D et al (2013) Archived formalin-fixed paraffin-embedded (FFPE) blocks: a valuable underexploited resources for extraction of DNA, RNA, and protein. Biopreserv Biobank 11:101–106
26. Knoppers BM, Isasi R (2010) Stem cell banking: between traceability and identifiability. Genome Med 2:73
27. Bravo E, Napolitano M, Santoro F et al (2013) The Italian Hub of Population Biobanks as a potential tool for improving public health stewardship. Biopreserv Biobank 11:173–175
28. Rahm AK, Wrenn M, Carroll NM et al (2013) Biobanking for research: a survey of patient population attitudes and understanding. J Community Genet 4:445–450
29. Harris JR, Burton P, Knoppers BM et al (2012) Toward a roadmap in global biobanking for health. Eur J Hum Genet 20:1105–1111
30. Gerrits RJ, Lunney JK, Johnson LA et al (2005) Perspectives for artificial insemination and genomics to improve global swine populations. Theriogenology 63:283–299
31. Tukas E, Korotiji A, Maros-Szabo Z et al (2012) Model requirements for Biobank Software Systems. Bioinformation 8:290–292
32. Arias-Diaz J, Martin-Arribas MC, Garcia del Pozo J et al (2012) Spanish regulatory approach for biobanking. Eur J Hum Genet 21:708–712
33. Meslin EM, Garba I (2011) Biobanking and public health: is a human rights approach the tie that binds? Hum Genet 130:451–463
34. Watson PH, Wilson-McManus JE, Barnes RO et al (2009) Evolutionary concepts in biobanking—the BC BioLibrary. J Transl Med 7:95
35. Kiehntopf M, Krawczak M (2011) Biobanking and international interoperability: samples. Hum Genet 130:369–376
36. Moore HM, Compton CC, Lim MD et al (2009) Biospecimen research network symposium: advancing cancer research through biospecimen science. Cancer Res 69:6770–6772
37. Marko-Varga G (2013) BioBanking as the central tool for translational medicine CTM issue. Clin Transl Med 2:4

Chapter 5

Biological Specimen Collection and Processing for Molecular Analysis

Susan Sanchez and Holly Sellers

Abstract

This chapter provides a standardized best practice approach to sample collection and handling for the purpose of nucleic acid (NA) extraction and PCR. These methods are described through text and clearly illustrated figures. Furthermore, for those cases in which transportation of samples cannot be accomplished due to the inability to maintain the cold chain or limitations on the import of live disease agents in diagnostic samples, the chapter describes the use of FTA cards for collection transport and NA preparation of samples for PCR. This chapter also makes emphasis in the best safety practices for handling of samples/tissues to avoid unnecessary disease exposures to laboratory personnel. Finally, NA extraction best practices and methods will be briefly outlined.

Key words Tissue, Swab, Culture, Virus, Bacteria, Fungi, Protozoa, Nucleic acid, Animals, Disease, Organs, FTA card, Polymerase chain reaction, PCR, Typing, DNA extraction, RNA extraction

1 Introduction

Sample collection is the first and most important step for accurate diagnostic testing. The sample must be appropriate for the test that is going to be performed. In this chapter, the primary focus will be on sampling and sample preparation for molecular analyses. The molecular analysis will most commonly be a polymerase chain reaction (PCR)-based test. Because the pathogens affecting both farm and companion animals are varied and include viral, bacterial, protozoal, and fungal pathogens, the processing of the samples outlined in this chapter will allow for both DNA and/or RNA extraction. Therefore, nucleic acid extraction (NA) will be used as an encompassing term that will be applicable to any pathogen.

PCR requires nucleic acid extraction from the diagnostic sample. Understanding the location of the pathogen in the host during an infection (this may vary during the course of the disease), as well as the duration of the infection, will improve the success of detecting the causative agent. It is also important to note that surveillance

Mónica V. Cunha and João Inácio (eds.), *Veterinary Infection Biology: Molecular Diagnostics and High-Throughput Strategies*, Methods in Molecular Biology, vol. 1247, DOI 10.1007/978-1-4939-2004-4_5, © Springer Science+Business Media New York 2015

Table 1
Examples of clinical signs and tissue samples that should be collected from chickens

Clinical signs	Sample to submit for testing
Hepatitis	Liver
Drop in egg production	Feces/large intestines, vaginal swabs
Lameness	Synovial fluid, tendons, heart, liver
Respiratory	Tracheas, tracheal swabs, feces, cloacal swabs, vaginal swabs (if also present with decreased egg production)
Dyspnea	Tracheal swabs, tracheas, eyelids, lungs
Nephritis, swollen kidneys, flushing	Kidneys
Tumors	Heparinized whole blood, tumor, plasma
Immunosuppression	Bursa, thymus, spleen, bone marrow
Skin lesions	Scab
Fowlpox	Pock lesion for cutaneous disease or trachea if diphtheritic disease
Neurological signs	Brains
Enteritis, malabsorption	Intestines, duodenal loop, feces
Proventriculitis	Proventriculus

These samples will allow for accurate molecular testing of virus and bacteria

(asymptomatic animals) and diagnosis of disease (sick animals) may call for different sample types. The methods described in detail in this chapter are more suited for disease diagnosis than for surveillance. For example, doing surveillance of foot-and-mouth disease in pigs can be accomplished by testing oral fluids present on rope samples; this allows for testing of a group, while the individual sick animal will require for confirmation the testing of the vesicular fluid. Similar case can be made with porcine circovirus type 2 and porcine reproductive and respiratory syndrome [1–3].

Many text books, commodity industries, and world organizations have published detailed information on sample selection for attaining the best results when diagnosing the many diseases that affect animals [4–10]. The intent of this chapter is not to repeat these details, but to address the important factors of sample collection and preparation using poultry as an example that can be applied to other animal groups (Table 1). Choosing the correct sample to send to the laboratory will allow for a fruitful diagnosis and a happy client.

Swabs, fluids, flushes, feces, and blood are convenient and appropriate samples to collect from live animals as are biopsies from affected sites. Fresh tissues or tissue scrapings are normally obtained from dead animals at necropsy. Unfixed tissue samples are the best specimens for pathogen detection. Nevertheless, most laboratories find them difficult to deal with due to the need for processing before nucleic acid extraction. This tissue processing is messy and must be performed consistently for repeatable and comparable results. Fixed tissues are sometimes the only sample available for analysis. The type of fixative and the time elapsed from fixation make these samples very unreliable, although useful for pathogen molecular detection if no other samples are available [11].

The method of choice for each laboratory must be based on the diagnostic needs, cost/benefit, and workload.

Nucleic acid-based molecular tests are some of the most versatile, as they are capable of detecting the pathogen directly in the sample and can be performed on a variety of sample types. Of course, the quality and quantity of the sample are of paramount importance for optimal results. Samples for PCR should be obtained with care to avoid contamination from other sites, the environment, other animals, etc., and shipped to the testing laboratory as soon as possible in sterile individual containers. The samples should be kept cold during shipping and moist with sterile saline. After their arrival to the laboratory, fluids, swabs, and flushes do not require processing prior to NA extraction and can be added directly to the lysis buffer of the nucleic acid extraction kit at the volume recommended by the manufacturer. Occasionally, these samples may be enriched or diluted in selective or enrichment media before processing, but in most cases this is not necessary. Tissues, however, always require processing prior to nucleic acid extraction.

If transport to the laboratory must be delayed, samples can be placed in RNA Later solution (there are many different suppliers of this product such as Ambion Inc., Austin, TX; Life Technologies, Grand Island, NY; Qiagen, Hilden, Germany) or DNA/RNA Shield (Zymo Research, Irvine, CA). The solutions containing nucleic acid preservatives inactivate viruses and nucleases and allow the storage of samples for up to a month at room temperature. Samples can also be refrigerated overnight or frozen at −20 or −80 °C for longer holding periods, until ready for shipment. The samples should be shipped frozen with enough ice to ensure that they arrive frozen to the testing laboratory. It is not always possible to maintain the cold chain; however, the use of FTA™ cards (Whatman, GE Healthcare, Piscataway, NJ) is a viable alternative for sample preservation. One drawback of this method is that the samples are then only useful for NA detection, but not culture, cytology, direct antigen detection, etc. [12–14].

The use of FTA™ cards has greatly facilitated the collection, handling, and shipment of samples for nucleic acid testing worldwide. FTA™ is an acronym for *Flinders Technology Associates* and the cards were originally developed in the 1980s by Burgoyne and Fowl at Flinders University, in Australia, as a method for protecting nucleic acid samples from degradation by nucleases and other processes. The patented FTA™ cards contain proprietary chemicals, integrated within a filter paper matrix, that lyse cells, denature proteins, and immobilize and preserve nucleic acids from just about any sample type. Samples can be stored and shipped at room temperature without special handling. The integrity of the samples is optimized when cards are stored in an airtight pouch with a desiccant. The cards are available in several formats including the FTA™ Indicator Card with a color indicator that changes from pink to white following sample application, making it ideal for application of colorless samples. Nucleic acids can be purified from just a couple of punches excised from the FTA™ card. We will describe later how to apply fluids and tissues on FTA™ cards for preservation of NA and shipping to the laboratory.

In this chapter, we will describe several methods to prepare tissues in a standardized manner, as well as describe the application of several sample types to FTA™ cards. Finally, the chapter will address FTA™ card processing for nucleic acid amplification. The Figs. 1, 2, 3, and 4 included for these processes are intended to be self-explanatory and easy to follow and give the operator well-defined visuals for sample processing. The figures are the result of many years of experience in busy laboratories with a heavy caseload.

2 Materials

2.1 Fresh Tissue Processing

2.1.1 Manual and Mechanical Grinder Common Materials Needed

1. Brain heart infusion broth (BHI).
2. Disposable weigh dish.
3. Scalpel and scalpel blades.
4. Sterile forceps.
5. Sterile pipette tips.
6. Pipette able to dispense 2 ml, 3 ml, and 200 μl.
7. Gloves.
8. Laboratory dedicated wear.

2.1.2 Manual Grinder Specific Material Needed

1. Small manual tissue grinder. Many manufacturers provide disposable grinders in sterile packages. Nevertheless, pestle and mortar or other similar manual instruments can be used. The advantage of the disposable is the fact that they have a plastic sleeve that will protect the user from splashes enhancing safety as well as minimize sample to sample contamination. *See* Fig. 1b for an example of a disposable manual grinder.

2.1.3 Mechanical Grinder Specific Material Needed

1. Mechanical grinder. There are several mechanical grinders from different manufacturers. Some examples are Bullet Blender (Next Advance Averill Park, USA), TissueLyser (Qiagen), and Tissue Homogenizer (Precellys, Bertin Technologies). In our

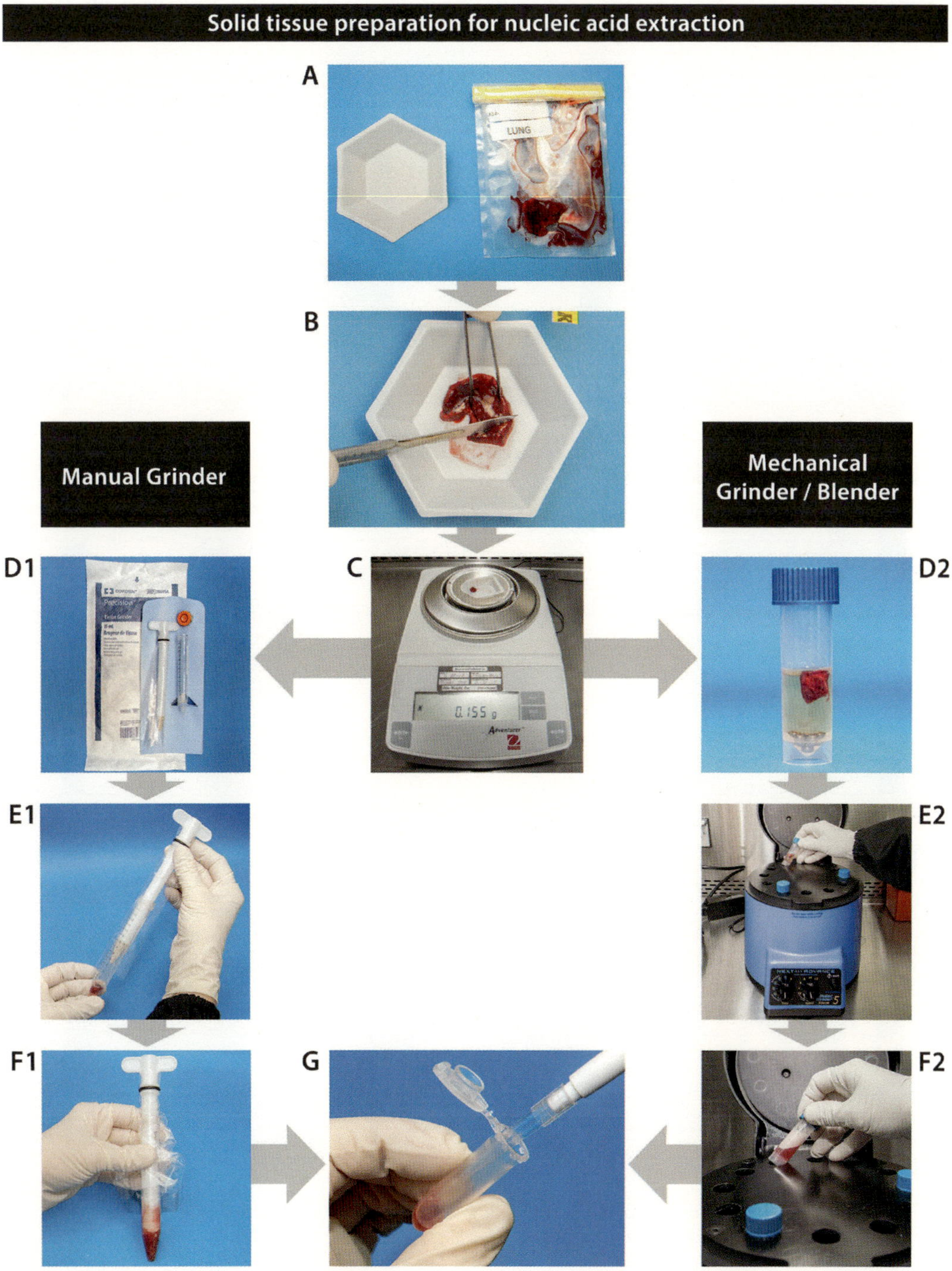

Fig. 1 Solid tissue preparation for nucleic acid extraction (*see* Subheading 3 for further information)

laboratory we use Bullet Blender preferentially. The protocol described here is for using this specific equipment.

2. Stainless steel beads 0.35 mm. Optimal for all tissue types of 0.150–0.200 g. Other bead sizes may be necessary based on the

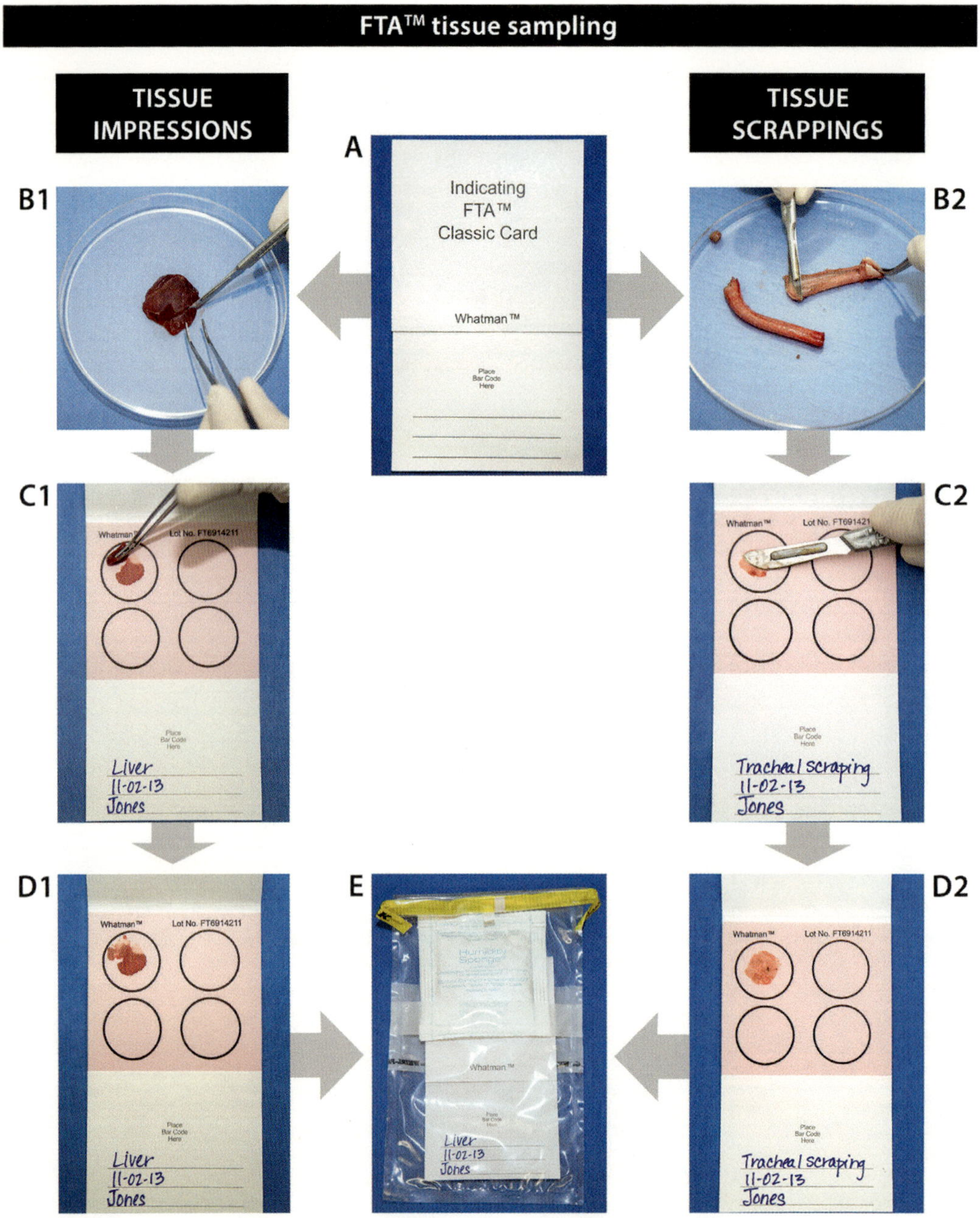

Fig. 2 FTA™ tissues and tissues scraping sampling (*see* Subheading 3 for further information)

size and type of tissue that will be processed. The manufacturer of the blender will likely carry beads of many different sizes, made of many materials in their catalog, available for purchase. Decide which ones are appropriate for your application and laboratory.

3. 5 ml sturdy tubes.

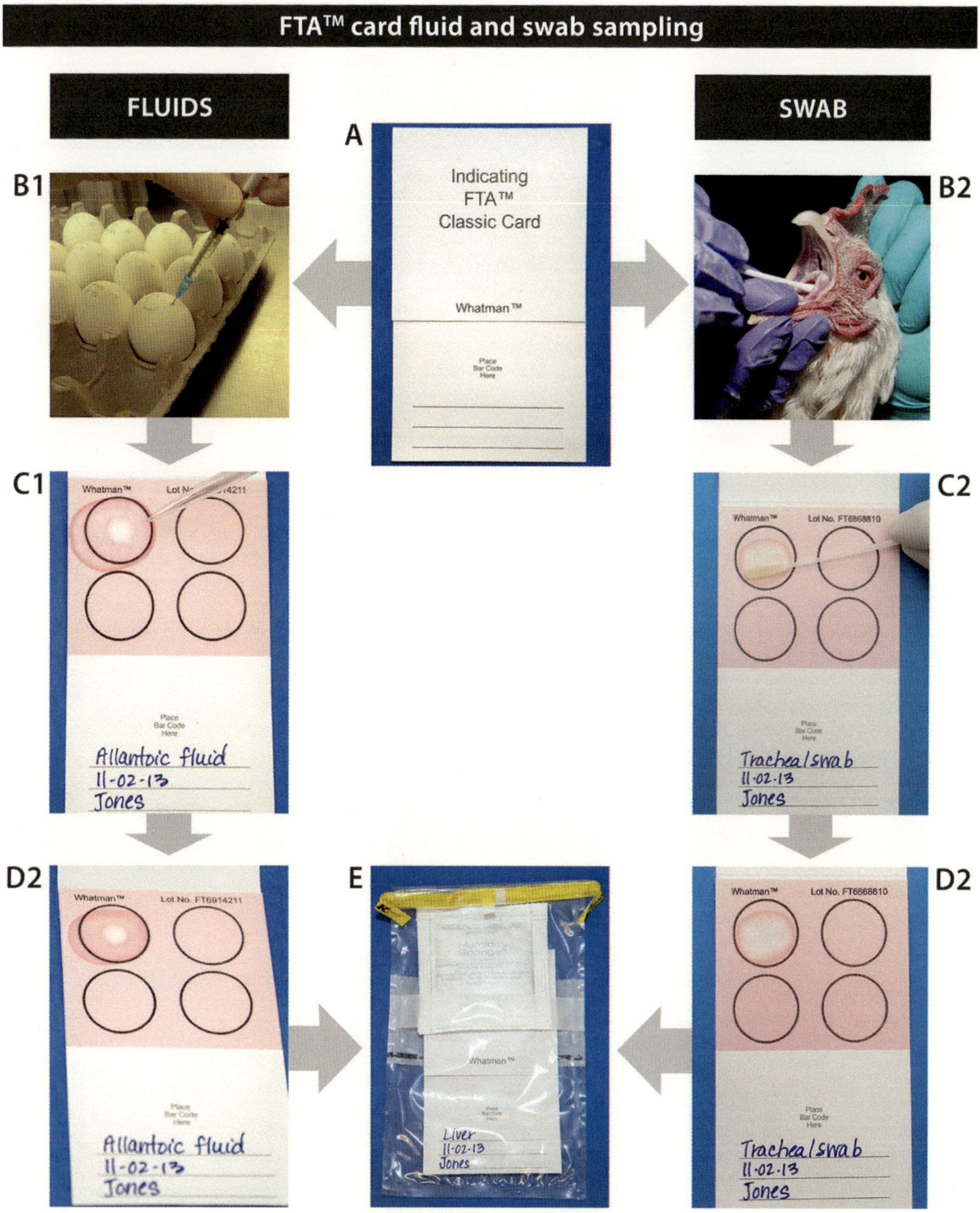

Fig. 3 FTA™ fluid and swab sampling (*see* Subheading 3 for further information)

2.2 Materials List for Sample Collection for FTA™ Cards

1. FTA™ cards (Classic or Indicating card—www.whatman.com).
2. Whirl pack bag or similar air tight storage pouch.
3. Desiccant packet.
4. Pipette (50–250 μl).
5. Sterile, RNAse-/DNAse-free pipette tips.

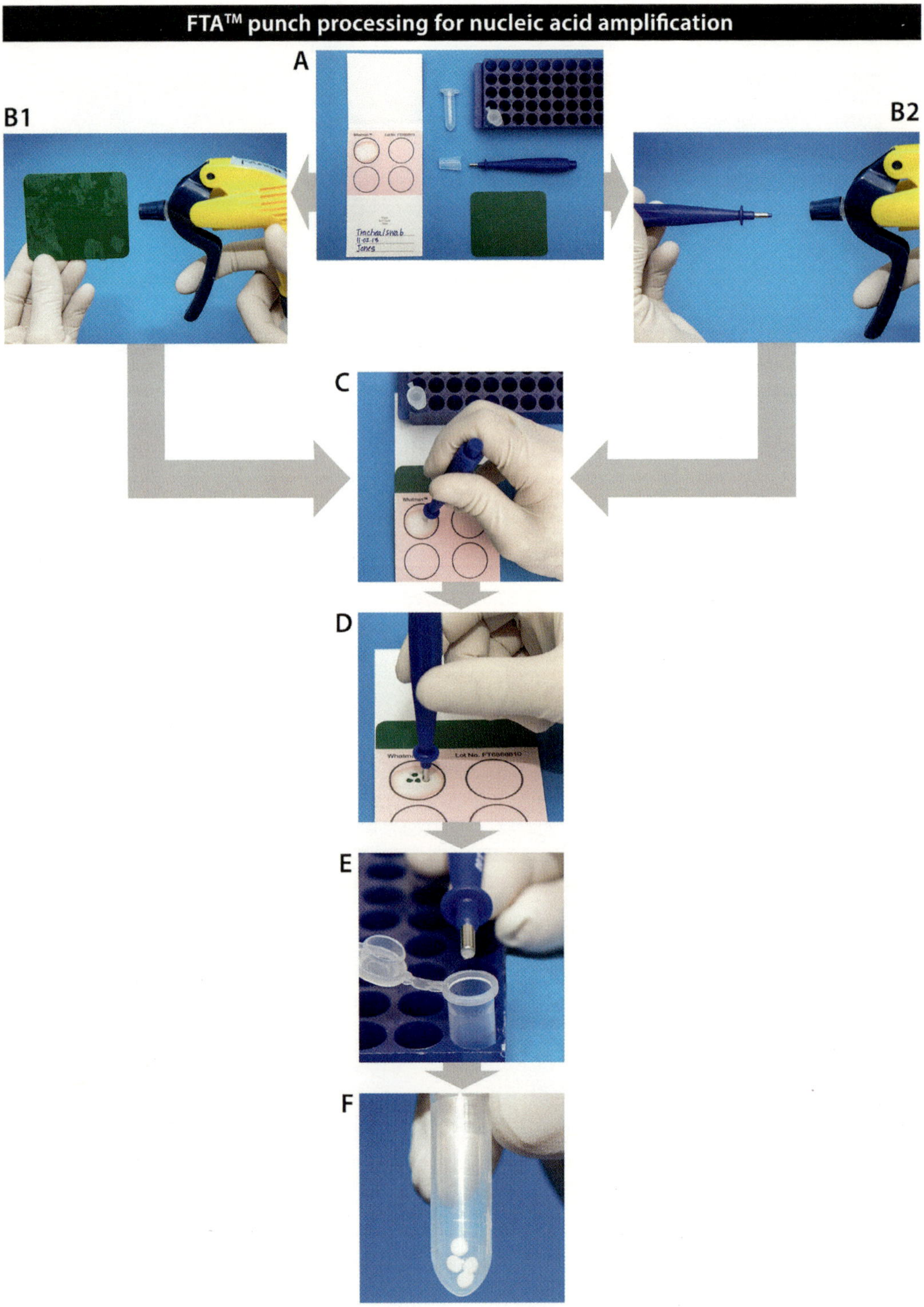

Fig. 4 FTA™ punch processing for nucleic acid amplification (*see* Subheading 3 for further information)

6. Dacron, polyester, or flocked sterile swabs.
7. Sterile scalpel.
8. Sterile scissors and forceps.
9. Sterile petri dish.
10. Gloves.

2.3 Materials List for FTA™ Card Punch Collection (Fig. 4a)

1. Harris Uni-Core punch (or similar).
2. Cutting mat.
3. 70 % Ethanol.
4. Sterile forceps.
5. RNAse-/DNAse-free microcentrifuge tube.
6. Gloves.

3 Methods

3.1 Tissues Preparation (Fig. 1; See Notes 1, 2, and 5)

3.1.1 Manual Grinder

1. Label a sterile bead tube with the sample identification number.
2. Using a sterile scalpel cut a small piece (~1 cm^3) of affected tissue and place in a weigh boat (Fig. 1b).
3. Weigh tissue to ≥0.150 g and no more than 0.200 g (Fig. 1c).
4. Transfer the tissue sample aseptically to the labeled tube of the disposable pestle (Fig. 1d1).
5. Add 1 ml of BHI to the tube; place the plastic sleeve over the top of the container (Fig. 1e1).
6. Push the pestle down the tube making sure that the tissue is at the bottom and twist it 180° in both directions at least twice. At this time the tissues will be mostly homogenized (Fig. 1f1).
7. Remove and discard the pestle/grinder.
8. Bring to a total volume of 3 ml by adding 2 ml of BHI to homogenate.
9. Transfer the required amount (normally 200 μl) to a microcentrifuge tube for further nucleic acid extraction processing (Fig. 1g).
10. Grinder tubes with homogenate can be stored frozen for later testing. Viral and bacterial cultures are possible from these samples.

3.1.2 Mechanical Grinder

1. Label a sterile bead tube with the sample identification number.
2. Using a sterile scalpel cut a small piece (~1 cm^3) of affected tissue and place in a weigh boat (Fig. 1b).
3. Weigh tissue to ≥0.150 g and no more than 0.200 g (Fig. 1c).

4. Transfer the tissue sample aseptically to the labeled tube. Add 3.0 ml of BHI broth (Fig. 1d2).
5. Tightly screw the tube closed and place in the grinder. A minimum of three tubes have to be used in the blender, spaced so that they are balanced. If fewer than three samples are to be blended, water filled tubes must be used to balance. Do not reuse the balance tubes more than five times due to the risk of tube breakage. These instructions are specific for the Bullet Blender, but most other equipment also requires balancing the loads. Regardless of the equipment, all tubes will break after multiple uses (Fig. 1e2).
6. Set the controls for speed 9 and time 4 min. Close the lid and press the start button (speed and times mentioned here are for the Bullet Blender; other equipment may require other speeds and times; check manufacturer's instructions and protocols).
7. After completion of grinding cycle visually inspect the samples (Fig. 1f2). Not all tissue samples are alike. Skin samples are usually tougher and, therefore, more difficult to homogenize. If samples are not sufficiently homogenized, repeat grinding process (*see* **Note 3**).
8. After homogenization is complete, transfer the required amount (normally 200 μl) to a microcentrifuge tube for further nucleic acid extraction processing (Fig. 1g).
9. Grinder tubes with homogenate can be stored frozen for later testing. Viral and bacterial cultures are possible from these samples.

3.2 FTA™ Card Tissue Sampling (Fig. 2; See Notes 1, 2, and 4)

3.2.1 Solid Tissue

1. Label the FTA™ card with sample identification, date, and other pertinent information (Fig. 2a).
2. Use a sterile scalpel to cut a cross section of the tissue (Fig. 2b1).
3. Make several tissue impressions with cut side of tissue to one circle on FTA™ card (Fig. 2c1).
4. Close the card and place in sealed pouch with desiccant (Fig. 2e).
5. Store at room temperature to −80 °C until nucleic acid extraction or shipment.
6. For shipment of the FTA™ card, place the pouch containing the FTA™ card and desiccant into an envelope and ship.

3.2.2 Tissue Scrapings

1. Label the FTA™ card with sample identification, date, and other pertinent information (Fig. 2a).
2. Use a sterile scalpel to scrape the surface of the tissue (Fig. 2b2).
3. Apply the tissue scrapings from the scalpel to one circle on the FTA™ card (Fig. 2c2).

4. Allow the spot to dry completely (this can take up to 1 h) (Fig. 2d2).
5. Close the card and place in a sealed pouch with desiccant (Fig. 2e).
6. Store at room temperature to −80 °C until nucleic acid extraction or shipment.
7. For shipment of the FTA™ card, place the pouch containing the FTA™ card and desiccant into an envelope and ship.

3.2.3 FTA™ Card Fluid and Swab Sampling (Fig. 3)

Fluids

1. Label the FTA™ card with sample identification, date, and other pertinent information (Fig. 3a).
2. Collect the fluid (e.g., allantoic fluid) samples (Fig. 3b1).
3. Pipette 250 μl of fluid dropwise onto the center of one circle on the FTA™ card (Fig. 3c1).
4. Allow the spot to dry completely (this can take up to 1 h) (Fig. 3d2).
5. Close the card and place in a sealed pouch with desiccant (Fig. 3e).
6. Store at room temperature to −80 °C until nucleic acid extraction or shipment.
7. For shipment of the FTA™ card, place the pouch containing the FTA™ card and desiccant into an envelope and ship.

Swabs

1. Label the FTA™ card with sample identification, date, and other pertinent information (Fig. 3a).
2. Use a Dacron, polyester, or flocked swab to obtain the sample from the patient (Fig. 3b2).
3. Roll and press the swab with the sample onto the circle of the FTA™ card, expressing as much sample as possible from swab (Fig. 3c2).
4. Allow the spot to dry completely (this can take up to 1 h) (Fig. 3d2).
5. Close the card and place in a sealed pouch with desiccant (Fig. 3e).
6. Store at room temperature to −80 °C until nucleic acid extraction or shipment.
7. For shipment of the FTA™ card, place the pouch containing the FTA™ card and desiccant into an envelope and ship.

3.3 FTA™ Cards Punch Collection (Fig. 4; See Notes 1 and 2)

1. Sanitize the Harris Uni-Core punch and mat with 70 % ethanol and allow to dry prior to use (Fig. 4b1, b2).
2. Place the mat under the FTA™ card circle to be punched (Fig. 4c).

3. Using the Harris Uni-Core punch, press down on the FTA™ card circle containing the sample. The paper disc will be retained in the core punch (Fig. 4c).
4. Repeat core sampling until the desired number of discs has been obtained. Discs will remain within the core punch. The punch can hold up to 8–10 discs (Fig. 4d).
5. Open an RNAse-/DNAse-free 1.8–2.0 ml microcentrifuge tube and depress the release button on the top of the Uni-Core punch to dispense discs into the tube (Fig. 4e).
6. Close the cap of the microcentrifuge tube.
7. Sanitize the punch and mat again with 70 % ethanol and allow to dry before obtaining another sample.
8. Punch is ready for PCR. Place the punch in your mastermix (Fig. 4f). There is no need for nucleic acid extraction from the punches. PCR is conducted suing the punch as template.

4 Notes

1. *Safety considerations*
   (a) Always wear a clean laboratory outer garment when working with diagnostic samples.
   (b) Wear protective glasses to avoid splashes to the eyes.
   (c) Wear gloves when handling animal tissues.
   (d) Fresh tissue manipulations should be carried out inside a biosafety cabinet.
   (e) Do not use the mechanical grinder if working with nonhuman primate tissues, non-captive marine mammals, and tissues suspect of any Risk Group 3 agents. There is a small risk that tubes may break.
2. *Quality assurance*
   The standardization of procedures is critical for the credibility of all diagnostic laboratories. Results should be repeatable; this is hampered occasionally by the type and volume of the samples received. Therefore, standardizing the sample of tissue by weighing, resuspending in standard volumes, and applying standard amounts to FTA™ cards is critical for your molecular diagnostic laboratory. Too much tissue or tissues that are not properly homogenized can lead to false positives or negatives. The protocols described here have been quality tested; this means that multiple tissue samples have been serially tested to determine the best procedure to yield positives and negatives consistently. It is always good practice to check the quality of

your procedure with known positive and known tissue samples and determine if repeated sampling yields consistent results.

3. *Important considerations for mechanical grinder use*
   (a) If homogenization is unsatisfactory, run for another 3 min at speed 10 (speed and times for the Bullet Blender; other equipment may require other speeds and times; check manufacturer's instructions and protocols). As a general rule, use more speed and less time. Be sure that lids are screwed on tightly.
   (b) Do not wash and reuse tubes.
4. *Important considerations for sampling on FTA™ cards*
   (a) Always wear gloves when handling FTA™ cards and avoid touching the area within the indicator circle to avoid contamination of samples.
   (b) Use FTA™ indicator cards for colorless samples so that the area to be sampled is easily identified by the color change once sample is applied. If an indicator card is not available, apply the sample to the card and circle the area of sample application with a pencil.
   (c) For tissue impressions or scrapings, allow complete absorption of sample, but do not leave additional pieces of tissue or scrapings on the card. All of the sample should be completely absorbed by the FTA™ paper.
   (d) Allow FTA™ cards to dry completely; otherwise, sample can transfer to other portions of the paper cassette. It may take up to 2–3 h for samples to dry completely on card.
   (e) Store dried FTA™ cards in sealed pouch preferably with desiccant pack.
5. *Important considerations about nucleic acid extraction*

   The steps to a diagnostic PCR test are as follows: Sample collection → sample processing → cell disruption → NA purification/concentration/inhibitor control → PCR → storage.

   Once the correct site for sampling has been determined, then any sample from that site collected using a swab or the sample itself (bodily fluids, tissues, etc.), as long as they are fresh, will be suitable for NA extraction, provided they have been handled appropriately after collection and they are not too old and kept at inappropriate temperature that allow for the degradation of the pathogen NA (RNA degrades faster than DNA). Formalin-fixed tissues can be used, but success is more variable mostly depending on the size of the product that will be targeted for amplification. The first step for the extraction is to break apart the bacteria, fungi, or viral target (also the host cells they may be invading) to release their DNA/RNA. Such methods vary from physical to chemical and/or combinations followed by the NA extraction through filtration/affinity columns or precipitation. Some samples such as fecal material have high levels of inhibitors that need to be controlled (eliminated/diluted) during the NA extraction to avoid nonspecific inhibition of the PCR tests [15–18]. Although we may think that noncommercial extractions are more economical than their commercial counterparts, they do not account for the cost of the labor and the quality control (QC) tests that have to be associated with making sure the extractions work just as efficiently every time with every batch of new reagents. Commercial tests are developed to be better than the company's previous rendition and better than their competitors [18]. They are sold as kits, where all the reagents are included, and they all have gone through rigorous QC. Every time a box is open, you are guaranteed that their efficiency will be the same as the one before and the same as the next one. Furthermore, they have been optimized for the use of high-throughput equipment making them very suitable for testing large numbers of samples; this is a common scenario in veterinary medicine herd health [19]. Current kits from many manufacturers decrease inhibitors, some also come with internal controls, and are able to isolate from the same sample, both DNA and RNA with high efficiency. The cost is relatively modest per sample, although they are sold in large packages that may be expensive. Nevertheless, they allow for easier validation of the extraction/PCR protocols for each of the matrices that will be use for disease diagnosis (feces, tissue, urine, etc.). A good NA extraction is a powerful adjunct to a good PCR test; the sensitivity of any PCR test will be dependent on how good the NA extraction is. No matter how well tuned your PCR is, if there are not enough copies of NA or there are inhibitors present, the sensitivity of the PCR will suffer. Commercial kits because they will maintain their quality across laboratories will allow for standardization across of PCR tests [20]. Much is written about NA extraction, and we recommend to check the current literature, check what is commercially available and you can afford, determine if you will require high throughput now or in the near future, and validate the method you choose to use comparing it with a gold standard for each of the matrices first and then with known positive clinical samples. Finally, always maintain strict quality control protocols that will allow for the reproducibility and reliability of the extraction method you decide to use and works best for your PCR test. "One extraction does not fit all PCR or matrices."

Acknowledgments

Photography credits to Christopher B. Herron, Digital Media Coordinator, College of Veterinary Medicine, The University of Georgia, Athens, USA; art credits to Kip Carter, Chief of Medical Illustration Services, College of Veterinary Medicine, The University of Georgia, Athens, USA.

References

1. Vosloo W, Morris J, Davis A et al (2013) Collection of oral fluids using cotton ropes as a sampling method to detect foot-and-mouth disease virus infection in pigs. Transbound Emerg Dis. doi: 10.1111/tbed.12196
2. Prickett J, Simer R, Christopher-Hennings J et al (2008) Detection of porcine reproductive and respiratory syndrome virus infection in porcine oral fluid samples: a longitudinal study under experimental conditions. J Vet Diagn Invest 20:156–163
3. Committee on Foreign and Emerging Diseases of the United States Animal Health Association (2008) Foreign animal diseases, 7th edn. USHAA, St. Joseph, MO
4. Dufour-Zavala L (ed) (2008) A laboratory manual for the isolation, identification and characterization of avian pathogens, 5th edn. American Association of Avian Pathologists, Madison, WI
5. Saif YM, Fadly AM, Glisson JR, McDougald LR, Nolan L, Swayne DE (eds) (2008) Diseases of poultry, 12th edn. Blackwell Publishing Professional, Ames, IA
6. Greene CE (2012) Infectious diseases of the dog and cat, 4th edn. Elsevier/Saunders, St. Louis, Mo
7. Lo YMD, Chiu RWK, Chan KCA (2006) Clinical applications of PCR, 2nd edn. Humana, Totowa, NJ
8. Radostits OM, Done SH (2007) Veterinary medicine: a textbook of the diseases of cattle, sheep, pigs, goats, and horses, 10th edn. Elsevier Saunders, New York, NY
9. Smith BP (2009) Large animal internal medicine, 4th edn. Mosby Elsevier, St. Louis, MO
10. Zimmerman JJ (2012) Diseases of swine, 10th edn. Wiley-Blackwell, Chichester
11. Granato A, Giantin M, Ariani P et al (2014) DNA and RNA isolation from canine oncologic formalin-fixed, paraffin-embedded tissues for downstream "-omic" analyses: possible or not? J Vet Diagn Invest 26:117–124
12. Burgoyne LA (1996) Solid medium and methods for DNA storage. US patent 54,965, 496,562
13. Rogers CDG, Burgoyne LA (2000) Reverse transcription of an RNA genome from databasing paper (FTA®). Biotechnol Appl Biochem 31:219–224
14. Seah LH, Burgoyne LA (2000) DNA databasing on FTA® paper: biological assault and techniques for measuring photogenic damage. In: Sensabaugh GF, Lincoln PJ, Olaisen B (eds) Progress in forensic genetics 8. International Congress Series. 1193, 74–77
15. Saunders NA, Lee MA (2013). Real-time PCR: advanced technologies and applications. Caister Academic
16. Schuller M, Carter IWJ, James GS et al (2010) PCR for clinical microbiology: an Australian and international perspective. Springer
17. Tang Y-W (2012) Advanced techniques in diagnostic microbiology. Springer, New York, NY
18. Yang G, Erdman DE, Kodani M et al (2011) Comparison of commercial systems for extraction of nucleic acids from DNA/RNA respiratory pathogens. J Virol Methods 171:195–199
19. Gaumann R, Muhlemann K, Strasser M et al (2010) High-throughput procedure for tick surveys of tick-borne encephalitis virus and its application in a national surveillance study in Switzerland. Appl Environ Microbiol 76:4241–4249
20. Iker BC, Bright KR, Pepper IL et al (2013) Evaluation of commercial kits for the extraction and purification of viral nucleic acids from environmental and fecal samples. J Virol Methods 191:24–30

Chapter 6

Validation of Molecular Diagnostic Assays and Quality Assurance and Control in the Veterinary Laboratory

Nick Saunders and Ian Sharp

Abstract

This chapter describes the process of validating in-house molecular assays although the principles described are equally relevant to all diagnostic assays. The best practice principles described below are based on the In Vitro Diagnostic Medical Devices Directive (IVDD) and associated documentation. Although compliance with these regulations is not required for diagnostic reagents used on animals, the principles are equally relevant to validation of all diagnostic assays, whatever their purpose.

Key words Validation, In-house, Molecular assays, Quality assurance, Quality control

1 Introduction

The introduction of new or modified diagnostic tests for veterinary application is associated with significant risks, and a consistent approach to assay validation and verification is therefore a requirement (Fig. 1).

In vitro diagnostics (IVDs) for human use come under statutory regulations in most jurisdictions (e.g., the US Food and Drug Administration (FDA), the European Commission (EC)), and although veterinary IVDs are generally free of these controls, there is a responsibility, and usually a commercial necessity, to ensure that tests are fit for purpose. Both in-house and commercial assays (commercial kits used in modified form or for off-label applications fall within the in-house status) need to be backed by the same level of evidence supporting their performance against a specification.

Once an assay has been introduced, systematic quality assurance (QA) activities are essential to ensure that the assay continues to perform according to the requirements of the specification and fulfills its purpose.

Mónica V. Cunha and João Inácio (eds.), *Veterinary Infection Biology: Molecular Diagnostics and High-Throughput Strategies*, Methods in Molecular Biology, vol. 1247, DOI 10.1007/978-1-4939-2004-4_6, © Springer Science+Business Media New York 2015

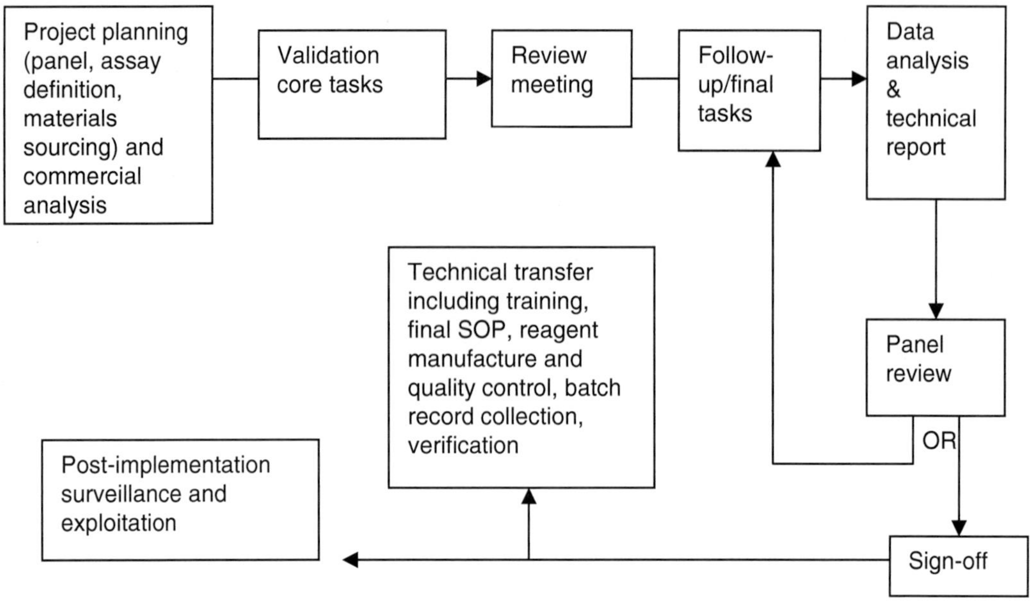

Fig. 1 Assay development and validation plan

Quality control (QC) procedures must also be applied to maintain the uniformity of the procedures and materials used to perform the assay. Output data monitoring using multi-rule criteria is a useful aspect of QC.

2 Validation of Molecular Diagnostics

This chapter refers to all nucleic acid-based (i.e., molecular) assays including those designed for diagnostic and reference purposes.

The World Organisation for Animal Health (OIE) has developed a register of diagnostic kits certified by the OIE as validated as fit for purpose [1]. Examples of the most common purposes are to:

1. Demonstrate freedom from infection in a defined population (country/zone/compartment/herd): (1a) "free" with and/or without vaccination and (1b) reestablishment of freedom after outbreaks.
2. Certify freedom from infection or presence of the agent in individual animals or products for trade/movement purposes.
3. Eradication of disease or elimination of infection from defined populations.
4. Confirmatory diagnosis of suspect or clinical cases (includes confirmation of positive screening test).

5. Estimate prevalence of infection or exposure to facilitate risk analyses (surveys, herd health status, disease control measures).
6. Determine immune status of individual animals or populations (post-vaccination).

These purposes are broadly inclusive of many narrower and more specific applications of assays. Such specific applications and their unique purposes need to be clearly defined within the context of a fully validated assay.

The term "validation" is often used very loosely and can cover a variety of different processes. From the manufacturing industry, "Validation is a quality assurance process of establishing evidence that provides a high degree of assurance that a product, service, or system accomplishes its intended requirements. This often involves acceptance of fitness for purpose with end users and other product stakeholders." Validation is an evidence-based process that requires proper planning in order to ensure that newly developed assays comply with laboratory standard systems. There are a number of stages in this process, including planning and inception, assay development and optimization, assay validation, rollout and verification (i.e., a quality control process that is used to evaluate whether the assay complies with its specification), and finally implementation. Method validation can be used to judge the quality, reliability, and consistency of analytical results. It is therefore an integral part of any good analytical practice. Annex 15 to the European Union (EU) Guide to Good Manufacturing Practice [2] which deals with qualification and validation provides a useful context.

Analytical methods need to be validated before their introduction into routine use and revalidated whenever the conditions under which the original validation was done change (e.g., use of an instrument with different characteristics or samples within a different carrier matrix) and whenever the method is changed or modified beyond the original specification. The changes to a protocol that may be considered significant and that therefore require assay revalidation with adequate evidence for equivalent performance depend on the specific details of the test. Validation may be extensive, for example, in the case of a newly developed in-house assay, or narrow in scope, for example, in the case of a commercial assay already in use which has had minor modifications. Various situations are likely to arise in which it is appropriate to repeat only a subset of validation tasks. For example, if the extraction method is changed, it may not be necessary to carry out specificity checks, but the sensitivity will require reassessment. It is essential to provide documentary evidence that any assay is suitable for its intended purpose.

The laboratory may already have in-house or commercial assays in use for which no specific evidence of previously undertaken validation or verification is available. Almost certainly, this work would have been performed, but historically there may not have been a good culture of record keeping. It is important to provide documentary evidence of fitness for purpose. It is not normally necessary to repeat validation and verification work, and in practice, it may not be possible to retrospectively undertake this. It may be sufficient to prepare a file referring to existing evidence, such as results from interlaboratory comparisons or other studies undertaken, copies of published papers, internal quality control (IQC) and external quality assessment (EQA) results, etc. However, the process of reviewing validation data may highlight factors that require confirmation.

3 Quality Assurance

Quality assurance is the process whereby the quality of laboratory reports can be guaranteed and comprises all the different measures taken to ensure the reliability of investigations. It is not limited to the technical procedures performed in the laboratory. Therefore, although procedures within the laboratory that ensure that the testing procedures (the analytical phase) are reliable are important, consideration must also be given to the pre- and post-analytical phases, where the majority of the errors in the entire testing pathway occur.

The laboratory does not have control of many of the preanalytical steps, such as what and how specimens were taken, labeling (of samples and request forms), and transportation. However, it can influence these activities by providing guidance in the form of a user manual. This provides details of those key factors related to the specimen which are known to affect the performance of the test or the interpretation of the results and instructions for transportation of samples, including any special handling needs. The laboratory should also have a procedure which defines the criteria for specimen rejection. It is good practice to notify the user concerning rejected specimens.

Many veterinary laboratories are accredited by the national accreditation body to the international standard ISO 17025 [3]. Accreditation is a means of assessing the technical competence of the laboratory and provides assurance to the laboratory and its customers that its service is fit for purpose.

The key elements of accreditation are competency of staff; use of documented, validated procedures; appropriate management and use of equipment and reagents; and a system of evaluation and quality improvement, involving internal audit, recording, and management of user complaints and nonconformities.

There is a much used saying among "quality" professionals, "If it isn't written down it didn't happen." Good record keeping is essential, for audit purposes (internal and external), to aid identification of root causes when problems are identified (e.g., determining which reagents or instruments might be responsible for a poor performing test) and evidence of due diligence if the quality of testing is questioned by a customer.

The most important aspect of quality is the culture of the organization. Some organizations regard accreditation as a tick box exercise. For these, compliance with accreditation standards will always be a burden. The efforts required getting ready for assessment visits by the accreditation body, to update standard operating procedures overdue review, to carry out audits, and to close nonconformities that should have been dealt with weeks or months ago, become a last minute struggle. For such organizations, the quality management system (QMS) is in place to maintain accreditation and not to ensure best practice. Another well-known saying is that "Quality starts at the top." If senior management recognize the value of the QMS, resource it appropriately, attend quality management meetings, and support quality related activities, then the culture of the organization will be enhanced as will be its performance.

4 Quality Control

Quality assurance of test methods will be provided by a combination of internal quality control (IQC), internal quality assessment (IQA), and external quality assessment (EQA).

4.1 Internal Quality Control

IQC is the analysis of material of known content in order to determine in real time if the procedures are performing within predetermined specifications. It is primarily the day-to-day monitoring of reproducibility or precision designed to detect errors in any single days analytical procedure. Performance of control material within predefined limits is essential for technical validation of a diagnostic test. The type of control used will depend on the type of assay. For qualitative assays, controls may just consist of a positive or negative sample. For quantitative assays, quality requirements of controls need to be determined for high and/or low clinical decision limits, depending on the analyte. A good understanding of the assay is essential in order to ensure that the appropriate controls are used. There is further discussion on the use of controls for polymerase chain reaction (PCR) assays later in this chapter. A number of papers have been published on the use and interpretation of controls in veterinary laboratories [4, 5].

Commercial assays will include assay controls but the laboratory should not rely on kit controls alone. Manufacturers adjust controls from batch to batch to give consistent results although assay sensitivity may vary between batches. This consistency is an obvious aid to the user, but it does mean that if you only use the controls that come with the kit, you will not detect any batch to batch variation. Therefore, it is recommended that the laboratory also use independent internal quality control materials, either purchased from a commercial source or prepared in-house.

Use of the same internal control material over an extended period monitors batch to batch variation.

Internally prepared controls must:

- Behave like real samples
- Have sufficient to last for a period of time, ideally at least a year
- Be stable over the period of use
- Be appropriately apportioned for convenient use
- Vary little in concentration between aliquots
- Operate within the linear region of the assay

A series of QC results may be plotted as run charts, also known as Levey Jennings or Shewhart charts. These show the values plotted against the mean and usually the 1, 2, and 3 standard deviation (SD) values. Westgard rules [6, 7] may then be used to define specific performance limits and detect both random and systematic errors. Three of the six commonly used Westgard rules are warning rules, the violation of which should trigger a review of test procedures, equipment calibration, and reagent performance. Three are mandatory rules which, if broken, should result in the rejection of results in that assay run.

It is important to note that a system of quality control is unlikely to improve a method that is fundamentally unsound. Performing quality control does not by itself improve the quality of any assay. It is the interpretation of the data obtained and appropriate actions taken that will lead to quality improvement.

4.2 Internal Quality Assessment (IQA)

IQA is the repeat testing of a percentage (typically 0.5–1 % of workload) of routine test samples to determine the laboratory's ability to obtain reproducible results. IQA is a commonly used tool in clinical microbiology laboratories but less so in other disciplines. Consistency is an important measure of quality assurance, so repeat tests continually giving the same results as the original show a system that is in control. The fact that IQA is performed on so many samples throughout the year means that the results obtained are statistically significant.

A specimen is split in two on arrival into the laboratory, and while one part is put through the test procedure in the normal way, the other one is given an IQA number and a new request form is created. The IQA sample is then tested and reported in the normal way, except that the report is sent to a member of staff rather than a requesting clinician. The IQA result is then compared with the original result and any discrepancies noted. Discrepancies are normally classed as either minor or major. Minor ones show variation but would not affect the result, whereas major discrepancies are likely to lead to a different result. All discrepancies should be investigated and major ones are likely to require repeat testing and may result in an amended report being issued.

IQA requires the repeat sample to be booked in, for tests to be selected and then performed, results to be validated, and a report to be produced, with interpretive comments included. Therefore, IQA assesses important aspects of the pre- and post-analytical phase which take place within the laboratory as well as the analytical phase itself. Although on its own, IQA does not prove that the laboratory is actually getting the right result, it is a good test of the system and, when combined with other quality control measures, is helpful in evaluating process control.

4.3 External Quality Assessment (EQA)

External quality assessment is usually an externally organized function that monitors the efficacy of quality assurance procedures. It compares the performance of different testing sites by allowing the analysis of an identical specimen at many laboratories, followed by comparison of individual results with those of other sites and with the correct answer. EQA acts as a check on the efficacy of internal quality control procedures.

EQA is performed on a limited number of samples, and the process is inevitably retrospective, providing an assessment of performance rather than a true control for each test performed. It gives participants an insight into their routine performance so that they can take action to achieve improvements. EQA is an educational tool. To achieve the greatest benefit from EQA, samples must be treated the same way as routine samples.

The diagram in Fig. 2 is a good illustration of how to interpret QC results in terms of assay performance. The correct EQA result

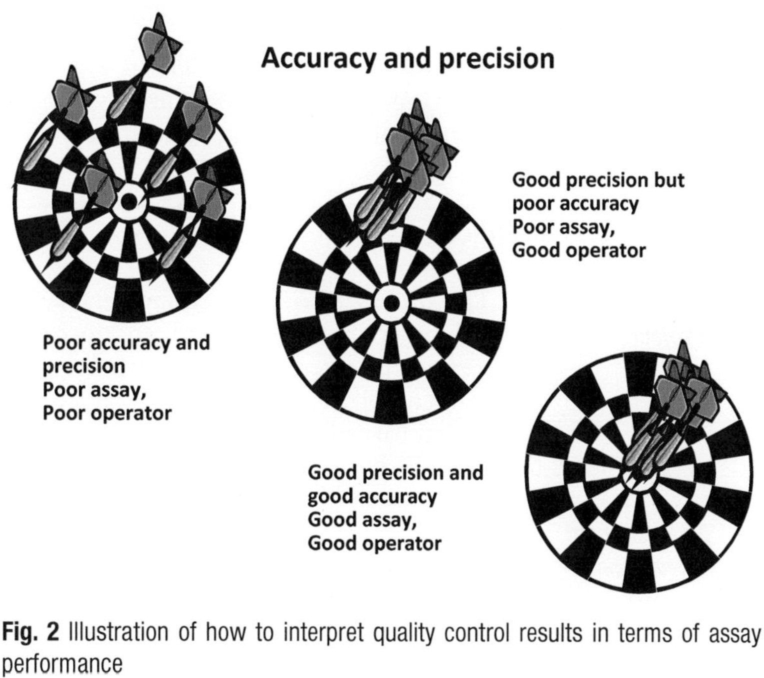

Fig. 2 Illustration of how to interpret quality control results in terms of assay performance

could be the dart closest to the bull's eye in the first dartboard on the left. Therefore, the correct EQA result does not show that the laboratory is capable of getting consistent results or of getting the correct result consistently. If IQA results are consistently the same as the original test results, they show good precision as shown in dart boards 2 and 3 but do not distinguish between these two options, i.e., show good process control but not whether the assay is good. If IQC results are consistently accurate (mean close to expected value of the control and small SD values), then this shows good precision and a good assay, as indicated by dartboard 3. However, only the examination phase is assessed by IQC.

Clearly, EQA, IQA, and IQC all have their role to play. EQA allows comparison with results obtained by all other laboratories participating in the scheme. IQA shows whether or not the laboratory has the pre-examination, examination, and post-examination activities in control, and IQC shows whether or not the actual results are correct. By performing EQA, IQA, and IQC and reviewing the data obtained, you get a powerful indication whether or not you have a well-controlled process (and competent operator) and also a good assay.

4.4 Personnel

All personnel involved with the validation, quality assurance, and quality control of diagnostic tests must have clearly defined lines of accountability and be equipped with appropriate knowledge, competency, and experience. Records of their qualifications must be available.

4.5 Equipment

All equipment used in the assay validation exercise must be maintained, serviced, calibrated, and monitored as appropriate to ensure that it is suitable for use. This is essential to ensure that all conditions can be reproduced accurately during subsequent routine production of reagents and performance of the assay.

5 Planning and Inception

5.1 Establishment of the Project

The drivers for introduction of new diagnostics are most commonly gaps in capability and capacity or opportunities for improved service presented by new knowledge and technology. During the planning phase, the aim is to produce a clear, agreed project plan. A vital part of the process is to ensure that the project is properly resourced.

5.2 Establishment of a Review Team

A suitable panel ("review team") should then be established to review the plan. This panel will also review the progress of the validation work, evidence that the test is fit for purpose and that plans for monitoring of test performance are in place. It is important to note that the size and composition will depend on the complexity of the project. The principle of having a review team will apply however simple the project. However, a straightforward revalidation following a minor change may be undertaken and overseen by just one person. However, final sign-off of the project must be undertaken by an appropriate senior member of staff.

The project leader and project manager roles may be performed by a single individual. The project manager, who has overall responsibility for the completion of the validation project and responsibility for signing off the completed validation file and the documented standard operating procedure (SOP) for performance of the assay, should, most appropriately, be at least at team leader level (however described). The project leader has responsibility for the project work, including laboratory activity needed for the validation, data analysis, compilation of the validation file, report writing, presentation of data to review meetings, writing and maintaining the SOP, and training of staff to carry out the procedure described in the new SOP.

One member of the review team should be responsible for ensuring that all documents relating to the project (i.e., the contents of the project dossier) are brought to the attention of senior management. This person must also ensure that the management are informed of the key project events (i.e., project inception and funding, development work successful in meeting design requirements, project abandonment, validation study completion, declaration that the test is fit for purpose and plans for deployment). An example of a suitable team would be two laboratory scientists, at least one clinical representative and the local quality representative. It is highly desirable that one or more of the members of the team should be a potential end user of the assay, as this will be useful in providing input to the validation parameters to ensure clinical utility. It is recommended that at least one of the members of the team has statistical expertise, but alternatively a statistician should be consulted to give advice on the validation study design. The project manager or project leader, but preferably not both, unless both roles are held by a single person, may be members of the review team.

The review team has the following responsibilities:

1. To assess how the assay will improve or fill gaps in the current testing repertoire. This should include identification of the diagnostic need, the currently available alternatives, the end users, and any other stakeholders.
2. To compile a register of risks associated with project success or failure and implementation of the assay (e.g., users might use inappropriate specimen types or misinterpret the results). The register should specify design actions to be taken in mitigation of the specified risks.
3. To ensure that laboratory safety issues associated with the test and the validation program have been assessed.

4. To ensure that the engagement of collaborative partners to provide expertise or share costs has been considered.
5. To ensure that training and other human resources issues are addressed.
6. To ensure that the means for efficient project management have been established, including the nomination of advisors and reviewers as necessary.
7. To approve the assay validation plan and then, when complete, to review the validation study data and decide whether the assay is suitable for deployment.
8. To review the assay deployment and post-deployment plans.
9. To ensure that the project dossier is maintained.

6 Assay Validation Plan

The objective of the assay validation plan is to ensure that the assay conforms to the required specification. The specification may be broad, for example, requiring that the assay accurately and reliably measures only the analyte of interest in clinical samples with the required level of sensitivity. Ensuring test reliability will include the need to control the uniformity of the assay procedure and reagents over time and the maintenance of full result traceability.

The review panel and project leader should conduct planning meetings, perform literature searches, appraise options, and, where possible, consult with other centers that carry out the same or similar assays. The project plan documentation should be version controlled. When the project plan has been agreed, the project leader will be responsible for performance of the laboratory tasks. When the agreed project milestones have been reached, a review panel meeting should be held with the project leader presenting the data. Any follow-up work and/or analysis, if necessary, will be agreed, following which the project lead will generate the technical report. The technical report is then circulated to the review panel, which will then either sign off the assay as ready for rollout for routine use (technical transfer including training of routine diagnostic staff) or request further work that is carried out before the assay can be signed off as suitable.

The technological details of the proposed assay, including information on the platforms, reagents, controls, and protocol to be used, should be specified in the validation plan. Sample preparation methods form an integral part of the diagnostic test for validation purposes.

The plan should specify the sample types to be evaluated and both the essential (i.e., minimum) and optimal sample volumes.

7 Validation Design

The project leader should prepare the validation plan including the following points that are based on the STARD initiative [8] and external literature including MIQE [9]:

1. Define the purpose and objectives of the validation study. For example, the study may be intended to validate the performance of a new assay or may aim to demonstrate that a significantly modified assay or protocol variant gives results within the tolerance of the original.
2. Identify any training requirements to ensure everyone involved in the validation has suitable levels of competency. Ensure training records are up to date for procedures being carried out.
3. Identify any risk assessments which need to be reviewed or written.
4. Identify the available standards or reference materials. These act as controls to allow the assay to be standardized, facilitate assay comparison, and permit stability of the assay to be determined over time.
5. Identify the assay to be used for comparison with the assay undergoing validation. This should be the currently accepted "gold standard" where one is available.
6. Design an analytical validation study to test the sensitivity and specificity of the assay using control materials, extracts from a wide range of strains/variants of the target organism, specimens spiked with the target organisms, and a range of unrelated strains or species that could be present in a sample, but that should not give a positive result.
7. Design a clinical validation study appropriate to the clinical context (e.g., surveillance, screening, clinical diagnosis). Choose the study group including species, case definitions, inclusion/exclusion criteria, and study settings.
8. Identify the types (i.e., specimen, method of sampling, transport and processing) and numbers of samples to be tested. Consider the need to include known positives, known negatives, low and high positives, and samples which are known or likely to be problematic (e.g., containing inhibitors or possibly cross-reactive markers).
9. Select appropriate statistical tools for determination of an appropriate sample size and to avoid bias. It is essential to consider statistical requirements to ensure that results are statistically significant. The sample size needed to ensure statistically significant results depends on a number of variables. Some guidance is given in Tables 1 and 2. The validation design should avoid discrepant analysis bias. Some samples may give discordant

Table 1
Relationship between sample size and 95 % confidence interval

Number of infected (noninfected) subjects required[a]	Estimated test sensitivity (or specificity)[b]					
	50 %	60 %	70 %	80 %	90 %	95 %
50	13.9 %	13.6 %	12.7 %	11.1 %	8.3 %	–
100	9.8 %	9.6 %	9.0 %	7.8 %	5.9 %	4.3 %
150	8.0 %	7.8 %	7.3 %	6.4 %	4.8 %	3.5 %
200	6.9 %	6.8 %	6.4 %	5.5 %	4.2 %	3.0 %
500	4.4 %	4.3 %	4.0 %	3.5 %	2.6 %	1.9 %
1,000	3.1 %	3.0 %	2.8 %	2.5 %	1.9 %	1.4 %

[a]As defined by the reference standard test
[b]95 % confidence interval around the estimated sensitivity or specificity (± value in table)

results with the new test compared to a "gold standard." If only these samples are retested, bias is introduced as there is a probability that the second analysis will give concordant results for some of these samples. Both concordant and discrepant samples should be retested to avoid bias.

10. Consider documenting an assessment of assay usability including method practicability, user feedback, and barriers to implementation.
11. Plan to review the validation study in a timely manner. The review meetings should have minutes detailing attendees and agreed actions.
12. Ensure that all SOPs related to the modified or new kits or reagents are current. It may be necessary to maintain new or revised SOPs as working drafts while their contents are being validated, ensuring risk assessments are up to date. SOPs should be controlled documents.
13. Where assays are designed to diagnose diseases for which relevant clinical material is hard to obtain or rare (e.g., the viral hemorrhagic fevers), their use may be justifiable due to their potential diagnostic value, even though the full validation criteria described here are not met. Deficiencies in assay validation should be documented in the development dossier, together with justification for each instance where the data are inadequate. In such cases, a plan for completion of satisfactory validation should be outlined. For example, it may be possible to obtain samples post-implementation, or it may be reasonable to place greater reliance on the use of carefully designed simulated specimens.

Table 2
Design parameters for validation experiments

Parameter	Design
Analytical sensitivity	Four different assay runs with at least three replicates per dilution of the sample
Diagnostic sensitivity	Testing of samples (that have been tested using the "gold-standard" or appropriate alternative assay) from cases with the defined clinical profile(s). The minimum numbers of samples to be tested (to give a required level of reliability of the sensitivity measurement) will depend on the prevalence of disease and can be calculated from the minimum sensitivity levels and the 95 % CI shown in Table 1
Analytical specificity	Testing of DNA extracted from as many variants as possible of the target organism, genetically related organisms and organisms likely to be found in positive and negative cases (>100) with the defined clinical profile(s)
Diagnostic specificity	Testing of >50 samples that were positive and >50 samples that were negative using the gold-standard assay
Efficiency (quantitative assays)	Test tenfold dilutions of a positive sample or control in triplicate. Dilution range to give C_qs from <12 to >35 cycles
Linearity (quantitative assays)	Test tenfold dilutions of a positive sample or control in triplicate. Dilution range to give C_qs from <12 to >35 cycles
Measurement range	Test tenfold dilutions of a positive sample or control in triplicate. Range to extend from lowest practical dilution to tenfold beyond highest dilution giving a positive result
Precision (quantitative assays)	Three samples (high, medium, and low positive) assayed at least four times or more in one run and over at least four different runs on different days
Reproducibility (quantitative assays)	Three samples (high, medium, and low positive) assayed at least four times or more in one run and in at least four different runs on different days. These to be run in different laboratories or using different reagent batches or different instruments
Analytical accuracy (quantitative assays)	Three analytical standards (high, medium, and low positive) assayed at least four times or more in one run and over at least four different runs on different days
Clinical accuracy (quantitative assays)	Three clinical standards (high, medium, and low positive) assayed at least four times or more in one run and over at least four different runs on different days
Reference intervals	Testing of >100 samples (that have been tested using the gold-standard assay) from cases with the defined clinical profile(s)
Clinical validation	Analysis of samples from cases with the defined clinical profile(s) with follow-up. This is on-going audit of assay performance
Shelf life	Samples from three batches stored at the designed storage temperature. Aliquots used to assay three samples (high medium and low positive) at least four times or more in one run and in at least two different runs on different days

8 Performing the Validation

8.1 General Principles

With appropriate planning, much of the data required for validation can be collected in relatively few assay runs with, for example, the same run used to produce data on accuracy and reproducibility in concert.

Diagnostic accuracy can be assessed through sensitivity and specificity, positive and negative predictive values (PPV and NPV), or positive and negative diagnostic likelihood ratios. The determination of accuracy requires that the true condition (i.e., as determined by a gold standard where one exists) of the sample is known as indicated in Table 3, which defines these terms. Where possible, the study should include high, medium, and low positives (i.e., reactive samples), as well as negative samples. It is likely that misleading results will be produced if only high positives are used to test diagnostic sensitivity.

Table 1 gives guidance on the acceptable sample numbers used in validation experiments. Interpretation of the acceptability of an assay based on its validation data will necessarily depend upon the performance relative to alternative tests and upon the diagnostic situation, for example, a very high NPV will be required for a screening test.

8.2 Controls

False negatives in molecular diagnostic assays, particularly the ones based on the PCR, may arise due to problems encountered at various stages of the diagnostic cycle. Although some of the problems are generic, also relating to other testing methods, some are specific to the design and use of diagnostic PCR. The problems of diagnostic PCR that are most intractable in terms of false-negative results are extraction failure and reaction inhibition.

Table 3
Definitions

		Reference test results (gold standard)	
		Positive	Negative
New test results	Positive	TP	FP
	Negative	FN	TN

TP number of true-positive specimens, *FP* number of false-positive specimens, *FN* number of false-negative specimens, *TN* number of true-negative specimens

Sensitivity = TP/(TP + FN)

Specificity = TN/(TN + FP)

Diagnostic accuracy = (TP + TN)/(TP + FP + TN + FN)

Positive predictive value = TP/(TP + FP)

Negative predictive value = TN/(FN + TN)

Positive diagnostic likelihood ratio = sensitivity/(1 − specificity)

Negative diagnostic likelihood ratio = (1 − sensitivity)/specificity

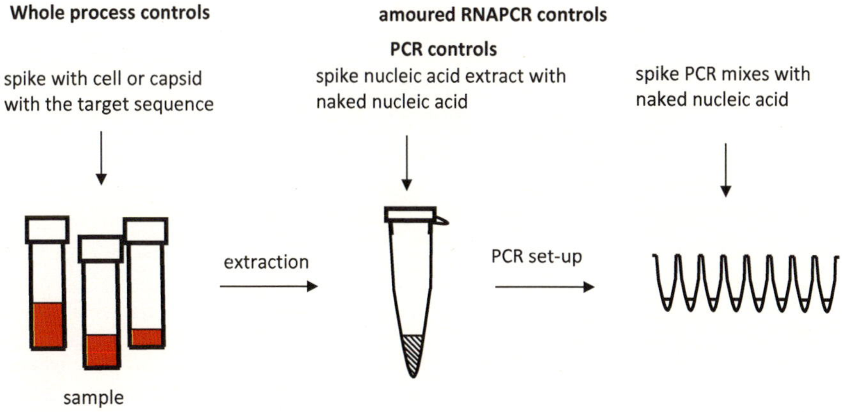

Fig. 3 PCR controls

The use of an appropriate internal control aids in identifying false-negative results and greatly reduces the risk of incorrect diagnosis and reporting. Consequently, it is best practice to include a whole process internal control (i.e., one capable of detecting both extraction failure and amplification inhibition). Figure 3 illustrates the difference between whole process and amplification controls.

External controls (i.e., where reference materials are tested in a parallel PCR reaction containing the sample) are less satisfactory although they are simple to design and implement. The risk that false negatives remain undetected, though greatly reduced, remains. However, for quantitative PCR it is advantageous that the control reaction cannot interfere with test accuracy.

It is essential to use an appropriate RNA or DNA control depending on target amplified. Figure 4 shows a selection of control materials. The internal control should be designed so that any adverse effect on the sensitivity of the assay is minimized. It should also be demonstrated that the internal control and target PCRs are similarly affected by the presence of potential inhibitory substances. This can be achieved by spiking the PCR reaction with potential inhibitors, such as hemoglobin or reagents, such as ethanol or phenol that may be carried over from the extraction process. The shift in crossing threshold values can be used to assess the relative impact of inhibition on the amplification of both the internal control and target organism.

8.3 Determination of Analytical Sensitivity (Detection Limits)

The analytical sensitivity of an assay is its ability to detect a low concentration of a given substance in a biological sample. This type of sensitivity is expressed as a concentration (e.g., as copies, colony-forming units (cfu), plaque-forming units (pfu), or genome equivalents per ml or per g of sample material) in acceptable units. A lower detectable concentration shows a greater analytical sensitivity.

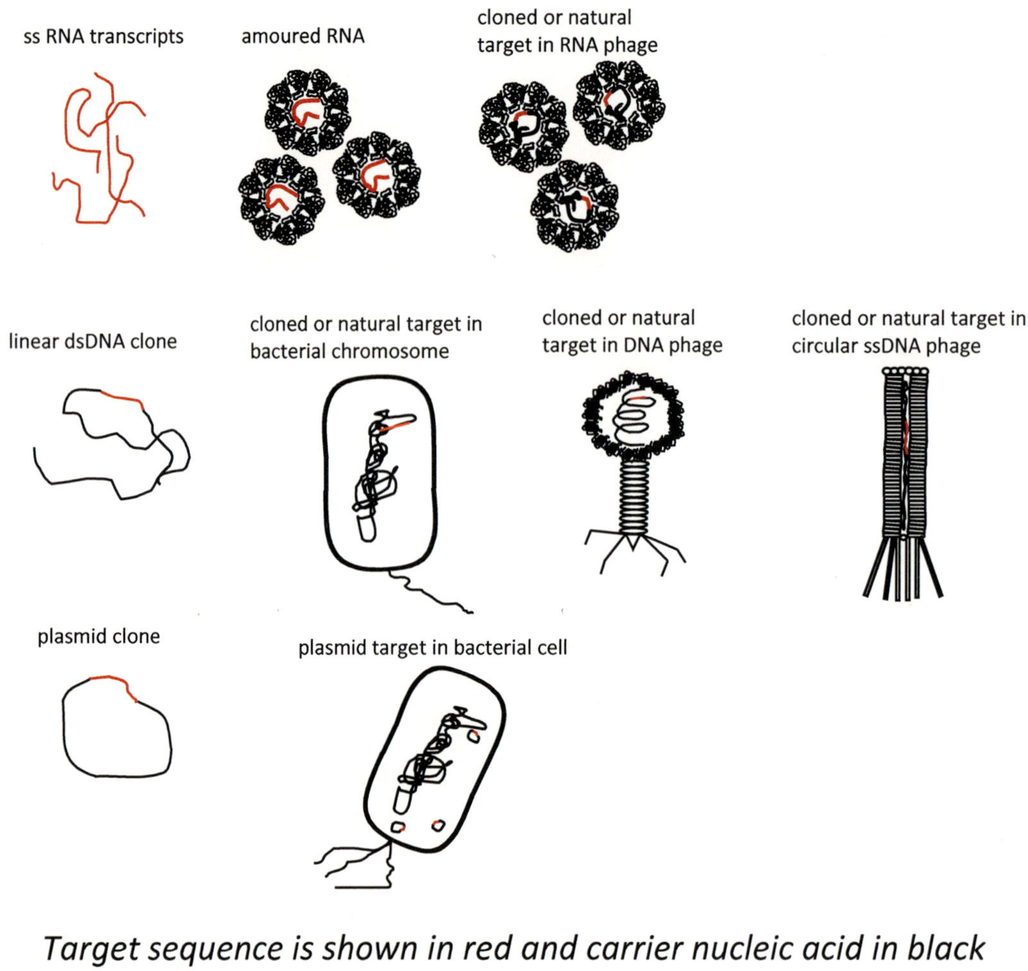

Fig. 4 Nucleic acid control targets for PCR

Analytical sensitivity is directly related to the limit of detection (LoD), also known as the minimal detectable concentration, which is the lowest quantity of a substance that can be distinguished from the absence of that substance (i.e., a blank value). Conventionally, the LoD is reported as the estimate of the detection limit that can be achieved with 95 % confidence. This determination requires probit analysis involving testing of replicate samples around the end point of the assay and the processing the detection rate at each level through statistical analysis software [10].

For validation purposes it is essential that the analytical sensitivity is determined by the final version of the assay, once development and optimization are complete. When reference controls are available, they should be used directly or indirectly via calibration of commercial or in-house working controls. The indirect route is only acceptable when the reference control material is derived from a true biological source that has restricted availability to calibration purposes only. When an international standard has been established, the units should be calibrated against this reagent.

Ideally, international reference standards, containing a known concentration of analyte, are the reagents to which all assays are standardized. Such standards are prepared and distributed by international reference laboratories. National reference standards are calibrated by comparison with an international standard reagent whenever possible; they are prepared and distributed by a national reference laboratory. In the absence of an international reference standard, a national reference standard becomes the standard of comparison for the candidate assay. These standard reagents are highly characterized through extensive analysis, and preferably the methods for their characterization, preparation, and storage have been published in peer-reviewed publications.

The analytical sensitivity should be measured over at least four different assay runs, with three replicates per assay. If the method is to be used to detect a range of sample types, the sensitivity with all types must be determined.

8.4 Determination of Analytical Specificity

Analytical specificity is the ability of an assay to exclusively identify a target substance or organism rather than similar but different substances (e.g., rabies rather than another lyssavirus) in a sample or specimen. For validation, appropriate materials (i.e., cells or virions) containing nucleic acid targets likely to be encountered in relevant samples should be tested. The widest, feasibly obtainable, variety of differing strains containing the target sequence should be included. In addition, nucleic acid containing material that should be negative or not detectable in the assay but that is likely to be encountered in samples should be tested.

8.5 Determination of Diagnostic Sensitivity (DSe) and Diagnostic Specificity (DSp)

The diagnostic sensitivity of an assay is the ability to detect the infection of interest in a population, expressed as a proportion or percentage (see Table 3). Diagnostic sensitivity of the assay depends on the ability to obtain the target substance in a processed sample from an animal that has the condition, as well as the ability to detect very low concentrations of a substance.

The diagnostic specificity of an assay is the ability to correctly identify an animal that does not have the infection in question and will ideally refer to a particular comparator group. The diagnostic specificity is expressed as the probability that a test will produce true negative results when used on a noninfected population.

The sampling design must be chosen to allow estimation of DSe and DSp. The designated number of known positive and known negative samples will depend on the likely values of DSe and DSp of the candidate assay and the desired confidence level for the estimates (Table 1). A rather large number of samples is required to achieve a very high confidence for DSe and DSp when a minimal amount of error in the estimate is desired. Logistical and financial limitations may require that less than an optimal number of samples will be evaluated. Sample size also may be limited by the fact that reference populations and gold standards may be lacking. It may, therefore, be necessary to use a suboptimal number of samples initially. It is, however, essential to improve the quality of the DSe and DSp estimates by testing samples as they become available.

8.6 Quantitative Assays

Additional criteria are relevant to the assessment of quantitative assay performance (e.g., when using quantitative real-time PCR assays). The slope (used to determine the PCR efficiency), the linear range, and the *X* and *Y* intercepts of the standard curve formed using dilutions of control material are key measures. The coefficients of variation across the linear range should be determined based on quantitative values (i.e., target copy numbers). Alternatively, it may be more helpful to calculate standard deviations of the quantification cycle (C_q) values. These values are essential in order to judge whether variation between clinical results is significant and to establish the reliable quantitative range for an assay.

International standards, where available, should be used for the calibration of quantitative assays. The use of commercially available quantified standards may also be appropriate, but the values assigned will not have the same standing as international standards. Quantified material can be generated synthetically (e.g., in plasmids) or by purification from the target organism. These standards are usually quantified by spectroscopy (i.e., from absorbance at 260 nm, A_{260}) or, if greater sensitivity is required, by fluorometry (i.e., using intercalating fluorescent dyes).

Results should not be extrapolated beyond the established linear dynamic range of the assay. Consequently, the quantitative range of the assay should ideally encompass the range expected from clinical samples. The standard curve should include a minimum of four points and the upper and lower values of the standards should be within one log of the top and bottom, respectively, of the reported quantitative range. When positive results that are above or below the quantitative range are obtained, these should be reported as "positive, greater than xx copies/mL" or "positive, less than xx copies/mL," respectively.

Appropriate quantified controls that may be used to monitor the performance of assays should be established. The levels of target molecule within controls should be set so that the assay is reliably positive. However, the concentration should not be significantly higher than that of a typical clinical sample (e.g., as an indication the control might be designed to give a C_q value of 30 in a typical real-time PCR reaction). Test controls allow assay performance to be monitored over time and assessed by Westgard rules [6, 7].

8.7 Linearity

The linearity of an analytical procedure is its ability (within a given range) to obtain test results which are directly proportional to the concentration of analyte in the sample. Ideally a linear relationship should be maintained across the range of the analytical procedure. Linearity may be assessed by testing dilutions of a quantified standard and then plotting C_q values as a function of analyte concentration. Results should be evaluated by appropriate statistical methods, for example, by calculation of a regression line by the method of least squares.

8.8 Measurement Range

The range of an analytical procedure is the interval between the upper and lower limits (e.g., concentration, number of organisms or number of DNA copies) in the sample for which it has been demonstrated that the analytical procedure has a suitable level of precision, accuracy, and linearity. This is normally derived from linearity studies and depends on the intended application of the procedure. It is established by confirming that the analytical procedure provides an acceptable degree of linearity, accuracy, and precision when applied to samples containing amounts of analyte within or at the extremes of the specified range of the analytical procedure.

8.9 Precision

The precision of an analytical procedure can be expressed as the variance, standard deviation, or coefficient of variation of a series of measurements.

Precision can be determined by repeat testing of samples. The precision of an analytical procedure expresses the closeness of agreement (degree of scatter) between a series of measurements obtained from multiple sampling of the same homogeneous sample under the prescribed conditions. Note: precision is not the same as accuracy since an assay may be precise but inaccurate.

Precision may be considered at three levels: repeatability, intermediate precision, and reproducibility. "Repeatability" is the agreement between replicates within and between assay runs by the same operator over a short period of time. "Intermediate precision" measures variation within a laboratory to include, for example, tests performed on different days, by different analysts and using different equipment. "Reproducibility" includes the agreement between replicate tests performed in different laboratories. Reproducibility studies are necessary if the diagnostic method is to be used in more than one laboratory.

Precision should be investigated using homogeneous, authentic samples, i.e., behaving as much like real samples as possible. However, if it is not possible to obtain a homogeneous sample, it may be investigated using artificially prepared samples or a sample solution. Known positive samples should give the same acceptable range of results if assayed four times or more in one run and over at least four different runs on different days. This validation is not an assessment of reproducibility, which is the closeness of agreement between independent results obtained with the same method on identical test material but under different conditions (i.e., different operators, different apparatus, different laboratories, and/or after different intervals of time). Reproducibility is measured as the standard deviation qualified with the term "reproducibility" (i.e., reproducibility standard deviation). Since there is less control of possible variables when determining reproducibility compared to repeatability, it should be expected that the reproducibility standard deviation will be higher than repeatability standard deviation. A comparison of precision between platforms should be considered, especially if more than one platform (i.e., for extraction and/or amplification) is an option, e.g., for contingency purposes such as during machine breakdown or surge capacity.

8.10 Analytical Accuracy

To assess analytical accuracy, known negative and positive samples (i.e., with known reference or accepted reference test values) should be extracted and assayed four or more times in one run. At least four replicate runs should be performed to allow intra-assay reproducibility to be measured, and these should each occur on different days. With sensible planning, this task can be achieved when performing analytical sensitivity testing. The acceptable range of results will depend upon the application.

8.11 Clinical Accuracy

The validation of clinical accuracy requires comparison of the assay to an appropriate "gold-standard" method using sequential clinical samples obtained in real clinical situations. The number of samples tested will vary depending on the availability of suitable clinical material. They should, wherever possible, include a wide range of concentrations of positive samples as well as negative samples. It may be helpful to consult a specialist statistician to determine the appropriate treatment of the data.

8.12 Robustness

The robustness of the assay may be evaluated by deliberately deviating aspects of the protocol that are perceived as being sensitive to the outcome, for example, by simulating pipetting errors affecting critical components, such as enzyme and Mg^{2+} or by extending the storage of PCR reaction mix at room temperature or at 4 °C before amplification. Such data are likely to be useful for troubleshooting if this is required.

8.13 Reference Intervals

The reference intervals, also referred to as the reference range, normal range, or reference limits, are the upper and lower levels of analyte that you would expect to see in a normal population. Any values above or below that range are outside normal limits. Reference intervals are important when the purpose of the assay is to determine whether the test subject or the sample is in or outside the normal range. Generally, reference intervals are not relevant for the quantification of infectious agents by real-time PCR since there is no infection in the normal population.

8.14 Control of Known Interferences

The presence of interferences may be identified during assay development and/or validation. When it is known that samples might contain materials that potentially interfere with the test result, the SOP should be modified, wherever possible, to introduce a suitable sample pretreatment. However, the complete removal of interfering substances cannot be guaranteed, and it is therefore essential to include appropriate positive controls to ensure that this problem is detected.

8.15 Limitations of the Method

The limitations of the assay, whether based on general experience or identified during validation, should be documented and made available to users. Examples of limitations include any lack of sensitivity compared to another method, low sensitivity for certain specimen types, and the possibility of false results in contaminated specimens.

8.16 Clinical Validation and Implementation in Diagnostic Pathways

While analytical validation is designed to show that the test chemistry reliably detects the target, diagnostic validation ensures that the test detects the target in clinical specimens. The clinical sensitivity and specificity of a test refer to its ability to detect the disease accurately. Clinical validation can be carried out retrospectively or prospectively. Often it is useful to establish an additional post-implementation prospective evaluation to add data to the file.

The next step is to integrate the test into routine as part of a clinical diagnostic pathway. Workflows are established to ensure that the test is performed at an appropriate point in the diagnostic cycle, that performance is triggered by specific clinical questions, and that the results are interpreted in a way that feeds back into the management of disease. The validation file should include information on the situations that would trigger use of the test and the appropriate clinical interpretation of the results in relation to identification of the pathogen. Details of appropriate reporting comments in relation to the results in particular scenarios should be provided. High and low positives in various samples and in different clinical contexts may have different implications. Thorough clinical validation should provide insight into the relevance of the test results.

8.17 Shelf Life of Materials

It is important to know how long the reagents used in diagnostic assays remain active when stored under specified conditions. All commercially purchase reagents have use by dates, which have been determined though shelf-life studies. It is not common for shelf life to be determined for in-house assays, but the same principles apply and it is best practice to do so.

The signal to noise ratio of the assay may decline gradually, and this may be difficult to detect without rigorous application of multi-rule run QC (i.e., Westgard [6]) since positive controls may give acceptable results while the assay is performing suboptimally.

The principle of shelf-life studies is straightforward. Batches of vials of the reagent are stored at the required temperature and samples are tested at different times using a known QC sample. The European Standard Stability testing of in vitro diagnostic reagents BS EN 13640 [11] recommends that shelf-life testing is performed on samples from three batches.

While shelf-life studies determine the stability of the reagents under specified conditions, reagents may be treated differently during their life. It is best practice to consider conditions that the reagents might be subjected to and recreate them in the laboratory to determine whether their performance is affected. For example, if the reagents might be freeze-thawed several times during their life aliquots should be subjected to freeze-thaw cycles and retested. Samples may be tested after each cycle or collected and tested in a single run. Where reagents are to be transferred between laboratories, they may, during transit, be stored overnight in a warm warehouse. It is recommended that easily envisaged scenarios such as this are simulated in the laboratory to test the effect on the assay. It is acceptable to perform stress studies on only one batch of a reagent.

If stress studies reveal that reagents are not stable under defined conditions, then instructions for use must clearly state this. For example, if reagents are found to be impaired following several freeze-thaw cycles, the SOP should require that freeze-thawing is limited to a number of cycles at which the level of impairment is acceptable, e.g., instructions for reagents that need to be stored frozen may need to dictate that the vial is discarded after first use.

9 Risk Assessment

To minimize the hazards to both users of the assay and to test subjects, a risk assessment should be performed prior to using any reagent in a diagnostic test [12]. The risk assessment should consider the infection risk of test materials that contain biological substances and take into account all combinations for use, for example, different platforms or ancillary reagents. The risks of an incorrect diagnosis, either false positive or negative, should also be assessed. Depending on what risks are identified, further action may be required to ensure that appropriate control measures are implemented. These might include treatments to inactivate infectious agents, a review of the scope of stress studies, a review of the reagent storage conditions, the provision of additional information in the instructions for use or revision of the guidance, or the interpretation of results or limitations of the assay.

10 Data Analysis and Composition of the Technical Report

The validation work should be completed in accordance with the study design. The technical report and validation file should summarize assay validation, results, and recommendations. The recommendations should include the multi-rule run QC criteria established using positive control results. For in-house assays, the validation should be supported by the work carried out during assay development. Workbook records can be cross-referenced in the validation report if appropriate.

To avoid bias, validation results should be analyzed as defined in the study design and then compared with expected values to determine whether or not the kit or reagent is suitable for use. The comparison of sensitivity and specificity may be with results obtained using alternative reagents or commercial kits.

11 Review of Technical Report and Sign-Off

Although validation should be completed in a timely manner, the need to meet deadlines must not compromise thoroughness. A report on the validation data should be presented to the reviewers who make the decision on whether the assay is fit for purpose guided by the assay definition. The panel's conclusion should be documented and include, as appropriate, a formal declaration, signed by the project leader and the project manager, that the assay is suitable for diagnostic or reference work. Any use prior to completion of the validation and sign-off must be reported as "research use only."

12 Instructions for Use and Labeling

Assays should be supplied with clear instructions for use. These may be in the form of an SOP or as a product information sheet (PIS). The IVDD [13] may be a good guide to the details of what should be included in the PIS, although some of the requirements are less relevant for in-house reagents. A minimum requirement for labels is that the reagent name, batch number, and expiry date are clearly identifiable.

13 Monitoring the Performance of Assays and Maintenance of the Validation File

It is good practice to retain batch records for reagents used in assays for an extended period of time. The international standard ISO 13485 [14], written specifically for medical devices but equally applicable for veterinary reagents, states that batch records must be retained for the lifetime of the reagent and not less than 2 years from the date of batch release. In practice, most laboratories retain records for considerably longer than this.

Batch records include details of the purchase and manufacture of every reagent, including reagent lot numbers, details of what equipment was used, how the reagent was made, and all treatment undertaken. All reagents must be manufactured, stored, and used under the control of the laboratory's quality system and sufficient records taken to allow a full audit trail to be undertaken.

Once satisfactory validation has been completed using a defined SOP, it is essential that the assay is performed according to the SOP. Minor changes to the method that are immaterial to the performance specification of the assay should, as far as possible, be accommodated within the SOP, provided evidence is available. For example, it may be better to specify the use of distilled, deionized, or molecular grade water rather than a particular brand of molecular grade water. Similarly, it may be reasonable to avoid specifying the particular model of PCR instrument to be used.

When changes to the protocol that fall outside of the SOP must be made, revalidation is required. Revalidation will vary from a single run showing that C_q values are unchanged for a range of reference samples (e.g., as might be appropriate for a change to a buffer) to full revalidation (e.g., for use of an alternative sample preparation method or primer change).

Assays that are currently in use with validation records that do not comply with the recommendations of this guidance should be retrospectively provided with a compliant validation file wherever practical. It may be necessary to implement appropriate data collection from continuing use to provide supportive information. Historical records should be reviewed and summarized to provide evidence that the assay is fit for purpose and a validation checklist should be used to cross-reference these documents. A conclusion based on the information obtained from the historical data should be documented including a formal declaration that the assay is suitable for use.

Documents relating to assay development and performance monitoring should be filed in a retrievable and auditable manner. All pages of documents should be numbered. The header or footer should show the document version number and a reference date.

14 Production of Reagents

Staff involved in the preparation of reagents must be suitably trained and have documented evidence of competency.

Following the development of a satisfactory assay, it is essential that the procedures for production of reagents for routine use are clearly defined to ensure that the assay continues to be fit for purpose when further batches are made. SOPs that describe the production process in detail, including specific information about the reagents, equipment, and conditions of storage and use, are required. Where appropriate, worksheets should be used to record manufacturing information. A complete reconstruction of the manufacturing process for every batch should be possible. SOPs should include details of how any interim and final products are quality controlled, including batch release criteria, prior to batch release. A worksheet should be prepared to allow recording of quality control results and should include a final batch release sign-off by a responsible person.

15 "Rollout" of Assays

The collection of diagnostic validation data will necessarily involve limited technical "rollout" within the developing laboratory. Full adoption of the new assay into clinical use will include consideration of the reagent supply chain and arrangements for quality assessment, including participation in external quality assessment (EQA) schemes wherever appropriate. If the test is required to meet the needs of a range of end users, rollout should be considered. A rollout plan should include the timeline, equipment, personnel, and risk management proposals.

Following rollout, an assay verification study and continuing quality assessment should be performed. This is usually best organized by the developing laboratory. Verification should involve the testing of validation panels or be limited in scope to a few well-characterized samples and standards. In some circumstances, it may be desirable that validation materials are sourced from laboratories other than that of the developer. Round-robins may be useful in ensuring continuing attention to quality.

16 "Post-Deployment" Surveillance and Verification

Post-deployment is the equivalent of "post-marketing," which is the term used in the IVDD and other regulatory literature to refer to the time following "rollout." Once the assay has been validated and put into use, information on its performance should continue to be gathered. However, through a validation it is not possible to include all sample types and less common problems may not be identified. Details of any problems, e.g., poor performance and false positives or negatives, should be documented. All problems should be investigated and appropriate corrective action implemented. Timely communication with users of the assay or similar assays is very important, both to make them aware of any problems and as part of the root cause corrective action. If necessary, the risk assessment should be reviewed in light of the new information.

It is possible that the assay may need to be modified to prevent the problem recurring. All information must be included in the project dossier with the assay development and validation documentation. The full project dossier should be available to all laboratories performing the test.

The assay should be reviewed periodically to highlight performance compared to alternative assays, whether commercial or in-house, and thus ensure continued improvement. Reviews should include the relevant scientific literature which may highlight alternative assay technologies or the emergence of novel strains.

An assay validation process checklist is presented in Table 4.

Table 4
Assay validation checklist

Name of assay			
Specific targets (pathogens and genes) of the assay			
Project manager			
Project leader			
Staff performing the hands-on development work			
Section: planning and inception			
Subsection	**Contributor**	**Deadline**	**Completion**
Setting purpose and objective for new assay			
Setting up a project risk register			
Health and safety issues			
Business analysis			
Commercial analysis			
Regulatory compliance			
Human resources aspects			
Project planning and initiation			
Section: assay validation			
Subsection	**Contributor**	**Deadline**	**Completion**
Design of validation study			
Setting benchmarks and performance measures			
Identification of gold standards			
Identification of reference material and reagents			
Preparation of specific SOPs (MIQE compliant)			
Assessment of analytical performance			

(continued)

Table 4
(continued)

Choice of study population			
Choice of sample type			
Sample size calculation			
Performance of clinical validation			
Data analysis and interpretation			
Assessment of usability			
Reagent stability studies			
Further optimization if required			
Production of documentation			
Sign-off process			
Section: rollout and verification			
Subsection	**Contributor**	**Deadline**	**Completion**
Review of needs and users			
Planning of rollout			
Field verification studies			
Provision of validation panels			
Interlaboratory comparison			
Section: implementation			
Subsection	**Contributor**	**Deadline**	**Completion**
Implementation in laboratory work flows			
Implementation in diagnostic pathways			
Implementation in clinical pathways			
Post-marketing assessment			
Long-term data collection			
Periodic QC/QA			
Periodic proficiency testing			
Production aspects of implementation			
Periodic reassessment of fitness for purpose			

17 Conclusions

With the advent of molecular biology, opportunities for development of new diagnostic assays have increased significantly. Molecular assays are faster, more sensitive, and more specific than we could have dreamed of even a decade ago. This has encouraged laboratory scientists to develop new molecular assays, either to replace existing non-molecular ones or to identify new markers. We expect commercial assays to have been rigorously developed and validated extensively to ensure that they meet their specification and are fit for purpose when we use them in the laboratory. We have a responsibility for ensuring that assays developed in-house provide the same level of assurance as commercial assays. It is salutary to remember that if an in-house assay is not fit for purpose or there is insufficient evidence that it is, it is the laboratory which must take legal responsibility if a diagnostic result leads to an adverse event.

Once developed, it is equally important that rollout and routine use of newly developed assays are carefully managed. An assay which works perfectly in the expert hands of an individual scientist who has carefully developed it must work just as well in routine use. Therefore, good quality assurance must be embedded at all stages of the process, i.e., during assay development, validation, and rollout and finally in routine use.

If the guidance provided within this chapter is followed, the developer will gain an excellent understanding of the performance of the new assay and should have every confidence that it is fit for purpose.

Glossary of Terms

Fitness for purpose "Fit for purpose" means that the kit has to be validated to such a level to show that the kit's results can be interpreted to have a defined meaning in terms of diagnosis or another biological property being examined (see www.oie.int/our-scientific-expertise/certification-of-diagnostic-tests/the-register-of-diagnostic-tests).

In-house Any assay developed within the laboratory or commercial assay which is modified or used off label, i.e., used in a different way, for a different purpose or using a different sample type from that recommended by the manufacturer.

Validation Confirmation, through the provision of objective evidence, that the requirements for a specific intended use or application have been fulfilled [ISO 9000:2000]. Validation is normally performed by the manufacturer (whether commercial or in-house).

Verification Confirmation, through the provision of objective evidence, that specified requirements have been fulfilled [ISO 9000:2000]. Verification is normally performed by the user prior to introduction of a validated assay to determine if the assay achieves the required specification in their hands.

References

1. OIE (2013) Register of diagnostic kits certified by the OIE as validated as fit for purpose. http://www.oie.int/our-scientific-expertise/certification-of-diagnostic-tests/the-register-of-diagnostic-tests. Accessed 30 December 2013
2. Working Party on Control of Medicines and Inspections (2001) Annex 15 to the EU guide to good manufacturing practice. http://ec.europa.eu/health/files/eudralex/vol-4/pdfs-en/v4an15_en.pdf. Accessed 30 December 2013
3. General requirements for the competence of testing and calibration laboratories (BS EN ISO/IEC 17025:2005)
4. Freeman KP, Gruenwaldt J (1999) Quality control validation in veterinary laboratories. Vet Clin Pathol 28:150–155
5. Farr AJ, Freeman KP (2008) Quality control validation, application of Sigma metrics, and performance comparison between two biochemistry analyzers in a commercial veterinary laboratory. J Vet Diagn Invest 20:536–544
6. Westgard JO, Barry PL, Hunt MR, Groth T (1981) A multi-rule Shewhart chart for quality control in clinical chemistry. Clin Chem 27:493–501
7. http://www.westgard.com/westgard-rules
8. Bossuyt PM, Reitsma JB, Bruns DE et al (2003) Standards for Reporting of Diagnostic Accuracy. Toward complete and accurate reporting of studies of diagnostic accuracy: the STARD initiative. Clin Chem 49:1–6
9. Bustin SA, Benes V, Garson JA et al (2009) The MIQE guidelines: minimum information for publication of quantitative real-time PCR experiments. Clin Chem 55:611–622
10. Burd EM (2010) Validation of laboratory-developed molecular assays for infectious diseases. Clin Microbiol Rev 23:550–576
11. Stability testing of in vitro diagnostic reagents (BS EN 13640. 2002)
12. Medical devices. Application of risk management to medical devices (BS EN ISO 14971. 2009)
13. Directive 98/79/EC of the European Parliament and of the Council of 27 October 1998 on in vitro diagnostic medical devices (1998-12-07 OJ No L 331/1). In vitro diagnostic medical devices. European Standards 1998
14. Medical devices. Quality management systems. Requirements for regulatory purposes (BS EN ISO 13485:2012)

Part II

Molecular Detection and Identification of Animal Pathogens in Laboratorial Settings

Chapter 7

Molecular Approaches to Recognize Relevant and Emerging Infectious Diseases in Animals

Fredrik Granberg, Oskar E. Karlsson, Mikael Leijon, Lihong Liu, and Sándor Belák

Abstract

Since the introduction of the first molecular tests, there has been a continuous effort to develop new and improved assays for rapid and efficient detection of infectious agents. This has been motivated by a need for improved sensitivity as well as results that can be easily communicated. The experiences and knowledge gained at the *World Organisation for Animal Health (OIE) Collaborating Centre for Biotechnology-based Diagnosis of Infectious Diseases in Veterinary Medicine, Uppsala, Sweden*, will here be used to provide an overview of the different molecular approaches that can be used to diagnose and identify relevant and emerging infectious diseases in animals.

Key words Infectious diseases, Pathogen detection, Molecular diagnosis, Transboundary animal diseases, Endemic diseases, Zoonoses, PCR, Isothermal amplification, Hybridization, Proximity ligation assay (PLA), Microarrays, Nanotechnology

1 Introduction

The increased occurrence and emergence of devastating infectious diseases, in both domestic and wildlife animal populations, are causing very serious socioeconomic losses at both global and regional levels. This increase has been attributed to several contributing factors, the most prominent being the accelerated movements of humans and animals due to increased globalization and international trade, the climatic changes, and the larger and larger populations kept together in animal husbandry and breeding. Some of these diseases, termed *transboundary animal diseases* (TADs), such as foot-and-mouth disease and classical swine fever, have a high capacity to spread very rapidly over countries and borders, having a devastating impact on animal productivity and trade, as well as causing other losses in the animal husbandries and in wildlife. Other diseases, such as anthrax, bovine tuberculosis, and rabies, have more *endemic* character,

Mónica V. Cunha and João Inácio (eds.), *Veterinary Infection Biology: Molecular Diagnostics and High-Throughput Strategies*, Methods in Molecular Biology, vol. 1247, DOI 10.1007/978-1-4939-2004-4_7, © Springer Science+Business Media New York 2015

establishing themselves in limited areas and showing slower tendency of spread. Considering their importance, many of these infectious diseases are listed by the World Organisation for Animal Health (OIE) as notifiable animal diseases, collectively referred to as OIE-listed diseases. The OIE is also determining and updating the *international animal disease status* on a regular basis. The current OIE-listed diseases and the latest disease status reports are available at the OIE website (www.oie.int).

Zoonoses, veterinary, and human public health. Of special importance among the animal infectious diseases are the ones that have the capacity to cross the species barriers and establish infections in a wider range of hosts including humans, causing *zoonotic infections.* It has been estimated that approximately 75 % of the new and emerging human infectious diseases over the past 10–20 years have been caused by pathogens originating from animals or from products of animal origin [1, 2]. Many of these diseases have the potential to spread through various means, over long distances, and to become global problems.

Accurate and rapid diagnosis. Considering the extremely high direct and indirect losses and other consequences caused by the TADs and the other infectious diseases, it is very important to develop and apply a wide range of diagnostic methods. These should preferably allow rapid detection and identification of the infectious agent(s), with high specificity and sensitivity, while still being affordable and readily available. When outbreaks do occur, rapid and accurate diagnosis is needed to screen susceptible populations and monitor the spread of the infectious pathogens, therefore helping with epidemiological investigation and implementation of necessary control measures, such as vaccination, stamping out, and quarantine restrictions, in order to prevent further spread.

Collection of clinical samples and sample preparation. Identification of the relevant groups of animals, showing clinical signs or at stages of infection when the presence of infectious agents is likely to be sufficiently high, and correct sampling are the first two crucial steps in the diagnostic process. The next steps of great importance are the sample preparation procedures, such as cleanup and target enrichment, which are performed in order to reduce possible contaminants and retain concentrated materials from the target agents, most commonly nucleic acid and/or proteins, for further analysis. If any of these steps are not properly considered and carried out, all diagnostic methods, even the most powerful and sensitive, will be unable to detect and identify the infectious agents, and this is leading to false diagnosis, which could have very serious consequences.

The OIE Collaborating Centre (OIE CC) for Biotechnology-Based Diagnosis of Infectious Diseases in Veterinary Medicine. Since the authors' institutes in Uppsala, Sweden, are well-recognized centers of excellence in molecular diagnostics, the OIE has granted them the mandate to work together as its only collaborating center focused on biotechnology-based diagnostics (www.sva.se/en/About-SVA/OIE-Collaborating-Centre). In this chapter, the experiences and knowledge gained at the OIE CC will be used to provide an overview of the molecular approaches capable of recognizing relevant and emerging infectious diseases in animals.

Detection and identification of the infectious agents. The diagnostic laboratories can apply two basic ways for a proper diagnosis: (a) *direct detection and identification* and (b) *indirect detection and identification* methods. *Direct detection and identification* means that the infectious agents and/or their components, such as nucleic acids or proteins, are detected in the collected samples. Commonly used *classical diagnostic methods* for direct detection include identification of microorganisms by culture techniques and immunofluorescence, and the most widely applied *molecular diagnostic methods* are the various assays of nucleic acid hybridization, e.g., polymerase chain reaction (PCR) and isothermal amplification methods, such as the loop-mediated isothermal amplification (LAMP), among others. When running *indirect diagnosis and identification*, the immune responses of the host are investigated, looking for antibodies against various infectious agents, which indicate the occurrence of the infections in the hosts. In this chapter we focus on *direct diagnosis*, with special regard to *molecular diagnostic methods*, as well as some considerations regarding the interpretation, understanding, and communication of the diagnostic results.

2 PCR-Based Approaches

Molecular approaches become increasingly important in infectious disease diagnostics and, with the exception of isolation by culturing, may supersede all other direct detection methods. The main reasons are that a unique signature of every microorganism is encoded in its genome, which in principle enables perfect specificity, and that various enzymatic mechanisms can be utilized to manipulate and amplify the genetic material, yielding an exquisite sensitivity of the molecular DNA-based assays. While bacteria have their genome encoded in the form of DNA, some viral genomes are composed of RNA, and an initial reverse transcription step is therefore required before further manipulations and amplification can be carried out. Enzymes typically utilized are polymerases, reverse transcriptases, ligases, glycosylases, and nucleases. Of these, the polymerases require a pair of sequence-specific primers, which enables selective target amplification.

2.1 PCR Assays

PCR employs thermostable polymerases to enable amplification by continuous thermocycling and is currently the most commonly used method for amplification of genetic material [3]. The highly charged phosphodiester backbone of DNA makes the PCR product amenable to high-resolution visualization on agarose gel electrophoresis utilizing DNA-binding fluorescent dyes such as ethidium bromide. Electrophoresis both provides a means for detection by band visualization and enables at least a tentative verification of specificity by estimation of the amplicon length.

Shortly after the introduction of PCR, attempts were made to enhance sensitivity of detection of target nucleic acid sequences by running a second PCR assay targeting the internal region of the amplicon resulting from the first reaction, so-called nested PCR [4, 5]. The greater sensitivity has been attributed to both a dilution effect of any inhibitory compounds present in the sample, since only a minor fraction of the first reaction volume is used in the second reaction, and the fact that the primer-driven reaction is run twice, using four specific primers, rather than two. An intermediate situation is obtained if one of the primers from the first reaction is retained in the second, which yields a semi-nested PCR format.

The drawback of using PCR, and in particular the nested PCR formats, is that conserved regions must exist on the genome, and this might be a serious problem for highly variable RNA viruses. Although more recently the convenient and less laborious real-time PCR methods have been developed (*see* below) and are mostly used today in clinical practice, nested PCR assays are still used due to their high sensitivity and robustness.

2.2 Real-Time PCR Assays

Gel-based PCR is a heterogeneous, relatively laborious, detection method. Furthermore, it only reflects the end point of the PCR and, for this reason, doesn't allow the determination of the initial quantity of the detected material, e.g., determination of the viral load. Since it lacks specific markers for the targeted amplicon, unspecific amplification yielding similar product sizes may lead to false positive detection. Nested PCR has the further disadvantage of being prone to cross-contaminations since reaction tubes with potentially very high quantities of target DNA are opened between the two reactions. Many of these drawbacks were solved by the advent of real-time PCR [6]. With this technique, the PCR product is monitored in the course of the reaction using DNA-binding moieties that alter their fluorescence upon binding to the amplified DNA. This allows a closed tube, homogeneous assay format, which reduces the risk for cross-contamination and also removes the laborious gel electrophoresis step. In addition, the cycle number where the fluorescence reaches a defined threshold level will depend on the initial quantity of target DNA or RNA (before reverse transcription).

Three main approaches have been taken to monitor fluorescence alteration in real time due to the buildup of the PCR product, which can be ordered according to the level of specificity the methods provide. The simplest method is to add a fluorescent dye to the PCR mixture with the property that the fluorescence intensity changes upon DNA binding. Typical dyes are asymmetric cyanine dyes, such as SYBR green or tiazole orange, that exhibit a fluorescence increase when bound to DNA [7, 8]. These types of real-time PCR have no better specificity than gel-based PCR, rather the opposite, since no information is provided about the product length. New possibilities are given by tethering the dye to one of the PCR primers that are constructed so that incorporation of the primer into the amplicon leads to an alteration of dye fluorescence. Several chemistries have been devised to this end, for example, scorpion primers [9], LUX primers [10], and Plexor primers [11]. Although in principle not providing a better specificity in regard to spurious amplification than the pure dye approach, fluorescent primers enable multiplexing by co-adding several primer pairs, each with a distinct fluorophore. The third approach includes addition of a third fluorescently labeled oligonucleotide, located between the primers, called a probe. The probe can also be labeled with a quencher (dual-labeled probe) but not always, e.g., not for the LightUp probes [7] or in the PriProET approach [12, 13]. Prominent examples of methods based on dual-labeled probes include TaqMan [14] and molecular beacons [15].

The signal that can be obtained from a probe-based real-time PCR experiment is often limited by the competing reannealing of the double-stranded PCR amplicon. Asymmetric PCR can be used to overcome this problem since it allows preferential amplification of one strand in a double-stranded DNA template. This is achieved by manipulating primer properties, most critically concentration, as well as other factors influencing primer melting temperature, such as length and nucleotide sequence. In the LATE-PCR method [16], asymmetric PCR has been combined with molecular beacons for readout to achieve a detection format that allows quantification from the end-point fluorescence. This format is suitable for simpler portable PCR instruments designed for detection in the field and has recently been commercialized by various companies.

The application of real-time PCR techniques and other methods in molecular diagnostics in veterinary medicine have recently been extensively reviewed [17, 18] and will be further discussed later in this section. To conclude this subsection, it is suitable to mention a recently developed method for the rapid molecular pathotyping of avian influenza [19] and Newcastle disease [20] viruses that combines several of the themes discussed here. This technique employs a three level semi-nested PCR format that utilize Plexor [11] fluorogenic primers as a detection mechanism. Furthermore, the assay format allows a highly multiplex interrogation of the sample by using primers in two vastly different concentration regimes. Instead of, as hitherto has been the case, requiring nucleotide sequencing over the hemagglutinin and fusion protein genes of avian influenza and Newcastle disease viruses, a much faster diagnosis can be obtained by a simple PCR-based method. This method could even be implemented on field PCR instruments for rapid on-site diagnosis and thereby providing means for faster containment of disease outbreaks.

3 Isothermal Amplification

Isothermal amplification of nucleic acids is an alternative method to PCR. The reaction is performed at a constant temperature in simple devices, such as water baths or heating blocks, which eliminates the need for high-end equipment and system maintenance. It can be used to test for infections in regions where resources are limited and logistic chains are impossible, but a rapid answer is needed. Isothermal amplification normally takes about an hour or less to complete, providing a fast specimen-to-result diagnosis at the point of care (POC). To make the best use of isothermal amplification, a system should ideally integrate the upstream sample preparation and the downstream detection steps and be operated by personnel without extensive training. Several platforms utilizing isothermal technology are commercially available or close to market [21].

Recently, the field of isothermal amplification technologies has advanced dramatically, resulting in several different amplification systems. These have been summarized by Niemz et al. [21] and include transcription-mediated amplification (TMA) [22], helicase-dependent amplification system [23], loop-mediated isothermal amplification (LAMP) [24], and rolling-circle amplification [25]. Of those methods, LAMP has gained the greatest interest because of its high specificity, efficiency, and rapidity. By addition of a reverse transcriptase in the reaction, RNA targets can also be amplified and detected by LAMP, which is referred to as RT-LAMP. The LAMP utilizes four primers that bind to six distinct regions of the target DNA to specifically amplify a short region and is catalyzed by *Bst* DNA polymerase with strand-displacement activity [24]. Addition of loop primers may accelerate the reaction [26]. As of 8 February 2014, PubMed listed 990 publications with the search term "loop-mediated isothermal amplification." LAMP technology has been applied for the detection of viral pathogens such as classical swine fever virus [27] and foot-and-mouth disease virus (FMDV) [28], bacteria such as *Clostridium difficile* [29], and parasites such as malaria [30]. Commercial developments have progressed: a total of eight LAMP kits are approved in Japan for the detection of SARS coronavirus, *Mycobacterium tuberculosis* (TB), *Mycoplasma pneumoniae*, *Legionella* species, influenza A virus, H1 pdm 2009 influenza virus, H5 influenza virus, and human papilloma virus, as reviewed by Mori et al. [31]. Future development would need to consider simplification of sample preparations, reaction mix in a dried down formation and integration of all three steps in a compact, disposable, and inexpensive system.

4 Detection by Hybridization-Based Approaches

Identification and classification of bacteria and viruses using DNA hybridization-based approaches rely on the use of oligonucleotide probes that selectively bind to target sequences based on the degree of complementarity. This was early utilized in fluorescence in situ hybridization (FISH), which became a valuable tool for localization of infectious agents in clinical samples without cultivation [32]. However, to overcome limitations in multiplex capacity, sensitivity, and signal intensity, there has been an ongoing development of the initial approach. This has resulted in high-throughput methods such as DNA arrays but also interesting new hybridization-based methodologies combined with signal amplification, such as padlock probe (PLP) [33] and proximity ligation assay (PLA) [34]. PLP belongs to the methodologies of genomic partitioning where one specific region of the genome is massively replicated, and thereby detectable, even though it normally is masked by the presence of other genomes or in too low amount to be detected. PLA relies on the primary detection of antigens followed by oligonucleotide amplification and subsequent detection by fluorescent probes or by RT-PCR.

4.1 DNA Array Technologies

With the development of DNA macro- and microarray technologies, it became possible to detect and characterize a wide variety of bacteria and viruses through simultaneous hybridization against large numbers of DNA probes immobilized on a solid support [35, 36].

The probes represent known sequences that may serve as markers for identification and/or genotyping of bacterial strains, resistance genes, viruses, etc. These are commonly arranged in an ordered array of spots (or features), and hybridization with a labeled target, i.e., the sample to be investigated, will therefore result in a hybridization profile in which individual probe results also can be assessed. As the names imply, the main difference between macro- and microarrays is the number and size of spots on the support. Macroarrays typically have larger and fewer spots and have proven particularly effective for detecting smaller subsets of genes, such as genes involved in antibiotic resistance [37]. Microarrays can contain thousands, and even up to many *hundred thousands*, of spots with different oligonucleotide probes and have successfully been used for detection and genotyping of bacterial and viral pathogens [38, 39]. The main advantages of microarray technology are high throughput, parallelism, miniaturization, and speed. However, microarrays are still considered to be an expensive technology and usually require large amounts of nucleic acid targets. Furthermore, unless it has been completely automated, the data analysis procedure might be time-consuming, and the results can be difficult to translate into information that is clearly communicable and decision supportive.

4.2 Genomic Partitioning

Genomic partitioning refers to the methodologies used for capture and enrichment of target regions. Within these methodologies, PLP has been used repeatedly for genotyping, localization, and array-based diagnostics. The earliest version of PLP consisted of two oligonucleotide probes of 20 nt connected by a linker region of 40 nt [33]. As the probes hybridize towards the target, the construct is ligated into a circular detector that can be replicated isothermally by Phi29 polymerase [40]. The detection can then be performed through incorporation of fluorophore tagged nucleotides. The PLP concept was further expanded with the introduction of the molecular inversion probe (MIP) technology. Where PLP leaves no gap after hybridization to the target region, MIP aims at leaving a single nucleotide gap. This gap is then filled in by addition of a single type of nucleotide into the assay. This approach enables substitutions on nucleotide level to be detected using just four reactions easily set up in a normal lab environment. It also provides a possibility of highly multiplexed designs of assays [41, 42]. Building on the same principle as PLP and MIP, the connector inversion probe (CIPer) technology extends the gap up to a few hundred nucleotides. Using DNA polymerase to fill the gap generates a product that can be sequenced, revealing the content of the target region [43]. Applications of PLP methodology and its derivatives for infectious diseases in animals include detection of all hemagglutinin and neuraminidase subtypes of AIV [44], as well as multiplex detection of FMDV, swine vesicular disease virus (SVDV), and vesicular stomatitis virus (VSV) [45]. In addition, by designing different probes for the genomic and replicative form of the virus, it is possible to not only detect a virus but also localize it in relation to the host cells and perform semiquantitative analysis of the amount of replicative viruses, as demonstrated with porcine circovirus type 2 [46].

4.3 Proximity Ligation Assay

Although PLA is designed for detection of protein interactions and localization using antibodies for target recognition, hybridization events are required to generate a detectable signal [34]. Two sets of antibodies are designed: one targets the protein/s of interest and the other target the first set. The antibodies in the second set carry short oligonucleotide strands that can hybridize with special connector oligonucleotides and thereby enable the formation of circular DNA constructs. These are amplified and detected by PCR and fluorescent probes. The methodology combines dual antibody specificity with the signal amplification power of DNA amplification to produce a versatile and sensitive method for detection of very low amounts of targets. It also enables in situ localization studies of protein targets within cells [47]. Furthermore, PLA requires little to no sample preparation, making it ideally suitable for screening of massive amounts of samples, and can be used with a solid support to capture antigens for detection, similar to ELISA. The use of a solid support may also facilitate the removal of contaminants from the sample, thereby enabling PCR-based detection without the problem of inhibition. By combining the solid-support approach with RT-PCR detection, great sensitivity was demonstrated in a study of avian influenza virus [48]. Other applications of PLA technology include detection of several viruses, among them FMDV, with detection levels close to those of RT-PCR and 100-fold more sensitive than ELISA [49], as well as localization of influenza virus proteins within cells [50].

5 Further Trends, New Tools in Molecular Diagnostics

In the development of new molecular diagnostic methods, there has been a continuous effort to enable efficient and rapid detection of infectious agents from ever-smaller volumes of complex fluids without the need for a skilled operator. As a result, microfluidic analysis systems and nanotechnology-based detection devices have gained increased popularity, as previously reviewed [51, 52]. These systems and devices have been employed to construct a *wide range of integrated tools*, capable of semiautomated complex diagnostic procedures, which also allow rapid, portable field-based testing [53].

5.1 Microfluidic Analysis Systems

Several sequential laboratory procedures are usually required to detect infectious agents in clinical samples, such as concentration, lysis, extraction, purification, amplification, and product detection. Recent progress in microfluidic technology has allowed multiple procedures to be incorporated in sequence for one-step sensing or in parallel for high-throughput screening [54, 55]. These integrated systems with use in molecular diagnostics are more commonly known as biochip or lab-on-a-chip (LOC) devices. Since they usually consist of fluid channels and sensing chambers with dimensions of a few to hundreds of microns, very small amounts of sample can be analyzed, requiring only low consumption of reagents. The use of materials that can be easily functionalized, such as glass and plastic, allows the inner surfaces to be coated with different capture and sensing agents, e.g., antibodies and nucleic acids. Although this makes microfluidic analysis systems versatile tools for pathogen detection, the main application involves systems based on the recognition of target nucleic acids.

As discussed above, the detection of target nucleic acid from a pathogenic microorganism or virus can be achieved either by direct probing or by first introducing an amplification step. *Amplification-based detection* usually gives higher sensitivity and has successfully been implemented on microfluidic chips using both PCR and alternative amplification methods, such as nucleic acid sequence-based amplification (NASBA) [56]. However, regardless of amplification method, it is first necessary to concentrate and lyse the sample material to extract and purify the nucleic acid. As described in the review by Heo et al. [57], a variety of alternative solutions have been developed to perform these sequential steps on a microfluidic chip. Popular strategies for sample concentration include magnetic beads [58] and dielectrophoresis [59]. The lysis of enriched samples can then be achieved by various methods, such as thermal energy, optothermal energy, mechanical force, and chemicals [60]. For the purification of extracted nucleic acid, packed silica beads, microfabricated structures, and magnetic beads have all proved to be useful solutions [61]. After amplification, the detection of products is most commonly performed with fluorescence or electrochemical methods, which easily can be miniaturized. A classification into three categories was suggested for microfluidic chips that use amplification-based detection by Mairhofer et al. [52]. These categories included microfluidic chips with (1) a stationary chamber as nano-/picoliter reservoir for conventional thermocycling, (2) a continuous flow where the sample is moved between individual temperature zones at different locations for cycling, and (3) a droplet-based system where each amplicon is individually amplified within a water-in-oil droplet. Examples of fully implemented amplification-based systems include devices for detection of different viruses, such as dengue virus and enteroviruses [62], as well as various bacteria, most notably *Bacillus anthracis* [63, 64].

5.2 Nanotechnology-Based Detection

Nanotechnology has extended the limits of molecular diagnostics to the nanoscale (one-billionth of a meter), allowing diagnostic assays to take advantage of the unique electrical, magnetic, luminescent, and catalytic properties of nanomaterials. This has contributed to the development of innovative assays that provide rapid detection of infectious agents with improved sensitivity and limit of detection (LOD) [65]. Because of the small scale, nanotechnology can also be used to create high-density arrays of sensors for high-throughput detection without increased sample requirements. Moreover, the use of sensitive nanoscale sensors has the potential to eliminate the need for sample preparation and target amplification, making it possible to construct assays for direct detection in opaque media, like blood and milk [51].

There has also been a special focus to develop affordable nanotechnology-based devices that provide fast and reliable results in simple and user-friendly formats for use even in rural areas of developing nations [66].

Most sensor systems for diagnostic use are comprised of two components, one receptor for target recognition by specific binding and one transducer that convert receptor readings into a signal that can be measured, such as an electronic or optical signal [67]. Nanoscale sensors are usually comprised of biological recognition elements coupled to different nanomaterials for signal transduction and detection. These nanomaterials include noble metal nanoparticles, nanobarcodes, quantum dots, and magnetic nanoparticles [68–71]. Nanowires and nanotubes can also be coated with biological recognition elements to be used as nanosensors, and binding events are measured as a change in their electrical conductance [72]. Another example is silicon-based cantilever sensors functionalized with biomolecules such as DNA for target recognition. These sensors are often combined into high-density arrays for high-throughput screening [73]. Applications of nanoscale sensors for detection of infectious agents include multiplex detection of both viruses and bacteria [74, 75].

6 Summary and Final Remarks

As detailed above, numerous molecular methods have been developed for the detection and characterization of infectious agents in the field of veterinary and human medicine. Among them, PCR has been the most commonly used technology. When considering the development of new technologies, a general trend can be observed towards robust and affordable automatic systems that also integrate sample preparation steps for rapid and highly sensitive multiplex detection of an easily enlarged panel of pathogens, both bacterial and viral. Although few, if any, of the novel systems have successfully incorporated all of these properties, they still represent important technological advancements towards more sensitive and efficient detection. Even so, only a limited number have so far been developed into commercial diagnostic kits, and only a few molecular tests are offered by veterinary diagnostic laboratories. The full potential and impact of molecular diagnosis is therefore yet to be realized. A possible explanation may be that most new published assays are only analytical validated and not properly evaluated in accordance with the appropriate criteria for field validation. New molecular tests might also not comply with current accreditation standards.

For the interpretation and understanding of the diagnostic results, it is very important to put the molecular diagnostic methods in the context of the complex scenario of infectious diseases, i.e., to follow not only the technical rules and procedures of the molecular methods but also simultaneously acquire sufficient medical understanding in order to gain a more complete picture. A "PCR positive result" by itself, without analyzing the complex scenario, can be unreliable, even misleading, and may cause serious problems for the veterinary and human medical health authorities during implementation of eradication programs. To avoid such problems and to provide a reliable diagnosis, it is important to obtain a complete medical understanding of the disease scenario. Reliable diagnoses can be reached, of course, even on the basis of single PCR assays, if they are raising the right questions and the results are professionally communicated. On the other hand, there are many cases of infectious diseases where the diagnosis is more reliable if a range of various methods, both direct and indirect approaches, are applied simultaneously. It should therefore be emphasized that in certain cases, the simultaneous application of novel molecular diagnostic methods and classical approaches, such as isolation by culturing, is required for a fully reliable diagnosis.

Another important, but often neglected, aspect is the communication of diagnostic results. The successful control and eradication of infectious diseases is strongly accelerated and enhanced if the diagnostic laboratories are able to communicate the results rapidly and properly towards the practitioners and the health authorities. It is very important to pay sufficient attention even to this task, because a rapid and clear two-way communication between the laboratories and the practitioners, as well as the decision-making authorities, is essential in order to assure the success of the control and eradication programs.

The authors' institutes that constitute the OIE CC have been early developers and adopters of new diagnostic technologies and approaches, from the first PCR-based assays until today's plethora of various molecular methods, closely following and participating in the ongoing effort to develop improved tests. More recently, this has resulted in the adaptation and evaluation of PLP and PLA for detection of veterinary important pathogens, as well as a new PCR-based multiplex platform for molecular pathotyping of viruses, among other contributions. The OIE CC has had an important role in the development of novel molecular diagnostic methods, in international standardization and validation, as well as in international dissemination of results, outreach, and training. These activities are done with the support of the OIE, our home institutes SVA and SLU, and in collaboration with large international and national consortia of various EU projects, such as LAB-ON-SITE, ASFRISK, CSFV_goDIVA, AniBioThreat, RAPIDIA-FIELD, and Epi-SEQ. National grant agencies are also supporting this work, such as the Formas BioBridges Strong Research Environment project No. 2011-1692, which is supporting the diagnostic developments for the improved diagnosis of a wide range of poultry pathogens, many of which have zoonotic features, in the spirit of the One World, One Health concept.

Acknowledgments

This work was supported by Epi-SEQ, a research project under the 2nd joint call for transnational research projects by EMIDA ERA-NET (FP7 project nr. 219235), the European Union FP7 project RAPIDIA-FIELD (FP7-289364), the Formas Strong Research Environments "BioBridges" project (No. 2011-1692), the Award of Excellence (Excellensbidrag) provided to SB by the Swedish University of Agricultural Sciences (SLU), and executed in the framework of the EU-project AniBioThreat (Grant Agreement: Home/2009/ISEC/AG/191) with the financial support from the Prevention of and Fight against Crime Programme of the European Union, European Commission, Directorate General Home Affairs. This publication reflects the views only of the authors, and the European Commission cannot be held responsible for any use, which may be made of the information contained therein. The funders had no role in study design, data collection and analysis, decision to publish, or preparation of the manuscript.

References

1. Cleaveland S, Laurenson MK, Taylor LH (2001) Diseases of humans and their domestic mammals: pathogen characteristics, host range and the risk of emergence. Philos Trans R Soc Lond B Biol Sci 356:991–999
2. Taylor LH, Latham SM, Woolhouse ME (2001) Risk factors for human disease emergence. Philos Trans R Soc Lond B Biol Sci 356: 983–989
3. Saiki RK, Gelfand DH, Stoffel S et al (1988) Primer-directed enzymatic amplification of DNA with a thermostable DNA polymerase. Science 239:487–491
4. Gouvea V, Glass RI, Woods P et al (1990) Polymerase chain reaction amplification and typing of rotavirus nucleic acid from stool specimens. J Clin Microbiol 28:276–282
5. Kemp DJ, Smith DB, Foote SJ et al (1989) Colorimetric detection of specific DNA segments amplified by polymerase chain reactions. Proc Natl Acad Sci U S A 86:2423–2427
6. Higuchi R, Fockler C, Dollinger G, Watson R (1993) Kinetic PCR analysis: real-time monitoring of DNA amplification reactions. Bio/Technology (N Y) 11:1026–1030
7. Leijon M, Mousavi-Jazi M, Kubista M (2006) LightUp probes in clinical diagnostics. Mol Aspects Med 27:160–175
8. Zipper H, Brunner H, Bernhagen J, Vitzthum F (2004) Investigations on DNA intercalation and surface binding by SYBR Green I, its structure determination and methodological implications. Nucleic Acids Res 32:e103
9. Whitcombe D, Theaker J, Guy SP, Brown T, Little S (1999) Detection of PCR products using self-probing amplicons and fluorescence. Nat Biotechnol 17:804–807
10. Nazarenko I, Lowe B, Darfler M et al (2002) Multiplex quantitative PCR using self-quenched primers labeled with a single fluorophore. Nucleic Acids Res 30:e37
11. Sherrill CB, Marshall DJ, Moser MJ et al (2004) Nucleic acid analysis using an expanded genetic alphabet to quench fluorescence. J Am Chem Soc 126:4550–4556
12. McMenamy MJ, McKillen J, Hjertner B et al (2011) Development and comparison of a Primer-Probe Energy Transfer based assay and a 5′ conjugated Minor Groove Binder assay for sensitive real-time PCR detection of infectious laryngotracheitis virus. J Virol Methods 175: 149–155
13. Rasmussen TB, Uttenthal A, de Stricker K, Belák S, Storgaard T (2003) Development of a novel quantitative real-time RT-PCR assay for the simultaneous detection of all serotypes of foot-and-mouth disease virus. Arch Virol 148: 2005–2021
14. Holland PM, Abramson RD, Watson R, Gelfand DH (1991) Detection of specific poly-

merase chain reaction product by utilizing the 5'-3' exonuclease activity of *Thermus aquaticus* DNA polymerase. Proc Natl Acad Sci U S A 88:7276–7280

15. Tyagi S, Kramer FR (1996) Molecular beacons: probes that fluoresce upon hybridization. Nat Biotechnol 14:303–308
16. Sanchez JA, Pierce KE, Rice JE, Wangh LJ (2004) Linear-after-the-exponential (LATE)-PCR: an advanced method of asymmetric PCR and its uses in quantitative real-time analysis. Proc Natl Acad Sci U S A 101:1933–1938
17. Belák S, Thorén P, LeBlanc N, Viljoen G (2009) Advances in viral disease diagnostic and molecular epidemiological technologies. Expert Rev Mol Diagn 9:367–381
18. Hoffmann B, Beer M, Reid SM et al (2009) A review of RT-PCR technologies used in veterinary virology and disease control: sensitive and specific diagnosis of five livestock diseases notifiable to the World Organisation for Animal Health. Vet Microbiol 139:1–23
19. Leijon M, Ullman K, Thyselius S et al (2011) Rapid PCR-based molecular pathotyping of H5 and H7 avian influenza viruses. J Clin Microbiol 49:3860–3873
20. Yacoub A, Leijon M, McMenamy MJ et al (2012) Development of a novel real-time PCR-based strategy for simple and rapid molecular pathotyping of Newcastle disease virus. Arch Virol 157:833–844
21. Niemz A, Ferguson TM, Boyle DS (2011) Point-of-care nucleic acid testing for infectious diseases. Trends Biotechnol 29:240–250
22. Hofmann WP, Dries V, Herrmann E et al (2005) Comparison of transcription mediated amplification (TMA) and reverse transcription polymerase chain reaction (RT-PCR) for detection of hepatitis C virus RNA in liver tissue. J Clin Virol 32:289–293
23. Jeong YJ, Park K, Kim DE (2009) Isothermal DNA amplification in vitro: the helicase-dependent amplification system. Cell Mol Life Sci 66:3325–3336
24. Notomi T, Okayama H, Masubuchi H et al (2000) Loop-mediated isothermal amplification of DNA. Nucleic Acids Res 28:E63
25. Johne R, Müller H, Rector A, van Ranst M, Stevens H (2009) Rolling-circle amplification of viral DNA genomes using phi29 polymerase. Trends Microbiol 17:205–211
26. Nagamine K, Hase T, Notomi T (2002) Accelerated reaction by loop-mediated isothermal amplification using loop primers. Mol Cell Probes 16:223–229
27. Zhang XJ, Sun Y, Liu L, Belák S, Qiu HJ (2010) Validation of a loop-mediated isothermal amplification assay for visualised detection of wild-type classical swine fever virus. J Virol Methods 167:74–78
28. Yamazaki W, Mioulet V, Murray L et al (2013) Development and evaluation of multiplex RT-LAMP assays for rapid and sensitive detection of foot-and-mouth disease virus. J Virol Methods 192:18–24
29. Lalande V, Barrault L, Wadel S et al (2011) Evaluation of a loop-mediated isothermal amplification assay for diagnosis of *Clostridium difficile* infections. J Clin Microbiol 49:2714–2716
30. Polley SD, Mori Y, Watson J et al (2010) Mitochondrial DNA targets increase sensitivity of malaria detection using loop-mediated isothermal amplification. J Clin Microbiol 48: 2866–2871
31. Mori Y, Kanda H, Notomi T (2013) Loop-mediated isothermal amplification (LAMP): recent progress in research and development. J Infect Chemother 19:404–411
32. Amann RI, Ludwig W, Schleifer KH (1995) Phylogenetic identification and in situ detection of individual microbial cells without cultivation. Microbiol Rev 59:143–169
33. Nilsson M, Malmgren H, Samiotaki M et al (1994) Padlock probes—circularizing oligonucleotides for localized DNA detection. Science 265:2085–2088
34. Fredriksson S, Gullberg M, Jarvius J et al (2002) Protein detection using proximity-dependent DNA ligation assays. Nat Biotechnol 20:473–477
35. Garaizar J, Rementeria A, Porwollik S (2006) DNA microarray technology: a new tool for the epidemiological typing of bacterial pathogens? FEMS Immunol Med Microbiol 47: 178–189
36. Hacia JG (1999) Resequencing and mutational analysis using oligonucleotide microarrays. Nat Genet 21(1 Suppl):42–47
37. Zhang SL, Shen JG, Xu PH et al (2007) A novel genotypic test for rapid detection of multidrug-resistant *Mycobacterium tuberculosis* isolates by a multiplex probe array. J Appl Microbiol 103:1262–1271
38. Ballarini A, Segata N, Huttenhower C, Jousson O (2013) Simultaneous quantification of multiple bacteria by the BactoChip microarray designed to target species-specific marker genes. PLoS One 8:e55764
39. Wang D, Coscoy L, Zylberberg M et al (2002) Microarray-based detection and genotyping of viral pathogens. Proc Natl Acad Sci U S A 99:15687–15692
40. Banér J, Nilsson M, Mendel-Hartvig M, Landegren U (1998) Signal amplification of

padlock probes by rolling circle replication. Nucleic Acids Res 26:5073–5078

41. Akhras MS, Thiyagarajan S, Villablanca AC et al (2007) PathogenMip assay: a multiplex pathogen detection assay. PLoS One 2:e223
42. Novais RC, Borsuk S, Dellagostin OA, Thorstenson YR (2008) Molecular inversion probes for sensitive detection of *Mycobacterium tuberculosis*. J Microbiol Methods 72:60–66
43. Akhras MS, Unemo M, Thiyagarajan S et al (2007) Connector inversion probe technology: a powerful one-primer multiplex DNA amplification system for numerous scientific applications. PLoS One 2:e915
44. Gyarmati P, Conze T, Zohari S et al (2008) Simultaneous genotyping of all hemagglutinin and neuraminidase subtypes of avian influenza viruses by use of padlock probes. J Clin Microbiol 46:1747–1751
45. Banér J, Gyarmati P, Yacoub A et al (2007) Microarray-based molecular detection of foot-and-mouth disease, vesicular stomatitis and swine vesicular disease viruses, using padlock probes. J Virol Methods 143:200–206
46. Henriksson S, Blomström AL, Fuxler L et al (2011) Development of an in situ assay for simultaneous detection of the genomic and replicative form of PCV2 using padlock probes and rolling circle amplification. Virol J 8:37
47. Soderberg O, Gullberg M, Jarvius M et al (2006) Direct observation of individual endogenous protein complexes in situ by proximity ligation. Nat Methods 3:995–1000
48. Schlingemann J, Leijon M, Yacoub A et al (2010) Novel means of viral antigen identification: improved detection of avian influenza viruses by proximity ligation. J Virol Methods 163:116–122
49. Nordengrahn A, Gustafsdottir SM, Ebert K et al (2008) Evaluation of a novel proximity ligation assay for the sensitive and rapid detection of foot-and-mouth disease virus. Vet Microbiol 127:227–236
50. Munir M, Zohari S, Berg M (2011) Non-structural protein 1 of avian influenza A viruses differentially inhibit NF-kappaB promoter activation. Virol J 8:383
51. Kaittanis C, Santra S, Perez JM (2010) Emerging nanotechnology-based strategies for the identification of microbial pathogenesis. Adv Drug Deliv Rev 62:408–423
52. Mairhofer J, Roppert K, Ertl P (2009) Microfluidic systems for pathogen sensing: a review. Sensors (Basel) 9:4804–4823
53. Yager P, Edwards T, Fu E et al (2006) Microfluidic diagnostic technologies for global public health. Nature 442:412–418
54. Cady NC, Stelick S, Kunnavakkam MV, Batt CA (2005) Real-time PCR detection of *Listeria monocytogenes* using an integrated microfluidics platform. Sens Actuators B Chem 107: 332–341
55. Easley CJ, Karlinsey JM, Bienvenue JM et al (2006) A fully integrated microfluidic genetic analysis system with sample-in-answer-out capability. Proc Natl Acad Sci U S A 103: 19272–19277
56. Compton J (1991) Nucleic acid sequence-based amplification. Nature 350:91–92
57. Heo J, Hua SZ (2009) An overview of recent strategies in pathogen sensing. Sensors (Basel) 9:4483–4502
58. Beyor N, Seo TS, Liu P, Mathies RA (2008) Immunomagnetic bead-based cell concentration microdevice for dilute pathogen detection. Biomed Microdevices 10:909–917
59. Lapizco-Encinas BH, Simmons BA, Cummings EB, Fintschenko Y (2004) Dielectrophoretic concentration and separation of live and dead bacteria in an array of insulators. Anal Chem 76:1571–1579
60. Kim J, Johnson M, Hill P, Gale BK (2009) Microfluidic sample preparation: cell lysis and nucleic acid purification. Integr Biol 1: 574–586
61. Wen J, Legendre LA, Bienvenue JM, Landers JP (2008) Purification of nucleic acids in microfluidic devices. Anal Chem 80: 6472–6479
62. Lien K-Y, Lee WC, Lei HY, Lee GB (2007) Integrated reverse transcription polymerase chain reaction systems for virus detection. Biosens Bioelectron 22:1739–1748
63. Belgrader P, Benett W, Hadley D et al (1998) Rapid pathogen detection using a microchip PCR array instrument. Clin Chem 44: 2191–2194
64. Higgins JA, Nasarabadi S, Karns JS et al (2003) A handheld real time thermal cycler for bacterial pathogen detection. Biosens Bioelectron 18:1115–1123
65. Jain KK (2003) Nanodiagnostics: application of nanotechnology in molecular diagnostics. Expert Rev Mol Diagn 3:153–161
66. Hauck TS, Giri S, Gao Y, Chan WC (2010) Nanotechnology diagnostics for infectious diseases prevalent in developing countries. Adv Drug Deliv Rev 62:438–448
67. Vo-Dinh T, Cullum B (2000) Biosensors and biochips: advances in biological and medical diagnostics. Fresenius J Anal Chem 366: 540–551
68. Gu H, Xu K, Xu C, Xu B (2006) Biofunctional magnetic nanoparticles for protein separation

and pathogen detection. Chem Commun 2006(9):941–949

69. Li Y, Cu YT, Luo D (2005) Multiplexed detection of pathogen DNA with DNA-based fluorescence nanobarcodes. Nat Biotechnol 23: 885–889

70. Medintz IL, Uyeda HT, Goldman ER, Mattoussi H (2005) Quantum dot bioconjugates for imaging, labelling and sensing. Nat Mater 4:435–446

71. Thaxton CS, Georganopoulou DG, Mirkin CA (2006) Gold nanoparticle probes for the detection of nucleic acid targets. Clin Chim Acta 363:120–126

72. Stoltenberg RM, Woolley AT (2004) DNA-templated nanowire fabrication. Biomed Microdevices 6:105–111

73. Ziegler C (2004) Cantilever-based biosensors. Anal Bioanal Chem 379:946–959

74. Yang L, Li Y (2006) Simultaneous detection of *Escherichia coli* O157:H7 and *Salmonella* Typhimurium using quantum dots as fluorescence labels. Analyst 131:394–401

75. Shanmukh S, Jones L, Driskell J et al (2006) Rapid and sensitive detection of respiratory virus molecular signatures using a silver nanorod array SERS substrate. Nano Lett 6: 2630–2636

Chapter 8

Real-Time Reverse Transcriptase PCR for the Detection of Bluetongue Virus

Carrie Batten, Lorraine Frost, and Chris Oura

Abstract

In recent years, real-time reverse transcription polymerase chain reaction (rRT-PCR) has become one of the most widely used methods for the diagnosis of infectious pathogens. The combined properties of high sensitivity, specificity, and speed, along with a low contamination risk, have made real-time PCR technology a highly attractive alternative to more conventional diagnostic methods. Numerous robust rRT-PCR systems have been developed and validated for important epizootic diseases of livestock, and in this chapter we describe an rRT-PCR protocol for the detection of bluetongue virus. The assay uses oligonucleotide primers to specifically amplify target regions of the viral genome and a dual-labeled fluorogenic (TaqMan®) probe which allows for the assay to be performed in a closed-tube format, thus minimizing the potential for cross-contamination.

Key words Bluetongue virus, Molecular biology, Real-time reverse transcriptase PCR, TaqMan®, Diagnosis

1 Introduction

Techniques based on the amplification of specific nucleic acid sequences by polymerase chain reaction (PCR) are highly sensitive and specific. Real-time polymerase chain reaction (rPCR) is currently one of the most widely used methods in the field of molecular diagnostics and research. The rPCR technique avoids the use of agarose gel electrophoresis, thus reducing the risks of contamination, and enables the amplification of nucleic acids and the detection of the amplified products in "real" time. The technique is fast and simple to perform and can be carried out in a 96-well format, making it suitable for large-scale testing and epidemiological screening. Portable real-time PCR machines are now available, enabling the application of molecular technologies in the "field" with prospects for radically changing diagnostic approaches in the future.

Mónica V. Cunha and João Inácio (eds.), *Veterinary Infection Biology: Molecular Diagnostics and High-Throughput Strategies*, Methods in Molecular Biology, vol. 1247, DOI 10.1007/978-1-4939-2004-4_8, © Springer Science+Business Media New York 2015

In real-time PCR, the detection of amplified target sequences is carried out by monitoring the fluorescence generated by intercalating dyes, fluorophore-labeled primers, or sequence-specific probes. Target sequences can be quantified by determining the number of amplification cycles required to reach the fluorescence threshold at the beginning of the exponential phase of the PCR. This is known of as the threshold cycle or Ct value.

The real-time reverse transcription PCR (rRT-PCR) protocol described in this chapter for the detection of bluetongue virus (BTV) uses a sequence-specific hydrolysis probe (commercially called TaqMan® probes) to generate fluorescence. Hydrolysis probes are dual-fluorophore-labeled oligonucleotides with a fluorescent reporter at one end and a quencher of fluorescence at the opposite end of the probe. The close proximity of the reporter to the quencher prevents detection of its fluorescence. The probe has a high melting temperature (*Tm*) and hybridizes to complementary sequences present on the amplicon prior to the extension step of the PCR. During primer extension, both fluorophores are subsequently released as a result of the 5′ to 3′-exonuclease activity of a suitable DNA polymerase (e.g., *Taq* polymerase). Once the labels are separated, the increase in reporter fluorescence that arises due to the lack of the adjacent quencher is monitored by a real-time PCR instrument. An increase in the product targeted by the probe at each PCR cycle therefore causes a proportional increase in fluorescence due to the breakdown of the probe and release of the reporter [1–3].

Recent outbreaks of bluetongue (BT) in northern Europe have highlighted the necessity to develop high-throughput, sensitive, and specific assays in order to rapidly detect BTV. When designing group-specific primers and probes for the detection of BTV, it is important to select regions of the genome that are sufficiently conserved to enable the detection of all known BTV serotypes and related topotypes but also sufficiently divergent from other orbiviruses so there are no cross-reactions between closely related viral species. This is not a simple task due to the high diversity of BTV which is evolving continuously by genetic drift, recombination, and gene reassortment. Many different rRT-PCR assays for the detection of BTV have been developed in recent years [4]; however, the World Organization for Animal Health (OIE) and European Union Reference Laboratory (EURL) for BTV at the Pirbright Institute consider that the assay described in this chapter [5, 6] is currently the group-specific BTV assay of choice as it is able to detect all recognized serotypes of BTV that are currently known to be circulating.

Table 1
Primers and probe sequences

Oligo name	Sequence (5′–3′)	Working concentration (μM)
Primer Hofm_BTV_IVI_F2	TGG AYA AAG CRA TGT CAA A	20
Primer Hofm_BTV_IVI_R2	ACR TCA TCA CGA AAC GCT TC	20
Probe Hofm_BTV_IVI_P[a]	*FAM*-ARG CTG CAT TCG CAT CGT ACG C-*Tamra*	5

[a]Probe labeled with FAM (carboxyfluorescein) fluorophore and *Tamra* quencher

2 Materials

2.1 Reagents and Consumables

1. Optical reaction plates and caps, 96-well PCR plate, or PCR strips/tubes.
2. DNA decontamination solution (e.g., DNA*Zap*™ solutions 1 and 2, Invitrogen).
3. Microcentrifuge tubes.
4. Disposable gloves.
5. Nuclease-free water.
6. Appropriate one-step reverse transcriptase real-time PCR kit (we describe the use of the Invitrogen Superscript III RT-PCR kit; however, the assay can be adapted to use other manufacturers' commercial systems).
7. Forward primer, reverse primer, and fluorogenic probe (Table 1; *see* **Note 1**). Primers and probes must be diluted to a working concentration (Table 1) in nuclease-free water and kept at 1–8 °C. Stock primers and probe (and additional aliquots of working concentrations of primers) are stored at −5 to −30 °C.
8. Aerosol-resistant pipette tips.
9. Adhesive PCR film.
10. Marker pens (waterproof) and adhesive labels.

2.2 Equipment

1. PCR cabinet.
2. Calibrated pipettes.
3. Freezer (−5 to −30 °C).
4. Refrigerator (1–8 °C).
5. Ice bucket with ice.
6. Large capacity centrifuge.
7. Real-time PCR machine.

Table 2
Composition of the master mix for one-step real-time RT-PCR

Master mix composition	Volume for 1 reaction (µl)
2× Superscript III RT-PCR reaction mix	12.5
Primer Hofm_BTV_IVI_F2 (20 µM)[a]	0.5
Primer Hofm_BTV_IVI_R2 (20 µM)[a]	0.5
Probe Hofm_BTV_IVI_P (5 µM)[a]	1.0
RNase-free water	2.5
2.5 µM ROX l	0.5
50 mM $MgSO_4$	1.0
Superscript III RT/Platinum Taq	0.5
Total volume	19

[a]The final concentration of the primers and probe per reaction is 0.4 µM and 0.2 µM, respectively

3 Methods

3.1 Sample Preparation

1. dsRNA from BTV test samples should be prepared as per standard methods (e.g., Qiagen/Roche viral nucleic acid extraction kits) and stored at −50 to −90 °C. BTV negative and positive control samples of known origin should also be prepared (*see* **Note 2**).

3.2 Assay Setup

1. In a PCR clean room, prepare the one-step real-time RT-PCR reaction master mix according to Table 2. Sufficient volume of the master mix should be prepared to allow for testing of the required number of samples (*see* **Note 3**).
2. Working in a clean laminar flow cabinet (*see* **Note 4**), add all reagents to a suitable container (e.g., microcentrifuge tube) allowing for the total volume of reagents (*see* **Note 5**). Mix the reagents gently with a pipette. Once outside the PCR clean room, maintain the master mix on ice and shielded from light.
3. In a class II safety cabinet, carefully aliquot 6 µl of extracted RNA for both samples and controls into an optical reaction PCR plate following a planned layout (*see* **Note 6**). Alternatively, use PCR strips/tubes that are suitable for a real-time PCR machine.
4. Seal the PCR plate containing the aliquoted RNA with a PCR adhesive film (or carefully close the caps on the PCR plate/strips/tubes, hereinafter referred to as PCR plate), and heat denature the RNA (*see* **Note 7**) for 5 min at 95 °C using a

Table 3
Thermal cycling program

Step	Temperature	Duration	Number of cycles
Reverse transcription	48 °C	30 min	1
Reverse transcriptase inactivation/*Taq* activation	95 °C	2 min	1
PCR	95 °C	15 s	45
	56 °C	30 s	
	72 °C	30 s	

thermocycler as a heating block. Label the remaining RNA samples and store at −50 to −90 °C.

5. When the denaturation is complete, ensure that the samples are not condensed on the adhesive film/optical cap/lids, hereinafter referred to as seal. If so, centrifuge the plate for 1 min at approx. 150 ×*g* to collect the sample at the bottom of the plate.
6. Working in a class II safety cabinet, carefully remove the PCR seal (*see* **Note 8**) and change gloves to avoid contamination.
7. Pipette 19 μl of the master mix (a multichannel pipette can be used) into the wells of the PCR plates containing the denatured RNA samples and controls. Cover each well of the PCR plate containing the reaction components firmly with a new seal (*see* **Note 9**).
8. Centrifuge for 1 min at approx. 150 ×*g* in a benchtop centrifuge.

3.3 Amplification and Detection

1. For instructions to set up the real-time PCR machine and how to use the software refer to the relevant manufacturers' manual. Amplification should be performed using the thermal profile outlined in Table 3.
2. Negative test controls should have "No Ct" as their final result (*see* **Note 10**).
3. All positive control values should fall within a predefined range (*see* **Notes 2**, **11**, and **12**).
4. Samples with Ct values are considered positive (*see* **Note 11**). Samples with Ct values of "No Ct" are considered negative.

4 Notes

1. The primer and probe set described target BTV genome segment 10 and are specific for BTV. This primer and probe set will detect BTV serotypes 1–26 [5, 6]. Primers and probe

arrive from a supplier in a solution or lyophilized state; all primers and probes should be HPLC purified. All primers and probes will be accompanied by a "Technical Data Sheet" which gives detailed information for the individual primers and probe. This information will also detail the volume of RNase-free water to be added to the lyophilized primer and probe in order to resuspend it to a concentration of 100 μM. In the case of a reagent in solution, the concentration of the solution will be given. Once resuspended, this solution should be considered the "stock solution" of primers and probe. Aliquots should be made and labeled appropriately (with the name, batch number, and concentration) to prevent repetitive freeze-thaw. Aliquots should not be freeze-thawed more than approximately five times. Stock solution of primers and probes should be stored at −30 to −5 °C. From the stock solution, a working concentration of primer and probe should be prepared by resuspending in RNase-free water. Those should be appropriately labeled with the name, batch number, concentration, and date and stored at 1–8 °C for no longer than six months.

2. Where possible, RNA should be extracted from known BTV negative and positive samples to act as controls. If feasible, a single batch of negative and positive control samples should be prepared and aliquoted for this purpose. Negative and positive samples should be extracted with each test. The Ct value for the positive control should be recorded and monitored between runs. Ideally a positive control should have a Ct value of approximately 28.
3. Generally, when preparing the master mix, make enough volume for the number of samples being tested plus 10 % to allow for possible pipetting errors.
4. All laminar flow cabinets, pipettes, and work surfaces should be cleaned regularly using a DNA contamination solution such as DNA*Zap*™ solutions 1 and 2, Invitrogen, or other similar product. This will ensure that there is no contamination from other master mix preparations, reducing the risk of false-positive results.
5. When using real-time RT-PCR kits, the *Taq* polymerase should be added to the master mix last, as the enzymes are labile at room temperature.
6. Great care should be taken to avoid the creation of aerosols and other potential routes of contamination. Use barrier pipette tips and change tip for each sample.
7. BTV has a dsRNA genome; therefore, the dsRNA needs to be separated to ssRNA prior to reverse transcription and PCR amplification in order for the reverse transcriptase enzyme to function. This is achieved by heat denaturation for 5 min at 95 °C.

8. Placing the plate in a 96-well rack stabilizes the plate and makes it easier to remove the seal. The bottom of the plate should be free from moisture, as this can evaporate leaving calcium deposits on the bottom of the plate during thermocycling. Calcium fluoresces, and this may interfere with the fluorescence captured during amplification. The same applies when using PCR strips/tubes.
9. A roller can be used to aid in sealing the PCR plate. Touching the seal with gloves or fingers may leave marks which affect the fluorescence detection.
10. A late Ct in a negative control with a sigmoidal character may indicate cross-contamination.
11. Positive controls and positive samples should generate clean, sigmoidal curves.
12. Raw data should be inspected if there are any samples/controls generating a non-sigmoidal curve. This may indicate a problem with the computer selecting a baseline, inhibition from inefficiencies during the extraction phase, or a fault with the real-time PCR machine.

References

1. Gibson UEM, Heid CA, Williams PM (1996) A novel method for real time quantitative RT PCR. Genome Res 6:995–1001
2. Heid CA, Stevens J, Livak KJ, Williams PM (1996) Real time quantitative PCR. Genome Res 6:986–994
3. Livak KJ, Flood SJA, Marmaro J, Giusti W, Deetz K (1995) Oligonucleotides with fluorescent dyes at opposite ends provide a quenched probe system useful for detecting PCR product and nucleic-acid hybridization. PCR Methods Appl 4:357–362
4. Hoffmann B, Beer M, Reid SM et al (2009) A review of RT-PCR technologies used in veterinary virology and disease control: sensitive and specific diagnosis of five livestock diseases notifiable to the World Organisation for Animal Health. Vet Microbiol 139:1–23
5. Hofmann M, Griot C, Chaignat V, Perler L, Thur B (2008) Bluetongue disease reaches Switzerland. Schweiz Arch Tierheilkd 150: 49–56
6. Chaignat VGW, Scherrer N, Hilbe M et al (2009) Toggenburg orbivirus, a new bluetongue virus: initial detection, first observations in field and experimental infection of goats and sheep. Vet Microbiol 138:11–19

Chapter 9

Nested and Multiplex Real-Time PCR Using Dual-Labeled Probes: Detecting and Discriminating *Mycobacterium tuberculosis* Complex Members in Cultures and Animal Tissues

Pedro Costa, Isabel Couto, Miguel Viveiros, and João Inácio

Abstract

Members of the *Mycobacterium tuberculosis* complex (MTC) are causative agents of tuberculosis (TB) in both humans and animals. In the last two decades, the accumulating knowledge of the nucleotide sequences of several genes, and of the whole genomes, of MTC members has allowed the development of novel molecular assays able to detect and discriminate between these species. However, despite the significant advances in the development of molecular assays for detecting MTC members in human samples, only a few assays have been described for detecting these agents in animal tissues. In this chapter we describe the use of two *TaqMan*®-based real-time PCR approaches, highly sensitive and specific and easy to perform, to detect and identify veterinary-relevant MTC species in both animal tissue samples and cultures.

Key words *Mycobacterium tuberculosis* complex, *Mycobacterium bovis*, Bovine tuberculosis, Real-time PCR

1 Introduction

Members of the *Mycobacterium tuberculosis* complex (MTC) are causative agents of tuberculosis (TB) in both humans and animals. This complex encompasses several closely related pathogenic species, notably *M. tuberculosis*, the main agent of human TB, *M. bovis*, primarily linked to bovine TB but also often isolated from a wide range of other domestic and wild animals, and *M. caprae*, mostly associated to caprine TB [1–3]. Other less frequently found MTC species associated to TB disease in animals are *M. pinnipedii*, *M. microti*, *M. mungi*, and *M. orygis* [4–10]. Finally, *M. canetti* and *M. africanum* complement the known list of MTC species, being these last two closely related with *M. tuberculosis* and almost always restricted to human tuberculosis, in spite of some sporadic reports of infections caused by *M. tuberculosis* also in domestic and wild animals [1, 8].

Mónica V. Cunha and João Inácio (eds.), *Veterinary Infection Biology: Molecular Diagnostics and High-Throughput Strategies*, Methods in Molecular Biology, vol. 1247, DOI 10.1007/978-1-4939-2004-4_9, © Springer Science+Business Media New York 2015

Bacteriological culture, followed by biochemical and/or molecular identification, remains the gold-standard method to confirm MTC infection, a time-consuming process due to the extremely fastidious growth of these mycobacteria. Also, the conventional laboratory diagnosis does not routinely differentiate between the species of the MTC.

In the last two decades, the accumulating knowledge of the nucleotide sequences of several genes, and of the whole genomes, of MTC members has allowed the development of novel molecular assays able to detect and discriminate between these species [11–17]. For example, the insertion element IS*6110* has become one of the most used DNA targets for developing molecular diagnostic tools for the detection of MTC species, since it is found exclusively within the members of this complex [18]. Comparative genomic analysis also evidenced that modern MTC species probably evolved from a common ancestor through the accumulation of sequential and irreversible genomic deletions, named regions of difference (RDs) [1, 2, 19–22]. The pattern of the presence or absence of these RDs in the genome of MTC members provides a highly specific molecular signature that can accurately discriminate among these mycobacteria [1, 2, 8, 18, 23].

In spite of the significant advances in the development of molecular assays for the detection of MTC species in human samples, only a few assays have been described for detecting these agents in animal tissues, particularly in fresh tissues from livestock [24–28]. Most of these PCR-based assays only yield a moderate sensitivity, particularly when testing tissues without the characteristic TB lesions or detectable acid-fast bacilli [24–26, 29, 30]. This limitation is most probably related to the inefficiency of mycobacterial DNA extraction procedures from affected animal tissues [18, 24, 30].

In this chapter we describe the use of two *TaqMan*®-based real-time PCR assays to detect and identify veterinary-relevant MTC species. These two approaches can be used complementarily to improve the laboratorial diagnosis of TB in animals, particularly of bovine TB. In the first approach an IS*6110*-targeted nested real-time PCR allows the direct detection of MTC members in fresh animal tissue samples with very high sensitivity and specificity. In the second approach, multiplex real-time PCR assays allow the identification of the MTC members most commonly associated with TB in livestock and other animals, based on genomic deletion analysis. Both approaches can be incorporated at the veterinarian mycobacteriology routine diagnostic algorithm or can be used for specific purposes in particular situations to obtain accurate confirmation of MTC infections and species identification.

2 Materials

1. Animal tissue samples (e.g., lymph nodes, liver, spleen, or lung tissue samples from TB-suspect animals such as bovine, wild boar, or deer).
2. Reference strains (e.g., *M. tuberculosis* ATCC 25177; *M. bovis* AN5; *M. bovis* BCG ATCC 27291) and clinical isolates of MTC.
3. Materials for homogenization and DNA extraction from tissues: pestle and mortar; zirconium beads; DNA extraction kit (e.g., the QIAamp DNA Mini Kit, Qiagen).
4. Phosphate-buffered saline (PBS) buffer: 137 mM of NaCl, 2.7 mM of KCl, 8 mM of Na_2HPO_4, 1.5 mM of KH_2PO_4, pH 7.2. Weigh all components into a glass beaker and dissolve in 800 ml water. Adjust the pH to 7.2 with HCl and NaOH solutions. Add distilled water to a total volume of 1 l, dispense the solution into aliquots, and sterilize by autoclaving (20 min, 121 °C). Store at room temperature.
5. TE buffer: 10 mM of Tris–HCl, pH 8.0, 1 mM of EDTA.
6. *TaqMan®* probes and primers (Table 1) (*see* **Note 1**).
7. Reagents for standard PCR amplification: *Taq* DNA polymerase and respective 10× reaction buffer; deoxynucleotide triphosphates (dNTPs); $MgCl_2$.
8. Reagents for real-time PCR amplification (e.g., the SsoFast supermix, BioRad).
9. Homogenizer/bead shaker (e.g., the FastPrep FP120 Bio101, Savant Instruments Inc., Holbrook, NY).
10. Centrifuge.
11. Standard and real-time PCR equipment (e.g., the CFX96 real-time PCR instrument, BioRad).

3 Methods

To prevent the risk of human infection, the manipulation of MTC cultures and TB-suspect tissues must be performed in a confined biosafety level 3 laboratory.

3.1 DNA Extraction from Reference and Clinical MTC Cultures

The culture supernatants can be processed using a rapid and simple boiling-based DNA extraction procedure.

1. Grow the MTC strains using standard liquid culture media and procedures for these organisms.
2. After incubation, centrifuge 10 ml of culture at 3,800 ×*g* for 30 min.

Table 1
Sequences of primers and probes

Primer/probe	Sequence (5′–3′)	Complementary target
F_Actin	GGC TCY ATY CTG GCC TC	*β-actin* gene of mammals[a]
R_Actin	GCA YTT GCG GTG SAC RAT G	
P_Actin[b]	Cy5.5-TAC TCC TGC TTG CTG ATC CAC ATC-BHQ2	
F_IS*6110*	GGG TCG CTT CCA CGA TG	IS*6110* element of MTC species[c]
FN_IS*6110*	CTC GTC CAG CGC CGC TTC GG	
R_IS*6110*	GGG TCC AGA TGG CTT GC	
P_IS*6110*[d]	FAM-CGC GTC GAG GAC CAT GGA GGT-BHQ1	
F_16SrDNA	CCG CAA GGC TAA AAC TCA AA	Mycobacterial 16S rDNA[e]
R_16SrDNA	TGC ACA CAG GCC ACA AGG GA	
P_16SrDNA[f]	TET-TCG ATG CAA CGC GAA GAA CCT TAC-BHQ1	
F-*esat6*	AGG CGT ACC AGG GTG TC	RD1 (Rv3875 locus, *esat6* gene)
R-*esat6*	CGA AGC CAT TGC CTG ACC	
P-*esat6*[b]	Cy5.5-ACAACGCGCTGCAGAACC TGG-BHQ2	
F-Rv1510	CCT GCA AGA AAC GAC CCG	RD4 (Rv1510 locus)
R-Rv1510	GCGACGGTGCCAATCATC	
P-Rv1510[f]	TET-CCATCGTACCCATCCGCT GCG-BHQ1	
F-Rv2073c	AGTCGGTGTGCACGATGG	RD9 (Rv2073c locus)
R-Rv2073c	CGC TCG TTG CCG AGC AC	
P-Rv2073c[g]	Texas Red-CTG GTC GCC GAG TAT CCC GAA G-BHQ2	

[a]Probes and primers described by Costa et al. [18]
[b]Probe labeled with Cy5.5 fluorophore and BHQ-2 quencher
[c]Probes and primers described by Restrepo et al. [33] and Costa et al. [18]
[d]Probe labeled with carboxyfluorescein (FAM) fluorophore and BHQ-1 quencher
[e]Probes and primers described by Richardson et al. [34], Kirschner et al. [35], and Costa et al. [18]
[f]Probe labeled with TET (tetrachlorofluorescein) fluorophore and BHQ1 quencher
[g]Probe labeled with Texas red fluorophore and BHQ2 quencher

3. Discard the supernatant, wash the pellet in 10 ml of PBS, and centrifuge again at 3,800 × *g* for 30 min.
4. Discard the supernatant and suspend the pellet in 250 μl of TE buffer.
5. Heat the suspension in a water bath at 95 °C for 25 min.
6. Centrifuge at 15,000 × *g* for 5 min.

7. Transfer a 150 μl aliquot of the supernatant (containing the DNA) to a sterile microtube and store at −20 °C until further use.
8. Stock DNA suspensions are diluted ten times in distilled water before its use as template for PCR assays.

3.2 DNA Extraction from Animal Tissue Samples

1. Homogenize the tissue sample using a clean, sterilized pestle and mortar (the addition of a small volume of PBS buffer and sterilized powdered glass, silica, or sand can help the homogenization process).
2. Transfer 450 μl of tissue suspension to screw-cap microcentrifuge tubes.
3. Inactivate the tissue sample in a water bath at 100 °C for 5 min.
4. Centrifuge the samples in a bench centrifuge at 15,000 × *g* for 2 min.
5. Discard the supernatant and add 80 μl of PBS buffer and an equivalent volume of 100 μl of zirconium beads.
6. Proceed to the mechanical disruption of the mycobacterial cells (e.g., FastPrep FP120 Bio101 bead shaker at 6.5 m/s for 45 s, three times).
7. Cool the suspensions on ice for 15 min.
8. Proceed to the DNA extraction using a commercially available kit, according to the manufacturer's instructions (e.g., the tissue protocol of the QIAamp DNA Mini Kit).
9. Store the genomic DNA suspensions at −20 °C until further use.
10. Stock DNA suspensions are diluted ten times in distilled sterile water before its use as template for PCR assays.

3.3 Detection of MTC in Tissue Samples by Nested Real-Time PCR

The nested IS*6110*-targeted real-time PCR assay consists of two steps: (1) a first standard PCR using primers FN_IS*6110* and R_IS*6110* and (2) a second duplex real-time PCR using the previous amplification product as template and a mixture of IS*6110* and *β-actin* gene-targeted *TaqMan*® probes (P_IS*6110* and P_Actin, respectively) and the corresponding flanking primers (F_IS*6110*/R_IS*6110* and F_Actin/R_Actin, respectively) (Table 1) (*see* **Notes 2** and **3**).

1. For the first standard PCR, each amplification reaction is prepared for a final volume of 25 μl, including the addition of 5 μl of template DNA sample.
2. Prepare a reaction mixture for all the DNA samples to test, including the positive (DNA from a reference strain culture) and negative (distilled sterile water) amplification controls, containing 400 μM of dNTPs, 1 U of *Taq* DNA polymerase and 1× of the respective buffer, 3.5 mM of $MgCl_2$, and 0.8 μM

of each primer (FN_IS*6110* and R_IS*6110*), completing to 80 % of the final volume with PCR-grade water (*see* **Note 4**).

3. Distribute 20 μl of the reaction mixture by individual 0.2 ml microtubes.
4. Label each tube and add 5 μl of the correspondent DNA sample and controls.
5. Proceed to the amplification step using the following program: (a) initial denaturation step at 95 °C for 10 min; (b) 45 cycles of 30 s at 95 °C, 30 s at 65 °C, 30 s at 72 °C; and (c) a final extension step of 10 min at 72 °C.
6. Store the products at 4 °C until their use for the second duplex real-time PCR step (*see* **Note 5**).
7. For the second nested duplex real-time PCR, each amplification reaction is prepared for a final volume of 20 μl, including the addition of 5 μl of the previous amplification product (including for the correspondent positive and negative amplification controls).
8. Prepare a reaction mixture for all the DNA samples to test containing: 1× SsoFast supermix, 0.4 μM of each primer (F_IS*6110*, R_IS*6110*, F_Actin, and R_Actin), and 0.15 μM of each *TaqMan*® probe (P_IS*6110* and P_Actin), completing to 75 % of the final volume with PCR-grade water.
9. Distribute 15 μl of the reaction mixture by individual 0.2 ml microtubes.
10. Label each tube and add 5 μl of the correspondent DNA sample (product of **step 6**) and controls.
11. Proceed to the amplification step using the following program: 1 cycle at 95 °C for 2 min, followed by 45 cycles at 95 °C for 5 s, and 60 °C for 10 s. The increase of fluorescence and amplification curves for each sample should be recorded and assessed according to the instructions of the manufacturer of the real-time PCR instrument. Only samples containing MTC DNA should yield positive amplification results with the IS*6110*-targeted probe (*see* **Note 2** and Fig. 1).

3.4 Identification of MTC Strains by a Two-Step Multiplex Real-Time PCR Algorithm

The identification algorithm of MTC strains consists of two steps: (1) a first duplex real-time PCR targeting the mycobacterial 16S rDNA and the MTC-specific IS*6110* and (2) a second triplex real-time PCR targeting the Rv3875-*esat6* (RD1), Rv1510 (RD4), and Rv2073c (RD9) genomic regions of MTC (*see* **Notes 3, 6–8**).

1. For the first duplex real-time PCR, each amplification reaction is prepared for a final volume of 20 μl, including the addition of 5 μl of template DNA sample.
2. Prepare a reaction mixture for all the DNA samples to test (extracted from MTC cultures to identify), including the positive

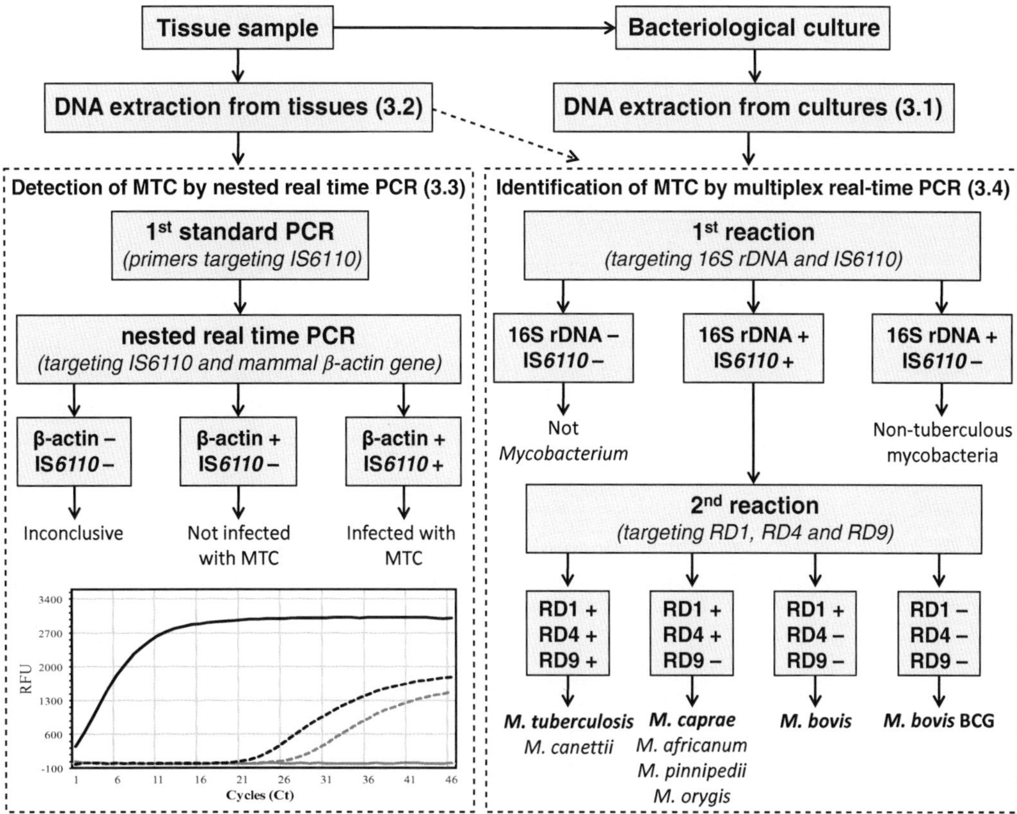

Fig. 1 Schematics of the detection and identification algorithm for MTC species most commonly associated with TB in livestock and other animals. DNA directly extracted from tissues can be used as template for the detection of MTC by nested real-time PCR targeting the IS*6110* (*left dashed box*). The amplification of the mammal β-actin gene is used as control for the occurrence of inhibitors of the reactions. The inset in the bottom illustrates the amplification results usually obtained by the nested duplex real-time PCR assay of an MTC-infected (*black lines*) and non-infected (*gray lines*) tissues samples for the amplification targeting the IS*6110* (*solid lines*) and the mammal β-actin gene (*dashed lines*) (RFU-relative fluorescence units). DNA extracted from cultures can be used as template for the identification of MTC by multiplex real-time PCR (*right dashed box*). The DNA extracted directly from tissues can be also used as template for these multiplex assays, but the sensitivity for the detection of MTC is lower than when using the nested real-time PCR assay. In the first amplification step, the isolate will be assigned as an MTC member (by detecting the presence of the IS*6110* element) or, alternatively, as a non-MTC *Mycobacterium* species. The subsequent RDs-targeted triplex PCR allows the identification of the most veterinary-relevant MTC members to the species level as *M. bovis* (or *M. bovis* BCG), *M. caprae*, or *M. tuberculosis*, according to their distinct patterns of presence or absence of RD1, RD4, and RD9. Other MTC members such as "*M. canettii*," *M. africanum*, *M. pinnipedii*, and *M. orygis* may present similar RDs profiles, but these species are rarely found in domestic (particularly livestock) and big game animals. Due to specific deletions spanning at least part of the region RD1, other less frequently found MTC species of *M. microti* and *M. mungi* present the alternative profile RD1 (–), RD4 (+), and RD9 (–)

and negative (water) amplification controls, containing 1× SsoFast supermix, 0.4 μM of each primer (F_16SrDNA, R_16SrDNA, F_IS*6110*, and R_IS*6110*), and 0.15 μM of each *TaqMan*® probe (P_16SrDNA and P_IS*6110*), completing to 75 % of the final volume with PCR-grade water.

3. Distribute 15 μl of the reaction mixture by individual 0.2 ml microtubes.
4. Label each tube and add 5 μl of the correspondent DNA sample and controls.
5. Proceed to the amplification step using the following program: 1 cycle at 95 °C for 2 min, followed by 45 cycles at 95 °C for 5 s, and 60 °C for 10 s. The increase of fluorescence and amplification curves for each sample should be recorded and assessed according to the instructions of the manufacturer of the real-time PCR instrument (*see* **Note 9**).
6. For the second triplex real-time PCR, each amplification reaction is prepared for a final volume of 20 μl, including the addition of 5 μl of template DNA sample.
7. Prepare a reaction mixture for all the DNA samples to test, including the positive and negative (water) amplification controls, containing 1× SsoFast supermix; 0.25 μM of F-*esat6*, R-*esat6*, F-Rv1510, and R-Rv1510 primers; 0.4 μM of F-Rv2073c and R-Rv2073c primers; 0.15 μM of P-*esat6* and P-Rv1510 *TaqMan*® probes; and 0.25 μM of P-Rv2073c *TaqMan*® probe, completing to 75 % of the final volume with PCR-grade water.
8. Distribute 15 μl of the reaction mixture by individual 0.2 ml microtubes.
9. Label each tube and add 5 μl of the correspondent DNA sample and controls.
10. Proceed to the amplification step using the following program: 1 cycle at 95 °C for 2 min, followed by 45 cycles at 95 °C for 5 s, and 60 °C for 10 s. The increase of fluorescence and amplification curves for each sample should be recorded and assessed according to the instructions of the manufacturer of the real-time PCR instrument.
11. The interpretation of the amplification results should be performed according to Fig. 1 (*see* **Note 10**).

4 Notes

1. Probes and primers are frequently delivered lyophilized and need to be diluted with sterile water according to the manufacturer's instructions. Stock solutions can be prepared at a standard concentration of 100 pmol/μl and stored at −20 °C.

Aliquots of working solutions of each probe and primer are prepared from stock solutions in water and stored also at −20 °C. Prepare small aliquots of working solutions (up to 100 μl) and avoid continuous freeze and thaw of the solutions. Keep labeled probes protected from light.

2. The amplification of the *β-actin* gene serves as control to detect inhibition of the PCR reactions when using DNA extracted from tissues as template [18].
3. The MTC-specific IS*6110*-targeted primers and probe used were shown to be highly efficient for detecting tuberculous mycobacteria in animal tissue samples [18]. It has recently been found that IS*6110*-like elements may be present in other non-MTC mycobacteria such as *M. smegmatis* [31]. However, the probe and respective flanking primers used show no relevant complementary regions with these IS*6110*-like nucleotide sequences [18].
4. The use of a nested amplification assay for MTC detection presents an associated increased risk of cross contamination of samples. Therefore, we should emphasize the need of working in a laboratory harboring good practice standard conditions for molecular analysis, which include working in separate clean rooms and the use of positive and negative controls.
5. The standard PCR step amplifies an MTC-specific 199 bp fragment of the IS*6110*. The amplified products can be analyzed in a 2 % agarose gel electrophoresis, according to standard protocols.
6. The complementary regions of the P-*esat6*, F-*esat6*, and R-*esat6* probe and flanking primers, respectively, are located in the 6 kDa early secretory antigenic target gene (*esat6*, Rv3875 locus), included in the RD1 genomic region, which is present in most MTC members with the exception of the vaccine *M. bovis* BCG strains.
7. The complementary regions of the P-Rv1510, F-Rv1510, and R-Rv1510 probe and flanking primers, respectively, are located in the Rv1510 locus, coding a conserved probable membrane protein, included in the RD4 genomic region, which is present in all MTC members with the exception of *M. bovis*. However, a recent study reported that RD4 may be also absent, at least in part, from some *M. caprae* isolates [32].
8. The complementary regions of the P-Rv2073c, F-Rv2073c, and R-Rv2073c probe and flanking primers, respectively, are located in the Rv2073c locus coding a probable short chain dehydrogenase, included in the RD9 genomic region, which is present in *M. tuberculosis* but absent from *M. bovis* and other MTC species.

9. The first step allows the identification of the cultures as MTC members, by targeting their IS*6110* element, or as a mycobacterial species, if only a 16S rDNA product is detected in the duplex amplification reaction.
10. The second amplification step allows assessing the presence or absence of the Rv3875-*esat6* (RD1), Rv1510 (RD4), and Rv2073c (RD9) loci in the MTC strains. The correspondent pattern allows inferring the species of the isolate as *M. tuberculosis*, if all loci are present, as *M. caprae*, if only the Rv3875-esat6 (RD1) and Rv1510 (RD4) loci are present, as *M. bovis*, if only Rv3875 (RD1) locus is present, and as *M. bovis* BCG, if all the previous loci are absent.

Acknowledgments

This work was partially funded by the project PTDC/CVT/111634/2009 from "Fundação para a Ciência e a Tecnologia."

References

1. Brosch R, Gordon SV, Marmiesse M et al (2002) A new evolutionary scenario for the *Mycobacterium tuberculosis* complex. Proc Natl Acad Sci U S A 99:3684–3689
2. Mostowy S, Cousins D, Brinkman J, Aranaz A, Behr MA (2002) Genomic deletions suggest a phylogeny for the *Mycobacterium tuberculosis* complex. J Infect Dis 186:74–80
3. Michel AL, Müller B, van Helden PD (2010) *Mycobacterium bovis* at the animal-human interface: a problem, or not? Vet Microbiol 140:371–381
4. van Soolingen D, de Haas PE, Haagsma J et al (1994) Use of various genetic markers in differentiation of *Mycobacterium bovis* strains from animals and humans and for studying epidemiology of bovine tuberculosis. J Clin Microbiol 32:2425–2433
5. Aranaz A, Cousins D, Mateos A, Dominguez L (2003) Elevation of *Mycobacterium tuberculosis* subsp. *caprae* Aranaz et al. 1999 to species rank as *Mycobacterium caprae* comb. nov., sp. nov. Int J Syst Evol Microbiol 53:1785–1789
6. Cousins DV, Bastida R, Cataldi A et al (2003) Tuberculosis in seals caused by a novel member of the *Mycobacterium tuberculosis* complex: *Mycobacterium pinnipedii* sp. nov. Int J Syst Evol Microbiol 53:1305–1314
7. Mostowy S, Cousins D, Behr MA (2004) Genomic interrogation of the dassie bacillus reveals it as a unique RD1 mutant within the *Mycobacterium tuberculosis* complex. J Bacteriol 186:104–109
8. Huard RC, Fabre M, de Haas P et al (2006) Novel genetic polymorphisms that further delineate the phylogeny of the *Mycobacterium tuberculosis* complex. J Bacteriol 188: 4271–4287
9. Alexander KA, Laver PN, Michel AL et al (2010) Novel *Mycobacterium tuberculosis* complex pathogen, *M. mungi*. Emerg Infect Dis 16:1296–1299
10. van Ingen J, Rahim Z, Mulder A et al (2012) Characterization of *Mycobacterium orygis* as *M. tuberculosis* complex subspecies. Emerg Infect Dis 18:653–655
11. Niemann S, Harmsen D, Rusch-Gerdes S, Richter E (2000) Differentiation of clinical *Mycobacterium tuberculosis* complex isolates by *gyrB* DNA sequence polymorphism analysis. J Clin Microbiol 38:3231–3234
12. Parsons LM, Brosch R, Cole ST et al (2002) Rapid and simple approach for identification of *Mycobacterium tuberculosis* complex isolates by PCR-based genomic deletion analysis. J Clin Microbiol 40:2339–2345
13. Huard RC, Lazzarini LC, Butler WR, van Soolingen D, Ho JL (2003) PCR-based method to differentiate the subspecies of the *Mycobacterium tuberculosis* complex on the basis of genomic deletions. J Clin Microbiol 41:1637–1650

14. Djelouadji Z, Raoult D, Daffé M, Drancourt M (2008) A single-step sequencing method for the identification of *Mycobacterium tuberculosis* complex species. PLoS Negl Trop Dis 2:e253
15. Pinsky BA, Banaei N (2008) Multiplex real-time PCR assay for rapid identification of *Mycobacterium tuberculosis* Complex members to the species level. J Clin Microbiol 46: 2241–2246
16. Costa P, Amaro A, Botelho A, Inácio J, Baptista PV (2010) Gold nanoprobe assay for the identification of mycobacteria of the *Mycobacterium tuberculosis* complex. Clin Microbiol Infect 16:1464–1469
17. Halse TA, Escuyer VE, Musser KA (2011) Evaluation of a single-tube multiplex real-time PCR for differentiation of members of the *Mycobacterium tuberculosis* complex in clinical specimens. J Clin Microbiol 49:2562–2567
18. Costa P, Ferreira AS, Amaro A et al (2013) Enhanced detection of tuberculous mycobacteria in animal tissues using a semi-nested probe-based real-time PCR. PLoS One 8:e81337
19. Mahairas GG, Sabo PJ, Hickey MJ, Singh DC, Stover CK (1996) Molecular analysis of genetic differences between *Mycobacterium bovis* BCG and virulent M. bovis. J Bacteriol 178: 1274–1282
20. Brosch R, Gordon SV, Billault A et al (1998) Use of a *Mycobacterium tuberculosis* H37Rv bacterial artificial chromosome library for genome mapping, sequencing, and comparative genomics. Infect Immun 66:2221–2229
21. Gordon SV, Brosch R, Billault A et al (1999) Identification of variable regions in the genomes of tubercle bacilli using bacterial artificial chromosome arrays. Mol Microbiol 32:643–655
22. Behr MA, Wilson MA, Gill WP et al (1999) Comparative genomics of BCG vaccines by whole genome DNA microarray. Science 284:1520–1523
23. Warren RM, Gey van Pittius NC, Barnard M et al (2006) Differentiation of *Mycobacterium tuberculosis* complex by PCR amplification of genomic regions of difference. Int J Tuberc Lung Dis 10:818–822
24. Parra A, García N, García A et al (2008) Development of a molecular diagnostic test applied to experimental abattoir surveillance on bovine tuberculosis. Vet Microbiol 127:315–324
25. Taylor MJ, Hughes MS, Skuce RA, Neill SD (2001) Detection of *Mycobacterium bovis* in bovine clinical specimens using real-time fluorescence and fluorescence resonance energy transfer probe rapid-cycle PCR. J Clin Microbiol 39:1272–1278
26. Taylor GM, Worth DR, Palmer S, Jahans K, Hewinson RG (2007) Rapid detection of *Mycobacterium bovis* DNA in cattle lymph nodes with visible lesions using PCR. BMC Vet Res 3:12
27. Coetsier C, Vannuffel P, Blondeel N et al (2000) Duplex PCR for differential identification of *Mycobacterium bovis*, *M. avium*, and *M. avium* subsp. *paratuberculosis* in formalin-fixed paraffin-embedded tissues from cattle. J Clin Microbiol 38:3048–3054
28. Roring S, Hughes MS, Skuce RA, Neill SD (2000) Simultaneous detection and strain differentiation of *Mycobacterium bovis* directly from bovine tissue specimens by spoligotyping. Vet Microbiol 74:227–236
29. Thacker TC, Harris B, Palmer MV, Waters WR (2011) Improved specificity for detection of *Mycobacterium bovis* in fresh tissues using IS*6110* real-time PCR. BMC Vet Res 7:50
30. Liébana E, Aranaz A, Mateos A et al (1995) Simple and rapid detection of *Mycobacterium tuberculosis* complex organisms in bovine tissue samples by PCR. J Clin Microbiol 33:33–36
31. Coros A, DeConno E, Derbyshire KM (2008) IS*6110*, a *Mycobacterium tuberculosis* complex-specific insertion sequence, is also present in the genome of *Mycobacterium smegmatis*, suggestive of lateral gene transfer among mycobacterial species. J Bacteriol 190:3408–3410
32. Domogalla J, Prodinger WM, Blum H et al (2013) Region of difference 4 in alpine *Mycobacterium caprae* isolates indicates three variants. J Clin Microbiol 51:1381–1388
33. Restrepo BI, Gomez DI, Shipley GL, McCormick JB, Fisher-Hoch SP (2006) Selective enrichment and detection of mycobacterial DNA in paucibacillary specimens. J Microbiol Methods 67:220–229
34. Richardson ET, Samson D, Banaei N (2009) Rapid identification of *Mycobacterium tuberculosis* and nontuberculous mycobacteria by multiplex, real-time PCR. J Clin Microbiol 47: 1497–1502
35. Kirschner P, Springer B, Vogel U et al (1993) Genotypic identification of mycobacteria by nucleic acid sequence determination: report of a 2-year experience in a clinical laboratory. J Clin Microbiol 31:2882–2889

Chapter 10

A Real-Time PCR Assay for the Diagnosis of Gastrointestinal Nematode Infections of Small Ruminants

Florian Roeber, Aaron R. Jex, and Robin B. Gasser

Abstract

The diagnosis of gastrointestinal nematode infections in small ruminants is central to studying the biology and epidemiology of these parasites and underpins their control. Traditional methods of diagnosis are inaccurate, time-consuming and laborious. Here, we describe a step-by-step protocol for the molecular-based diagnosis of infections by real-time PCR.

Key words Livestock parasites, Strongylid nematodes, Diagnosis, PCR, Real-time PCR

1 Introduction

Parasitic worms of livestock cause diseases of major socioeconomic impact worldwide. The current financial losses caused by parasites to agriculture have a substantial impact on farm profitability around the world [1, 2]. Parasitic roundworms (nematodes) of livestock animals are mainly controlled by treatment with antiparasitic drugs (anthelmintics) [3]. Even with optimally timed, strategic treatments, this type of control is expensive. The excessive and uncontrolled use of anthelmintics has resulted in substantial and widespread problems with resistance in nematodes against these compounds [4, 5]. Given the significant problems with parasitic diseases and drug resistance, there is an urgent need for an increased focus on integrated control, which includes the use of diagnostic methods. Unfortunately, traditional parasitological methods of diagnosis are often unreliable and/or time-consuming to carry out [6]. These limitations relate to their inability to accurately identify parasite stages (eggs or larvae) from fecal samples to species and also to the time that it takes to allow eggs to develop to larvae (via "coproculture") for subsequent microscopic identification [7]. Recently, a DNA approach was developed to overcome

Mónica V. Cunha and João Inácio (eds.), *Veterinary Infection Biology: Molecular Diagnostics and High-Throughput Strategies*, Methods in Molecular Biology, vol. 1247, DOI 10.1007/978-1-4939-2004-4_10, © Springer Science+Business Media New York 2015

these limitations. Using genetic markers in the second internal transcribed spacer (ITS-2) of nuclear rRNA genes, we established a rapid and highly effective real-time PCR assay for the specific diagnosis of infections by nematodes, including *Haemonchus contortus*, *Teladorsagia circumcincta*, *Trichostrongylus* spp., *Chabertia ovina* and *Oesophagostomum venulosum*, of sheep [8]. This real-time PCR involves the incorporation of a specific fluorescent dye (SYTO-9®) into the PCR, which binds to produced double-stranded molecules and enables the detection of accumulating DNA. The change of fluorescence during the thermocycling is directly related to the initial starting number of target sequences. The fewer the cycles required to produce a detectable fluorescence, measured as cycle threshold or C_t value, the greater the number of target sequences present. Published evidence [9, 10] shows clearly that this assay outperforms traditional methods used for the diagnosis of gastrointestinal nematode infections in small ruminants, and can be employed for routine diagnostic application or as an epidemiological tool. Here we describe a step-by-step protocol for this PCR assay (Fig. 1).

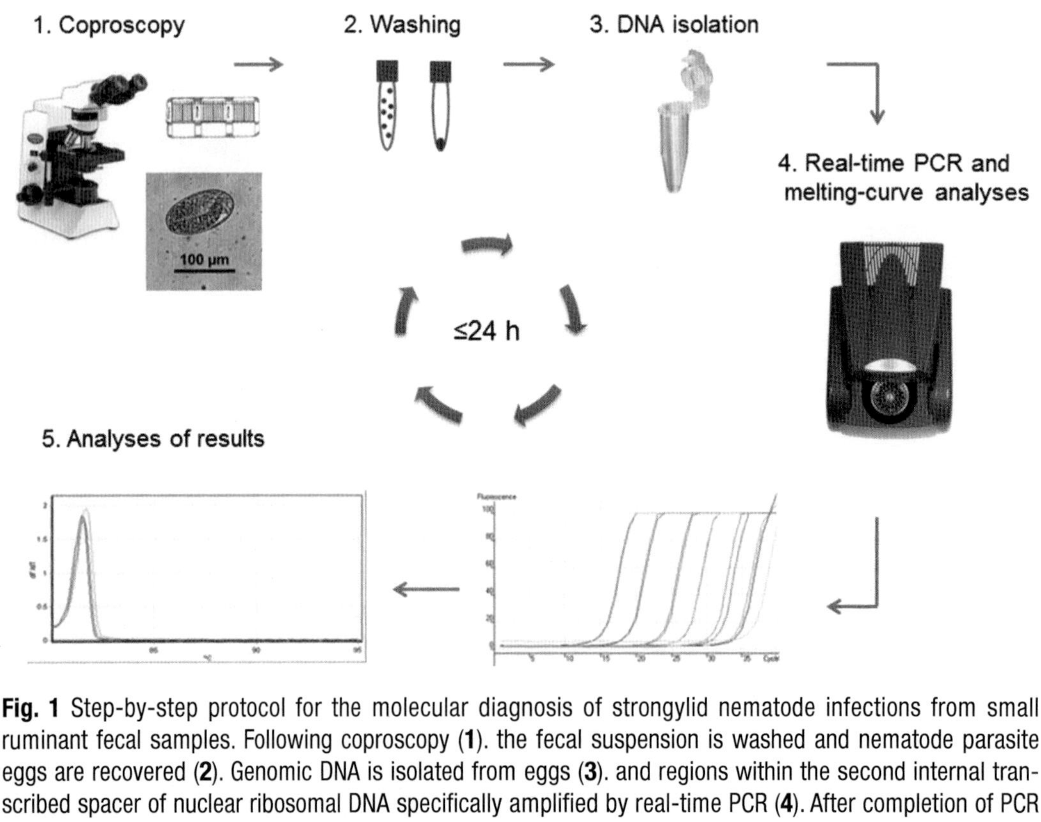

Fig. 1 Step-by-step protocol for the molecular diagnosis of strongylid nematode infections from small ruminant fecal samples. Following coproscopy (**1**). the fecal suspension is washed and nematode parasite eggs are recovered (**2**). Genomic DNA is isolated from eggs (**3**). and regions within the second internal transcribed spacer of nuclear ribosomal DNA specifically amplified by real-time PCR (**4**). After completion of PCR and melting-curve analysis (**5**). an estimate of the contribution of individual nematode species or genera to the egg count is estimated

2 Materials

2.1 For Fecal Flotation and the Enumeration of Nematode Eggs

1. Saturated sodium nitrate flotation solution: Fill a beaker with 1 l of hot water and add 400 g of sodium nitrate salt. Continuously stir the suspension until the salt is fully dissolved. Check specific gravity of 1.300 with a hydrometer (*see* **Note 1**).
2. McMaster parasite egg counting chambers.
3. Metal spatula.
4. Metal sieve (aperture of 250 μm).
5. 60 ml plastic container.
6. Pipette with sieve top.
7. Weight (±0.05 g accuracy).
8. 50 ml tubes with conical bottom.

2.2 For the Isolation of Nucleic Acids from Nematode Eggs

1. Standard pipettes and tips (1 ml, 200 μl and 20 μl).
2. Vortex.
3. RNase/DNase-free microcentrifuge tubes (1.5 ml).
4. Refrigerator (4 °C).
5. Centrifuge for 50 ml tubes; minimum of 2,000 × *g* at room temperature.
6. Microfuge.
7. Adequate DNA extraction kit (e.g., PowerSoil® DNA Isolation Kit, MO BIO Laboratories Inc., USA).

2.3 For the Amplification of Nucleic Acids by Real-Time PCR

1. Oligonucleotide primers targeting the ITS-2 region of the most relevant nematode parasites (Table 1) and the conserved primers NC1 (5′-ACG TCT GGT TCA GGG TTG TT-3′) and NC2 (5′-TTA GTT TCT TTT CCT CCG CT-3′) [8, 11].
2. Real-time PCR thermal cycler and respective software (*see* **Note 2**).
3. Commercial PCR mixture containing standard reaction buffer, heat-activated DNA polymerase, dNTPs, and 6 mM $MgCl_2$ (*see* **Note 3**).
4. SYTO®9 green fluorescent nucleic acid stain (Life Technologies, USA) (*see* **Note 4**).

3 Methods

3.1 Preparation of Fecal Samples and Enumeration of Nematode Eggs

1. Collect feces from the rectum of sheep using a disposable plastic glove. Invert the glove to capture the sample, expel air, tie a knot in the glove and label with a permanent marker (*see* **Note 5**).

Table 1
Parasite-specific primers used in the real-time PCR assays

Primer[a]	Sequence (5′–3′)	Start position in ITS-2 region[b]	Amplicon length (bp)[c]	Melting temperature of target sequence (°C)	Target species
HAE	CAA ATG GCA TTT GTC TTT TAG	41	265	78.81	*H. contortus*
TEL	TAT GCA ACA TGA CGT ACG ACG G	98	218	78.15	*Te. circumcincta*
TRI	TCG AAT GGT CAT TGT CAAA	40	267–268	77.87	*Trichostrongylus* spp.
CHO	GTG ATG ACC TCG TTG TCA CCG TG	143	162	82.12	*C. ovina*
OEV	TGA AAT GAG ACA ACC GTA GTC G	222	105	79.38	*O. venulosum*

[a]According to Bott et al. [8]
[b]Using the sequences with the GenBank access numbers for *H. contortus* (accession no. X78803), *Te. circumcincta* (accession no. X86026), *Trichostrongylus axei*, *Tr. colubriformis*, *Tr. vitrinus*, *Tr. rugatus* (accession nos. X78065, X78063, X78064 and Y14818) *Oe. venulosum* (accession no. Y10790) and *C. ovina* (accession no. Y10789) as references
[c]When combined with the conserved NC2 reverse primer at the 5′ axei end of the large subunit of rDNA

2. Homogenize the entire fecal sample and transfer 4 g to a 60 ml container (*see* **Note 6**).
3. Add 50 ml of sodium nitrate solution and homogenize (*see* **Note** 7).
4. Pour suspension through a sieve and collect run-through in a clean container.
5. Pour suspension into a 50 ml tube and make up to 50 ml with sodium nitrate solution. Close the tube and invert three times. Immediately open the tube, aspirate 1.5 ml with a sieve-top pipette and fill three chambers of the McMaster slide.
6. Count thin-shelled strongylid nematode eggs (i.e., <100 μm in length and <50 μm in width) in each of the three chambers and calculate the mean number from the three counts. Every egg counted equates to 30 eggs per gram in a 4 g sample.

3.2 Concentration of Nematode Eggs from the Fecal Sample

1. Centrifuge the suspension at 1,000 × *g* at 22–24 °C for 5 min to float the eggs to the top of the suspension.
2. Decant 5 ml from the supernatant into a fresh 50 ml tube and fill with tap water. Centrifuge again at 2,000 × *g* for 5 min to pellet the eggs in the bottom of the tube (*see* **Note 8**).
3. Discard the supernatant without dislodging the pellet. Completely resuspend the pellet in 5 ml of water by vortexing, add 45 ml of water and then centrifuge again at 2,000 × *g* for 5 min.

4. Discard the supernatant. Add 250 μl of water and aspirate using a pipette and transfer the suspension (0.5–1.5 ml) to a 1.5 ml microcentrifuge tube, freeze (−20 °C) or use directly for genomic DNA isolation.

3.3 DNA Isolation from Fecal Pellet

1. Transfer 250 μl of the suspension to a PowerSoil® DNA isolation tube and perform isolation of nucleic acids according to the manufacturer's instructions.
2. Use DNA samples immediately for molecular analysis or store frozen (−70 °C).

3.4 Real-Time PCR, Melting Curve, and Analyses of Results

1. Five primer pairs HAE-NC2, TEL-NC2, TRI-NC2, CHO-NC2 and OEV-NC2 are used in separate reactions for the specific amplification of the ITS-2 region of *H. contortus*, *Te. circumcincta*, *Trichostrongylus* spp., *C. ovina* and *O. venulosum*, respectively, from strongylid egg DNA from fecal samples. In addition, primer pair NC1-NC2 [8, 11] is used to assess inhibition in, and amplification efficiency for, individual genomic DNA samples.
2. Perform each PCR reaction in a volume of 25 μl, containing 12.5 μl Sensimix dT Mastermix, 0.2 μM of forward and reverse primer and 8 μM of SYTO-9® fluorescent dye [9, 10]. Samples without genomic DNA (no-DNA controls) are included in each PCR run. Also included in each run is a serial titration (1 ng, 100 pg, 10 pg and 1 pg) of ITS-2 sequences of each *H. contortus*, *Te. circumcincta*, *T. vitrinus*, *C. ovina* and *O. venulosum*, cloned into the vector pGEM-T (Promega), as calibrated "reference positive" controls (to provide standard curves) (*see* **Note 9**).
3. PCR is performed under the following conditions: 95 °C for 10 min, followed by 35 cycles of 95 °C for 15 s (denaturation), 55 °C for 30 s (annealing) and 72 °C for 5 s (extension). To verify their specificity, all amplicons are subjected to melting-curve analysis (75–85 °C at 0.1 °C/s) (*see* **Note 10**).
4. Test-positive samples are identified on the basis of a single melt peak, which is consistent with that of the homologous control for each PCR (*see* **Note 11**). The specificity of the amplicons can also be verified by selective sequencing, employing an established approach [11] (*see* **Note 12**).

4 Notes

1. It is critical to use a salt solution of this specific gravity to achieve maximum flotation of nematode eggs.
2. We use the Rotor-Gene 3000 thermal cycler (Qiagen, USA) and the respective software.

3. We use the Sensimix dT Mastermix (Bioline, UK).
4. SYTO®9 is light sensitive, and exposure to light must be minimized. It is supplied in 100 μl volumes and can be made up to a stock solution (1 ml) by mixing 19 μl of dye with 981 μl of molecular grade water. From this stock solution, use 2 μl in a 25 μl PCR reaction to achieve a final dye concentration of 8 μM. Repeated thawing of the stock solution and exposure to light can result in reduced signal in real-time PCR assays and should therefore be kept to a minimum.
5. Fill sampling jar or bag as much as possible and seal airtight to provide oxygen-poor environment (to delay development and hatching of eggs). Store samples refrigerated (4 °C) and send for diagnosis within 1 day [12]. Development and hatching of eggs may have impact on the quantification of nematode eggs and should therefore be reduced.
6. If feces are dry, add 0.5 ml of water to facilitate homogenization. Thorough homogenization of fecal matter is essential to release the nematode eggs from the fecal mass and helps to disperse the eggs evenly throughout the sample.
7. If a spatula is used for homogenization, clean with bleach solution (3 %) [13] to avoid possible transfer of eggs from sample to sample.
8. If the supernatant contains a significant amount of debris (e.g., fecal and plant), sieve through one layer of surgical gauze.
9. To prepare a standard curve for quantification in real-time PCR, the concentration of the reference DNA sample has to be determined spectrophotometrically. Typically, a DNA concentration of 25–100 ng/μl can be expected from a single nematode. From this stock solution, take a specific volume (e.g., 4 μl) and mix into molecular grade water (e.g., 96 μl) to prepare a dilution of 1 ng/μl. This solution can be further diluted in tenfold dilution steps (using 10 μl of the previous dilution and mixing it into 90 μl of water) to obtain reference controls of 1 ng, 100 pg, 10 pg and 1 pg. Instead of using parasite DNA as reference controls, target sequences can be cloned into a plasmid vector (pGEM-T-Easy, Promega, USA) and then grown in *Escherichia coli*, according to the manufacturer's protocol. In brief, 8 μl of purified amplicon containing the insert sequence are ligated into the vector and incubated at 4 °C overnight. The ligation product is mixed with competent *E. coli* and cultured on Luria Bertani agar plates at 37 °C for 12–16 h. Screening and selection can be performed by PCR using primers specific to the cloned insert. Successfully transformed colonies can be further grown in a liquid broth and preserved frozen as 30 % glycerol stocks. The cloned DNA inserts can be serial titrated with molecular grade water, to determine the dilution or concentration of template required

to achieve the same or a similar amplification characteristic and standard curves as for genomic DNA reference samples.

10. We use Rotor-Gene v.1.7.87 software, and apply the normalization option and a confidence threshold of 96 %.
11. Any suspected inhibition in PCR, likely linked to fecal components (e.g., humic acids, phenolic compounds and/or polysaccharides) can be assessed. In brief, aliquots (2 μl) of samples that are test negative by PCR but shown to contain strongylid eggs by coproscopic examination are spiked with a limiting amount (1 pg) of genomic DNA from *H. contortus* or an alternative strongylid nematode. The amplification from spiked sample aliquots is compared directly (in the same experiment) with that from 1 pg of *H. contortus* DNA alone and a sample without DNA (no-template control).
12. Based on the findings from previous studies [9, 10], this PCR assay can replace inaccurate and time-consuming classical diagnostic procedures. This assay achieves specific or generic diagnosis and takes less than 1 day to perform, compared with at least 1 week for larval culture, thus significantly reducing delays and response times for the treatment or control of clinical cases of parasitic disease. The assay has high diagnostic performance (i.e., sensitivity and specificity) [9, 10] and has broad applicability, in that it can be used to conduct large-scale epidemiological studies, to support the diagnosis of drug resistance and will be applicable or adaptable to other parasites and/or hosts. This PCR tool has the potential to replace the conventional technique of larval culture and can be extended to include the testing of other parasites or pathogens, depending on where the assay is to be deployed. Current evidence [14] shows that this assay is adaptable to an automated PCR platform (*Easy*-Plex, AusDiagnostics Pty. Ltd.), allowing the development of a range of next-generation diagnostic tools to underpin the control of socioeconomically important infectious diseases of animals. The routine application of such automated diagnostic platforms for pathogens of veterinary importance provides major scope for better disease surveillance, detailed epidemiological or ecological studies, and shorter response times to tackle and control disease outbreaks.

Acknowledgments

This research was supported through funds from the Australian Research Council (RBG and ARJ). Other support from Melbourne Water Corporation, the National Health and Medical Research Council, and the Alexander von Humboldt Foundation is gratefully acknowledged (RBG). FR was the recipient of scholarships from the University of Melbourne.

References

1. Perry BD, Randolph TF (1999) Improving the assessment of the economic impact of parasitic diseases and of their control in production animals. Vet Parasitol 84:145–168
2. Sackett D, Holmes P (2006) Assessing the economic cost of endemic disease on the profitability of Australian beef cattle and sheep producers. Meat and Livestock Australia, Report No. ISBN: 1741910021, Sydney, Australia
3. Hoste H, Torres-Acosta JF (2011) Non chemical control of helminths in ruminants: adapting solutions for changing worms in a changing world. Vet Parasitol 180:144–154
4. Wolstenholme AJ, Fairweather I, Prichard R, Samson-Himmelstjerna GV, Sangster NC (2004) Drug resistance in veterinary helminths. Trends Parasitol 20:469–476
5. Kaplan RM (2004) Drug resistance in nematodes of veterinary importance: a status report. Trends Parasitol 20:477–481
6. Gasser RB, Bott NJ, Chilton NB, Hunt P, Beveridge I (2008) Towards practical, DNA-based diagnostic methods for parasitic nematodes of livestock-bionomic and biotechnological implications. Biotechnol Adv 26:325–334
7. Roeber F, Jex AR, Gasser RB (2013) Next-generation molecular-diagnostic tools for gastrointestinal nematodes of livestock, with emphasis on small ruminants: a turning point? Adv Parasitol 83:267–333
8. Bott NJ, Campbell BE, Beveridge I, Chilton NB, Rees D, Hunt PW et al (2009) A combined microscopic-molecular method for the diagnosis of strongylid infections in sheep. Int J Parasitol 39:1277–1287
9. Roeber F, Jex AR, Campbell AJD, Campbell BE, Anderson GA, Gasser RB (2011) Evaluation and application of a molecular method to assess the composition of strongylid nematode populations in sheep with naturally acquired infections. Infect Genet Evol 11:849–854
10. Roeber F, Larsen JWA, Anderson N, Campbell AJD, Anderson GA, Gasser RB et al (2012) A molecular diagnostic tool to replace larval culture in conventional faecal egg count reduction testing in sheep. PLoS One 7:e37327
11. Gasser RB, Hu M, Chilton N, Campbell BE, Jex AR, Otranto D et al (2006) Single-strand conformation polymorphism (SSCP) for the analysis of genetic variation. Nat Protoc 1: 3121–3128
12. Taylor MA, Coop RL, Wall RL (2007) The laboratory diagnosis of parasitism. Chapter 15. In: Taylor MA, Coop RL, Wall RL (eds) Veterinary parasitology, 3rd edn. Blackwell, Oxford, UK, p 798
13. Kemp B, Smith D (2005) Use of bleach to eliminate contaminating DNA from the surface of bones and teeth. Forensic Sci Int 154:53–61
14. Roeber F, Jex AR, Campbell AJ, Nielsen R, Anderson GA, Stanley KK et al (2012) Establishment of a robotic, high-throughput platform for the specific diagnosis of gastrointestinal nematode infections in sheep. Int J Parasitol 42:1151–1158

Chapter 11

Improved Detection of *Mycobacterium bovis* in Bovine Tissues Using Immunomagnetic Separation Approaches

Irene R. Grant and Linda D. Stewart

Abstract

Immunomagnetic separation (IMS) represents a simple but effective method of selectively capturing and concentrating *Mycobacterium bovis*, the causative agent of bovine tuberculosis (bTB), from tissue samples. It is a physical cell separation technique that does not impact cell viability, unlike traditional chemical decontamination prior to culture. IMS is performed with paramagnetic beads coated with *M. bovis*-specific antibody and peptide binders. Once captured by IMS, *M. bovis* cells can be detected by either PCR or cultural detection methods. Increased detection rates of *M. bovis*, particularly from non-visibly lesioned lymph node tissues from bTB reactor animals, have recently been reported when IMS-based methods were employed.

Key words *Mycobacterium bovis*, Lymph node tissue, Immunomagnetic separation (IMS), Isolation, Detection, IMS-PCR, IMS-culture

1 Introduction

Bovine tuberculosis (bTB), caused by *Mycobacterium bovis*, continues to be a significant animal health issue in many countries of the world [1]. The single intradermal comparative cervical tuberculin (SICCT) test, more commonly known as the tuberculin "skin test," is used in many countries to identify bTB "reactor" animals, which are then compulsorily slaughtered. At the time of slaughter, meat inspectors look for visible lesions typical of bTB in the lymph nodes of the head and chest and in the lungs of these animals and excise tissue samples to be sent to the bTB testing laboratory to allow confirmation of *M. bovis* infection status. Tissues are also taken from bTB reactor animals displaying no visible lesions (NVL). Currently, confirmation of diagnosis of bTB is reliant on successful isolation of *M. bovis* by culture, but this approach can be problematic for a variety of reasons. There may be small numbers of mycobacteria present in the selected tissues, at or below the detection limit of culture, so

Mónica V. Cunha and João Inácio (eds.), *Veterinary Infection Biology: Molecular Diagnostics and High-Throughput Strategies*, Methods in Molecular Biology, vol. 1247, DOI 10.1007/978-1-4939-2004-4_11,

false-negative culture results may be obtained. Chemical decontamination of the tissues (typically with oxalic acid) prior to culture on solid and liquid media is known to significantly reduce the viability of *M. bovis* in vitro [2], which may also lead to false-negative culture results. The time to confirm the presence or absence of *M. bovis* in clinical samples by culture can be up to 8 weeks, and any delay in confirmation, as well as false-negative culture results for NVL tissues, has consequences for disease control programs [3].

Immunomagnetic separation (IMS) is a sample preparation technique that aids the selective separation and concentration of target bacterial cells from complex food and veterinary sample matrices such as milk, feces, blood, and tissues [4]. It effectively selects the desired bacterium out of the sample background microflora and sample components by use of microscopic paramagnetic beads coated with antibodies (or other appropriate binders) specific for the bacterium of interest. Numbers of target bacterial cells may also be concentrated from the test sample by resuspending beads in a smaller volume after IMS. IMS has a longer history of being employed for food testing [5] than in the veterinary diagnostic laboratory context, but it is becoming more widely used for veterinary testing. Several IMS methods for *M. bovis* have been published in recent years [6–9]. However, Stewart et al. [9] attempted to optimize the IMS method by evaluating a range of novel *M. bovis* binders (polyclonal and monoclonal antibodies, as well as phage display-derived 12-mer *M. bovis*-specific peptide binders) they had produced, in order to identify the best bead-binder combination to achieve maximal *M. bovis* cell capture (Fig. 1). Dynabeads® MyOne™ Tosylactivated dually coated with a

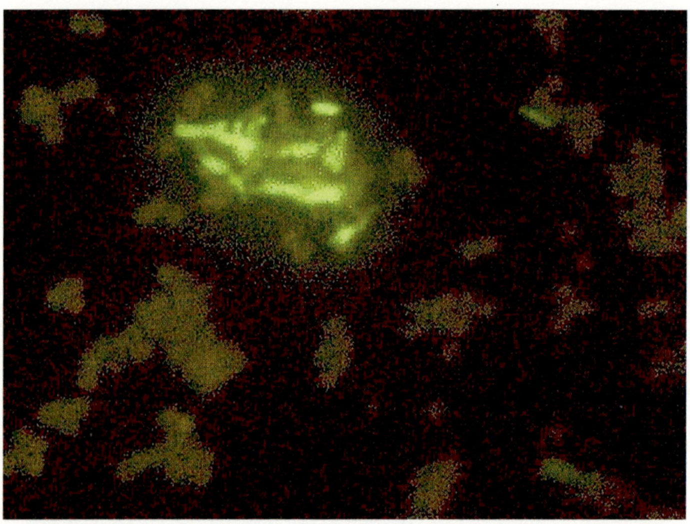

Fig. 1 *Mycobacterium bovis* cells captured by monoclonal antibody and biotinylated 12-mer peptide-coated Dynabeads® MyOne™ Tosylactivated—a large clump of *M. bovis* cells and an individual cell are clearly seen attached to the beads. Bead suspension after IMS was stained by auramine O fluorescent acid-fast stain

monoclonal IgM antibody and a biotinylated 12-mer peptide was found to perform best [9]. The optimized *M. bovis* IMS protocol was subsequently used to test a large number of bovine lymph node tissues from bTB reactor animals demonstrating either visible lesions (VL) or non-visible lesions (NVL), and *M. bovis* cells captured on the magnetic beads were subsequently detected by touchdown PCR targeting IS*6110* and MGIT™ liquid culture [10]. Results of this survey indicated that the IMS-based approaches confirmed *M. bovis* infection in more lymph node samples, particularly in NVL tissues from bTB skin test reactor animals, than the existing oxalic acid decontamination and solid and liquid culture approach. Here, the optimized IMS approaches for isolation and detection of *M. bovis* in bovine tissues will be described.

2 Materials

1. Purified mouse anti-*Mycobacterium bovis* IgM monoclonal antibody (11G3) (*see* **Note 1**).
2. N-terminally biotinylated 12-mer peptide (EEA302) with amino acid sequence NFRVSIDVVKSR (10 mg/ml in sterile distilled water), custom synthesized by any peptide synthesis company.
3. Dynabeads® MyOne™ Tosylactivated (Life Technologies): bead diameter 1.08 μm, bead concentration 100 mg beads/ml (approx. 10^{12} beads/g), surface area 8 m^2/g (*see* **Note 2**).
4. Coating buffer: 0.1 M sodium borate buffer pH 9.5, prepared by dissolving 6.183 g H_3BO_3 (MW 61.83) in 800 ml distilled water, adjusting pH to 9.5 using 5 M NaOH and then adjusting volume to 1,000 ml with distilled water.
5. 3 M ammonium sulfate: prepared in coating buffer by dissolving 39.6 g $(NH_4)_2SO_4$ (MW 132.1) in 0.1 M sodium borate (pH 9.5), adjusting pH (if necessary) and then adjusting volume to 100 ml.
6. Phosphate buffered saline pH 7.4 (PBS): 0.01 M phosphate buffered saline composed of 0.138 M sodium chloride and 0.0027 M potassium chloride, pH adjusted to 7.4.
7. Washing and storage buffer for beads (PBS/BSA/T20): phosphate buffered saline pH 7.4 (PBS) with 0.1 % (w/v) bovine serum albumin and 0.05 % (w/v) Tween 20 added.
8. Wash buffer for IMS (PBS/T20): phosphate buffered saline pH 7.4 (PBS) with 0.05 % (w/v) Tween 20 added.
9. Tris-EDTA buffer (pH 8.0): 10 mM Tris–HCl and 1 mM disodium EDTA, pH adjusted to 8.0.
10. Reagents for conventional PCR reactions (for post-IMS detection of *M. bovis* by PCR): DNA polymerase enzyme and

respective 10× buffer, primers INS1 (5′-cgt gag ggc atc gag gtg gc-3′) and INS2 (5′-gcg tag gcg tcg gtg aca aa-3′) [11], $MgCl_2$ (25 mM), dNTPs (25 mM), and distilled PCR-grade water. In this protocol, a PCR SuperMix is employed for PCR reactions (Platinum® Blue PCR SuperMix, Life Technologies).

11. BBL™ MGIT™ culture tubes for *M. bovis* previously supplemented with BBL™ MGIT™ OADC and BBL™ MGIT™ PANTA supplements (Becton Dickinson) (for post-IMS detection of *M. bovis* by culture).
12. Equipment and other supplies: centrifuge; magnetic rack; Stuart rotator mixer (or similar); Dynal BeadRetriever™ and respective tube and tip strips (Life Technologies) (not necessary if using the manual IMS procedure); thermal cycler, electrophoresis apparatus, and UV transilluminator (for post-IMS detection of *M. bovis* by PCR); MGIT 960 instrument (Becton Dickinson) (for post-IMS detection of *M. bovis* by culture); sterile mortar, sterile sand, and pestle.

3 Methods

3.1 Coating Dynabeads® MyOne™ Tosylactivated with Phage Display-Derived Peptide and Monoclonal IgM Antibody

This coating procedure is essentially as described in the pack insert accompanying Dynabeads® MyOne™ Tosylactivated (*see* **Note 2**).

1. Transfer 250 μl of uncoated Dynabeads® MyOne™ Tosylactivated to a sterile microcentrifuge tube.
2. Wash beads twice with 1 ml of coating buffer, separating on a magnetic rack for 2 min between washes.
3. Resuspend beads in 100 μl of coating buffer and vortex thoroughly.
4. Premix 50 μl of N-terminally biotinylated 12-mer peptide and 50 μl of purified mouse anti-*M. bovis* monoclonal IgM antibody (*see* **Notes 1** and **3**); add to activated beads and mix by vortexing.
5. Add a further 735 μl of coating buffer and mix again by vortexing.
6. Add 415 μl of 3 M ammonium sulfate and mix by vortexing.
7. Incubate overnight at 37 °C with "end-to-end" mixing on a Stuart rotator mixer (or similar) at 10 rpm.
8. Wash freshly coated beads twice with 1 ml of washing buffer, separating on a magnetic rack for 2 min between washes.
9. Resuspend coated beads in 500 μl storage buffer, which is twice the original volume of uncoated beads used. This final volume is sufficient for 50 IMS reactions when 10 μl of coated beads are used per 1 ml test sample.

10. The Dynabeads® MyOne™ Tosylactivated are now coated and ready for use. They should be stored at 2–8 °C until required (*see* **Note 4**).

3.2 Lymph Node Preparation for IMS

For health and safety reasons all procedures involving bovine tissues containing, or potentially containing, *M. bovis* must be carried out in a class 1 biological safety cabinet located in a containment level 3 laboratory facility.

1. Transfer approx. 3 g of cubed lymph node material to a sterile mortar, add sterile sand, and grind thoroughly with pestle.
2. Add 4.5 ml of sterile phosphate buffered saline pH 7.4 (PBS) and grind further (=1:1.5 dilution).
3. Transfer sample to centrifuge tube and centrifuge at 300 × *g* for 3 min to sediment sand and tissue particulates.
4. Make a 1:10 dilution of clarified lymph node tissue supernatant in sterile PBS (*see* **Note 5**) and use 1 ml of this dilution (=1:15 dilution of original lymph node sample) for immunomagnetic separation (IMS).

3.3 Immunomagnetic Separation

3.3.1 Automated Immunomagnetic Separation (IMS) Using Dynal BeadRetriever™

1. Add 10 μl of dually coated (Mab 11G3 and biotinylated peptide EEA302) Dynabeads® MyOne™ Tosylactivated to first well of BeadRetriever™ tube strip, 1 ml of PBS/T20 buffer in the next 2 wells, and an appropriate volume of buffer, depending on subsequent endpoint detection method (PCR or culture; *see* later), to 4th well.
2. Transfer 1 ml of the 1:10 dilution of the clarified lymph node tissue supernatant to the 1st well of the BeadRetriever™ tube strips. Fifteen samples can be processed at the same time.
3. Transfer tube rack containing samples to BeadRetriever™ machine.
4. Pre-wet BeadRetriever™ tip strips (magnet covers) by dipping each tip briefly in PBS/T20 and slide into place in BeadRetriever™ machine (*see* **Note 6**).
5. Perform automated IMS using "environmental" program. This preloaded IMS program consists of a 35-min incubation period in well 1 of the bead retriever strip with mixing at a medium speed throughout. The beads are then captured and transferred to well 2 and washed for 1 min at a medium speed. During the next stage, the beads are transferred to well 3 and washed again for 1 min at medium speed. Finally, the beads are transferred to well 4 (*see* **Note 7**) where they are released using a 10-s high-speed mix into an appropriate buffer, depending on which endpoint detection method is going to be applied (*see* below).

3.3.2 Manual IMS Using Magnetic Rack

In the absence of a Dynal BeadRetriever™, IMS may be performed manually (*see* **Note 8**) using 1.5 ml microcentrifuge tubes and a suitable magnetic rack (*see* **Note 9**).

1. Distribute 10 μl of dually coated (Mab 11G3 and biotinylated peptide EEA302) Dynabeads® MyOne™ Tosylactivated into sufficient sterile microcentrifuge tubes for the number of samples to be tested (*see* **Note 10**).
2. Dispense 1 ml of 1:10 dilution of clarified lymph node tissue supernatant into tubes containing beads, vortex briefly, and then place on Stuart rotator mixer (or similar rotating mixer) at room temperature for 30 min at 10 rpm.
3. Transfer tubes to a suitable magnetic rack and separate beads for 10 min before removing supernatants carefully with pastettes and discarding into suitable disinfectant. Keep magnet in place throughout and be careful to avoid loss of beads with sample (*see* **Note 11**).
4. Dispense 1 ml PBS/T20 into each tube, remove magnet from rack, and shake samples thoroughly.
5. Replace magnet for 2 min to capture beads then remove and discard spent PBS/T20.
6. Repeat **steps 4** and **5** again (=second wash step).
7. Resuspend beads in a buffer appropriate for subsequent detection by PCR or culture (*see* below).

3.4 *M. bovis* Detection Options Post-IMS

3.4.1 Touchdown IS6110 PCR (See Note 12)

1. Resuspend beads after IMS in 100 μl Tris-EDTA buffer (pH 8.0), transfer bead suspension from well 4 of tube strip to screw-capped microcentrifuge tube, and boil for 25 min at 100 °C in a water bath to inactivate bound *M. bovis* cells and release DNA. Centrifuge tubes briefly to sediment cell debris and beads and use supernatant as template DNA.
2. Each PCR reaction consists of 45 μl Platinum® Blue PCR SuperMix (*see* **Note 13**) plus 1 μM of primers INS1 and INS2 [11], 2 mM $MgCl_2$, and 5 μl of template DNA.
3. Perform touchdown PCR amplification on a thermal cycler with an initial denaturation step of 96 °C for 3 min, followed by 8 cycles of denaturation at 96 °C for 1 min, annealing temperatures starting at 72 °C for 1 min (decreasing by 1 °C/cycle), and 72 °C for 1 min for extension. This step is followed by 30 cycles of 96 °C for 1 min, 65 °C for 1 min, 72 °C for 2 min, and a final extension at 72 °C for 8 min before holding at 4 °C.
4. Visualize PCR products using 2 % agarose gel electrophoresis and ethidium bromide staining.

3.4.2 MGIT™ (Mycobacteria Growth Indicator Tube) Culture

1. Resuspend beads after IMS in 100–300 μl (*see* **Note 14**) of PBS and inoculate into a BBL™ MGIT™ tube previously supplemented with BBL™ MGIT™ OADC and BBL™ MGIT™ PANTA as per usual practice for *M. bovis* culture.
2. Incubate MGIT™ culture tubes in MGIT 960 instrument for up to 8 weeks at 37 °C.
3. Examine any IMS-MGIT™ culture that indicates growth positive on the MGIT™ system throughout the incubation period for the presence of acid-fast bacteria typical of *M. bovis* by Ziehl-Neelsen (ZN) staining. A subsample of each acid-fast positive IMS-MGIT™ culture should be sent for genotyping (by spoligotyping) after boiling in a screw-capped microcentrifuge tube for 25 min at 100 °C in a water bath (to render samples safe to be taken out of containment level 3 laboratory).
4. At the end of the 8-week incubation period, a subsample (100 μl) of all IMS-MGIT™ cultures that have not indicated growth positive on the MGIT™ 960 system, or have indicated growth positive but tested ZN negative (*see* **Note 15**), is transferred to screw-capped microcentrifuge tubes and boiled for 25 min at 100 °C in a water bath (to render samples safe to be taken out of containment level 3 laboratory) and then subjected to touchdown IS*6110* PCR (as described above) in order to detect the presence of low numbers of viable *M. bovis* which may not have reached detection threshold of either MGIT™ system or ZN staining.

4 Notes

1. The monoclonal antibody (11G3) was jointly produced by Queen's University Belfast and the Agri-Food and Biosciences Institute for Northern Ireland [9]. Other anti-*M. bovis* polyclonal or monoclonal antibodies may be available commercially or may have been generated in-house by other research groups. Any such antibody could potentially be used to coat Dynabeads® MyOne™ Tosylactivated for IMS purposes; however, there is no guarantee that capture of *M. bovis* will be as good as when monoclonal antibody 11G3 is used in conjunction with the 12-mer peptide. An experiment to assess the detection sensitivity of such coated beads should be carried out, as described by Stewart et al. [9], to verify good *M. bovis* capture capability before adoption of an alternative IMS protocol.
2. Other types and sizes of surface-activated magnetic beads are commercially available. If a different type of bead is employed, then the bead coating protocol may differ, so follow the manufacturer's instructions accordingly.

3. This combination of *M. bovis* binders with Dynabeads® MyOne™ Tosylactivated was empirically shown to be the best bead-binder combination for maximal capture of *M. bovis* from buffer and animal tissue homogenates [9].
4. If the coated beads are not used within 2–3 weeks, it is recommended to "refresh" the storage buffer by separating beads on magnetic rack, removing spent storage buffer, and adding freshly prepared storage buffer.
5. This 1:10 dilution of the clarified lymph node supernatant proved necessary to permit beads to associate freely with *M. bovis* cells within the tissue sample during capture phase of IMS.
6. This is an important step because if not pre-wetted, the beads tend to stick to the plastic tips which may reduce the number of beads recoverable.
7. Automated IMS achieves greater cleanup of beads because beads move from well to well, leaving original sample behind in well 1.
8. Manual IMS achieves capture of target bacterium but, as beads stay in same tube throughout all steps in the process, the same degree of cleanup of beads is not achieved as when automated BeadRetriever™ protocol is used.
9. Larger sample volumes (10–50 ml) could be tested if magnetic racks for 10 ml or 50 ml tubes are available; however, in our experience larger sample volumes and racks are more difficult to work with. Beads tend not to be held as securely at the magnet interface when using the larger volume racks, so there is more risk of losing them and hence bound *M. bovis* cells during the washing steps.
10. Vortex and coated beads thoroughly immediately before use to ensure uniform dispersal and equal numbers of beads added per test sample.
11. The beads may visibly slide down back of tube and could easily be aspirated (and any bound *M. bovis* lost) when initial removal of sample takes place, so care must be exercised at this point. However, as washing steps proceed, the beads will be observed to be more tightly held by the magnet.
12. A published touchdown PCR specific for *M. tuberculosis* complex [11] was employed by Stewart et al. [10]. However, any *M. bovis*-specific PCR method, such as Taylor et al. [12], could potentially substitute the touchdown PCR described here.
13. A PCR SuperMix was used because, when so many samples were being processed, we found it easier and quicker than pipetting out each component of the PCR reaction.
14. Volume of buffer to resuspend beads in will be dictated by whether only a MGIT tube is being inoculated or a MGIT

tube plus two slopes of a solid culture medium. Remember, only if you resuspend beads in a smaller volume after IMS will concentration of the *M. bovis* cells from the original sample be achieved (e.g., 1 ml of sample volume subjected to IMS and beads resuspended in 100 μl of buffer or broth = 10× concentration of *M. bovis* numbers).

15. Stewart et al. study [10] demonstrated that if only ZN staining is relied upon to confirm presence of *M. bovis* in MGIT cultures, then some samples containing low numbers of viable *M. bovis* will be missed (false-negative culture result). Hence, we advocate that all MGIT cultures should undergo final PCR check before disposal. There was also some suspicion that the presence of the beads may have interfered with the MGIT™ 960 detection system, although this is not proven currently.

Acknowledgement

This work was supported by a grant from the UK Department of Environment, Food and Rural Affairs (Project SE3262).

References

1. Office International des Epizooties (2011) Chapter 2.4.7. Bovine tuberculosis. Manual of diagnostic tests and vaccines for terrestrial animals 2009. https://www.oie.int/fileadmin/Home/eng/Health_standards/tahm/2.04.07_BOVINE_TB.pdf. Accessed 15 Aug 2013
2. Corner LA, Trajstman AC, Lund K (1995) Determination of the optimum concentration of decontaminants for the primary isolation of *Mycobacterium bovis*. N Z Vet J 43:129–133
3. de la Rua-Domenech R, Goodchild T, Vordermeier M et al (2006) Ante mortem diagnosis of Bovine Tuberculosis: the significance of unconfirmed test reactors. Gov Vet J 16:65–71
4. Stevens KA, Jaykus LA (2004) Bacterial separation and concentration from complex sample matrices: a review. Crit Rev Microbiol 30:7–24
5. Benoit PW, Donahue DW (2003) Methods for rapid separation and concentration of bacteria in food that bypass time-consuming cultural enrichment. J Food Prot 66:1935–1948
6. Sweeney FP, Courtenay O, Ul-Hassan A et al (2006) Immunomagnetic recovery of *Mycobacterium bovis* from naturally infected environmental samples. Lett Appl Microbiol 2:460–462
7. Sweeney FP, Courtenay O, Hibberd V et al (2007) Environmental monitoring of *Mycobacterium bovis* in badger feces and badger sett soil by real-time PCR, as confirmed by immunofluorescence, immunocapture, and cultivation. Appl Environ Microbiol 73:7471–7473
8. Garbaccio SG, Cataldi AA (2010) Evaluation of an immunomagnetic capture method followed by PCR to detect *Mycobacterium bovis* in tissue samples from cattle. Rev Argent Microbiol 42:247–253
9. Stewart LD, McNair J, McCallan L et al (2012) Production and evaluation of antibodies and phage-display derived peptide ligands for immunomagnetic separation of *Mycobacterium bovis*. J Clin Microbiol 50:1598–1605
10. Stewart LD, McNair J, McCallan L et al (2013) Improved detection of *Mycobacterium bovis* infection in bovine lymph node tissue using immunomagnetic separation (IMS)-based methods. PLoS One 8:e58374
11. Zumárraga MJ, Meikle V, Bernardelli A et al (2005) Use of touch-down polymerase chain reaction to enhance the sensitivity of *Mycobacterium bovis* detection. J Vet Diagn Invest 17:232–238
12. Taylor GM, Worth DR, Palmer S et al (2007) Rapid detection of *Mycobacterium bovis* DNA in cattle lymph nodes with visible lesions using PCR. BMC Vet Res 3:12

Chapter 12

Detection of Fish Pathogens by Loop-Mediated Isothermal Amplification (LAMP) Technique

Hatem Soliman, Mona Saleh, and Mansour El-Matbouli

Abstract

Rapid detection of fish pathogens is mandatory for applying the crucial preventive and control measures to reduce fish losses and, consequently, minimize the economic impact of diseases on the fish farm owners. The currently used molecular diagnostic tools of fish infectious agents, such as PCR and RT-PCR, are sensitive and specific but still have some drawbacks. These tools are usually time consuming and laborious, need skilled persons, and require sophisticated devices to be performed. Therefore, next-generation tools for rapid diagnosis of fish infectious diseases were developed to conquer these shortages. One of these novel tools is the loop-mediated isothermal amplification (LAMP) technique. LAMP is considered a more advantageous tool than PCR because it needs only a heating block or a thermostatically controlled water bath as a source of constant temperature. It is considered to be more specific than the PCR assay as it uses 4–6 primers, which may diminish the occurrence of false-positive results. The time required for the amplification process by LAMP is ranging from 30 min to 1 h comparing to 3–5 h in the case of PCR. The visual detection methods coupled with the LAMP assay eliminates the post-run processing for detection of the amplification products. Its sensitivity is either comparable with the PCR or better than it. A variety of LAMP assays were developed for simple and rapid detection of a diversity of fish pathogens. Herein, we describe how to perform a LAMP assay and troubleshoot any potential problem arising during the process.

Key words Diagnosis of fish infectious diseases, *Bst* polymerase enzyme, Visual detection, Lateral flow strips, Loop primers, SYBR Green I stain, Fluorescent detection reagent (FDR), FITC-labeled DNA probe, Biotin-labeled primer

1 Introduction

In the past centuries, diagnosis of fish infectious diseases was conventional and based on clinical signs, postmortem examination, and isolation of the etiological agents, followed by phenotypic and serological confirmation or histopathological investigations [1, 2]. However, these techniques have some drawbacks, such as lack of specificity and inadequate sensitivity to detect pathogens present in low numbers or in the absence of the disease clinical signs [3]. Therefore, a new generation of diagnostic techniques was in

Mónica V. Cunha and João Inácio (eds.), *Veterinary Infection Biology: Molecular Diagnostics and High-Throughput Strategies*, Methods in Molecular Biology, vol. 1247, DOI 10.1007/978-1-4939-2004-4_12, © Springer Science+Business Media New York 2015

request. By discovery of nucleic acid amplification technologies, diagnosis of infectious diseases became more specific, rapid, and sensitive [4]. These techniques, as leading methods in detecting small quantities of nucleic acids, improved the detection of various kinds of pathogens [5]. Molecular research has demonstrated not only the ability to identify pathogenic species but also to identify particularly virulent strains [6]. The most extensively used tool for nucleic acid amplification of infectious agents is the polymerase chain reaction (PCR) [7]. However, PCR-based methods have some drawbacks, such as the need of thermal cycling sophisticated instruments for the amplification process, they are relatively time consuming, and usually request complicated post-run analysis for the detection of the amplified products [8]. A next-generation nucleic acids amplification technique was recently developed to overcome the PCR disadvantages and to offer an isothermal assay for the detection of infectious agents [9]. Loop-mediated isothermal amplification (LAMP) was developed as a simple, rapid technique for efficient amplification of nucleic acids using a heating block or a thermostatically controlled water bath, to provide a constant temperature, with high specificity and sensitivity [10]. LAMP is based on auto-cycling strand displacement activity of the *Bst* DNA polymerase large fragment for DNA synthesis [10, 11]. The assay is carried out at a constant temperature between 60 and 65 °C, usually within 1 h. Four specially constructed primers are necessary to perform LAMP assays [10]. The use of these primers improves the specificity of the assay as it recognizes six distinct regions on the target DNA [10]. By the use of one or two additional primers (loop primers), not only the duration of the assay will be reduced but also the specificity of the assay will be increased; as in this case the six primer sets will recognize eight different sequences on the target DNA, which may aid in the elimination of any false-positive results [12]. A valuable advantage of LAMP is the possibility of amplification of RNA templates through reverse-transcription loop-mediated isothermal amplification (RT-LAMP). In addition to the LAMP reagent mixture, a reverse transcriptase enzyme will be used under the same temperature and within the same time range [13]. The sensitivity of the LAMP assay is either comparable to that of PCR or sometimes is superior to it [14]. More recently, LAMP technology has been developed into commercial kits for detection of a variety of pathogens [15]. Detection of infectious agents with LAMP comprises three steps: sample preparation, amplification and detection of the amplified products. While the amplification step is already optimized to be carried out in 30 min to 1 h, still the sample preparation and detection steps may be time consuming. We tried to simplify the sample preparation step and reduce its processing time by using immunocapture and direct binding approaches to replace the DNA extraction procedures [16]. These new techniques reduced not only the processing time to 15–30 min but also the cost of the sample preparation step as there is no need for nucleic acid extraction kits. LAMP yields a large amount of DNA and a pyrophosphate by-product, which enabled the development of simple visual detection methods of the amplicons without costly specialized equipments [17]. In addition to SYBR Green I, fluorescent detection reagent, and cationic polymers, nucleic acid lateral flow assays have been used for the visual detection of the LAMP products [14, 18]. LAMP and RT-LAMP have thus been used successfully for the detection of a variety of fish pathogens. Herein, we describe how can LAMP and RT-LAMP assays be performed correctly in order to help the veterinarians to reach a rapid and accurate field diagnosis with reduced costs.

2 Materials

2.1 Primers

1. LAMP uses a mixture of 4–6 primers, depending on the use of one or two additional loop primers (*see* **Note 1**). The primer designations are usually outer forward primer (F3), outer backward primer (B3), forward inner primer (FIP), backward inner primer (BIP), forward loop primer (FLP), and backward loop primer (BLP). *See* Table 1 for examples of LAMP primer sets that we have recently described for the detection of viral hemorrhagic septicemia virus (VHS), of infectious pancreatic necrosis virus (IPNV), and of Cyprinid herpesvirus-3 (CyHV-3).
2. Primers stock solutions: primers are ordered and come from the synthesis company with a specification sheet that usually contains all the information required to rehydrate the primers. For each of the LAMP primers, add the recommended amount of PCR-grade water and mix it well to get a primer stock solution of 100 pmol/μl. Prepare several aliquots from these stocks to avoid degradation by repeated freezing and thawing, and keep it at −20 °C until used.
3. Primers working solutions: the working concentrations of LAMP primers solutions may be as following—10 pmol/μl of F3 and B3; 80 pmol/μl of FIP and BIP; and 40 pmol/μl of FLP and BLP. Prepare 100 μl of each LAMP primer working solution as indicated below.

   Primers F3 and B3: mix 10 μl from the correspondent 100 pmol/μl primer stock solution with 90 μl of PCR-grade water.

   Primers FIP and BIP: mix 80 μl from the correspondent 100 pmol/μl primer stock solution with 20 μl of PCR-grade water.

   Primers FLP and BLP: mix 40 μl from the correspondent 100 pmol/μl primer stock solution with 60 μl of PCR-grade water.

Table 1

Sequences of LAMP primers targeting relevant viral fish pathogens

Target virus	Primer sequences (5′–3′)	References
VHS[a]	*F3*—GGS AAG CAA GGA YCA CGA G	[13]
	B3—CAG GTG TCC YTC TAG TGT TTC	
	FIP—GAT CCA CCG ATA CTG TTT TTG GGG TTT TCC CGT TCT TCC CTG AAC CC	
	BIP—ARG GGG TYT GCA CAR CCT CGC TTT TCG ACK YGG GRC AAK GGG C	
	FLP—GTT ATG TCC TTA TGG ACA TTG	
	BLP—GTC AAA CTC ATT GGC AGG G	
IPNV[b]	*F3*—CCA ATC TGC GGT GTA GAC AT	[14]
	B3—CAT CAG CTC TCC CAG GTA CT	
	FIP—CCT CCT CGT CCA CTC CTG GTT TTT CCA TCG CAG CCC ATG AAC	
	BIP—TGC GAA ACA CAT CCC TGG CCT TTT TCT TGT TGG AGC CCT TTG C	
	FLP—CGA TGA GTG GCA GCC CTT	
	BLP—GAT CCA GAC CGG AAC CCT G	
CyHV-3[c]	*F3*—TGC AGC AGC CCT TCA AG	[16, 18]
	B3—GAC ACA CCG CCT GGT AAG	
	FIP—TGC ACA CCG CCG TCA GCT CAG GTG ACG GCG TTG GT	
	BIP—GAA GTG CAA GAT GCG CGA CGA CTC GGC GCC TCC AA	
	FLP—GTC CAG CTT GTC CGC CAT G	
	BLP—CAC CCT TCA CCG TCA GAA TCT C	

[a]Viral hemorrhagic septicemia virus
[b]Infectious pancreatic necrosis virus
[c]Cyprinid herpesvirus-3

Primer mix: prepare the primer mix by thorough mixing of equal volumes from each LAMP primer working solution in a new microcentrifuge tube, and keep it at −20 °C until used (*see* **Note 2**).

2.2 Reagents and Other Materials for LAMP Reactions and Direct Product Detection

1. 10× LAMP reaction buffer: 20 mM Tris–HCl, pH 8.8, 10 mM KCl, 1.5 mM $MgSO_4$, 10 mM $(NH_4)_2SO_4$, 0.1 % Triton X-100 (e.g., 10× Thermopol® reaction buffer, New England BioLabs, GmbH, Frankfurt, Germany).
2. 5 M betaine solution.

3. 100 mM dNTPs mix solution.
4. 25 mM $MgSO_4$ (*see* **Note 3**).
5. *Bst* DNA polymerase, large fragment (New England BioLabs, GmbH, Frankfurt, Germany).
6. PCR-grade water.
7. Enhanced Avian Myeloblastosis Reverse Transcriptase (eAMV) (Sigma–Aldrich, GmbH, Schnelldorf, Germany).
8. SYBR Green I nucleic acid stain, 10,000× concentrate in DMSO. To prepare the working dilution (1:10 in DMSO), mix 1 μl of SYBR Green I nucleic acid stain 10,000× concentrate with 9 μl DMSO, and then make aliquots of 1 μl each and keep it at −20 °C until used.
9. Fluorescent detection reagent (FDR) (Eiken Chemical Co. Ltd., Japan).

2.3 Detection of LAMP Products Using Lateral Flow Strips

1. Lateral flow strips for nucleic acid detection (Milenia GenLine HybriDetect, Milenia Biotec GmbH, Bad Nauheim, Germany). It contains dipsticks and assay buffer.
2. 5′ end biotin-labeled FIP primer (prepared as in Subheading 2.1).
3. 5′ end FITC-labeled DNA probe (*see* **Note 4**).

3 Methods

LAMP reaction mixtures should be prepared on ice. After thawing, LAMP reagents and primers should be thoroughly mixed by vortexing and then spin-down and kept on ice until used. Carefully follow all waste disposal regulations when disposing waste materials.

3.1 Amplification of DNA Templates by LAMP

1. LAMP reactions are usually carried out in a total volume of 25 μl.
2. Prepare the master mix, which consists of all the reagents needed for one sample multiplied by the number of samples to test plus the positive and no-template controls and one additional sample to overcome eventual pipetting errors.
3. The reagents needed for one LAMP reaction are 2.5 μl of 10× reaction buffer, 8 μl of 5 M betaine solution, 0.7 μl of 100 mM dNTPs solution (*see* **Note 5**), 3 μl of primer mix (*see* **Note 6**), 2 μl of 25 mM $MgSO_4$ solution (*see* **Note 3**), 1 μl (8 units) of *Bst* DNA polymerase, and 5.8 μl PCR-grade water to complete the volume to 23 μl.
4. After mixing the reagents of the master mix, dispense 23 μl in each tube labeled with the sample number.

5. Add 2 μl of sample DNA to each tube (*see* **Note 7**). In the positive control tube, add 2 μl of the relevant DNA solution, while in the no-template control, add 2 μl of PCR-grade water.
6. Incubate the reaction tubes in a water bath or heating block at 65 °C for 1 h.
7. After incubation, inactivate the enzyme at 85 °C for 3 min and proceed to the products detection methods.

3.2 Amplification of RNA Template by RT-LAMP

1. Perform as described previously for the amplification of DNA templates (in Subheading 3.1) with the following modifications: the reaction mixture will contain 2.5 μl of 10× reaction buffer, 8 μl of 5 M betaine solution, 0.7 μl of 100 mM dNTPs solution (*see* **Note 5**), 3 μl of primer mix (*see* **Note 6**), 2 μl of 25 mM $MgSO_4$ solution (*see* **Note 3**), 1 μl (20 units) of eAMV reverse transcriptase (*see* **Note 8**), 1 μl (8 units) of *Bst* DNA polymerase, and 4.8 μl PCR-grade water to complete the volume to 23 μl.
2. After dispensing 23 μl of the master mix in each tube, add 2 μl of sample RNA (*see* **Note 7**). In the positive control tube, add 2 μl of the relevant RNA solution, while in the no-template control, add 2 μl of PCR-grade water.

3.3 Detection of LAMP Products

Visual inspection is the simplest and fastest method for detection of the LAMP products. Herein, we describe the close-to-field methods that may be used for this purpose.

3.3.1 Using SYBR Green I Nucleic Acid Stain

1. After termination of the LAMP reaction, spin-down the reaction tubes (*see* **Note 9**).
2. Add 1 μl of 1:10 diluted SYBR Green I stain to each reaction tube, mix by pipetting, and observe the results.
3. The reaction mixture will turn green in the presence of LAMP products while it will remain orange in their absence (Fig. 1).
4. The positive control must be green in color and the no-template control must be orange.

3.3.2 Using Fluorescent Detection Reagent (FDR)

1. During the preparation of the master mix, add 1 μl of FDR to the reaction mixture and reduce the amount of the PCR-grade water to 4.8 μl in the case of DNA amplification or 3.8 μl in the case of RNA amplification.
2. After completion of the LAMP reaction, expose the reaction tubes to the UV illumination (wavelength of 254 nm).
3. Samples containing LAMP products will yield a green fluorescence while negative samples will not yield any green fluorescence (Fig. 2).
4. The positive control must yield a green fluorescence and the no-template control will not produce any green fluorescence.

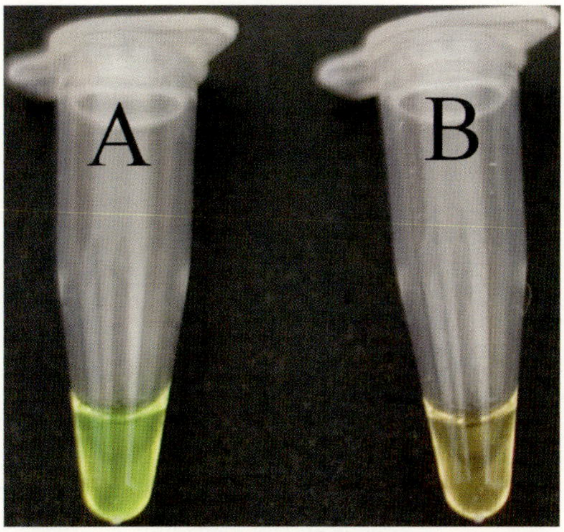

Fig. 1 Visual detection of LAMP products using SYBR Green I nucleic acid stain. In tube A, the color of the reaction mixture changed to *green*, indicating the presence of the LAMP product (*positive reaction*). In tube B, the color of the reaction mixture remained *orange*, indicating the absence of LAMP products (*negative reaction*)

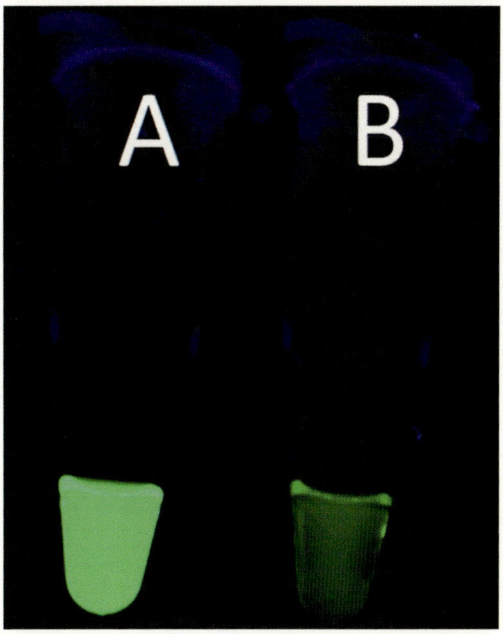

Fig. 2 Visual detection of LAMP products using fluorescent detection reagent (FDR). In tube A, the reaction mixture is emitting a green fluorescence under UV light (wavelength of 254 nm) indicating the presence of LAMP products (*positive reaction*). In tube B, the reaction mixture is not emitting green fluorescence, indicating absence of the LAMP products (*negative reaction*)

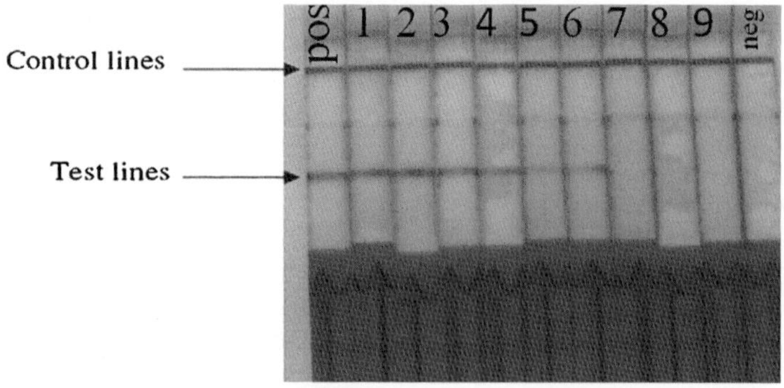

Fig. 3 Detection of LAMP products using nucleic acid lateral flow strips. The strip labeled as "pos" is the positive control showing two *purple bands* (*positive reaction*). Strips 1–6 correspond to positive samples, demonstrating two *purple bands* at both the control and test lines. Strips 7–9 correspond to negative samples showing only one *purple band* on the control line. Strip labeled as "neg" is the no-template control (Color figure online)

3.3.3 Using Lateral Flow Dipsticks

1. Replace the unlabeled FIP primer with the biotin-labeled FIP version in the preparation of the primer mix.
2. After finishing of the LAMP reaction, add 10 pmoles of the FITC-labeled DNA probe to the LAMP products (*see* **Note 10**), denature at 95 °C for 1 min, and then incubate at 60 °C for 5 min (*see* **Note 11**).
3. Mix 8 μl of the hybridized products with 150 μl of the assay buffer in a new tube, dip the lateral flow strip into the mixture, and observe the result.
4. Samples that produce two purple bands in the strip (*see* **Note 12**) are considered to be positive, meaning that specific LAMP products were amplified, while negative samples produce only one purple band, correspondent to the control line (Fig. 3).
5. The positive control must also produce two purple bands while the no-template control must produce one band.

4 Notes

1. Usually, four primers (F3, B3, FIP, and BIP) must be used to perform the LAMP assay. No LAMP products will be produced in the absence of these primers. One or two additional loop primers (FLP and BLP) may be used, depending on the target sequence used to construct the primers. Sometimes the target sequence does not enable the design of any loop primer or will enable the design of one (forward or reverse) or two loop primers. These primers, if present, will usually accelerate

the amplification process and increase its specificity. LAMP primers may be designed from target sequences using the software program (PrimerExplorer V4, Net Laboratory, Tokyo, Japan) from Eiken Chemical (https://primerexplorer.jp/e/). The program generates a huge number of primer sets (may reach 1,000 primer sets). Generated primer sets should be selected avoiding the potential formation of primer dimers and according to the stability of the primers ends which should be below –4 kcal/mol.

2. The preparation of a primer mix containing all of the 4–6 LAMP primers in only one solution will reduce pipetting procedures and potential errors and will make the preparation of the master mix easier.

3. $MgSO_4$ concentration is a key factor in the LAMP assay and must be optimized for each primer set. If the amount of $MgSO_4$ is not optimized in the reaction mixture, no LAMP products will be produced. As stated in the composition of the ThermoPol® reaction buffer, it contains already 1.5 mM of $MgSO_4$. To adjust the final $MgSO_4$ concentration in the reaction mixture, we know that the addition of 1 μl of the 25 mM $MgSO_4$ will increase its concentration by 1 mM, when the end volume of the reaction mixture is 25 μl. For example, for a final $MgSO_4$ concentration of 4.5 mM, we will have to add 3 μl of the 25 mM $MgSO_4$ solution to the reaction mixture.

4. One of the loop primers (FLP or BLP), if present, can be used as a probe, after labeling it with FITC at the correspondent 5′ end. In this case, the selected loop primer (unlabeled) should be omitted from the LAMP reaction mixture. This means that for a LAMP reaction if we have 6 primers (F3, B3, FIP, BIP, FLP, and BLP) and we select the FLP primer to be labeled at its 5′ end and used it as a probe so, the primer mix will be performed using the rest 5 primers only (F3, B3, FIP, BIP, and BLP).

5. The concentration of the dNTPs in the reaction mixture is much higher than in standard PCR reactions and may need to be optimized for each LAMP assay.

6. The amount of primer mix will depend on the number of primers included in the mix (*see* **Note 1**). If it contains 6 primers (when including both loop primers), 3 μl will be added to the reaction mixture; if it contains 5 primers (with only one loop primer), 2.5 μl will be added; finally, if it contains 4 primers (without loop primers), only 2 μl of the primer mix will be added to the reaction mixture. The amount of added PCR-grade water must be adjusted accordingly. Primers concentrations in the reaction mixture will be 0.2 μM of F3 and B3, 1.6 μM of FIP and BIP, and, if present, 0.8 μM of FLP and/or

BLP. The primer concentrations in the reaction mixture may need to be optimized for different primer sets. It is found that increasing the concentration of the FIP and BIP, and of the loop primers if present, may improve the sensitivity of the LAMP assays. However, increasing the concentrations of the F3 and B3 primers should have no effect on the sensitivity since these outer primers are only used for initiating the amplification reaction.

7. The full description of viral nucleic acid extraction procedures from biological fish samples is out of the scope of this chapter but several "in-house" and commercial approaches are available and widely described in the literature. Please also refer to our previous published work for examples of RNA and DNA extraction procedures from clinical fish samples [13, 14, 16, 18].
8. eAMV reverse transcriptase is preferable as it works under high temperatures (up to 65 °C), which is the same temperature of the LAMP reaction.
9. This procedure is needed to remove any droplets from the inner side of the lid, to prevent any contamination when opening the tubes.
10. The amount of added FITC-labeled DNA probe will have to be optimized for each LAMP reaction [18]. When setting up a new assay, the optimum amount of the probe can be determined by testing different concentrations. The hybridization of the probe with the amplification products may also be optimized under different temperatures and incubation times. The probe concentration that yields the highest intensity of the purple color band on the lateral flow strip, at the selected incubation temperature and time, will be chosen as the optimum concentration.
11. This incubation is for the hybridization between the probe and the complementary LAMP products.
12. This type of strips contains two marked lines (control and test lines). The control line (on top of the strip) should always yield a purple color, since it confirms that the capillary lateral flow of the products was correctly performed and that the strips are not expired. The test line will yield a purple color only in the presence of specific LAMP products. If the strip develops only a purple band in the test line, but without the correspondent control band, nonspecific reactions may have occurred and the assay did not performed correctly.

References

1. Bernardet JF, Campbell AC, Buswell JA (1990) *Flexibacter maritimus* is the agent of 'black patch necrosis' in Dover sole in Scotland. Dis Aquat Org 8:233–237
2. Pazos F, Santos Y, Macías AR et al (1996) Evaluation of media for the successful culture of *Flexibacter maritimus.* J Fish Dis 19: 193–197
3. Ambrosia RE, De Wall DT (1990) Diagnosis of parasitic disease. Rev Sci Tech 9:759–778
4. Craw P, Balachandran W (2012) Isothermal nucleic acid amplification technologies for point-of-care diagnostics: a critical review. Lab Chip 12:2469–2486
5. Gill P, Ghaemi A (2008) Nucleic acid isothermal amplification technologies: a review. Nucleosides Nucleotides Nucleic Acids 27:224–243
6. Cunningham CO (2002) Molecular diagnosis of fish and shellfish diseases: present status and potential use in disease control. Aquaculture 206:19–55
7. Walker P, Subasinghe R (2000) DNA-based molecular diagnostic techniques: research needs for standardization and validation of the detection of aquatic animal pathogens and diseases. In: Report and proceedings of the joint FAO/NACA/CSIRO/ACIAR/DFID expert workshop, Bangkok, Thailand, 7–9 February 1999. FAO fisheries technical paper, no. 395. FAO, Rome, pp 93
8. Parida M, Sannarangaiah S, Dash PK et al (2008) Loop mediated isothermal amplification (LAMP): a new generation of innovative gene amplification technique; perspectives in clinical diagnosis of infectious diseases. Rev Med Virol 18:407–421
9. Tomita N, Mori Y, Kanda H et al (2008) Loop-mediated isothermal amplification (LAMP) of gene sequences and simple visual detection of products. Nat Protoc 3:877–882
10. Notomi T, Okayama H, Masubuchi H et al (2000) Loop mediated isothermal amplification of DNA. Nucleic Acids Res 28:e63
11. Nagamine K, Watanabe K, Ohtsuka K et al (2001) Loop-mediated isothermal amplification reaction using a nondenatured template. Clin Chem 47:1742–1743
12. Nagamine K, Hase T, Notomi T (2002) Accelerated reaction by loop mediated isothermal amplification using loop primers. Mol Cell Probes 16:223–229
13. Soliman H, El-Matbouli M (2006) Reverse transcription loop-mediated isothermal amplification (RT-LAMP) for rapid detection of viral hemorrhagic septicaemia virus (VHS). Vet Microbiol 114:205–213
14. Soliman H, Midtlyng P, El-Matbouli M (2009) Sensitive and rapid detection of infectious pancreatic necrosis virus by reverse transcription loop mediated isothermal amplification. J Virol Methods 158:77–83
15. Mori Y, Notomi T (2009) Loop-mediated isothermal amplification (LAMP): a rapid, accurate, and cost-effective diagnostic method for infectious diseases. J Infect Chemother 15:62–69
16. Soliman H, El-Matbouli M (2009) Immunocapture and direct binding loop mediated isothermal amplification simplify molecular diagnosis of Cyprinid herpesvirus-3. J Virol Methods 162:91–95
17. Mori Y, Nagamine K, Tomita N et al (2001) Detection of loop-mediated isothermal amplification reaction by turbidity derived from magnesium pyrophosphate formation. Biochem Biophys Res Commun 289:150–154
18. Soliman H, El-Matbouli M (2010) Loop mediated isothermal amplification combined with nucleic acid lateral flow strip for diagnosis of cyprinid herpes virus-3. Mol Cell Probes 24:38–43

Chapter 13

Direct Detection of *Theileria annulata* in Bovine Blood Samples Using Standard and Isothermal DNA Amplification Approaches

Jacinto Gomes and João Inácio

Abstract

Tropical theileriosis is a tick-borne disease responsible for important health problems in cattle, caused by the hemoprotozoan *Theileria annulata*. Traditionally, detection of *Theileria* pathogens in infected animals requires the microscopic examination of stained-blood smears and serological methods. Molecular diagnostic assays have been developed for the detection of *Theileria* parasites, including PCR-based and reverse line blotting approaches, but these methods usually demand qualified personnel, complex instrumentation, and expensive materials. Loop-mediated isothermal amplification (LAMP) can facilitate the design of molecular assays independent of the use of sophisticated equipment. In this chapter we describe the application of two molecular assays for the direct detection of *T. annulata* in bovine blood samples, based in real-time PCR and LAMP, both targeting the *Tams1*-encoding gene of this parasite.

Key words *Theileria annulata*, Theileriosis, Molecular diagnostics, Real-time PCR, Loop-mediated isothermal amplification

1 Introduction

Tropical theileriosis is a tick-borne hemoprotozoan disease responsible for important health problems in cattle (*Bos taurus* and *Bos indicus*) and in Asian buffalo (*Bubalus bubalis*). The etiological agent is the apicomplexan parasite *Theileria annulata*, which occurs around the Mediterranean basin, Middle East, and Southern Asia [1–3]. The animals that survive the acute disease become carriers of *T. annulata* piroplasms and play an important role as a reservoir for the maintenance of the parasite life cycle [4]. Traditionally, detection of *Theileria* pathogens in infected animals requires the microscopic examination of stained-blood smears, which has low sensitivity and specificity. Serological methods are also available, but cross-reactions are common, current infections and previous exposures are not generally distinguished, and antibodies tend to disappear in long-term animal carriers [2, 5].

Mónica V. Cunha and João Inácio (eds.), *Veterinary Infection Biology: Molecular Diagnostics and High-Throughput Strategies*, Methods in Molecular Biology, vol. 1247, DOI 10.1007/978-1-4939-2004-4_13,

Molecular diagnostic assays have been developed for the detection of *Theileria* parasites, including PCR-based and reverse line blotting approaches [1, 4, 6–9]. However, these molecular assays usually demand qualified personnel, complex instrumentation, and expensive materials. For an effective and wider use in the routine diagnosis of animal diseases, especially in low-resource settings, these technologies should be simpler, standardized, affordable, field deployable, and disposable. Isothermal DNA amplification processes, such as loop-mediated isothermal amplification (LAMP) [10], could facilitate the integration of DNA-based methodologies into bench molecular diagnostics kits independent of the utilization of sophisticated equipments. LAMP relies upon an autocycling strand displacement DNA synthesis and is more tolerant to the presence of inhibitory substances such as blood, serum, plasma, or heparin [10]. The reaction runs very rapidly in the presence of template DNA and deoxynucleoside triphosphates, usually in less than 90 min at a constant temperature (e.g., 60–65 °C). LAMP provides high amplification efficiency and shows a detection limit and specificity comparable to those of standard PCR. The high potential of LAMP for the development of improved molecular diagnostic assays fully justifies the increasing number of reports on its application, including for the detection of *Theileria* parasites [11–15], namely, of *T. annulata* [16, 17].

In this chapter we describe the use of two molecular assays for the direct detection of *T. annulata* in bovine blood samples, based in standard real-time PCR and LAMP, both targeting the *Tams1*-encoding gene of this parasite.

2 Materials

1. Genomic DNA extracted from bovine blood samples to test (*see* **Note 1**).
2. Positive control of amplification: DNA extracted from a *T. annulata* positive sample (*see* **Note 2**).
3. PCR specific primers for *T. annulata* targeting the *Tams1*-encoding gene: Tams1_forw (5′-CAA ATT CGA GAC CTA CTA CGA TG-3′) and Tams1_rev (5′-CCA CTT RTC GTC CTT AAG CTC G-3′) (*see* **Notes 3–5**) [9].
4. LAMP specific primers for *T. annulata* targeting the *Tams1*-encoding gene: Tams1_F3 (5′-CCG TTA ATG CTG CAA ATG AGG-3′), Tams1_B3 (5′-CCA CTT ATC GTC CTT AAG CTC G-3′), Tams1_FIP (5′-GCT TAA GTT TGA ATG CCT KTA CTG GCC CTT AAG GTC GGA GAC AAG-3′), and Tams1_BIP (5′-GAT GTT CAA GAA GAA GGG AGA CAA GCC CTT GAA CAA GAC WTC ATC G-3′) (*see* **Notes 3**, **6**, and **7**) (Fig. 1).

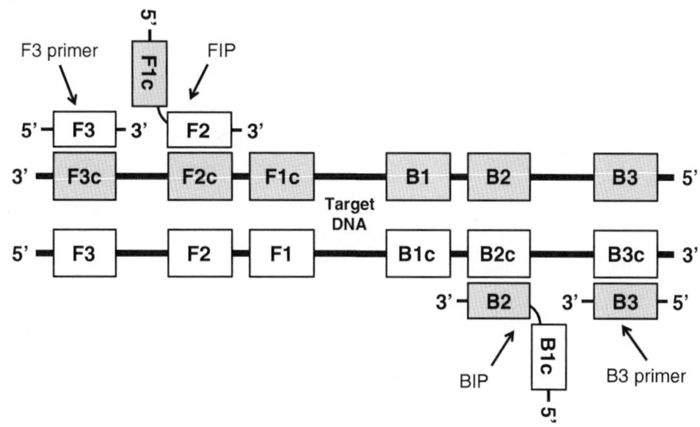

Fig. 1 Generic location of the six segments in the target DNA used to design LAMP primers. Forward (F3) and backward (B3) outer primers and forward (FIP) and backward (BIP) inner primers are indicated. The specially designed FIP and BIP primers contain two distinct sequences (F1c plus F2 and B1c plus B2, respectively) corresponding to sense and antisense segments of the target DNA, one for priming in the first stage and the other for self-priming in a subsequent amplification reaction stage

5. Reagents for performing real-time PCR amplifications (e.g., SsoFast™ Evagreen® Supermix, Bio-Rad, CA, USA).
6. Reagents for performing LAMP: *Bst* DNA polymerase large fragment and respective 10× reaction buffer (New England Biolabs), 25 mM of $MgCl_2$, 20 mM of dNTPs, and 5 M of betaine.
7. Reagents for performing gel electrophoresis: agarose, ethidium bromide, and 1× TBE buffer.
8. Standard and real-time PCR equipments (e.g., CFX96™ Real-Time PCR Detection System, Bio-Rad, CA, USA).
9. Standard equipment for performing agarose gel electrophoresis and the respective detection of the products under UV light.

3 Methods

3.1 Detection of *T. annulata* with Real-Time PCR

1. Each amplification reaction is prepared for a final volume of 20 μl, including the addition of 5 μl of template DNA sample.
2. Prepare a reaction mixture for all the DNA samples to test, including the positive and negative (water) amplification controls, containing 1× SsoFast™ Evagreen® Supermix, 0.3 μM of Tams1_forw primer and 0.15 μM of Tams1_rev primer, completing to 75 % of the final volume with PCR-grade water.

3. Distribute 15 μl of the reaction mixture by individual 0.2 ml microtubes.
4. Label each tube and add 5 μl of the correspondent DNA sample and controls.
5. Proceed to the amplification step using the following program: (1) one initial denaturing step for 2 min at 95 °C and (2) 45 cycles of denaturation for 15 s at 95 °C, annealing for 30 s at 55 °C and extension for 30 s at 72 °C (*see* **Note 8**). The increase of fluorescence and amplification curves for each sample should be recorded and assessed according to the instructions of the manufacturer of the real-time PCR instrument. Only samples containing *T. annulata* DNA should yield positive amplification results.
6. After the amplification step, an additional control step for the determination of the melting curve of the amplified fragments can be performed (if the real-time PCR instrument used has that feature). For this, at the end of the amplification program, add an additional step consisting of a 1 °C temperature increase every 5 s (beginning at 55 °C and ending at 95 °C) (*see* **Note 9**).

3.2 Detection of *T. annulata* with LAMP

1. Each isothermal amplification reaction is prepared for a final volume of 15 μl, including the addition of 5 μl of template DNA sample.
2. Prepare a reaction mixture for all the DNA samples to test, including the positive and negative (water) amplification controls, containing 4.8 U of the *Bst* DNA polymerase large fragment and 1× of the respective hybridization buffer, 6 mM of $MgCl_2$, 1,400 μM of each dNTP, 0.8 M of betaine, 1.6 μM of each Tams1_FIP and Tams1_BIP primers, and 0.2 μM of each Tams1_F3 and Tams1_B3 primers, completing to 66.7 % of the final volume with PCR-grade water (*see* **Note 10**).
3. Distribute 10 μl of the reaction mixture by individual 0.2 ml microtubes.
4. Label each tube and add 5 μl of the correspondent DNA sample and controls (*see* **Note 11**).
5. Proceed to the amplification step by incubating the tubes at 63 °C during 90 min (*see* **Note 12**).
6. Finalize the amplification step with an incubation at 80 °C during 2 min, to inactivate the enzyme.
7. Confirm the occurrence of positive amplification results by analyzing the products in a 1.5 % (w/v) agarose gel electrophoresis (in 1× TBE buffer, at 90 V for 90 min; with ethidium bromide staining) and visualization under UV light, using standardized protocols (*see* **Notes 13–16**) (Fig. 2).

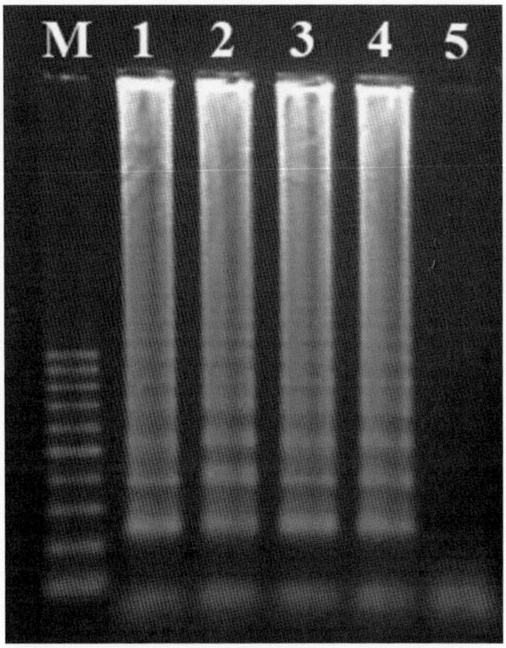

Fig. 2 Characteristic ladderlike appearance of LAMP products in an agarose gel electrophoresis. Lanes 1–4 correspond to positive amplification results and lane 5 corresponds to the non-template negative control. M—log scale 100 bp DNA Ladder (Jena Bioscience)

4 Notes

1. Blood samples may be collected from animals into sterile tubes with EDTA and the total genomic DNA extracted using commercially available kits or automated systems (e.g., we use a BioSprint®96 automated workstation and the BioSprint®96 Blood kit, Qiagen) [9]. The average total DNA yield in samples is around 35–40 ng/μl. Extracted DNA should be stored at −20 °C until further use.
2. As positive controls of amplification, we may use DNA samples extracted from *T. annulata*-infected macrophage cultures or directly from bovine blood samples for which *T. annulata* DNA was detected using other molecular tests such as reverse line blotting [9].
3. Primers are frequently delivered lyophilized and need to be diluted with sterile water according to the manufacturer's instructions. Stock solutions can be prepared at a standard concentration of 100 pmol/μl and stored at −20 °C. Aliquots of working solutions of each primer are prepared from stock solutions in water and stored also at −20 °C. Prepare small aliquots of working solutions (up to 100 μl) and avoid continuous freeze and thaw of the solutions.

4. These primers were designed with complementary targets in conserved segments of the *Tams1* gene, allowing the amplification of a fragment with about 319 bp. Alignments containing tens of *Tams1* gene sequences were analyzed for detecting these conserved nucleotide segments within *T. annulata*, providing also enough nucleotide differences when compared to homologous genes from other closely related species [9]. The homologous genes of the closely related species *T. lestoquardi*, *T. parva*, and *T. taurotragi* all present several mismatches in the complementary target region for both primers, rendering it highly specific for *T. annulata*.
5. *Tams1* is a *T. annulata*-specific gene encoding an immunodominant major merozoite/piroplasm surface antigen of this parasite. This gene is commonly used as genomic target for detecting this parasite [4, 8, 9, 18, 19].
6. LAMP uses a minimum of four primers (two inner primers, FIP and BIP, and two outer primers, F3 and B3) that recognize six distinct regions flanking the amplified DNA target sequence (Fig. 1). An adequate design of these primers is the most important key for the success of the LAMP approach. It may be necessary to design several primer sets before finding one that works efficiently in the LAMP reaction [20, 21]. Some useful tips when designing LAMP primers are as follows: (1) 5′ and 3′ ends of FIP and BIP inner primers should not be adenine and thymine (AT)-rich and the *Tm* for each domain (F1c, F2, B1c, and B2) should be between 55 and 65 °C; (2) the distance between the 5′ end of F2 and the 5′ end of F1 domains should be 40–60 bp (the same for the distance between the 5′ end of B2 and the 5′ end of B1 domains); (3) the distance between the F2 and F3 domains (as well as between the B2 and B3 domains) should be 0–20 bp; and (4) the total length of the amplified DNA segment (from F2 to B2 domains, including both these domains) should be <200 bp. Primers should be designed so as not to easily form secondary structures. Dedicated software for designing LAMP primers is freely available online: PrimerExplorer (http://primerexplorer.jp/e/).
7. The purity of the LAMP primers is important for obtaining reproducible amplification results. The use of HPLC-purified primers is recommended.
8. In order to improve the detection of lower levels of *T. annulata* in blood samples, we use 45 cycles in real-time PCR assays.
9. This step of melting temperature curve analysis allows confirmation that the detection of fluorescence is related to the

amplification of specific DNA targets from *T. annulata* (presenting melting temperatures between 79 °C and 83 °C), and not with the formation of artifacts such as primer dimmers (with melting temperatures around 73 °C). The distinct melting temperatures of *Tams1* gene fragments, amplified from different bovine blood samples, suggest that several *T. annulata* genotypes may be circulating in a region [9].

10. The reagents are stored at −20 °C and the preparation of the reaction mixtures should be conducted on ice. Mix well all reagents by pipetting or tapping with the cap closed, avoiding the formation of bubbles, and then spin down. Avoid violent mixing of the reagents as it may inactivate the *Bst* DNA polymerase.
11. LAMP is possible when using nondenatured DNA templates. Nevertheless, for attaining higher sensitivities, the use of prior denatured DNA template targets is recommended (e.g., by heating at 95 °C for 5 min) [20].
12. For incubation we may use, e.g., a thermoblock or a water bath.
13. To confirm the specificity of the amplified products, the DNA fragments may be digested with the restriction enzyme *Rsa*I, at 37 °C for 1 h, and subject to a 1.5 % (w/v) agarose gel electrophoresis and posterior visualization under UV light, after staining with ethidium bromide, using standardized protocols.
14. We use ethidium bromide to stain the LAMP amplified products when performing gel electrophoresis. We notice the occurrence of migration artifacts during the gel electrophoresis step of these complex mixtures of products when using alternative fluorescent dyes (e.g., SYBR Safe DNA Gel Stain, Life Technologies). Ethidium bromide is a known mutagen and should be handled as a hazardous chemical.
15. The final amplification products present stem-loop DNA structures, encompassing alternate inverted repeats of the target sequence with multiple loops, and appear with a ladderlike pattern in agarose gel electrophoresis (Fig. 2).
16. Due to the very high yield of DNA amplification and to the high sensitivity of LAMP, this method also presents a very high risk for contamination when handling amplified products. Therefore, opening and closing of the reaction tubes should be conducted in a different room from where the reaction mixtures are prepared, and the DNA extraction from samples is performed.

References

1. Gubbels JM, de Vos AP, van der Weide M et al (1999) Simultaneous detection of bovine *Theileria* and *Babesia* species by reverse line blot hybridization. J Clin Microbiol 37:1782–1789
2. García-Sanmartín J, Nagore D, García-Pérez AL, Juste RA, Hurtado A (2006) Molecular diagnosis of *Theileria* and *Babesia* species infecting cattle in Northern Spain using reverse line blot macroarrays. BMC Vet Res 2:16
3. Gomes J, Soares R, Santos M et al (2013) Detection of *Theileria* and *Babesia* infections amongst asymptomatic cattle in Portugal. Tick Tick Borne Dis 4:148–151
4. D'Oliveira C, van der Weide M, Habela MA, Jacquiet P, Jongejan F (1995) Detection of *Theileria annulata* in blood samples of carrier cattle by PCR. J Clin Microbiol 33: 2665–2669
5. Altay K, Aydin MF, Dumanli N, Aktas M (2008) Molecular detection of *Theileria* and *Babesia* infections in cattle. Vet Parasitol 158:295–301
6. Criado-Fornelio A, Buling A, Asenzo G et al (2009) Development of fluorogenic probe-based PCR assays for the detection and quantification of bovine piroplasmids. Vet Parasitol 162:200–206
7. Georges K, Loria GR, Riili S et al (2001) Detection of haemoparasites in cattle by reverse line blot hybridisation with a note on the distribution of ticks in Sicily. Vet Parasitol 99:273–286
8. Bilgic HB, Karagenç T, Shiels B et al (2010) Evaluation of cytochrome b as a sensitive target for PCR based detection of *T. annulata* carrier animals. Vet Parasitol 174:341–347
9. Santos M, Soares R, Costa P et al (2013) Revisiting the *Tams1*-encoding gene as a species-specific target for the molecular detection of *Theileria annulata* in bovine blood samples. Tick Tick Borne Dis 4:72–77
10. Notomi T, Okayama H, Masubuchi H et al (2000) Loop mediated isothermal amplification of DNA. Nucleic Acids Res 28:e63
11. Alhassan A, Thekisoe OM, Yokoyama N et al (2007) Development of loop-mediated isothermal amplification (LAMP) method for diagnosis of equine piroplasmosis. Vet Parasitol 143:155–160
12. Wang LX, He L, Fang R et al (2010) Loop-mediated isothermal amplification (LAMP) assay for detection of *Theileria sergenti* infection targeting the *p33* gene. Vet Parasitol 171:159–162
13. Liu A, Guan G, Du P et al (2013) Rapid identification and differentiation of *Theileria sergenti* and *Theileria sinensis* using a loop-mediated isothermal amplification (LAMP) assay. Vet Parasitol 191:15–22
14. Thekisoe OM, Rambritch NE, Nakao R et al (2010) Loop-mediated isothermal amplification (LAMP) assays for detection of *Theileria parva* infections targeting the PIM and p150 genes. Int J Parasitol 40:55–61
15. Salih DA, Ali AM, Liu Z et al (2012) Development of a loop-mediated isothermal amplification method for detection of *Theileria lestoquardi*. Parasitol Res 110:533–538
16. Liu A, Guan G, Du P et al (2012) Loop-mediated isothermal amplification (LAMP) assays for the detection of *Theileria annulata* infection in China targeting the 18S rRNA and ITS sequences. Exp Parasitol 131:125–129
17. Salih DA, Liu Z, Bakheit MA et al (2008) Development and evaluation of a loop-mediated isothermal amplification method for diagnosis of tropical theileriosis. Transbound Emerg Dis 55:238–243
18. Almeria S, Castellà J, Ferrer D et al (2001) Bovine piroplasms in Minorca (Balearic Islands, Spain): a comparison of PCR-based and light microscopy detection. Vet Parasitol 99:249–259
19. Aktas M, Altay K, Dumanli N (2006) A molecular survey of bovine *Theileria* parasites among apparently healthy cattle and with a note on the distribution of ticks in eastern Turkey. Vet Parasitol 138:179–185
20. Inácio J, Flores O, Spencer-Martins I (2008) Efficient identification of clinically relevant *Candida* yeast species by use of an assay combining panfungal loop-mediated isothermal amplification with hybridization to species-specific oligonucleotide probes. J Clin Microbiol 46:713–720
21. Enosawa M, Kageyama S, Sawai K et al (2003) Use of loop-mediated isothermal amplification of the IS900 sequence for rapid detection of cultured *Mycobacterium avium* subsp. *paratuberculosis*. J Clin Microbiol 41:4359–4365

Chapter 14

Reverse Line Blot Hybridization with Species-Specific Oligonucleotide Probes: Application to Piroplasm Detection

Ana Hurtado

Abstract

Reverse line blot (RLB) hybridization has become a well-established and widely used method for the multiplex identification of several *Babesia* and *Theileria* species in hosts and tick vectors. The procedure is based on the simultaneous PCR amplification of a polymorphic region of the 18S rRNA gene from different piroplasms followed by identification of the individual species by hybridization to species-specific oligonucleotide probes covalently linked to a nylon membrane in a macroarray format.

Key words PCR, RLB hybridization, *Babesia*, *Theileria*, Piroplasms, Ticks, Tick-borne disease

1 Introduction

Piroplasmosis are worldwide-distributed diseases caused by tick-borne intracellular apicomplexan parasites of the genera *Theileria* and *Babesia* [1, 2]. These diseases are of serious health and economic concern in extensive or semi-extensive production systems where livestock spend most of the year grazing in mountain pastures in contact with ticks. Specific and sensitive identification of piroplasms in infected animals and ticks is crucial in disease investigations and epidemiological surveys.

Reverse line blot (RLB) allows the simultaneous detection and identification of piroplasms in three steps: DNA purification (not described here), simultaneous PCR amplification of a polymorphic region of the 18S rRNA gene from the different piroplasm species, and identification of the individual species by hybridization to species-specific oligonucleotide probes bound to a nylon membrane. Simultaneous PCR amplification of the different *Babesia* and *Theileria* species is achieved by using generic primers (one of them biotinylated) that target conserved regions of the 18S rRNA gene. Species-specific oligonucleotide probes designed within variable regions of the amplicons are covalently linked to the carboxyl groups of a negatively charged nylon membrane through a C6

Mónica V. Cunha and João Inácio (eds.), *Veterinary Infection Biology: Molecular Diagnostics and High-Throughput Strategies*, Methods in Molecular Biology, vol. 1247, DOI 10.1007/978-1-4939-2004-4_14, © Springer Science+Business Media New York 2015

amino linker using a line-blotter apparatus. The membrane is then rotated 90° before adding the biotin-labeled PCR amplicons so that they come into contact with all the probes in a macroarray format. Biotin-labeled PCR products specifically hybridized to the oligoprobes are visualized by chemiluminescence; streptavidin-horseradish peroxidase (HRP) conjugate binds to the biotin-labeled amplicons and, after washing, bound conjugate acts on a chemiluminescent substrate (e.g., ECL or SuperSignal West Dura) to produce light that can be captured using an autoradiography film. A schematic representation of the process along with an example of the hybridization signal obtained is shown in Fig. 1. Amplicons can be stripped away and the entire blot used again in a new hybridization assay.

RLB hybridization is a highly specific and sensitive diagnostic tool that can be used to identify piroplasms in different sample types like blood and tissues from different animal hosts and ticks, both as single and mixed infections [3]. The use of generic 18S rRNA gene primers and the inclusion of a catchall *Theileria* and

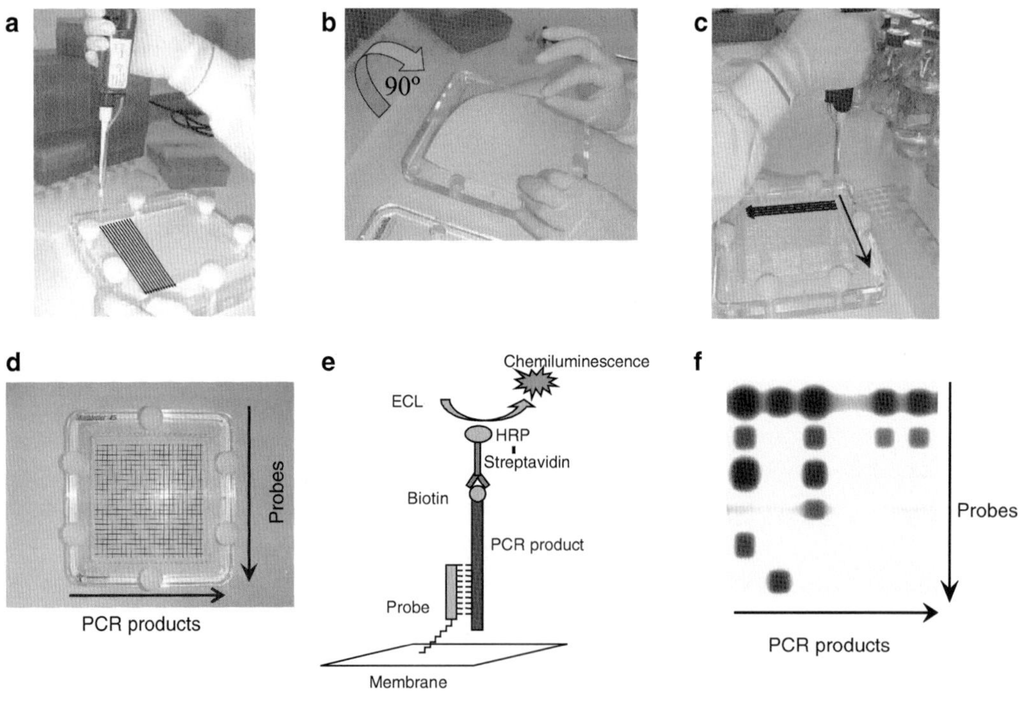

Fig. 1 Schematic representation of the RLB hybridization process. (**a**) Oligoprobes are covalently coupled to the membrane in lines using a line-blotter apparatus; (**b**) the membrane is then rotated 90°; (**c**) the PCR amplicons are added perpendicularly to the probes; (**d**) amplicons come into contact with all the probes in a macroarray format; (**e**) schematic representation of the hybridization and detection reactions; (**f**) example of the RLB hybridization signal on an autoradiography film

Babesia control probe allow for the discovery of novel species or genotypes; a generic hybridization signal with the catchall probe in the absence of species-specific hybridization signals would indicate that a new species or genotype is present. Sequencing analysis of the amplicon would then be needed to characterize it, and, if required, a new specific probe could be designed and added to the panel of probes used in the array. In fact, this strategy has helped in the description of novel species/genotypes [4–6].

RLB hybridization methods were first used for bovine piroplasm detection in 1999 [3] and soon extended to other piroplasm species [4, 5, 7, 8]. Nowadays, RLB hybridization has become the molecular technique of choice for the simultaneous detection and identification of several *Babesia* and *Theileria* species in hosts and tick vectors [9–15]. More recently, the piroplasm RLB membrane-based assay for bovine piroplasm detection has been transferred to a DNA bead-based suspension array test using the Luminex® xMAP technology that provides higher throughput screening and more flexibility in array preparation [16].

2 Materials

2.1 Equipment

1. PCR thermocycler.
2. *Miniblotter®* 45 line-blotter apparatus and foam cushions.
3. Hybridization oven, glass cylinders, and hybridization mesh sheets.
4. Shaking water bath.
5. Centrifuge.
6. Vacuum pump.
7. Orbital shaker.
8. Exposure cassette.
9. Plastic container (e.g., Tupperware).

2.2 PCR

1. Primer RLB-F2 [7]: 5′-GAC ACA GGG AGG TAG TGA CAA G-3′.
2. Primer RLB-R2 [7]: 5′-CTA AGA ATT TCA CCT CTG ACA GT-3′ (5′ biotin-labeled).
3. PCR Buffer, $MgCl_2$, and *Taq* polymerase.
4. dNTPs.
5. Molecular grade ultrapure water.

2.3 RLB

1. Negatively charged nylon membrane (e.g., Biodyne® C, Pall Corporation, NY, USA).
2. 16 % EDAC (1-ethyl-3-(3-dimethylaminopropyl)carbodiimide, hydrochloride): Weight 3.2 g of EDAC and add 20 ml of ultrapure water.

3. 20× SSPE: Weight and mix 175.3 g of NaCl, 27.6 g of NaH_2PO_4, and 7.4 g of EDTA. Add 800 ml of water, adjust the pH to 7.4 with 10 M NaOH, and bring volume to 1 L with water. Sterilize in the autoclave for 15 min at 121 °C.
4. 2× SSPE: Dilute 100 ml of 20× SSPE into 900 ml water.
5. 100 mM NaOH: Weight 4.2 g of NaOH and bring volume to 1 L with water.
6. 10 % SDS: Weight 100 g of SDS, add 800 ml of water, mix well, and bring volume to 1 L with water.
7. 1 % SDS: Dilute 100 ml of 10 % SDS into 900 ml of water.
8. 2× SSPE/0.1 % SDS: Mix 495 ml of 2× SSPE and 5 ml of 10 % SDS.
9. 2× SSPE/0.5 % SDS: Mix 950 ml of 2× SSPE and 50 ml of 10 % SDS.
10. 0.5 M EDTA: Weight 46.5 g of EDTA-Na_2 and bring volume to 250 ml with water.
11. 20 mM EDTA: Mix 960 ml of water and 40 ml of 0.5 M EDTA, and adjust pH to 8.0 with NaOH.
12. Indian ink: Make up a 1/100 dilution in 2× SSPE.
13. 500 mM $NaHCO_3$: Weight 4.2 g of $NaHCO_3$, add 90 ml of water, adjust pH to 8.4 with NaOH, and bring volume to 100 ml with water.
14. Streptavidin-horseradish peroxidase (HRP) conjugate.
15. Chemiluminescent substrate (e.g., ECL or SuperSignal West Dura): The substrate consists of two solutions to be mixed prior to incubation.
16. Film developer and fixer: Dilute with distilled water following manufacturer's instructions.
17. Autoradiography films 18 × 24 cm.
18. Oligonucleotide probes (*see* Table 1), containing a *N*-(trifluoroacetamidohexyl-cyanoethyl-*N,N-diisopropyl-phosphoramidite* [TFA])-C6 amino linker.

3 Methods

3.1 Generic PCR Targeting the V4 Region of the 18S rRNA Gene of Theileria and Babesia Species

1. *PCR reaction mix*: Reactions are performed in a final volume of 25 μl containing 50–100 ng of genomic DNA, 200 nM of each primer (RLB-F2 and 5′-biotin-labeled RLB-R2), 1× PCR buffer, 1.5 mM of $MgCl_2$, 200 μM of each dNTP, 1 U of *Taq* polymerase, and PCR-grade water to complete the volume (*see* **Notes 1** and **2**).

Table 1
Sequence and concentration of oligonucleotide probes used for piroplasm species identification by RLB

Target species	Sequence (5′–3′)[a]	Concentration (μM)	References
Catchall probe (*Theileria* spp. + *Babesia* spp.)	TAA TGG TTA ATA GGA (A/G)C(A/G) GTT G	8	[7]
B. bigemina	CGT TTT TTC CCT TTT GTT GG	8	[3]
B. bovis	CAG GTT TCG CCT GTA TAA TTG AG	8	[3]
B. caballi (genotype B)	GTT GCG TTG TTC TTG CTT TTT GCT T	32	[5]
B. caballi (genotype A)	CGG GTT ATT GAC TTC GCT TTT TCT T	8	[5]
B. canis subsp. *canis*	CGT TGA CGG TTT GAC CAT TTG GT	8	[11]
B. canis subsp. *vogeli*	GTG TTC GAG TTT GCC ATT CGT T	8	[11]
B. crassa	TTA TGG CCC GTT GGC TTA T	8	[8]
B. divergens	GTT AAT ATT GAC TAA TGT CGA G	8	[3]
B. gibsoni	TTG CCC GAC TCG GCT ACT TG	32	[11]
B. major	TCC GAC TTT GGT TGG TGT	8	[7]
B. microti	ATC TCG CTT CCG AGC GTT TTT T	16	[11]
B. motasi	ATT GGA GTA TTG CGC TTG CTT TTT	16	[4]
B. occultans	GTG TGC CTC TTT TGG CCC ATC	16	[17]
B. ovis	GCG CGC GGC CTT TGC GTT ACT	32	[4]
T. annae	CCG AAC GTA ATT TTA TTG ATT TGG C	8	[11]
T. annulata	CCT CTG GGG TCT GTG CA	8	[7]
T. buffeli	GGC TTA TTT CGG (A/T)TT GAT TTT	8	[3]
T. equi	TGG TTT TAG GAG CC(A/G) GAG	10	[18]
T. equi (genotype A)	GTT TCG ATT ATT CGT TTC CCG G	16	[5]
T. equi (genotype B)	GGG GCA TGT TTT CAT GAC TCG A	8	[5]
T. lestoquardi	ATT GCT TGT GTC CCT CCG	8	[8]
T. luwenshuni/OT1	ATC TTC TTT TTG ATG AGT TGG TGT	8	[4]
T. ovis	TTT TGC TCC TTT ACG AGT CTT TGC	8	[4]
Theileria sp. OT3	ATT TTC TCT TTT TAT ATG AGT TTT	32	[4]
Theileria sp. 3185/02	CGG TTA TAA AAT TTA TTT TAT TTC CG	32	[12]

Note: cross-reaction between the *T. lestoquardi* probe [8] and the amplicon generated from *T. annulata* and between the *T. annulata* probe [7] and the amplicon generated from *T. lestoquardi* can occur since targeted sequences in both species differ only in one nucleotide within the sequence of the probes

[a]Oligonucleotide probes contain a *N*-(trifluoroacetamidohexyl-cyanoethyl-*N*,*N*-diisopropyl phosphoramidite [TFA])-C6 amino linker at 5′ end

2. *Cycling conditions*: PCR conditions consist of an enzyme activation step of 4 min at 94 °C and 40 cycles of 30 s at 94 °C, 35 s at 51 °C, and 35 s at 72 °C.
3. *Gel electrophoresis (optional)*: Run 5 μl of the PCR product in a 1.5 % agarose gel to visualize bands of 385–450 bp.

3.2 Covalent Coupling of Oligonucleotide Probes to the Membrane

1. Dilute the probes to the concentration indicated in Table 1 in 160 ml of 500 mM $NaHCO_3$ pH 8.4 (*see* **Note 3**).
2. Cut a piece of negatively charged nylon membrane to a suitable size and activate it for 10 min at room temperature (RT) in 20 ml of freshly prepared 16 % EDAC (*see* **Note 4**).
3. Rinse the membrane in water.
4. Place a foam cushion on the miniblotter bottom part and place the membrane on top of it. Assemble the blotter tightening it with the screws and remove all remaining water from the slots by aspiration using the vacuum pump.
5. Fill the slots with ca. 150 ml of the diluted oligoprobes and incubate at RT for 5 min (*see* **Notes 5** and **6**).
6. Remove the oligoprobes from the slots by aspiration using the vacuum pump.
7. Remove the membrane from the blotter, place it into a plastic container, and incubate it at RT in 100 mM NaOH for 6–7 min to inactivate it (*see* **Note 7**).
8. Wash the membrane in 2× SSPE/0.1 % SDS at 60 °C for 5 min using a shaking water bath (*see* **Note 8**). The membrane is now ready for hybridization, but if it is to be stored at this point, follow next step.
9. Wash the membrane with 20 mM EDTA pH 8.0 for 15 min at RT with shaking using an orbital shaker before storage at 4 °C (*see* **Note 9**).

3.3 RLB Hybridization with the PCR Products and Detection

1. Add 130 μl of 2× SSPE/0.1 % SDS to the PCR products (*see* **Note 10**).
2. Denature the diluted PCR products by heating at 100 °C for 10 min and immediately cool on ice (*see* **Note 11**).
3. Incubate the membrane for 5 min at room temperature in 2× SSPE/0.1 % SDS in a plastic container.
4. Place the membrane onto the cushion in the miniblotter (rotated 90° so that the slots of the miniblotter are perpendicular to the oligoprobe lines) and aspirate remaining liquid from the slots with the vacuum pump.

5. Fill the slots with the denatured PCR products avoiding air bubbles (*see* **Note 12**) and incubate at 42 °C for 1 h in the prewarmed hybridization oven (do not shake).
6. Remove the PCR products from the slots by aspiration using the vacuum pump before removing the membrane from the miniblotter.
7. Cover the membrane (DNA side up) with the hybridization mesh and gently roll them into the shape of a cylinder. Place the covered membrane inside a hybridization glass cylinder.
8. Wash the membrane with 2× SSPE/0.5 % SDS into the glass cylinder while rotating it in the hybridization oven at 52 °C for 10 min (*see* **Note 13**).
9. Do a second wash.
10. Incubate the membrane with streptavidin-peroxidase in 2× SSPE/0.5 % SDS into the glass cylinder while rotating it in the hybridization oven at 42 °C for 30 min (*see* **Note 14**).
11. Wash the membrane with 2× SSPE/0.5 % SDS into the glass cylinder while rotating it in the hybridization oven for 10 min at 42 °C twice.
12. Remove the membrane from the glass cylinder, place it in a plastic container, and wash it with 2× SSPE for 5 min at RT twice agitating the fluid gently using an orbital shaker.
13. Blot the edge of the membrane against filter paper to remove excess liquid and add the mix of chemiluminescent substrate as per manufacturer's instructions. Incubate for 1 min (*see* **Note 15**).
14. Wrap the membrane in plastic wrap and place it in the expose cassette (*see* **Note 16**).
15. In the dark room place an autoradiography film on top of the membrane (*see* **Note 17**) and expose it as desired (*see* **Note 18**).
16. Develop the film.

3.4 Stripping of Hybridized Amplicons

1. Place the membrane in a closed plastic container.
2. Wash the membrane in 1 % SDS at 90 °C for 30 min in a shaking water bath.
3. Do a second wash in 1 % SDS at 90 °C for 30 min in a shaking water bath.
4. Incubate in 20 mM EDTA, pH 8.0 for 5 min at RT twice in an orbital shaker.
5. Store in 20 mM EDTA, pH 8.0 at 4 °C, and reuse it up to 8–10 times (*see* **Notes 9** and **19**).

4 Notes

1. Units of *Taq* polymerase can vary according to type and brand used.
2. Extraction controls and PCR negative (water) controls are included in each PCR run as negative controls.
3. Oligonucleotide probes are synthesized with a *N*-(trifluoroacetamidohexyl-cyanoethyl-*N,N-diisopropyl-phosphoramidite* [TFA])-C6 amino linker at the 5′ end. Resuspend lyophilized oligoprobes in water at a concentration of 100 μM upon arrival and store the stock solutions at −20 °C.
4. Always prepare fresh EDAC before use and incubate the membrane for just 10 min, not more.
5. Fill slots 1 and 45 with Indian ink diluted 1/100 in 2× SSPE for membrane orientation reference; the ink will indicate the direction of probes in the membrane.
6. To avoid membrane drying never leave empty slots, fill with 2× SSPE all the slots that are not filled with probes or ink.
7. Incubations longer than 10 min will produce weaker signals.
8. Pre-warm the 2× SSPE/0.1 % SDS at 60 °C in the oven or water bath before using it for membrane inactivation.
9. Seal membrane in plastic wrap or keep it in a closed container to avoid dehydration while stored.
10. Always include PCR negative and positive controls, the former to control contamination and the latter to control the process.
11. Quick spin the tubes after denaturing to pull down condensation.
12. To avoid membrane drying, never leave empty slots; fill empty slots with 2× SSPE/0.1 % SDS.
13. Make sure to set oven temperature in advance as required in each step and keep solutions pre-warmed at the required temperature.
14. When using ECL (Amersham) as chemiluminescent substrate, mix 3.8 μl streptavidin-peroxidase with 15 ml of 2× SSPE/0.5 % SDS (1:4,000 dilution); if using SuperSignal West Dura (Pierce), mix 1 μl streptavidin-peroxidase with 75 ml of 2× SSPE/0.5 % SDS (1:75,000 dilution).
15. Warm both detection reagents to room temperature before mixing them as per manufacturer's instructions. Make sure the membrane is well covered. This step does no need to be carried out in the dark.

16. Overhead transparency sheets can be used instead of wrapping paper for easier handling; however, if longer exposure times are to be used, wrapping paper is preferable to avoid membrane drying.
17. Place the film on top of the membrane in one quick and single movement, particularly if using SuperSignal West Dura (Pierce) which gives a very strong signal in the first minutes; otherwise, a moved image will be obtained.
18. Exposure time will depend on the number of uses of the membrane and the chemiluminescent substrate used. Use the positive controls to estimate the most adequate times.
19. Amplicons can be stripped and the membrane reused several times in a new hybridization assay; positive controls can be used to make sure that sensitivity is not compromised by re-hybridization.

Acknowledgments

This work was supported by the Department of Agriculture of the Basque Country Government, the Spanish National Institute for Agricultural and Food Research and Technology (INIA), and the European Regional Development Fund (ERDF).

References

1. Preston PM (2001) Theilerioses. In: Service MW (ed) Encyclopedia of arthropod-transmitted infections of man and domesticated animals. CABI Publishing, Wallingford, UK, pp 487–502
2. Uilenberg G (2001) Babesiosis. In: Service MW (ed) Encyclopedia of arthropod-transmitted infections of man and domesticated animals. CABI Publishing, Wallingford, UK, pp 53–60
3. Gubbels JM, de Vos AP, van der Weide M et al (1999) Simultaneous detection of bovine *Theileria* and *Babesia* species by reverse line blot hybridization. J Clin Microbiol 37:1782–1789
4. Nagore D, García-Sanmartín J, García-Pérez AL et al (2004) Identification, genetic diversity and prevalence of *Theileria* and *Babesia* species in a sheep population from Northern Spain. Int J Parasitol 34:1059–1067
5. Nagore D, García-Sanmartín J, García-Pérez AL et al (2004) Detection and identification of equine *Theileria* and *Babesia* species by reverse line blotting: epidemiological survey and phylogenetic analysis. Vet Parasitol 123:41–54
6. Oosthuizen MC, Allsopp BA, Troskie M et al (2009) Identification of novel *Babesia* and *Theileria* species in South African giraffe (*Giraffa camelopardalis*, Linnaeus, 1758) and roan antelope (*Hippotragus equinus*, Desmarest 1804). Vet Parasitol 163:39–46
7. Georges K, Loria GR, Riili S et al (2001) Detection of haemoparasites in cattle by reverse line blot hybridisation with a note on the distribution of ticks in Sicily. Vet Parasitol 99:273–286
8. Schnittger L, Yin H, Qi B et al (2004) Simultaneous detection and differentiation of *Theileria* and *Babesia* parasites infecting small ruminants by reverse line blotting. Parasitol Res 92:189–196
9. Altay K, Dumanli N, Aktas M (2007) Molecular identification, genetic diversity and distribution of *Theileria* and *Babesia* species infecting small ruminants. Vet Parasitol 147:161–165
10. García-Sanmartín J, Nagore D, García-Pérez AL et al (2006) Molecular diagnosis of *Theileria* and *Babesia* species infecting cattle in Northern Spain using reverse line blot macroarrays. BMC Vet Res 2:16

11. García-Sanmartín J, Barandika JF, García-Pérez AL, Hurtado A (2008) Distribution and molecular detection of *Theileria* and *Babesia* in questing ticks from Northern Spain. Med Vet Entomol 22:318–325
12. García-Sanmartín J, Aurtenetxe O, Barral M et al (2007) Molecular detection and characterization of piroplasms infecting cervids and chamois in Northern Spain. Parasitology 134:391–398
13. Kouam MK, Kantzoura V, Masuoka PM et al (2010) Genetic diversity of equine piroplasms in Greece with a note on speciation within *Theileria* genotypes (*T. equi* and *T. equi-like*). Infect Genet Evol 10:963–968
14. Oura CA, Bishop RP, Wampande EM et al (2004) Application of a reverse line blot assay to the study of haemoparasites in cattle in Uganda. Int J Parasitol 34:603–613
15. Silva MG, Marques PX, Oliva A (2010) Detection of *Babesia* and *Theileria* species infection in cattle from Portugal using a reverse line blotting method. Vet Parasitol 174:199–205
16. Ros-García A, Juste RA, Hurtado A (2012) A highly sensitive DNA bead-based suspension array for the detection and species identification of bovine piroplasms. Int J Parasitol 42:207–214
17. Ros-García A, M'ghirbi Y, Bouattour A, Hurtado A (2011) First detection of *Babesia occultans* in *Hyalomma* ticks from Tunisia. Parasitology 138:578–582
18. Ros-García A, M'ghirbi Y, Hurtado A, Bouattour A (2013) Prevalence and genetic diversity of piroplasm species in horses and ticks from Tunisia. Infect Genet Evol 17:33–37

Chapter 15

DNA Microarray-Based Detection of Multiple Pathogens: *Mycoplasma* spp. and *Chlamydia* spp.

Christiane Schnee and Konrad Sachse

Abstract

Rapid detection of slow-growing or non-culturable microorganisms, such as *Mycoplasma* spp. and *Chlamydia* spp., is still a challenge to diagnosticians in the veterinary field. In addition, as epidemiological evidence on the frequency of mixed infections involving two and more bacterial species has been emerging, detection methods allowing simultaneous identification of different pathogens are required. In the present chapter, we describe DNA microarray-based procedures for the detection of 83 *Mollicutes* species (*Mycoplasma* assay) and 11 *Chlamydia* spp. (*Chlamydia* assay). The assays are suitable for use in a routine diagnostic environment, as well as in microbiological research.

Key words DNA microarray, Rapid detection, *Mycoplasma* spp., *Chlamydia* spp., Multiple-species infection

1 Introduction

1.1 Mycoplasmas: Etiological Importance and Diagnosis

Microorganisms of the class *Mollicutes* commonly referred to as mycoplasmas exhibit a number of unique properties. These include the absence of a rigid cell wall, the capability of surface antigen variation and a small genome size, which is associated with a reduced number of metabolic pathways. These characteristics render the organisms well-adapted inhabitants of mucosal cell surfaces of mammals, birds, and other vertebrates. Their parasitic life style results in a balanced equilibrium with their hosts without causing clinical disease. However, several *Mycoplasma* species are significant pathogens and cause or contribute to infections of the respiratory or urogenital tracts. Mycoplasmoses typically take a chronic course with high morbidity and low mortality rates. The four economically most important mycoplasmoses are listed as notifiable diseases by the World Organization of Animal Health (OIE) [1] and include (1) contagious bovine pleuropneumonia (CBPP) caused by *Mycoplasma (M.) mycoides* subsp. *mycoides* and endemic in Sub-Saharan Africa, (2) contagious caprine pleuropneumonia

Mónica V. Cunha and João Inácio (eds.), *Veterinary Infection Biology: Molecular Diagnostics and High-Throughput Strategies*, Methods in Molecular Biology, vol. 1247, DOI 10.1007/978-1-4939-2004-4_15, © Springer Science+Business Media New York 2015

(CCPP) caused by *M. capricolum* subsp. *capripneumoniae*, (3) contagious agalactia caused by *M. agalactiae*, and (4) avian mycoplasmosis caused by *M. gallisepticum* or *M. synoviae*. Other relevant syndromes include mastitis in cows and pneumonia in calves (*M. bovis*), which predominantly occur in industrial cattle production in North America [2] and Europe [3]. Also ocular and respiratory infections in small ruminants caused by *M. conjunctivae* and *M. ovipneumoniae*, respectively, as well as enzootic pneumonia, arthritis, and anemia in swine caused by *M. hyopneumoniae*, *M. hyorhinis*, and *M. suis*, respectively, are of economic importance.

Sixteen different mycoplasmas have been found in humans [4]. While the majority of them represent commensals, *M. pneumoniae* in the oropharynx as well as *M. hominis*, *M. genitalium*, and *Ureaplasma* spp. in the urogenital tract are of clinical significance.

Furthermore, mycoplasma contamination of cell culture is a persistent problem in research laboratories and the pharmaceutical industry, because the unwanted presence of *Acholeplasma laidlawii*, *M. orale*, *M. arginini*, *M. fermentans*, and others affect growth and development of cell culture and can distort the results of in vitro tests [5].

The broad spectrum of mycoplasmas either directly involved in pathogenic processes or acting as commensals and interfering with detection assays presents a particular diagnostic challenge that is only insufficiently solvable through individual PCR tests (*see* Subheading 1.3). Therefore, in the last decade, a number of advanced tests based on generic PCR amplification and subsequent specific product analysis were developed, such as 16S rRNA-PCR/denaturing-gradient gel electrophoresis [6], PCR/high-resolution melting curve analysis [7], and PCR/microarray assay [8–10].

1.2 Chlamydiae: Etiological Importance and Diagnosis

A unique feature of the obligate intracellular bacteria commonly known as chlamydiae is their biphasic developmental cycle. As a result, permanent cell lines or embryonated chicken eggs are necessary to culture the strains. The procedure is laborious and requires experienced staff. In addition, some of the strains are extremely difficult to grow. A description of current state-of-the-art diagnostic assays is given in the OIE Manual [11, 12] and in a recent review [13].

Among the major pathogens are *Chlamydia (C.) psittaci*, the causative agent of avian chlamydiosis, which is transmissible to humans; *C. abortus* (ovine and human abortion); as well as the human pathogens *C. trachomatis* (genital and ocular diseases) and *C. pneumoniae* (community-acquired pneumonia).

Until recently, the taxonomy of the family *Chlamydiaceae* was the subject of controversy. The division into two genera *Chlamydia* and *Chlamydophila* as proposed by Everett at al. [14] did not find universal acceptance [15] and was finally reversed to the single genus *Chlamydia* [16].

Avian chlamydiosis (also known as psittacosis or ornithosis) is widespread and represents a major factor of economic loss to the poultry industry, as well as a permanent risk for zoonotic transmission to man [17]. The disease is notifiable in most European countries, as well as in Australia and the USA. Depending on the chlamydial strain and the avian host involved, the infection leads to pneumonia, air sacculitis, pericarditis, hepatitis, and/or splenitis, occasionally with fatal outcome, the major signs being fever, anorexia, lethargy, and diarrhea. Subclinical infection often leads to recurring manifestations and chronicity. Even in the absence of clinical signs, intermittent shedding of *C. psittaci* by carriers represents an important source of infection and also a challenge for diagnosticians [18, 19]. Apart from birds, the agent can also be encountered in cattle, goats, swine, and cats [20], as well as in sheep [21] and horses.

As a result of several studies in Germany, France, and Italy in the past 7 years, the list of chlamydial species is about to be extended. Phylogenetic studies of ribosomal RNA genes from 11 isolates and analysis of the first genome sequences led to the proposal of two new species [22]. *Chlamydia avium* sp. nov. has been found in pigeons and psittacine birds, some of which were cases of severe disease. *Chlamydia gallinacea* sp. nov. has been identified in domestic poultry hosts, so far from asymptomatic chicken, guinea fowl, and turkey. A zoonotic potential cannot be ruled out.

Ovine chlamydiosis or enzootic abortion of ewes is caused by *C. abortus*. Outbreaks of the disease result in major economic losses for the sheep industry. The abortion typically occurs in the last 2–3 weeks of pregnancy with the appearance of stillborn lambs and inflamed placentas [23]. Chlamydial abortion also occurs in goats and, less frequently, cattle, pigs, horses, and deer may be affected.

The main hosts of *C. pecorum* are cattle and small ruminants, where it may cause enteritis, pneumonia, polyarthritis, and abortions [24]. The agent also frequently occurs in swine.

C. suis is typically encountered in swine. Infections mostly remain asymptomatic, but an association with respiratory disease, diarrhea, and conjunctivitis seems likely under certain environmental and epidemiological conditions. The recent emergence of antibiotic resistance in this agent [25] deserves further attention.

C. caviae and *C. felis* are largely but not exclusively confined to their specific host, i.e., guinea pig and cat, respectively, eliciting conjunctivitis.

Besides being the most prevalent sexually transmitted human pathogen, *C. trachomatis* can also be found occasionally in animals [26, 27]. Likewise, certain biovars of *C. pneumoniae* can also be encountered in animals, such as horses, frogs, and koalas, where they are capable of causing respiratory disorders.

1.3 DNA Microarray Detection Assays: Principle and Potential

Rapid detection of bacterial pathogens remains a challenge to diagnosticians in veterinary medicine, particularly when slow-growing or non-culturable microorganisms are involved, as is the case with *Mycoplasma* spp. and *Chlamydia* spp. Early diagnosis of infection is crucial for the effectiveness of control measures to contain the spread of the infectious agent and prevent economic losses.

In the past two decades, the most significant advances in diagnostic technology were due to the broad application of nucleic acid amplification techniques, notably the polymerase chain reaction (PCR). Now that demands on quality, quantity, and rapidity of microbiological diagnosis are steadily increasing, the inherent limitations of PCR are becoming evident. The parallelity of PCR assays is very limited, i.e., usually a single agent is targeted, and even in multiplex assays the number of targets is lower than 10. This is a serious drawback as diagnosticians are increasingly becoming aware of dual and multiple infections. Furthermore, as soon as one has to deal with more subtle differences between species or strains, such as minor sequence variations up to single-nucleotide polymorphisms or multi-locus sequence features, PCR alone cannot provide the necessary resolution.

In this situation, a DNA microarray-based approach, which is capable of verifying the exact nucleotide sequence of a target region through hybridization, appears a promising alternative. Moreover, a DNA microarray assay can be designed to target a large number of genomic loci (limited only by the size of the array) to ensure discrimination between microbial species, strains, genotypes, serotypes, resistance types, etc.

The commercially available ArrayStrip™ (AS) platform represents an efficient system for processing low- and high-density DNA arrays (Alere Technologies, http://alere-technologies.com/products). An AS unit consists of eight connected plastic vessels in microtiter format, each one carrying a microarray chip of 3 × 3 mm size with an active area of 2.4 × 2.4 mm on the bottom. Hybridization and analysis can be conducted in an easy, rapid, and parallel fashion, largely using standard laboratory equipment (*see* Fig. 1 and **Note 1**).

Validated protocols for differentiation among 37 *Mollicutes* species [10] and nine *Chlamydia* spp. [28] have been published by our group. Other applications based on AS assays include DNA serotyping of *Salmonella enteric* [29], genotyping of methicillin-resistant *Staphylococcus aureus* [30], enterohemorrhagic *Escherichia coli* [31], and many more.

In the present chapter, we describe the procedure for detection of 83 *Mollicutes* species (*Mycoplasma* assay, *see* Table 1) and 11 *Chlamydia* spp. (*Chlamydia* assay). Basic principles of assay design and experimental features are given in **Notes 2** and **3**.

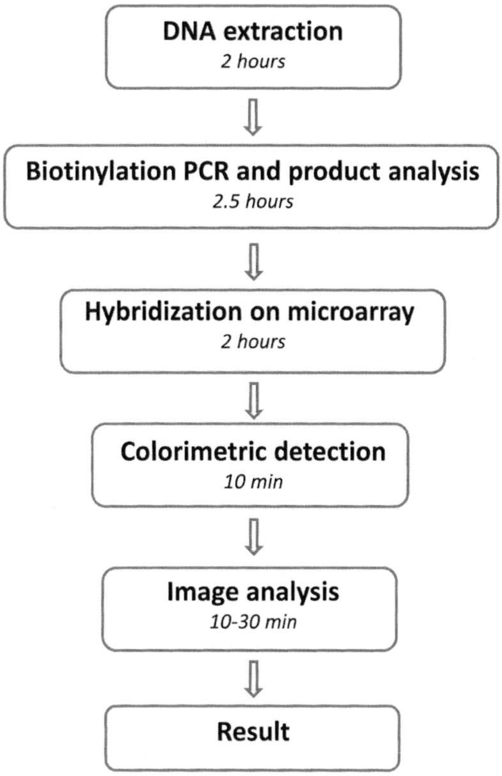

Fig. 1 General workflow and timeline of the *Mycoplasma* and *Chlamydia* assays

Table 1
Selection of important pathogenic animal and human mycoplasmas and cell culture contaminants that can be identified using the *Mycoplasma* microarray assay

Animal mycoplasmas	Human mycoplasmas	Mycoplasmas in cell culture
M. agalactiae	*M. genitalium*	*A. laidlawii*
M. bovigenitalium	*M. hominis*	*M. arginini*
M. bovis	*M. pneumoniae*	*M. fermentans*
M. californicum	*U. parvum*	*M. hyorhinis*
M. capricolum subsp. *capripneumoniae*[a]	*U. urealyticum*	*M. orale*
M. conjunctivae		*M. salivarium*
M. dispar		
M. felis		
M. gallisepticum		
M. hyopneumoniae		
M. mycoides subsp. *mycoides*[a]		
M. ovipneumoniae		
M. suis		
M. synoviae		

[a]Members of the *M. mycoides* cluster are identified at species but not at subspecies level

2 Materials

2.1 DNA Extraction

Commercial DNA extraction kit, e.g., High Pure PCR Template Preparation Kit (Roche Diagnostics, Mannheim, Germany) suitable for cultured strains and a wide range of tissue samples, e.g., nasal, vaginal and conjunctival swabs, mucus, bronchoalveolar lavage, organs, feces, and milk.

2.2 Biotinylation PCR

1. PCR-grade water.
2. PCR reagents. We use DyNAmo™ Flash SYBR™ Green qPCR Mastermix (Finnzymes Vantaa, Finland) for pre-hybridization amplification of mycoplasmal DNA and conventional *Taq* DNA polymerase, e.g., Native *Taq* Polymerase (Fermentas, St. Leon-Rot, Germany) or Phusion Green High-Fidelity DNA Polymerase (Thermo Scientific, Dreieich, Germany) with the corresponding buffer system and a dNTP mixture (2 mM of each nucleotide) for chlamydial samples.
3. Primers. The sequences of primer oligonucleotides are given in Table 2. The concentration of stock solutions is 100 pmol/μl and of working solutions 10 pmol/μl.
4. Internal amplification control pGEM-EGFP2rev [33]. Commercially available as INTYPE IC-DNA from Qiagen Leipzig, Germany.

Table 2
Primers for biotinylation PCR

Name	Sequence 5′–3′[a]	Target gene	Amplicon size	References
F1388	5′Bio-GTT TCC TGG GCA AGG TTC G-3′	*Mycoplasma* 23S rDNA	594 bp	[10]
R1982	5′Bio-CCG TTA TAG TTA CGG CCG CC-3′			
tuf-064F	5′Bio-ATG CCN CAA ACW MGW GAA CAC-3′	*Mycoplasma tuf*	614 bp	[10]
tuf-681R	5′Bio-TRT GAC KWC CAC CTT CWT CTT-3′			
U23F-19	5′Bio-ATT GAM AGG CGA WGA AGG A-3′	*Chlamydia* 23S rDNA	171 bp	[28]
23R-22	5′Bio- GCY TAC TAA GAT GTT TCA GTT C-3′			
EGFP-11F	5′Bio-CAG CCA CAA CGT CTA TAT CAT G-3′	Internal control	276 bp	[33]
EGFP-10R	5′Bio-CTT GTA CAG CTC GTC CAT GC-3′			

[a]All primers are labeled with biotin at their 5′ end

2.3 Electrophoresis

1. Agarose, molecular biology grade: 1.5 % (w/v) gels.
2. Tris-borate EDTA electrophoresis buffer (TBE): 0.09 M of Tris-borate, 0.002 M of EDTA, pH 8.0. For 1 L of 10× TBE, mix 108 g of Tris-base, 55 g of boric acid, and 80 mL of 0.25 M EDTA, make up with water. Dilute 1:10 before use.
3. Gel loading buffer (GLB): 20 % (v/v) of glycerol, 0.2 M of EDTA, 0.01 % (w/v) of bromophenol blue, 0.2 % (w/v) of Ficoll 400.
4. Ethidium bromide stock solution: 1 % (10 mg/mL) solution in water. *Caution*: the substance is presumed to be mutagenic. Avoid direct contact with skin. Wear gloves when preparing solutions and handling gels.
5. DNA size marker. We mostly use the O'RangeRuler ("100-bp ladder") (Fermentas, St. Leon-Rot, Germany).

2.4 DNA Microarray Hybridization

The Identibac™ Hybridisation Kit (Alere Technologies, Jena, Germany) is the most efficient and convenient option and contains all necessary reagents: hybridization buffer (C1), washing buffers (C2, C5), streptavidin-peroxidase conjugate (C3 + C4), and TMB substrate (D1). Alternatively, buffers can be prepared manually according to the protocol published previously [32].

2.5 General Equipment and Consumables

1. Benchtop centrifuge, e.g., 5402 (Eppendorf, Hamburg, Germany).
2. Vortex shaker, e.g., Vortex 1 (IKA Labortechnik, Staufen, Germany).
3. Set of pipettes covering the volume range from 0.1 to 1,000 μl and aerosol-resistant filter tips.
4. Sterile, DNAse and RNAse-free plastic tubes.
5. Thermal cycler. We use the Mx3000P with MxPro™ 4.10. software (Agilent, Waldbronn, Germany) for *Mycoplasma* assay and Mastercycler personal (Eppendorf, Hamburg, Germany) for *Chlamydia* assay.
6. Apparatus for horizontal gel electrophoresis.
7. UV transilluminator, 254 nm and/or 312 nm.
8. Video documentation or photographic equipment.
9. ArrayStrip™ or ArrayTube™ reaction vessels (Alere Technologies, Jena, Germany) with integrated DNA microarray chips for the *Mycoplasma* assay (layout Myc_05 or higher) or the *Chlamydia* assay (layout Chlam_gesamt_4_AS or higher). These arrays are commercially available from Alere. The company also has a service for ordering customized arrays. The sequences of the oligonucleotide probes immobilized on these arrays were previously published in Sachse et al. [32] (*Chlamydia* assay) and Schnee et al. [10] (*Mycoplasma* assay).

10. Heatable horizontal tube shaker. We recommend the BioShake iQ (Quantifoil Instruments, Jena, Germany; *see* **Note 4**).
11. ArrayMate transmission reader (Alere Technologies, Jena, Germany).
12. Iconoclust software, version 2.3 or higher (Alere Technologies, Jena, Germany).

3 Methods

3.1 DNA Extraction

Follow the protocol given by the commercial supplier of the DNA extraction kit.

3.2 Pre-hybridization Biotinylation PCR

3.2.1 *Mycoplasma* Assay

The two genomic targets in the 23S rRNA and *tuf* genes are amplified independently in two separate real-time PCRs. The former is amplified in a simplex reaction, and the latter is co-amplified with the internal control template, i.e., plasmid pGEM-EGFP2rev [33] (*see* **Note 5**).

1. Prepare master mixtures according to Table 3 as a multiple of 20 μl depending on sample numbers.

Table 3
Composition of the reaction mixtures for pre-hybridization real-time PCR in the *Mycoplasma* assay

Target	Components	Working concentration	Volume per reaction (total 20 μl)	Final concentration
23S rDNA	PCR-grade water	–	7 μl	–
	DyNAmoq PCR Mastermix	2×	10 μl	1×
	Primer F1388	10 pmol/μl	1 μl	500 nM
	Primer R1982	10 pmol/μl	1 μl	500 nM
	DNA template	–	1 μl	–
tuf	PCR-grade water	–	5.9 μl	–
	DyNAmoq PCR Mastermix	2×	10 μl	1×
	Primer tuf-064F	10 pmol/μl	1 μl	500 nM
	Primer tuf-681R	10 pmol/μl	1 μl	500 nM
	ctrl primer EGFP-11F	10 pmol/μ	0.5 μl	250 nM
	ctrl primer EGFP-10R	10 pmol/μl	0.5 μl	250 nM
	IC: pGEM-EGFP2rev[a]	10^5 copies/μl	0.1 μl	10^4 copies/rxn
	DNA template	–	1 μl	–

[a]IC internal control

2. Add template to each reaction vessel: 1 μl of DNA extract from your sample. If the DNA contents of the extract is low, up to 4 μl of sample DNA can be used and the amount of water be reduced accordingly.
3. In each series, include external amplification controls that contain DNA of mycoplasma reference strains, e.g., *M. bovis* PG45, as positive control, and water, instead of sample extract, as negative control.
4. Run real-time PCR under the following conditions: initial denaturation at 95 °C for 10 min, 40 cycles of denaturation at 95 °C for 30 s, annealing at 52 °C for 30 s, and elongation at 72 °C for 40 s.
5. For PCR product evaluation, proceed with dissociation curve analysis at real-time PCR cycler, from 55 °C to 95 °C with continuous recording of fluorescence. Melting curves of mycoplasma-specific *tuf* amplicons typically show peaks between 78 and 82 °C and 23S rDNA amplicons between 82 and 86 °C (*see* **Note 6**).

3.2.2 *Chlamydia* Assay

The chlamydia-specific target in the 23S rDNA is amplified alongside the internal control template pGEM-EGFP2rev in a conventional duplex PCR.

1. Prepare master mixtures according to Table 4 as a multiple of 20 μl depending on the number of samples.

Table 4
Composition of reaction mixtures for pre-hybridization PCR in the *Chlamydia* assay

Components	Working concentration	Volume per reaction (total 20 μl)	Final concentration
PCR-grade water	–	11.1 μl	–
PCR buffer	10×	2 μl	1×
$MgCl_2$	50 mM	0.6 μl	1.5 mM
dNTP	2 mM each	2 μl	200 nM
Primer U23F-19	10 pmol/μl	1 μl	500 nM
Primer 23R-22	10 pmol/μl	1 μl	500 nM
ctrl primer EGFP-11F	10 pmol/μl	0.5 μl	250 nM
ctrl primer EGFP-10R	10 pmol/μl	0.5 μl	250 nM
IC: pGEM-EGFP2rev[a]	10^5 copies/μl	0.1 μl	10^4 copies/rxn
Taq DNA polymerase	5 U/μl	0.2 μl	2 U
DNA template	–	1 μl	–

[a]IC internal control

2. Add template to each reaction vessel: 1 μl of DNA extract from your sample. If the DNA contents of the extract is low, up to 4 μl of sample DNA can be used and the amount of water be reduced accordingly.
3. In each series, include external amplification controls that contain DNA of a chlamydial reference strain, e.g., *C. psittaci* 6BC, as positive control, and water, instead of sample extract, as negative control.
4. Run PCR at conventional thermal cycler according to the following temperature-time profile: initial denaturation at 95 °C for 15 min, 40 cycles of denaturation at 94 °C for 30 s, primer annealing at 50 °C for 90 s, primer extension at 72 °C for 90 s, and final extension at 72 °C for 10 min.
5. Analyze PCR products by standard agarose gel electrophoresis. Expected fragment sizes are 171 bp for chlamydial DNA and 276 bp for internal control (*see* **Note 6**).

3.3 DNA Microarray Hybridization

1. For mycoplasma: transfer 0.5 μl of each PCR product from Subheading 3.2.1 into a 0.2 mL plastic tube and add 99 μl of hybridization buffer (buffer C1).

   For chlamydia: transfer 1 μl of the PCR product from Subheading 3.2.2 into a 0.2 mL plastic tube and add 99 μl of hybridization buffer (buffer C1).
2. Denature DNA by heating at 95 °C for 5 min. Cool down immediately by putting the tube on ice for 1 min. Spin down the liquid by centrifugation for 10 s.
3. Condition ArrayStrip™ by adding 100 μl of water to each well. Pipette the liquid up and down 4 times, and then discard it. Be careful not to touch the array chip surface.
4. Add 100 μl of C1 buffer to each well; shake on BioShake iQ at 50 °C and 550 rpm for 5 min. Remove liquid.
5. Hybridization. Add the hybridization mix (100 μl each) from **step 2** to AS wells. Incubate on BioShake iQ at 50 °C (*Mycoplasma* assay) or at 58 °C (*Chlamydia* assay) at 550 rpm for 60 min. Remove supernatant and discard it.
6. Add 200 μl of washing buffer C2 to each well; wash at 45 °C (*Mycoplasma* assay) and at 43 °C (*Chlamydia* assay) and 550 rpm for 10 min. Remove liquid and discard it.
7. Repeat **step 6**.
8. Combine 792 μl of C4 and 8 μl of C3 solutions (horseradish peroxidase conjugated with streptavidin) in a plastic tube, vortex and spin down. The amount is for a single AS, i.e., 8 wells. Add 100 μl of this mix to each well. Incubate at 30 °C and 550 rpm for 10 min. Remove supernatant.

9. Wash wells by adding 200 μl of washing buffer C5 and 4 times up-and-down pipetting at room temperature. Remove all the liquid thoroughly and completely.
10. Add 100 μl of D1 solution (peroxidase substrate) to each well; incubate at room temperature for 5 min.
11. Remove liquid and put the AS assay into the ArrayMate reader.

3.4 Data Processing and Interpretation

1. Conduct the reading process according to the instructions for the ArrayMate equipment.
2. Transfer the image files (bmp format) to your computer and process the data using the Iconoclust software.
3. Check signals of control probes: for a valid result, the signal of the biotinylated staining control probe should be higher than 0.7. Only negative results are validated with the internal amplification/hybridization control. The hybridization signal of at least one amplification/hybridization control probe should be higher than 0.6.
4. Identify *Mycoplasma* or *Chlamydia* species using the PatternMatch algorithm or perform manual species assignment as follows (*see* **Note 7**).

3.4.1 Manual Identification of Mollicutes Species

The following criteria need to be considered.

1. The intensity of all relevant signals must be higher than 0.2 (cutoff).
2. At least two species-specific hybridization signals at one target gene and, at least, one species-specific hybridization signal at the second target gene are required for a valid species assignment.
3. If two signals appear only at one target gene, the identification is regarded as ambiguous or doubtful.
4. Some species are only differentiable at one target gene and share a signal pattern with a sister species at the second target gene: *M. bovis/M. agalactiae*, *M. imitans/M. gallisepticum*, *and M. yeatsii/M. cottewii.*
5. The *Mycoplasma mycoides* cluster members can be differentiated only at species and not at subspecies level using the 23S rRNA and *tuf* target genes.

3.4.2 Manual Identification of *Chlamydia* spp.

A typical bar diagram of a sample examined with the *Chlamydia* assay is shown in Fig. 2. The following general rules will apply.

1. If all probes of a species show a hybridization signal intensity higher than 0.07 (cutoff), the assignment to this species is valid.
2. Species-specific and genus-specific signals must logically fit. This means that signals of probes "chlamydophila_1 + 2" have

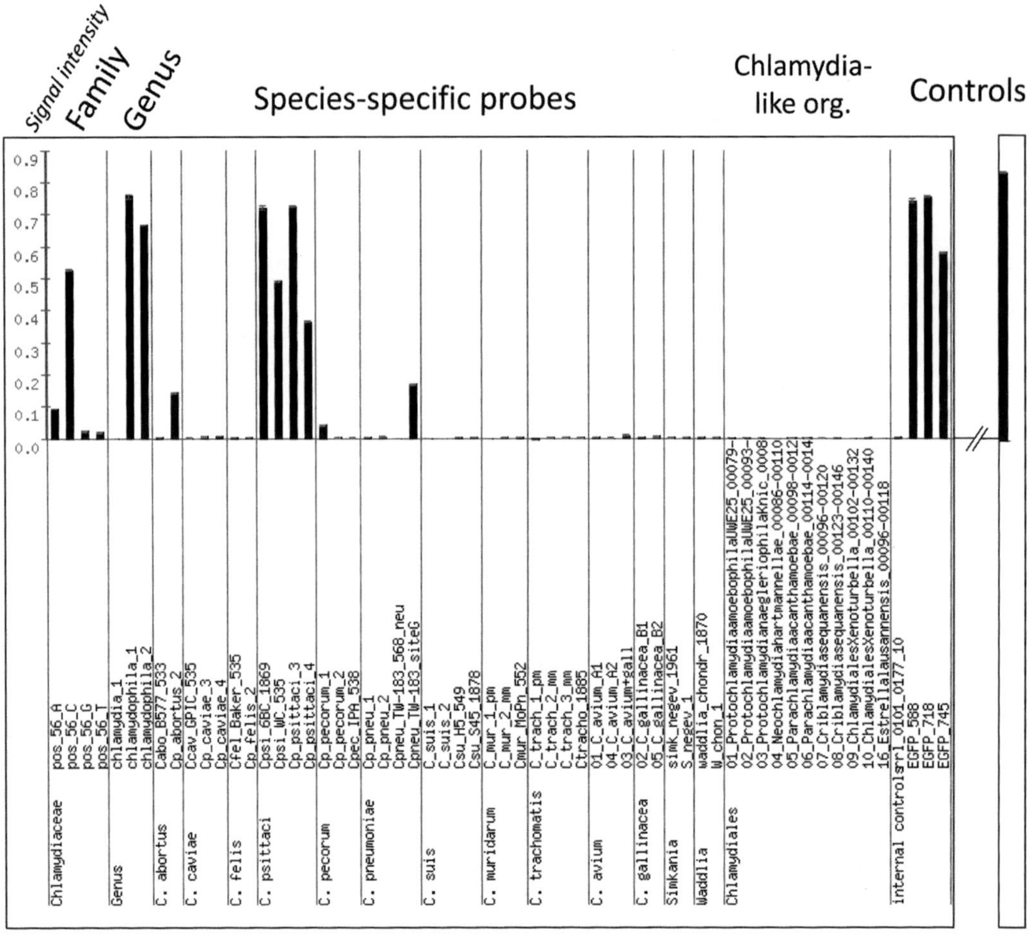

Fig. 2 Examination of a cell culture sample using the *Chlamydia* assay. The species *C. psittaci* was identified. The *bar diagram* reveals the following specific hybridization signals (*from left to right*): family *Chlamydiaceae* (two probes reacting), genus *Chlamydia* ("*Chlamydophila*" probes reacting), species *C. psittaci* (all four probes reacting). Control reactions on the right-hand margin: background control for spotting buffer negative, internal amplification/hybridization controls positive (three probes reacting), staining control positive. All other signals represent cross-hybridization or are below cutoff. As the microarray carries three more sectors of spotted *Chlamydia* probes, only the relevant parts are shown here

to appear alongside the species-specific signals of *C. abortus*, *C. caviae*, *C. felis*, *C. psittaci*, *C. pecorum*, *C. pneumoniae*, *C. avium*, or *C. gallinacea*, respectively. On the other side, the signal of probe "chlamydia_1" must appear together with the species-specific signals of *C. trachomatis*, *C. suis*, or *C. muridarum*, respectively. Please note that the designation of the genus-specific probes is historic and all three of them recognize the recently recombined genus *Chlamydia*.

3. If all relevant probes of two species show a reaction, one has to assume a mixed (dual) infection.
4. A sample will be regarded as negative when all signal intensities are below 0.07 or when the signal distribution contradicts the logical fit in point 2.

4 Notes

1. The *AS technology* is easy to handle as it mainly involves standard laboratory equipment and, unlike in more expensive microarray platforms, no sophisticated devices, such as hybridization chamber and fluorescence reader, are needed. In a positive reaction, oligonucleotide probes covalently linked to a glass surface will form a duplex with complementary target DNA strands carrying a biotin label. To visualize the hybridization signal, a streptavidin-horseradish peroxidase conjugate is added and allowed to cleave a tetramethylbenzidine-like substrate. As a result, dark blue precipitates will be formed at each reactive spot.

   The expenses for consumables are moderate, particularly when the high degree of parallelity is taken into account. This means that, for instance, a single AS test for *Chlamydia* spp. is equivalent to 11 different PCR tests for the individual species. Detection of mycoplasmas or chlamydiae using the AS assay can be accomplished within a working day (6–8 h). This technology is manageable in a high-throughput environment, with up to 40 samples per day and technician.
2. For mycoplasma identification, the 23S ribosomal (r) RNA and elongation factor Tu (*tuf*) gene loci were shown to be suitable target regions with a high discriminatory potential at species level but also with high intraspecific stability [10, 34]. The necessary discriminatory capacity and robustness of the assay have been attained through this combinatorial two-target approach. The current version of the mycoplasma microarray (no. 5) carries five genus-specific (*Mycoplasma* and *Ureaplasma*) and 142 species-specific oligonucleotide probes derived from the 23S rDNA target, as well as 157 species-specific probes from the *tuf* site, thus enabling identification of 83 *Mollicutes* species from animals, birds, man, and cell cultures. The major selection criterion for the hybridization probes was the specificity of the target sequence, i.e., at least two nucleotides difference to the second-best matching target. In rare cases where this criterion is not fulfilled, species assignment will be possible at the alternative target or by a combinatorial approach via analysis of more complex hybridization patterns. The selected oligonucleotides are sized between 20 and 36 nt, have an average

melting temperature of 59.2 °C and an average G+C content of 40 %, and are spotted twofold on the microarray glass surface. The array further includes three probes for the detection of the internal amplification and hybridization control (pGEM-EGFP2rev), a biotinylated oligonucleotide as staining control and spotting buffer as background control.

3. For differentiation among *Chlamydia* spp., we identified a discriminating site in domain I of the 23S rRNA gene [32] and derived all probes from there. The currently available version (no. 4) of the chlamydia array covers 11 different species of *Chlamydia* and includes four family-specific probes (*Chlamydiaceae*), three genus-specific (*Chlamydia/Chlamydophila*), and 38 probes for 11 *Chlamydia* spp. and the nearest relatives, i.e., *Waddlia chondrophila* and *Simkania negevensis*. In addition, 11 probes for some of the chlamydia-like organisms outside the family *Chlamydiaceae* are present. The oligonucleotides are sized between 19 and 32 nt (mean 25), the average *Tm* is 56.4 °C, and G+C is 41 %. Control probes are equivalent to those on the mycoplasma array. As an example, Fig. 2 shows the graphical output of a sample tested positive for *C. psittaci*.
4. For the sake of high specificity and stringency of the hybridization reaction, it is extremely important to ensure that the prescribed temperatures are actually attained in the AS vessel itself. This requires heat transfer from the heatable shaker to the liquid contents of the AS vessel to be very rapid and efficient. Most of the commercially available shakers are too slow, so that too much time is lost until the necessary in-tube temperature has been reached. In our hands, the BioShake iQ fulfills the criteria to be used in the hybridization process.
5. The pre-hybridization PCR is the crucial step of agent detection and identification in terms of sensitivity. While 23S rDNA primers were designed to exclusively amplify mycoplasmal or chlamydial DNA, *tuf* primers are not completely specific for the targeted *Mollicutes* species. They may also align to other bacterial sequences in clinical samples leading to a competition for PCR resources between mycoplasmal DNA and alternative targets and lowering the sensitivity for mycoplasma detection.
6. We recommend agarose gel electrophoresis of PCR products and, in the *Mycoplasma* assay, also dissociation curve analysis as control methods to check amplification products. Nevertheless, it is worth noting that samples exhibiting faint amplicon bands and ambiguous dissociation curves may also produce clear hybridization signals and valid hybridization patterns. As a rule of thumb, samples showing Ct < 33 reliably give valid hybridization signals, while those with Ct 33–36 will only occasionally produce positive signals.

7. The PatternMatch algorithm compares the experimentally obtained signal pattern with those of reference strains representing 83 different *Mollicutes* species or 11 *Chlamydia* spp., respectively. It provides combined bar diagrams of sample and reference, as well as two numerical parameters to assess the similarity of two patterns and the accuracy of identification. The matching score (MS) represents the sum of numerical differences between corresponding signal intensities of sample and theoretical and/or practical reference hybridization patterns. Thus, the MS value is a measure of the overall dissimilarity between two hybridization patterns. An ideal match of two patterns based on the same set of oligonucleotide probes will yield MS = 0, whereas values greater than 45 in the *Mycoplasma* assay or seven in the *Chlamydia* assay represent a poor match that does not allow reliable species assignment (note: these numerical limits may change when updated software versions will appear in the future). The arithmetic difference between best and second-best match, termed Delta MS, indicates the reliability of a given species assignment. Values of Delta MS ≥ 0.5 are regarded as representing a sufficient degree of distinction between best and second-best matches. Manual data interpretation and species assignment is possible, if PatternMatch software is not available, and is recommended for cases of dual- or multiple-species infection.

References

1. OIE (2013) OIE-Listed diseases, infections and infestations in force in 2013. http://www.oie.int/en/animal-health-in-the-world/oie-listed-diseases-2013
2. Maunsell FP, Woolums AR, Francoz D et al (2011) *Mycoplasma bovis* infections in cattle. J Vet Intern Med 25:772–783
3. Pfutzner H, Sachse K (1996) *Mycoplasma bovis* as an agent of mastitis, pneumonia, arthritis and genital disorders in cattle. Rev Sci Tech 15:1477–1494
4. Waites KB, Xiao L, Paralanov V, Viscardi RM, Glass JI (2012) Molecular methods for the detection of *Mycoplasma* and *Ureaplasma* infections in humans: a paper from the 2011 William Beaumont Hospital Symposium on molecular pathology. J Mol Diagn 14:437–450
5. Volokhov DV, Graham LJ, Brorson KA, Chizhikov VE (2011) *Mycoplasma* testing of cell substrates and biologics: review of alternative non-microbiological techniques. Mol Cell Probes 25:69–77
6. McAuliffe L, Ellis RJ, Lawes JR, Ayling RD, Nicholas RA (2005) 16S rDNA PCR and denaturing gradient gel electrophoresis; a single generic test for detecting and differentiating *Mycoplasma* species. J Med Microbiol 54:731–739
7. Rebelo AR, Parker L, Cai HY (2011) Use of high-resolution melting curve analysis to identify *Mycoplasma* species commonly isolated from ruminant, avian, and canine samples. J Vet Diagn Invest 23:932–936
8. Volokhov DV, George J, Liu SX et al (2006) Sequencing of the intergenic 16S-23S rRNA spacer (ITS) region of Mollicutes species and their identification using microarray-based assay and DNA sequencing. Appl Microbiol Biotechnol 71:680–698
9. Tonelli A, Sacchini F, Krasteva I et al (2012) One test microbial diagnostic microarray for identification of *Mycoplasma mycoides* subsp. *mycoides* and other *Mycoplasma* species. Mol Biotechnol 52:285–299
10. Schnee C, Schulsse S, Hotzel H et al (2012) A novel rapid DNA microarray assay enables identification of 37 *Mycoplasma* species and highlights multiple *Mycoplasma* infections. PLoS One 7:e33237

11. OIE (2012) Avian chlamydiosis. World organisation for animal health: manual of diagnostic tests and vaccines for terrestrial animals (chapter 2.3.1), vol. 1, 7th edn. Paris
12. OIE (2012) Enzootic abortion of ewes (ovine chlamydiosis). World organisation for animal health: manual of diagnostic tests and vaccines for terrestrial animals (chapter 2.7.7), vol. 1, 7th edn. Paris
13. Sachse K, Vretou E, Livingstone M et al (2009) Recent developments in the laboratory diagnosis of chlamydial infections. Vet Microbiol 135:2–21
14. Everett KD, Bush RM, Andersen AA (1999) Emended description of the order *Chlamydiales*, proposal of *Parachlamydiaceae* fam. nov. and *Simkaniaceae* fam. nov., each containing one monotypic genus, revised taxonomy of the family *Chlamydiaceae*, including a new genus and five new species, and standards for the identification of organisms. Int J Syst Bacteriol 49:415–440
15. Stephens RS, Myers G, Eppinger M, Bavoil PM (2009) Divergence without difference: phylogenetics and taxonomy of *Chlamydia* resolved. FEMS Immunol Med Microbiol 55:115–119
16. Kuo C-C, Stephens RS, Bavoil PM, Kaltenboeck B (2011) Genus *Chlamydia* Jones, Rake and Stearns 1945, 55. In: Krieg NR, Staley JT, Brown DR, Hedlund BP, Paster BJ, Ward NL, Ludwig W, Whitman WB (eds) Bergey's manual of systematic bacteriology, vol 4, 2nd edn. Springer, Heidelberg, pp 846–865
17. Anonymous (2002) Avian chlamydiosis as a zoonotic disease and risk reduction strategies. SCAHAW (Scientific Committee on Animal Health and Animal Welfare) European Commission, Health & Consumer Protection Directorate-General, SANCO/AH/R26/2002
18. Kaleta EF, Taday EM (2003) Avian host range of *Chlamydophila* spp. based on isolation, antigen detection and serology. Avian Pathol 32:435–461
19. Andersen AA, Vanrompay D (2000) Avian chlamydiosis. Rev Sci Tech 19:396–404
20. Pantchev A, Sting R, Bauerfeind R, Tyczka J, Sachse K (2010) Detection of all *Chlamydophila* and *Chlamydia* spp. of veterinary interest using species-specific real-time PCR assays. Comp Immunol Microbiol Infect Dis 33: 473–484
21. Lenzko H, Moog U, Henning K et al (2011) High frequency of chlamydial co-infections in clinically healthy sheep flocks. BMC Vet Res 7:29
22. Sachse K, Laroucau K, Riege K et al (2014) Evidence for the existence of two new members of the family *Chlamydiaceae* and proposal of *Chlamydia avium* sp. nov. and *Chlamydia gallinacea* sp. nov. Syst Appl Microbiol 37:79–88
23. Buxton D, Anderson IE, Longbottom D et al (2002) Ovine chlamydial abortion: characterization of the inflammatory immune response in placental tissues. J Comp Pathol 127:133–141
24. Reinhold P, Sachse K, Kaltenboeck B (2011) Chlamydiaceae in cattle: commensals, trigger organisms, or pathogens? Vet J 189:257–267
25. Di Francesco A, Donati M, Rossi M et al (2008) Tetracycline-resistant *Chlamydia suis* isolates in Italy. Vet Rec 163:251–252
26. Michel R, Daraoui A, Gorny M et al (2012) Iodine-129 and iodine-127 in European seawaters and in precipitation from Northern Germany. Sci Total Environ 419:151–169
27. Kauffold J, Melzer F, Berndt A et al (2006) Chlamydiae in oviducts and uteri of repeat breeder pigs. Theriogenology 66:1816–1823
28. Borel N, Kempf E, Hotzel H et al (2008) Direct identification of chlamydiae from clinical samples using a DNA microarray assay: a validation study. Mol Cell Probes 22:55–64
29. Braun SD, Ziegler A, Methner U et al (2012) Fast DNA serotyping and antimicrobial resistance gene determination of *Salmonella enterica* with an oligonucleotide microarray-based assay. PLoS One 7:e46489
30. Monecke S, Coombs G, Shore AC et al (2011) A field guide to pandemic, epidemic and sporadic clones of methicillin-resistant *Staphylococcus aureus*. PLoS One 6:e17936
31. Geue L, Schares S, Mintel B et al (2010) Rapid microarray-based genotyping of enterohemorrhagic *Escherichia coli* serotype O156:H25/H-/Hnt isolates from cattle and clonal relationship analysis. Appl Environ Microbiol 76:5510–5519
32. Sachse K, Hotzel H, Slickers P, Ellinger T, Ehricht R (2005) DNA microarray-based detection and identification of *Chlamydia* and *Chlamydophila* spp. Mol Cell Probes 19:41–50
33. Hoffmann B, Depner K, Schirrmeier H, Beer M (2006) A universal heterologous internal control system for duplex real-time RT-PCR assays used in a detection system for pestiviruses. J Virol Methods 136:200–209
34. Kamla V, Henrich B, Hadding U (1996) Phylogeny based on elongation factor Tu reflects the phenotypic features of mycoplasmas better than that based on 16S rRNA. Gene 171:83–87

Chapter 16

In Situ Hybridization with Labeled Probes: Assessment of African Swine Fever Virus in Formalin-Fixed Paraffin-Embedded Tissues

Maria Ballester and Fernando Rodríguez

Abstract

In situ hybridization (ISH) has become a very valuable molecular diagnostic tool to detect specific DNA or RNA sequences in biological samples through the use of complementary DNA- or RNA-labeled probes. Here, we describe an optimized in situ hybridization protocol to detect African swine fever virus (ASFV) DNA in formalin-fixed, paraffin-embedded tissues using digoxigenin-labeled probes.

Key words In situ hybridization, Nucleic acid, Formalin-fixed paraffin-embedded tissues, Digoxigenin, Molecular diagnostic tool, African swine fever virus

1 Introduction

In situ hybridization is a method that allows the precise location and/or quantification of specific DNA or RNA sequences in morphologically preserved chromosomes, tissues, or cell preparations. The principle of the technique is based on the remarkable stability of the double DNA helix through the hydrogen bonding of complementary strands, which can be broken (DNA denaturation or melting) with heat or chemicals and rejoined (DNA hybridization) under normal conditions. Thus, specific nucleotide-labeled probes are annealed to complementary sequences and visualized using different detection systems depending on the type of label used to tag the probe [1].

Since the first ISH experiment in the late 1960s [2], in which the method was applied to localize DNA/RNA hybrids in cytological preparations, the method has undergone many improvements to become an important tool for both research and diagnostic purposes.

Nowadays, there are a variety of ISH procedures with different applications [3–5] although the main steps are basically the same.

Mónica V. Cunha and João Inácio (eds.), *Veterinary Infection Biology: Molecular Diagnostics and High-Throughput Strategies*, Methods in Molecular Biology, vol. 1247, DOI 10.1007/978-1-4939-2004-4_16,

The purpose of this chapter is to describe an ISH protocol to detect African swine fever virus (ASFV) genome in formalin-fixed, paraffin-embedded tissues [6]. For this purpose, a double-stranded DNA-digoxigenin-labeled probe isolated from purified virions was used. The different steps of the protocol (probe preparation, permeabilization, hybridization, post-hybridization washes, and detection) have been adapted to lead to higher specificity and sensibility of virus detection in different tissues.

2 Materials

Prepare all the stock solutions using ultrapure water- and analytical-grade reagents and store them at room temperature (unless otherwise indicated). Please follow the lab security issues governed by your national regulations on good laboratory practices, check how to securely work with the chemicals described in this protocol, and follow all waste disposal regulations diligently.

2.1 Probes

1. Restriction enzyme: *Mbo*I (*see* **Note 1**).
2. Purification kit for small dsDNA fragments (*see* **Note 2**).
3. Digoxigenin DNA labeling system (*see* **Note 3**).
4. Competitor DNA (*see* **Note 4**).
5. 3 M sodium acetate, pH 5.5: Dissolve 24.609 g of sodium acetate trihydrate in 80 ml of water. Mix and adjust pH with glacial acetic acid and add water to 100 ml. Sterilize by autoclaving.
6. Absolute ethanol. Dilute with water to prepare also 70 % of ethanol.
7. Hybridization buffer: 50 % (v/v) of formamide (*see* **Note 5**), 2× of SSC, 10 % (w/v) of dextran sulfate, 1 % (v/v) of Tween-20. Prepare 1 L of 20× SSC, pH 6.3 stock solution by dissolving 175.3 g of NaCl, and 88.2 g of sodium citrate dihydrate in 800 ml of water. Adjust the pH with HCl and add water to 1 L. Sterilize by autoclaving. The final concentrations of the ingredients are 3 M of NaCl and 0.3 M of sodium citrate. To prepare 20 ml of hybridization buffer, use 10 ml of formamide, 2 ml of 20× SSC, 4 ml of 50 % (w/v) dextran sulfate solution, and 2 ml of 10 % (v/v) Tween-20 and make up with water to 20 ml. Store in small aliquots at −20 °C.

2.2 ISH

1. Automation buffer: 1× automation buffer was prepared in water from a 10× stock solution (GeneTex) (*see* **Note 6**).
2. Protease solution: 0.25 mg/ml of proteinase K in 2× SSC (*see* **Note 7**).
3. Denaturation solution: 70 % (v/v) of formamide in 2× SSC (*see* **Note 5**).

4. Humidified chamber or box (*see* **Note 8**).
5. Rubber cement.
6. Buffer 1: 100 mM of Tris–HCl, pH 7.5, 150 mM of NaCl. Prepare 1 L of buffer 1 by dissolving 12.11 g of Tris base and 8.765 g of NaCl in 900 ml of water and adjust the pH to 7.5 with HCl. Make up with water to 1 L. Sterilize by autoclaving.
7. Buffer 2: 100 mM of Tris–HCl, pH 9.5, 100 mM of NaCl, 50 mM of $MgCl_2$. Prepare 1 L of buffer 2 by dissolving 12.11 g of Tris base, 5.84 g of NaCl, and 10.17 g of magnesium chloride hexahydrate in 900 ml of water and adjust the pH to 9.5 with HCl. Make up with water to 1 L. Sterilize by autoclaving.
8. Buffer 3: 10 mM of Tris–HCl, pH 8, 1.27 mM of EDTA. Prepare 1 L of buffer 3 by dissolving 1.211 g of Tris base and 0.372 g of EDTA in 900 ml of water and adjust the pH to 8 with HCl. Make up with water to 1 L. Sterilize by autoclaving.
9. Wash solution 1: 0.5× SSC, 0.4 % (v/v) of Tween-20, 0.25 % of Brij-35. To prepare 50 ml of wash solution 1, add 200 μl of Tween-20, 125 μl of Brij-35, and 1250 μl of 20× SSC and make up with water to 50 ml (*see* **Note 9**).
10. Wash solution 2: 0.25× SSC, 0.4 % (v/v) of Tween-20, 0.25 % of Brij-35. To prepare 50 ml of wash solution 2, add 200 μl of Tween-20, 125 μl of Brij-35, and 625 μl of 20× SSC and make up with water to 50 ml (*see* **Note 9**).
11. Wash solution 3: 0.4 % (v/v) of Tween-20, 0.25 % of Brij-35. To prepare 50 ml of wash solution 3, add 200 μl of Tween-20 and 125 μl of Brij-35 and make up with buffer 2 to 50 ml (*see* **Note 9**).
12. Blocking solution: 1 % (v/v) of sheep serum, 0.3 % (v/v) of Triton X-100. To prepare 50 ml of blocking solution, add 500 μl of sheep serum, available commercially, and 150 μl of Triton X-100 and make up with buffer 1 to 50 ml (*see* **Note 9**).

2.3 Detection System and Counterstain

1. Anti-DIG solution: Anti-digoxigenin antibody conjugated to alkaline phosphatase diluted in blocking solution (*see* **Note 10**).
2. NBT/BCIP solution: Dilute 55 μl of NBT/BCIP stock solution (18.75 mg/ml of nitro blue tetrazolium chloride and 9.4 mg/ml of 5-bromo-4-chloro-3-indolyl phosphate, toluidine salt, in 67 % (v/v) of dimethyl sulfoxide; available commercially) in 2 ml of Wash solution 3.
3. Fast Green solution: To prepare 250 ml of Fast Green solution, add 3.75 g of Fast Green FCF dye and make up with water to 250 ml.

2.4 Special Equipment

Several ISH steps (post-hybridization washes and detection) can be performed in an automated workstation (e.g., MicroProbe Staining Station, Fisher Scientific) to handle the slides and minimize reagent consumption. However, all the steps can also be performed manually in coplin jars.

3 Methods

Carry out all the procedures at room temperature unless otherwise specified.

3.1 Probe Preparation

1. Digest total viral DNA, isolated from purified virions, with the appropriate restriction enzyme following the manufacturer instructions (*see* **Note 11**).
2. Purify the DNA after digestion using a DNA purification kit and quantify the concentration of digested DNA (*see* **Note 12**).
3. Run an agarose gel to assure the complete digestion of viral DNA by determining the length of the DNA fragments (Fig. 1) (*see* **Note 13**).
4. Label the DNA fragments using a DNA labeling system, following the instructions of the fabricant (*see* **Note 14**).
5. After DNA labeling, purify probes using a DNA purification kit and quantify the concentration of the labeled DNA (*see* **Note 12**).
6. Mix 300 ng of DNA-labeled probes (*see* **Note 15**) with 30 μg of competitor DNA and add water to obtain a precipitable volume (minimum volume of 30 μl).

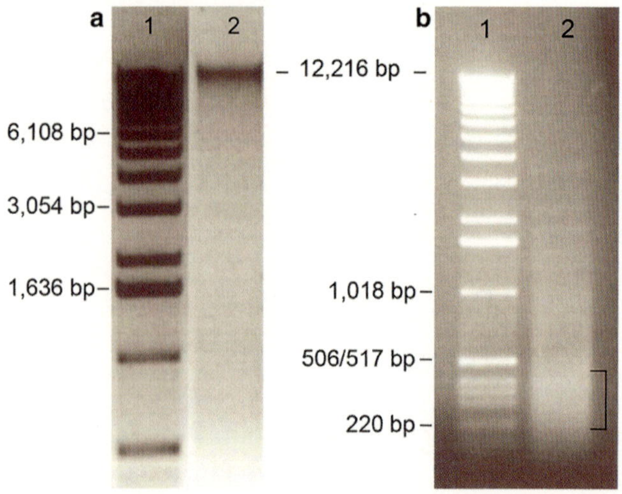

Fig. 1 ASFV viral DNA digested with restriction enzyme. (**a**) Lane 1: DNA ladder. Lane 2: two microliters (400 ng) of non-digested ASFV viral DNA. (**b**) Lane 1: DNA ladder. Lane 2: ten microliters (763 ng) of *MboI* digested ASFV viral DNA

7. Precipitate the mixed DNA using a standard ethanol precipitation protocol (*see* **Note 16**).
8. Resuspend the DNA probes in 33 μl of hybridization buffer (*see* **Note 17**) and store at −20 °C (*see* **Note 18**).

3.2 In Situ Hybridization

1. Dewax paraffin-embedded tissue sections 3 times in xylene, 6 min each time (*see* **Note 19**).
2. Rehydrate the tissue sections through an ethanol series (2 times in absolute ethanol, twice in 96 % ethanol, and once in water, 3 min each time) and wash in 1× automation buffer (*see* **Note 20**).
3. Digest the tissue sections with 25–30 μl of protease solution for 10 min at 37 °C (*see* **Note 21**) in a humidified box. Cover the sections with parafilm (*see* **Note 22**).
4. After the pretreatment with protease solution, wash all sections with 1× automation buffer.
5. Denature the DNA probes at 75 °C for 10 min and pre-anneal them at 37 °C for 90 min (*see* **Note 23**).
6. Denature the tissue sections at 75 °C for 10 min in denaturation solution (*see* **Notes 23** and **24**).
7. Following tissue sections denaturation, distribute the 33 μl of each DNA probe preparation over each section, cover them with coverslips, seal with rubber cement, and incubate in a humidified box at 37 °C overnight (*see* **Note 25**).
8. Following the overnight hybridization step, immerse the preparations in 2× SSC to allow the coverslips to drop off.
9. Wash the slides 2× with wash solution 1, 5 min each time.
10. Wash the slides with wash solution 2 at 37 °C for 5 min.
11. Block the slides 2× with blocking solution, 5 min each time (*see* **Note 26**).
12. Add anti-DIG solution and incubate for 1 h at 37 °C (*see* **Note 27**).
13. Rinse the slides 2–3 times with blocking solution.
14. Rinse the slides 3–4 times with 1× automation buffer.
15. Wash the slides with wash solution 3 for 5 min.
16. Add NBT/BCIP solution and incubate during 15–20 min at 37 °C in the dark (*see* **Notes 28** and **29**).
17. Rinse the slides 1–2 times with buffer 3 to stop the color reaction and deep the preparations into buffer 3 until the Fast Green counterstaining step.
18. Counterstain the preparations with Fast Green solution for 10 min.
19. Wash with distilled water.
20. Mount sections and examine by light microscopy (Fig. 2) (*see* **Notes 30** and **31**).

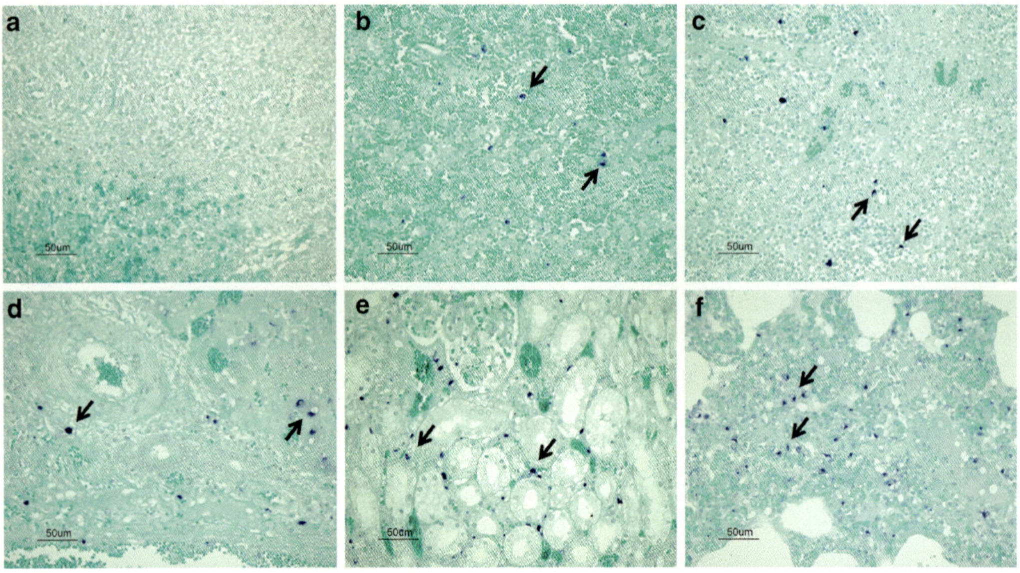

Fig. 2 ASFV-DNA detection using DIG-labeled probes in formalin-fixed paraffin-embedded tissues. (**a**) Negative lymph node. (**b–f**) Positive tissues, where *dark-blue dots* in the preparation correspond to the presence of viral nucleic acids (examples of positive labeling are indicated with *arrows*). (**b**) Spleen. Intense positive detection in red pulp macrophages and trabecular medullary areas. (**c**) Lymph node. Moderate positive detection in perifollicular macrophages (marginal zone). (**d**) Liver. Moderate to intense positive detection in sinusoidal and alveolar macrophages and Kupffer cells. (**e**) Kidney. Intense positive detection in circulating macrophages and renal endothelium. (**f**) Lung. Intense positive detection in pulmonary alveolar, vascular, and parenchymal macrophages

4 Notes

1. ISH experiments can be performed with different types of probes (DNA, cDNA, RNA, oligonucleotides, etc.). One of the limitations to overcome during the ISH procedure is the probe size. When using probes of dsDNA, the optimal probe size is between 200 and 500 bp. In our case, we are using all the ASFV viral genome (approx. 180 kb) and, for that reason, we choose a restriction enzyme, *Mbo*I, with a recognition site equal to 4 bases long (GATC) to cut ASFV genome very frequently. This enzyme generates medium ASFV-DNA fragment lengths of 300–500 bp (Fig. 1).
2. Any method or commercial kit which recovers small dsDNA fragments can be used here. We use Qiagen Nucleotide Removal Kit (Qiagen).
3. dsDNA probes prepared by random priming present higher yield of labeled probe compared with nick-translation method. We use DIG-High Prime system (Roche) for labeling dsDNA probes.

4. To avoid unspecific hybridization of labeled probes in the cellular cytoplasm or slides, add unlabeled competitor DNA. Usually, we use competitor DNA from different species, available from commercial companies, such as fish sperm DNA (100 μg of competitor DNA for each microgram of DNA probe).
5. Use deionized formamide. Wear appropriate gloves and safety glasses when handling solutions containing formamide. Formamide should be handled in a fume hood.
6. Alternatively, a PBS-Tween-20 buffer can be used: 1× PBS, 0.1 % (v/v) Tween-20. Add 1 ml of Tween-20 (take slowly) to 1 L of 1× PBS and stir for some time.
7. Prepare fresh solution immediately before use.
8. The humidified box consists of a closed plastic container (e.g., slide box) with paper towel at the bottom. Before use, humidify the paper towel with distilled water.
9. Prepare fresh solution and mix with a magnetic stirrer at low speed for 15 min before use.
10. We use anti-digoxigenin antibody conjugated to alkaline phosphatase (Fab fragments from sheep, Roche) diluted 1:500.
11. As stated in **Note 1**, there are different types of probes. Oligonucleotide probes have been successfully used to detect small viruses [7, 8], but it depends on some viral characteristics such us genome size, replication cycle, and/or the presence of envelope. For pathogens with large DNA genomes, we recommend the use of longer probes (up to 500 bp) which will cover more target sequences. We have previously tested three types of DIG-labeled probes (a pool of three oligonucleotide probes, a 18.5 kb restriction enzyme viral DNA fragment, and a complete viral genome probe) to detect ASFV in formalin-fixed paraffin-embedded tissues, and the genome full-length probe was the most sensitive one [6]. The description of the culture procedures and preparation of the purified virions is out of the scope of this chapter but can be assessed in Carrascosa et al. [9].
12. A spectrophotometric or any other available method can be used here for DNA quantification.
13. This step is very important to obtain probes with good penetration properties. If there is no available restriction enzyme, DNA can be digested with DNase or disrupted by sonication.
14. It is important to test different quantities of template DNA to obtain the highest yield of labeled probe. The amount of newly synthesized labeled DNA depends on the purity of the template DNA and varies also depending on the starting template DNA amount and the incubation time. We obtained the higher yield of DIG-labeled probe from 100 ng of template DNA and 20 h of incubation.

15. Test different quantities of DNA-labeled probes to obtain the optimal signal without increasing background. We have previously tested 150, 300, and 500 ng of DIG-labeled probes. While the former led to weak signals, we obtained the same sensitivity with the other two absolute quantities.
16. Add 1/10 volume of sodium acetate, 3 M, pH 5.5, and vortex. Next, add 2.5× volumes of absolute ethanol and vortex. Centrifuge at maximum speed (20,000 × *g*) for 15 min at 4 °C. Discard supernatant and rinse with 70 % ethanol. Centrifuge again for 5 min at 4 °C. Finally, discard supernatant and allow the DNA pellet to dry in air for 10 min.
17. Vortex and allow the pellet of DNA to be homogenously resuspended at room temperature for 90 min. Vortex the sample every 10–15 min during the incubation.
18. You can prepare and stock several DNA-labeled probes. They can be stored at −20 °C during several months.
19. In our experiments, tissues were fixed in 10 % neutral buffered formalin for 2 weeks. Prolonged fixation time is a critical step.
20. Tissue preparations can be maintained in 1× automation buffer during the preparation of the protease solution.
21. This pretreatment step is crucial to increase the efficiency of hybridization by increasing the target accessibility. The concentration of proteinase K and incubation time depend on tissue type and length of fixation. However, it is also important to consider the virus isolate, which may present different virulence, and the target infected tissues, when performing the protease treatment, because too much proteinase K can disintegrate the tissue totally. We recommend testing different concentrations and incubation times of proteinase K before performing the complete ISH protocol.

    Although other protease treatments such as the use of pepsin has been proved to be very efficient in formalin-fixed paraffin-embedded tissues, in our ISH experiments we obtained a higher and more intense signal with better tissue integrity and lower background using the proteinase K treatment [6].
22. Pre-warm the humidified box at 37 °C. Cut small pieces of parafilm and cover the tissue sections without pressing them.
23. Calculate the time of denaturation and pre-annealing to have the DNA probes ready to use after the tissue section denaturation step.
24. We perform this step in a closed coplin jar in a water bath. As the denaturation solution temperature is lower than the water bath temperature, it is necessary to increase the water bath temperature several degrees (5–10 °C) to reach the desired denaturation solution temperature. To assure no variations in the hybridization temperature, we measure directly the tem-

perature of the denaturation solution. Do not open and close the coplin jar very frequently to avoid temperature variations.

25. Before inserting the slides in the pre-warmed humidified box, let the rubber cement dry completely. This step is very important to facilitate the contact of the DNA-labeled probes with their target sequences.
26. This step can be done in the workstation by immersing the whole slides in blocking solution or adding a drop (100–150 μl) of blocking solution onto the slides.
27. This step can be done in the workstation filling by capillarity the interspace existing between two slides or adding a drop (100 μl) of anti-DIG solution onto the sections and incubating them in the humidified box following the same indications pointed out in **Note 22**.
28. This step can be done in the workstation filling by capillarity the interspace existing between two slides or adding a drop (100–150 μl) of NBT/BCIP solution onto the sections.
29. A positive signal may be seen after a few minutes depending of viral replication. The reaction time may be evaluated by checking microscopically the signal/noise ratio.
30. We use DPX mounting medium. Preparations are dehydrated through an ethanol series (once in 70 % ethanol, once in 96 % ethanol, and twice in absolute ethanol, 3 min each time) and 1× acetone-xylene (50:50) for 6 min, cleared twice for 6 min each in xylene and mounted in DPX.
31. Prepare negative controls by omitting the specific probes in the hybridization mix, using the specific probes in noninfected tissues or by using unrelated probes in infected tissues.

Acknowledgment

This work has been fully supported by the AGL2010-22229-C03-01 Project from the Ministerio de Economía y Competitividad, Spanish Government.

References

1. Jin L, Lloyd RV (1997) In situ hybridization: methods and applications. J Clin Lab Anal 11:2–9
2. Gall JG, Padue ML (1969) Formation and detection of RNA-DNA hybrid molecules in cytological preparation. Proc Natl Acad Sci U S A 63:378–383
3. Ballester M, Rodríguez-Cariño C, Pérez M et al (2011) Disruption of nuclear organization during the initial phase of African Swine Fever Virus infection. J Virol 85:8263–8269
4. Jehan Z, Uddin S, Al-Kuraya KS (2012) In-situ hybridization as a molecular tool in cancer diagnosis and treatment. Curr Med Chem 19:3730–3738
5. Wheeler G, Valoczi A, Havelda Z et al (2007) In situ detection of animal and plant microRNAs. DNA Cell Biol 26:251–255

6. Ballester M, Galindo-Cardiel I, Gallardo C et al (2010) Intranuclear detection of African swine fever virus DNA in several cell types from formalin-fixed and paraffin-embedded tissues using a new in situ hybridization protocol. J Virol Methods 168:38–43
7. Cubie HA, Grzybowski J, da Silva C et al (1995) Synthetic oligonucleotide cocktails as probes for detection of human parvovirus B19. J Virol Methods 53:91–102
8. Rosell C, Segalés J, Plana-Duran J et al (1999) Pathological, immunohistochemical, and in-situ hybridization studies of natural cases of postweaning multisystemic wasting syndrome (PMWS) in pigs. J Comp Pathol 120: 59–78
9. Carrascosa AL, del Val M, Santarén JF et al (1985) Purification and properties of African swine fever virus. J Virol 54:337–344

Chapter 17

Fluorescence In Situ Hybridization for the Tissue Detection of Bacterial Pathogens Associated with Porcine Infections

Henrik Elvang Jensen, Louise Kruse Jensen, Kristiane Barington, Susanne Elisabeth Pors, Thomas Bjarnsholt, and Mette Boye

Abstract

Fluorescence in situ hybridization (FISH) is an efficient technique for the identification of specific bacteria in tissue of both experimental and spontaneous infections. The method detects specific sequences of nucleic acids by hybridization of fluorescently labeled probes to complementary target sequences within intact cells. FISH allows direct histological localization of the bacteria in the tissue and thereby a correlation between the infection and the histopathological changes present. This chapter presents protocols for FISH identification of bacterial pathogens in fixed deparaffinized tissue samples mounted on glass slides. Two different methods are presented: one is illustrated with the use of peptide nucleic acid (PNA) that is carried out directly on glass slides (Method I), whereas the other is exemplified by using a DNA probe in a Shandon rack (Method II). In the two methods, both PNA and DNA probes can be used.

Key words Bacteria, DNA, PNA, FISH, Fluorescence, Hybridization, In situ, Porcine, rRNA, Tissue

1 Introduction

Fluorescence in situ hybridization (FISH) has proven effective for detecting specific species of bacteria in both experimental and spontaneous infections in pigs (Table 1). The method detects specific sequences of nucleic acids by hybridization of fluorescently labeled oligonucleotide probes to complementary target sequences within intact cells (Figs. 1 and 2) [1]. FISH can be used for the detection of DNA and RNA sequences [2]. For the identification of bacteria by the FISH technique, ribosomal RNA (rRNA)-targeting probes are most commonly applied because of the natural amplification of rRNA molecules [3]. Bacterial rRNA is present in all cells and highly conserved between species, but still contains variable sequences which serve as the target for identification at species level. Bacterial 70S ribosomes consist of a 50S subunit and a 30S subunit. The 50S subunit consists of two RNA molecules

Mónica V. Cunha and João Inácio (eds.), *Veterinary Infection Biology: Molecular Diagnostics and High-Throughput Strategies*, Methods in Molecular Biology, vol. 1247, DOI 10.1007/978-1-4939-2004-4_17, © Springer Science+Business Media New York 2015

Table 1
Panel of rRNA-targeting probes used for the detection of pathogenic bacteria by fluorescence in situ hybridization in porcine tissue samples

Target species	Tissue sample	Systematic name[a]	Probe sequence (5′–3′)	References
Actinobacillus pleuropneumoniae	Lung, ear, joints, bone, brain	S-S-Ap-0185-a-A-19	CCCACCCTTTAATCCATAG	[11–14]
Genus *Brachyspira*	Intestine	L-G-Serp-1410-a-A-19	GTCATTCCATCGAAACATA	[15–17]
Brachyspira hyodysenteriae	Intestine	L-S-S.hyo-1210-a-A-19	CTCACGATGAACCTTCGAC	[15, 17, 18]
Brachyspira murdochii	Intestine	L-S-B.murdoc-1219-a-A-18	CCGCCTTACGGCAAACCT	[17]
Brachyspira pilosicoli	Intestine	S-S-S.pilo-0209-a-A-18	GCTCATCGTGAAGCGAAA	[15–17]
Clostridium perfringens	Intestine	S-S-Cperfring-0185-a-A-18	TGGTTGAATGATGATGCC	[19, 20]
Clostridium difficile	Intestine	S-S-Cl.diff-0193-a-A-18	TGTACTGGCTCACCTTTG	[19]
Chlamydiales	Intestine	S-O-Chls-0523-a-A-18	CCTCCGTATTACCGCAGC	[21]
Chlamydiaceae	Intestine	S-F-Cla-0574-a-A-18	CTTTCCGCCTACACGCCC	[21]
Chlamydia	Intestine	S-G-Chla-0232-a-A-18	TAGCTGATATCACATAGA	[21]
Chlamydophila	Intestine	S-G-Chlph-0583-a-A-18	CTAACTTTCCTTTCCGCC	[21]
Enterococcus faecium	Intestine	L-S-Efaecium-0347-a-A-18	GTGTCTTCCACATTTCGT	[20]

Erysipelothrix rhusiopathiae	Heart	S-S-E.rhusiopathiae-0449-a-A-18	TCCCTCTTCCTATCGTTC	[22]
Escherichia coli	Intestine	L-S-Eco-1531-a-A-21	CACCGTAGTGCCTCGTCATCA	[23]
Klebsiella pneumoniae	Intestine	L-S-Kpneu-1705-a-A-18	TACACACCAGCGTGCCTT	[20]
Leptospira interrogans	Intestine	S-G-Leptospira-1414-a-A-18	CGGGTGCTCCCCACTCAG	[24]
Lawsonia intracellularis	Intestine	S-S-L.intrac-1148-a-A-20	AACCGGAGCAGTCTCTCTAG	[6, 25–28]
Mycoplasma hyopneumoniae	Lung, heart	S-S-M.hyop-0466-a-A-18	CCGTCAAGACTAGAGCAT	[29]
Mycoplasma hyosynoviae	Lung, heart, joints	S-S-M.hyos-0466-a-A-18	CCGTCAGTTCAGTTGCAT	[29]
Mycoplasma hyorhinis	Lung, heart	S-S-M.hyor-0193-a-A-18	GCTGTGAAGCTCCTTTCT	[29]
Pasteurella multocida	Lung, heart, kidney	S-S-Pmul-0449-a-A-20	CTATTTAACAACATCCCTTC	[30, 31]
Salmonella spp.	Intestine	L-S-Sal-1713-a-A-18	AATCACTTCACCTACGTG	[32, 33]
Streptococcus suis	Heart, brain	S-S-S.suis-0183-a-A-18	CCATGCGGTAAATACTGT	[22, 34]
Treponema spp.	Intestine	S-S-Treponema-0833-a-A-18	CCCAGTCCTCATGACCAG	[24]

[a]According to Alm et al. [35]

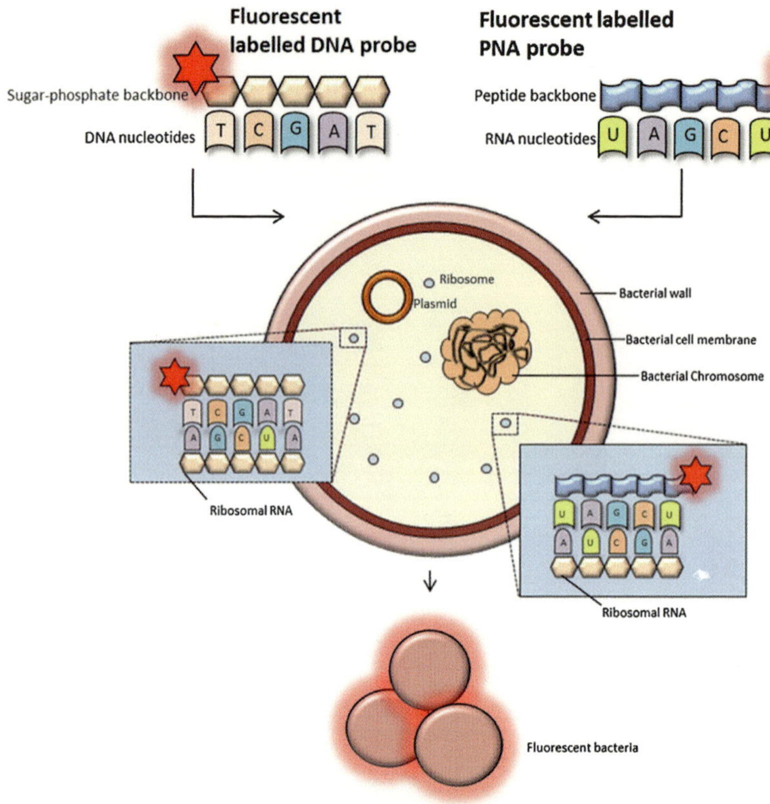

Fig. 1 FISH using oligonucleotide probes. FISH probes can be classified as DNA or PNA probes depending on the structure of the backbone. PNA probes are non-charged which allow a tighter and more specific binding to RNA nucleic acid targets. DNA probes must overcome a destabilizing electrostatic repulsion during hybridization. The fluorescently labeled probes target RNA of the bacterial ribosomes (rRNA). The 16S and 23S rRNA gene sequences contain hyper variable regions that can provide species-specific signature sequences useful for bacterial identification, which most often is utilized in FISH. *A* adenine, *T* thymine (DNA specific), *G* guanine, *C* cytosine, and *U* uracil (RNA specific)

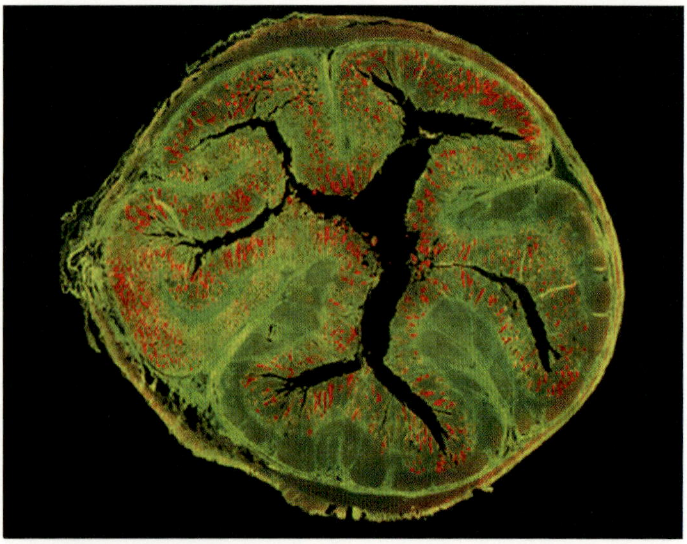

Fig. 2 Visualization of *Lawsonia intracellularis* (*red*) by in situ hybridization within a cross section of a porcine ileum. The tissue is *green* due to autofluorescence. From: Mølbak et al., 2008, Vet Microbiol, 128, 96–107 [25], with permission

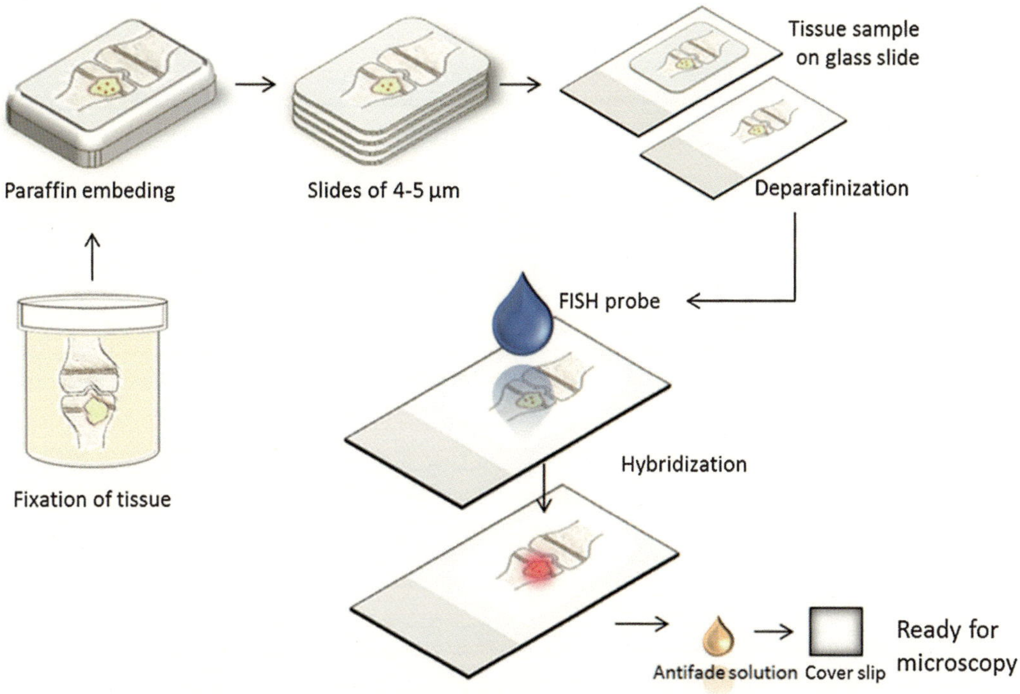

Fig. 3 A bone with osteomyelitis is fixated in formalin and afterward embedded in paraffin. The block of paraffin is cut with a microtome and the tissue is mounted on glass slides. It is necessary to remove the paraffin before the application of the FISH probe. Following hybridization, it is possible to see the fluorescent bacteria within the tissue using a microscope or a scanner equipped for fluorescence

(5S and 23S), while the 30S subunit consists of a single RNA molecule (16S). The 16S rRNA is the preferred target for the identification of specific bacteria due to its combination of conserved sites and variable regions [4]. The 23S rRNA subunit may be used as well; however, as it has not been sequenced in a number of bacteria, most probes are targeting specific 16S rRNA. The FISH technique is easy to apply and of a low cost [1]. When the probes have been designed and evaluated, the FISH technique can be completed in a few hours [5]. In addition, the technique allows the direct localization of the bacteria in the tissue and thereby a histological correlation between the bacteria the tissue morphology and the pathological changes present (Fig. 2). Predominantly, viable cells are detected as rRNA is fragile and rapidly disintegrates if the cell has suffered irreversible damage [6]. Because the identification of bacteria by FISH is dependent on the sequence of the probe, the technique will not identify unknown species [4]. However, universal (pan-bacterial) probes are useful for the initial screening of sections for contents of bacteria [1].

The FISH technique consists of four steps: (1) fixation and permeabilization of the sample, (2) hybridization, (3) removing unbound probe, and (4) detection of labeled cells (Figs. 2 and 3).

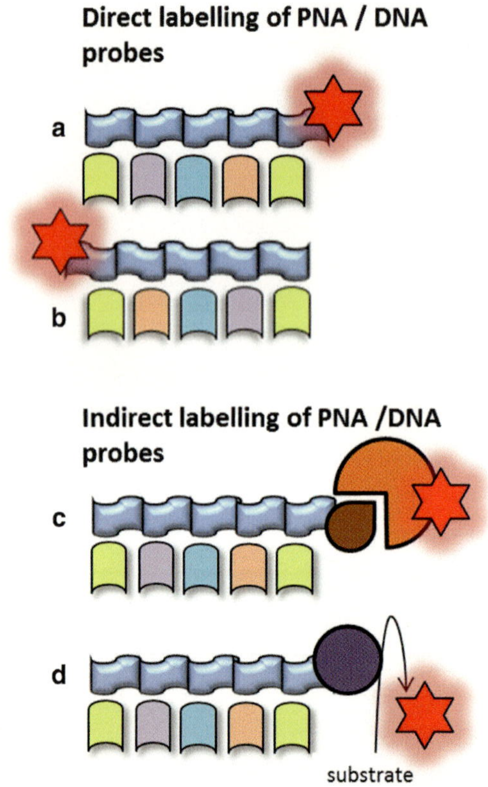

Fig. 4 (**a**) Direct labeling of the 3′ tail of the probe. (**b**) Direct labeling of the 5′ tail of the probe. (**c**) Labeling of the probe with a reporter molecule which is detected by a fluorescent antibody. (**d**) Labeling of the probe with horseradish peroxidase (HRP) using a substrate for an enzymatic signal amplification

Tissue samples must be fixed and permeabilized prior to hybridization to preserve nucleic acids and ensure that the fluorescently labeled probes can enter the cells. At hybridization, the probe binds to a specific sequence of rRNA inside the bacterial cells (Fig. 1). After removing any unbound probe by briefly rinsing, the tissue sample is ready for screening for reacting cells by fluorescence microscopy [3, 7].

The classical DNA probes consist of fluorescently labeled oligonucleotides or polynucleotides, targeting a specific sequence of microbial rRNA (Fig. 1) [3]. Moreover, peptide nucleic acid (PNA) probes have been developed (Fig. 1). The PNA probes, which are oligomers of single bases linked by a peptide backbone, are more stable to degradation and hybridize to complementary sequences with a higher affinity compared to the classical probes [1, 3, 7]. Probes can be labeled directly or indirectly (Fig. 4). Direct labeling of probes does not require further procedures after hybridization. Indirect labeling of probes uses a reporter molecule or an enzyme bound to the probe and will often result in a brighter signal (Fig. 4).

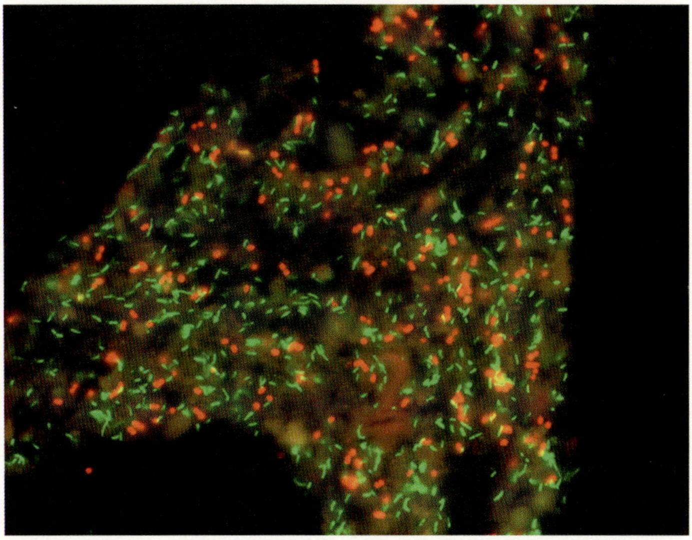

Fig. 5 Visualization of *Bifidobacterium* spp. (*green*) and *Megasphaera elsdenii* (*red*) by in situ hybridization in a formalin-fixed porcine colon tissue sample

After hybridization, a fluorescent antibody or substrate for enzymatic signal amplification is added depending on the type of labeling of the probe [1]. Identification of different bacterial species in a single tissue sample can be carried out by the application of different fluorophores labeled to each type of probe (Fig. 5).

A number of genus- and species-specific probes have successfully been designed and applied for the detection of bacteria of importance in the pig (Table 1), some being available commercially, e.g., *Staphylococcus aureus* [8].

In the following sections of materials and methods, two different methods (I and II) for FISH are included (Subheadings 2.4 and 3.5 for Method I and Subheadings 2.5 and 3.6 for Method II). Both methods require fixation of tissue (Subheadings 2.1 and 3.1; Fig. 3), deparaffinization (Subheadings 2.2. and 3.2; Fig. 3), and preparation of the probe solution (Subheadings 2.3, 3.3, and 3.4).

2 Materials

2.1 Fixation of Tissue (Fig. 3)

1. Tissue sample.
2. 10 % neutral-buffered formalin, pH 6.8 (formaldehyde, 37–40 %: 100 mL/L; distilled water 900 mL/L; sodium phosphate, monobasic 4.0 g/L; sodium phosphate, dibasic (anhydrous) 6.5 g/L).
3. 70 %, 96 %, and 99 % ethanol.
4. Xylene.

5. Paraffin wax.
6. Bowl of water.
7. Plastic container with a tight-fitting lid.
8. Tissue cool plate.
9. Microtome.
10. Adhesive glass slides, e.g., SuperFrost Plus slides (Gerhard Menzel GmbH, Braunschweig, Germany), poly-L-lysine-coated glass (Ted Pella, Inc., Redding, CA, USA), or Biobond Tissue Section Adhesive (AX-LAB, Copenhagen, Denmark).

2.2 Deparaffinization (Fig. 3)

1. Paraffin-embedded tissue sections on glass slides.
2. Xylene.
3. 96 % and 99.9 % ethanol.
4. Sterile water.
5. Incubator (60 °C).

2.3 Probe Solution

1. Probe in stock, PNA or DNA probes (*see* Table 1 for examples of probe sequences).
2. Hybridization buffer, 50 mL of 1 M Tris–HCl (pH 7.2), 90 mL of 5 M NaCl, 5 mL of 10 % (w/v) sodium dodecyl sulfate (SDS), and H_2O up to total volume of 500 mL (the final composition of the hybridization buffer is 100 mM of Tris–HCl (pH 7.2), 0.9 M of NaCl, and 0.1 % of SDS).
3. Crushed ice.
4. Styrofoam box.
5. Microcentrifuge tubes (1.5 mL).

2.4 Method I: Hybridization with PNA or DNA Probes on Tissue Sections Mounted on Glass Slides (Fig. 3)

1. Tissue sections on glass slides (deparaffinized).
2. Probe solution.
3. Coverslips, thickness 0.15 mm.
4. Pencil.
5. Heating block (55 °C) with a lid (*see* **Note 1**).
6. Washing buffer (55 °C), 50 mL of 1 M Tris–HCl (pH 7.2), 90 mL of 5 M NaCl, and H_2O up to total volume of 500 mL (the final composition of the washing buffer is 100 mM of Tris–HCl (pH 7.2) and 0.9 M of NaCl) (*see* **Note 1**).
7. Antifading mounting media, e. g., VECTASHIELD mounting media with 4′,6-diamidino-2-phenylindole (DAPI) (Vector Laboratories, Burlingame, CA, USA) or ImmunoSelect Antifading Mounting Medium (Dianova Gmbh, Hamburg, Germany).

8. Fluorescence microscope equipped with a 40–100× oil objective and a 100 W mercury lamp or similar, camera for fluorescence, and the correct filter sets for the chosen fluorescent-labeled probes to be used.
9. Nonfluorescent immersion oil for microscopy.

2.5 Method II: Hybridization with DNA or PNA Probes on Tissue Sections Mounted on Glass Slides Using a Shandon Rack (Fig. 6)

1. Tissue sections on glass slides (deparaffinized).
2. Probe solution.
3. Shandon rack (Thermo Shandon, Cheshire, United Kingdom).
4. Deionized water.
5. Washing buffer, 55 °C (*see* Subheading 2.4 and **Note 1**).
6. Tinfoil.
7. Incubator.
8. Hybridization buffer, 55 °C (*see* Subheading 2.3 and **Note 1**).
9. Coplin jar.
10. Clean lab napkin or open slide box.
11. MilliQ water.
12. Coverslips, thickness 0.15 mm.
13. Antifading mounting media (*see* Subheading 2.4).
14. Fluorescence microscope (*see* Subheading 2.4).
15. Nonfluorescent immersion oil for microscopy.

3 Methods

3.1 Fixation of Tissue (Fig. 3)

1. Fix the tissue samples by immersion in 10 % neutral-buffered formalin for 1–3 days in a plastic container with a tight-fitting lid (*see* **Note 2**).
2. After fixation, process the tissues through graded concentrations of ethanol (70 %, 96 %, and 99 %) and xylene and finally embed in paraffin wax.
3. Place the paraffin-embedded tissue blocks on a tissue cool plate (−5 °C) for a minimum of 5 min.
4. Cut sections at 4–5 μm thickness using a microtome and gently transfer to a bowl of water.
5. Mount the tissue sections on adhesive glass slides (by placing the slide beneath the tissue while it is still on the water surface and lifting it out of the water) (*see* **Note 3**).
6. Let the slides dry at room temperature (18–22 °C).

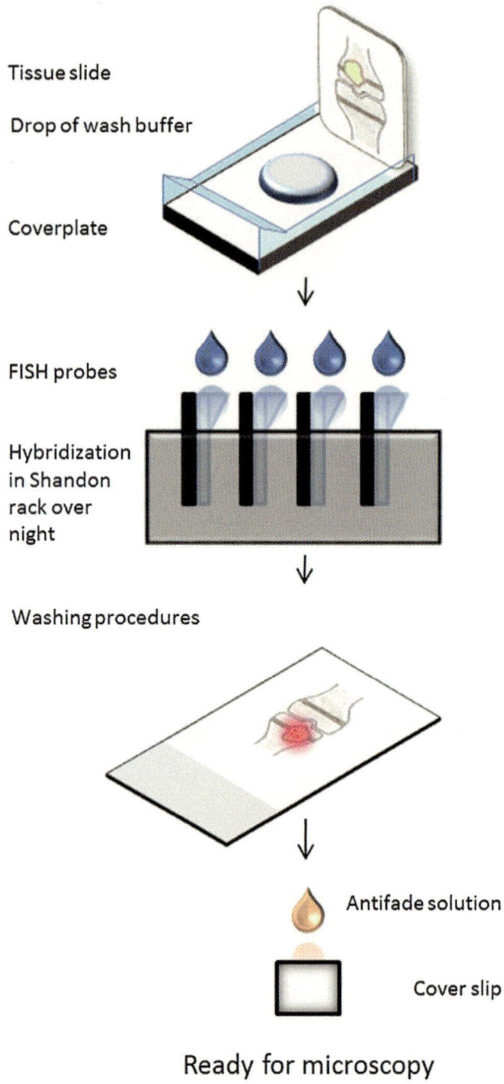

Fig. 6 Detection of bacteria with FISH in tissue mounted on glass slide using a Shandon rack

3.2 Deparaffinization (Fig. 3)

Prior to hybridization, paraffin wax must be removed and tissue sections rehydrated by completing the following six steps of deparaffinization:

1. Incubate the paraffin-embedded tissue sections on glass slides at 60 °C for 1 h.
2. Immerse the slides in xylene 2 times for 2–5 min.
3. Immerse the slides in 99.9 % ethanol 1–2 times for 2–3 min.
4. Immerse the slides in 96 % ethanol 1–2 times for 2–3 min.

5. Immerse the slides in sterile water 3 times for 3 min.
6. Air-dry the slides at room temperature (18–22 °C).
7. After deparaffinization, slides are ready for hybridization (*see* **Notes 4** and **5**).

3.3 Selecting a Probe

Nucleotide sequences of DNA and RNA can be found in online databases as, e.g., GenBank (http://www.ncbi.nlm.nih.gov/genbank/), DNA DataBank of Japan (http://www.ddbj.nig.ac.jp/), the European Molecular Biology Laboratory (http://www.embl.de/), SILVA rRNA database project (http://www.arb-silva.de/), and Greengenes (http://greengenes.secondgenome.com/). Complete nucleotide sequences of rRNA from various porcine pathogenic bacteria are available. Species-specific probes are designed by applying software such as ARB (Technische Universität München, Munich, Germany, http://www.arb-home.de/) on gene databases as those mentioned above. Labeled probes can be ordered by providing the nucleotide sequence of the specific sequence of rRNA at, e.g., GenScript USA Inc., Piscataway, NJ, USA; Tag Copenhagen, Copenhagen, Denmark; Eurofins MWG Operon AG, Ebersberg, Germany; and AdvanDx Inc., Woburn, Massachusetts, USA (*see* **Note 6**). Although a probe seems specific according to the software used, it is mandatory to have the specificity verified on a panel of well-characterized mono-bacterial tissue infections. One limiting issue when designing probes for FISH is that not all sites within the rRNA molecules are readily accessible for hybridization [9].

The method should be repeated with EUB338 and non-EUB338 as positive and negative controls, respectively, in hybridization experiments [10].

3.4 Probe Solution

1. PNA probes are typically received ready for use and are stored at 4 °C (*see* **Note 7**).
2. DNA probes are stored at −20 °C or −80 °C (*see* **Note 7**). If the probe is delivered as lyophilized, it should be dissolved in nuclease-free sterile water, e.g., to a stock concentration of 500 ng/μL.
3. Thaw the probes and keep them on ice within a Styrofoam box in the dark until preparing the probe solution. For each slide, 100 μL solution of probe should be used. Calculate with one extra slide in each hybridization solution. Calculate the total volume (V_{total}) of probe solution needed by using the following formula (where n_{slide} = number of slides):

$$V_{\text{total}} = 100\,\mu\text{L} \times \left(1 + n_{\text{slide}}\right)$$

4. The concentration of the probe in the solution should be 5 ng/μL for each probe. To calculate the volume needed from the probe in stock ($V_{\text{probe in stock}}$), use the following formulas:

$$m_{\text{probe}} = V_{\text{total}} \times 5\text{ng} / \mu\text{L}$$

$$V_{\text{probe in stock}} = \frac{m_{\text{probe}}}{C_{\text{probe in stock}}}$$

The m_{probe} is the mass of the probe needed in ng, while the $C_{\text{probe in stock}}$ is the concentration of the probe in stock in ng/μL. Calculate the volume of hybridization buffer ($V_{\text{hybridization buffer}}$) by using the following formula:

$$V_{\text{hybridization buffer}} = V_{\text{total}} - V_{\text{probe in stock}}$$

The calculated volumes of hybridization buffer ($V_{\text{hybridization buffer}}$) and probe in stock ($V_{\text{probe in stock}}$) are mixed in a microcentrifuge tube.

For example, preparing a probe solution for four slides and an extra slide:

$$V_{\text{total}} = 100\mu\text{L} \times (1+4) = 500\mu\text{L}$$

The concentration of the probe solution should be 5 ng/μL. If the concentration of the probe solution in stock is 13.5 ng/μL:

$$m_{\text{probe}} = 500\mu\text{L} \times 5\text{ng} / \mu\text{L} = 2{,}500\text{ng}$$

$$V_{\text{probe in stock}} = \frac{2{,}500\text{ ng}}{13.5\text{ng} / \mu\text{L}} = 185.2\mu\text{L}$$

$$V_{\text{hybridization buffer}} = 500\ \mu\text{L} - 185.2\ \mu\text{L} = 314.8\ \mu\text{L}.$$

185.2 μL of the probe solution in stock should be mixed with 314.8 μL of hybridization buffer to get at total volume of 500 μL with a concentration of 5 ng of probe per μL.

3.5 Method I: Hybridization with PNA or DNA Probes on Tissue Sections on Glass Slides (Fig. 3)

1. Place the slides with the tissue sections on a flat surface.
2. Add 50 μL (1 droplet) of the probe solution to each slide.
3. Place a coverslip on top of the material. Gently spread the probe under the slide and remove any bubbles by pressing the coverslip using a pencil.
4. Place the slide and coverslip on a heating block for hybridization at 55 °C for 90 min covered by a lid (*see* **Notes 1**, **7**, and **8**).
5. Remove the coverslip by dipping the slide in washing buffer.
6. Wash slides for 30 min at 55 °C in washing buffer (*see* **Notes 1** and **9**).

7. Apply antifading mounting media and add a coverslip to each slide. Gently press the slide with a pencil to spread the antifading mounting media and to remove bubbles.
8. Inspect slides by using a fluorescence microscope equipped with a camera and the appropriate filters for fluorescein isothiocyanate (FITC) (excitation/emission: 492–495 nm/520–525 nm), a Texas Red (excitation/emission: 591–596 nm/608–620 nm), and a DAPI (excitation/emission: 340–359 nm/461–488 nm). Also a dual FITC/Texas Red and a dual DAPI/Texas Red filter may be used (*see* **Notes 10** and **11**).

3.6 Method II: Hybridization with DNA or PNA Probes on Tissue Sections on Glass Slides Using a Shandon Rack (Fig. 6)

1. Open the Shandon rack by lifting the top rack. Pour 2–3 mL deionized water in the bottom container (*see* **Note 12**).
2. Place the rack lid bottom up on the bench. Lay the cover plate horizontally across the rack lid, front side up. Place a few drops of washing buffer on the cover plate.
3. Place the tissue slide on the cover plate; tissue section must face the front of the cover plate (*see* **Note 13**).
4. The tissue slide should be placed within the six stop notches on the cover plate. A hybridization chamber of about 80 μL is thereby formed between the cover plate and the slide.
5. Place the hybridization chamber upright in the Shandon rack chamber slot so that the rectangular stop notch in the slot fits exactly ("clicks" in place) into the rectangular hole in the middle of the spring clamp.
6. Apply 100 μL of probe solution to the hybridization chamber's top well.
7. Place the lid on the Shandon rack, wrap it in tinfoil, and incubate overnight at 55 °C. Place the buffers in the incubator together with the Shandon rack in order to equilibrate them to the washing temperature of 55 °C (*see* **Notes 1** and **9**).
8. On the second day, remove the tinfoil and the lid from the rack and place it back in the incubator. Apply warm (55 °C) hybridization buffer to the hybridization chamber's top well (*see* **Notes 1** and **14**). Let the buffer run through and repeat the procedure two times. Repeat this with the washing buffer.
9. Fill a Coplin jar with MilliQ water, remove the slide from the cover plate, and place it in the jar for 1–2 min at room temperature.
10. Remove the slides from the Coplin jar and place them in the incubator 55 °C on a clean lab napkin or in an open slide box until they air-dry (*see* **Note 1**).
11. Apply antifading mounting media and add a coverslip to each slide. Gently press with a pencil to spread the antifading mounting media under the slide and to remove bubbles.

12. Inspect slides by using a fluorescence microscope equipped with a camera and the appropriate filter sets for fluorescein isothiocyanate (FITC) (excitation/emission: 492–495 nm/520–525 nm), a Texas Red (excitation/emission: 591–596 nm/608–620 nm), and a DAPI (excitation/emission: 340–359 nm/461–488 nm). Also a dual FITC/Texas Red and a dual DAPI/Texas Red filter set may be used (*see* **Notes 10** and **11**).

4 Notes

1. The temperature of the hybridization buffer, washing buffer, heating block, and incubator when using DNA probes depends on the melting temperature (*Tm*) of the probe. This may vary from 35 °C to 60 °C. Preliminary specificity tests should be carried out at 10 °C below the *Tm* of the actual probe. PNA probes are always run at 55 °C.
2. Formalin is carcinogenic; therefore, only handle it when wearing nitrile gloves and in a fume hood. For ensuring maximum retention of nucleic acids, fixation should be carried out promptly. Apart from formalin, which is a cross-linking fixative, a number of other fixation techniques may be used, e.g., freezing, formaldehyde based on paraformaldehyde, and Carnoy's fixative, but also acetic acid and ethanol can be used before cryostat sectioning.
3. Paraffin-embedded tissue sections must not be folded when mounted on a glass slide. Changing the temperature of the water in the bowl can help unfold the tissue sections. For most tissues, 47 °C is optimal, but ±5 °C may solve folding problems. When mounting brain and skin tissue, a lower temperature of approximately 37 °C is often required.
4. Slides with tissue sections treated through **steps 1** to **3** in the deparaffinization process can be removed directly from 99.9 % ethanol (deparaffinization **step 3**) and left to air-dry on a clean paper napkin before hybridization.
5. In order to facilitate the penetration of the probe, pretreatment is necessary for some Gram-positive species before the FISH procedure. Lysozyme is used on streptococci and on staphylococci in FISH. This enzyme helps the oligonucleotide with the fluorescent dye molecule to enter the bacterial cell. Lysozyme pretreatment is done on the slide. We routinely use 3 mg/ml lysozyme solution in 100 mM Tris–HCL, 50 mM EDTA, pH 7.2, for 10 min. Lysozyme treatment is done after the ethanol series.
6. When a probe has been designed in silico, its specificity should be verified by looking up the sequence in other databases afterward.

7. Whenever possible, protect the probe solution and the glass slides with tissue samples from light. Fluorescent probes are degraded by light. If PNA probes are not received ready for use, the probe solution to be used can be prepared as described for the DNA probe.
8. The use of a coverslip may be omitted.
9. Make sure that you have enough hybridization (only for Method II) and washing buffers for the washing procedure. You will need 10–12 mL of each buffer per slide.
10. If there is green fluorescent protein (GFP), the sample should preferably be visualized immediately after it is prepared.
11. Autofluorescence may appear; make sure that the fluorescent signal is correlated to the size and morphology of the investigated cells (Fig. 2). The fluorescent signal should only appear when using the correct filter set, not in other spectra.
12. The Shandon rack must never contain more deionized water than the maximum volume marker on the inside of the container indicates.
13. In order to avoid air bubbles, moisten the tissue section with washing buffer before placing it on the cover plate.
14. A squirt flask can be used to apply warm (55 °C, *see* **Note 1**) hybridization buffer to the hybridization chamber's top well when using a Shandon rack.

References

1. Moter A, Gobel UB (2000) Fluorescence *in situ* hybridization (FISH) for direct visualization of microorganisms. J Microbiol Methods 41:85–112
2. Levsky JM, Singer RH (2003) Fluorescence *in situ* hybridization: past, present and future. J Cell Sci 116:2833–2838
3. Bottari B, Ercolini D, Gatti M et al (2006) Application of FISH technology for microbiological analysis: current state and prospects. Appl Microbiol Biotechnol 73:485–494
4. Fraher MH, O'Toole PW, Quigley EM (2012) Techniques used to characterize the gut microbiota: a guide for the clinician. Nat Rev Gastroenterol Hepatol 9:312–322
5. Wagner M, Haider S (2012) New trends in fluorescence *in situ* hybridization for identification and functional analyses of microbes. Curr Opin Biotechnol 23:96–102
6. Jensen TK, Christensen BB, Boye M (2006) *Lawsonia intracellularis* infection in the large intestines of pigs. APMIS 114:255–264
7. Amann R, Fuchs BM (2008) Single-cell identification in microbial communities by improved fluorescence *in situ* hybridization techniques. Nat Rev Microbiol 6:339–348
8. Johansen LK, Koch J, Frees D et al (2012) Pathology and biofilm formation in a porcine model of staphylococcal osteomyelitis. J Comp Pathol 147:343–353
9. Behrens S, Rühland C, Inácio J et al (2003) In situ accessibility of small-subunit rRNA of members of the domains *Bacteria*, *Archaea* and *Eucarya* to Cy3-labeled oligonucleotide probes. Appl Environ Microbiol 69:1748–1758
10. Wallner G, Amann R, Beisker W (1993) Optimizing fluorescent in situ hybridization with rRNA-targeted oligonucleotide probes for flow cytometric identification of microorganisms. Cytometry 14:136–143
11. Jensen TK, Boye M, Hagedorn-Olsen T et al (1999) *Actinobacillus pleuropneumoniae* osteomyelitis in pigs demonstrated by fluorescent *in situ* hybridization. Vet Pathol 36:258–261

12. Madsen L, Boye M, Jensen TK et al (2001) *Actinobacillus pleuropneumoniae* demonstrated *in situ* in exudative meningitis and nephritis. Vet Rec 149:746–747
13. Kvist P, Jensen E, Aalbaek B et al (2002) Evaluation of the pathology, pathogenesis and aetiology of auricular elephantiasis in slaughter pigs. J Vet Med A 49:517–522
14. Soerensen C, Holmskov U, Aalbaek B et al (2005) Pulmonary infections in swine induce altered porcine surfactant protein D expression and localization to dendritic cells in bronchial-associated lymphoid tissue. Immunology 115: 526–535
15. Boye M, Jensen TK, Moller K et al (1998) Specific detection of the genus *Serpulina*, *S. hyodysenteriae* and *S. pilosicoli* in porcine intestines by fluorescent rRNA *in situ* hybridization. Mol Cell Probes 12:323–330
16. Jensen TK, Moller K, Boye M et al (2000) Scanning electron microscopy and fluorescent *in situ* hybridization of experimental *Brachyspira (Serpulina) pilosicoli* infection in growing pigs. Vet Pathol 37:22–32
17. Jensen TK, Christensen AS, Boye M (2010) *Brachyspira murdochii* colitis in pigs. Vet Pathol 47:334–338
18. Jensen TK, Boye M, Moller K et al (1998) Association of *Serpulina hyodysenteriae* with the colonic mucosa in experimental swine dysentery studied by fluorescent *in situ* hybridization. APMIS 106:1061–1068
19. Sangild P, Siggers R, Schmidt M et al (2006) Diet- and colonization-dependent intestinal dysfunction predisposes to necrotizing enterocolitis in preterm pigs. Gastroenterology 130:1776–1792
20. Cilieborg MS, Boye M, Molbak L et al (2011) Preterm birth and necrotizing enterocolitis alter gut colonization in pigs. Pediatr Res 69:10–16
21. Pollmann M, Nordhoff M, Pospischil A et al (2005) Effects of a probiotic strain of *Enterococcus faecium* on the rate of natural chlamydia infection in swine. Infect Immun 73:4346–4353
22. Jensen HE, Gyllensten J, Hofman C et al (2010) Histologic and bacteriologic findings in valvular endocarditis of slaughter-age pigs. J Vet Diagn Invest 22:921–927
23. Gustavo Hermes R, Molist F, Francisco Perez J et al (2013) Casein glycomacropeptide in the diet may reduce *Escherichia coli* attachment to the intestinal mucosa and increase the intestinal lactobacilli of early weaned piglets after an enterotoxigenic *E. coli* K88 challenge. Br J Nutr 109:1001–1012
24. Molbak L, Klitgaard K, Jensen TK et al (2006) Identification of a novel, invasive, not-yet-cultivated *Treponema* sp. in the large intestine of pigs by PCR amplification of the 16S rRNA gene. J Clin Microbiol 44:4537–4540
25. Boye M, Jensen TK, Moller K et al (1998) Specific detection of *Lawsonia intracellularis* in porcine proliferative enteropathy inferred from fluorescent rRNA *in situ* hybridization. Vet Pathol 35:153–156
26. Molbak L, Johnsen K, Boye M et al (2008) The microbiota of pigs influenced by diet texture and severity of *Lawsonia intracellularis* infection. Vet Microbiol 128:96–107
27. Boutrup TS, Boesen HT, Boye M et al (2010) Early pathogenesis in porcine proliferative enteropathy caused by *Lawsonia intracellularis*. J Comp Pathol 143:101–109
28. Jensen TK, Boesen HT, Vigre H et al (2010) Detection of *Lawsonia intracellularis* in formalin-fixed porcine intestinal tissue samples: comparison of immunofluorescence and *in-situ* hybridization, and evaluation of the effects of controlled autolysis. J Comp Pathol 142:1–8
29. Boye M, Jensen TK, Ahrens P et al (2001) *In situ* hybridisation for identification and differentiation of *Mycoplasma hyopneumoniae*, *Mycoplasma hyosynoviae* and *Mycoplasma hyorhinis* in formalin-fixed porcine tissue sections. APMIS 109:656–664
30. Mbuthia P, Christensen H, Boye M et al (2001) Specific detection of *Pasteurella multocida* in chickens with fowl cholera and in pig lung tissues using fluorescent rRNA *in situ* hybridization. J Clin Microbiol 39: 2627–2633
31. Pors SE, Hansen MS, Bisgaard M et al (2011) Occurrence and associated lesions of *Pasteurella multocida* in porcine bronchopneumonia. Vet Microbiol 150:160–166
32. Nordentoft S, Christensen H, Wegener H (1997) Evaluation of a fluorescence-labelled oligonucleotide tide probe targeting 23S rRNA for *in situ* detection of *Salmonella* serovars in paraffin-embedded tissue sections and their rapid identification in bacterial smears. J Clin Microbiol 35:2642–2648
33. Martin-Pelaez S, Costabile A, Hoyles L et al (2010) Evaluation of the inclusion of a mixture of organic acids or lactulose into the feed of pigs experimentally challenged with *Salmonella Typhimurium*. Vet Microbiol 142:337–345
34. Boye M, Feenstra A, Tegtmeier C et al (2000) Detection of *Streptococcus suis* by *in situ* hybridization, indirect immunofluorescence, and peroxidase-antiperoxidase assays in formalin-fixed, paraffin-embedded tissue sections from pigs. J Vet Diagn Invest 12:224–232
35. Alm E, Oerther D, Larsen N et al (1996) The oligonucleotide probe database. Appl Environ Microbiol 62:3557–3559

Chapter 18

Identification of Animal *Pasteurellaceae* by MALDI-TOF Mass Spectrometry

Joachim Frey and Peter Kuhnert

Abstract

Species of the family *Pasteurellaceae* play an important role as primary or opportunistic, predominantly respiratory, pathogens in domestic and wild animals. Some of them cause severe disease with high economic losses in commercial animal husbandry. Hence, rapid and accurate differentiation of *Pasteurellaceae* is important and signifies a particular challenge to diagnostic laboratories. Identification and differentiation of *Pasteurellaceae* is mostly done using phenotypic tests or genetic identification based on sequence similarity of housekeeping genes, such as the *rrs* gene encoding the 16S ribosomal RNA (16S rRNA). Both approaches are time consuming, laborious, and costly, therefore often delaying the final diagnosis of disease or epidemics. Matrix-assisted laser desorption/ionization time-of-flight (MALDI-TOF) mass spectrometry represents an alternative rapid and reliable method for the differentiation of most members of the family *Pasteurellaceae*. It is able to differentiate within a few minutes the currently known 18 genera and most of the over 60 species and subspecies of *Pasteurellaceae* including many members encountered in veterinary diagnostic laboratories. A few closely related species and subspecies that cannot be discriminated by MALDI-TOF are easily identified further by complementary simple tests, such as hemolysis done simultaneously or routinely during pathogen isolation.

Key words MALDI-TOF MS, Bacterial identification, Veterinary diagnostics, Molecular identification, *Pasteurellaceae*, New taxa, Rapid diagnosis

1 Introduction

The family *Pasteurellaceae* represents Gram-negative, aerobic, coccoid- or rod-shaped, nonspore-forming, and nonmotile bacteria, currently consisting of 18 genera and more that 60 validly named species (J.P. Euzeby, www.bacterio.net) [1–3]. While most taxa appear as commensal bacteria on mucosal surfaces of animals, several species are of particular concern, either as persistent opportunistic or as primary pathogens in farm animals, such as *Actinobacillus pleuropneumoniae* in pigs, *Pasteurella multocida* and *Avibacterium paragallinarum* in poultry, *Mannheimia haemolytica* in cattle, or *Actinobacillus equuli* subsp. *haemolyticus* in horses. Phenotypic identification based on special growth media, detection of

Mónica V. Cunha and João Inácio (eds.), *Veterinary Infection Biology: Molecular Diagnostics and High-Throughput Strategies*, Methods in Molecular Biology, vol. 1247, DOI 10.1007/978-1-4939-2004-4_18, © Springer Science+Business Media New York 2015

metabolites, and biochemical tests, combined with knowledge of host specificity that is generally encountered for most pathogenic *Pasteurellaceae*, are normally used in routine diagnostics [4]. Commercial phenotypic identification systems frequently lack animal pathogens in their databases, where *Pasteurellaceae* typically are underrepresented. More recently, DNA sequence-based identification methods are applied in veterinary diagnostics [5, 6]. Although these latter methods are highly discriminatory, they request qualified personnel and are time consuming and costly.

Matrix-assisted laser desorption/ionization time-of-flight mass spectrometry (MALDI-TOF MS; shortly MALDI-TOF) has newly entered in the identification procedures of bacteria in research as well as in routine diagnostic laboratories [7–9]. Briefly, the sample to be analyzed, which may be composed of whole bacterial cells, is mixed with a matrix solution, applied onto a metal plate target slide, and irradiated with a laser. The matrix along with the sample analytes absorbs the laser light and vaporizes. Thereby, the various proteins gain an electrical charge (ionization), which enables electrical fields to accelerate them into the time-of-flight mass spectrometer where they are separated according to their mass to charge ratio and the respective abundance is measured, yielding a characteristic spectrum (Fig. 1). Differentiation of bacterial genera and species is mainly based on time-of-flight mass spectra of ribosomal proteins, which generate characteristic fingerprints. This is possible because ribosomes are highly abundant in bacteria at 20,000 copies in the average, and hence ribosomal proteins

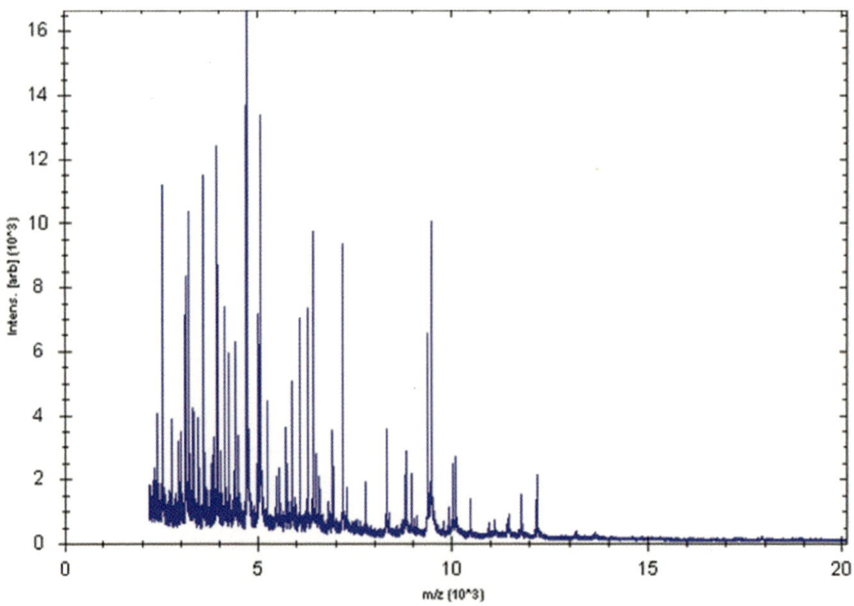

Fig. 1 MALDI-TOF spectrum of *Actinobacillus pleuropneumoniae* type strain S4074^T

contribute with the strongest signals to the MALDI-TOF spectra that can be resolved and finally constitute the fingerprints. The composition of ribosomal proteins also reflects evolutionary relations of bacterial species and hence mirrors to a large extent the phylogeny established with ribosomal RNA sequences. Moreover, the composition of ribosomal proteins in bacteria is stable under any conditions and represents the most characteristic biomarkers accessible in the analysis of intact organism without extraction, separation, or amplification. In this respect, ribosomal proteins are also to be considered as essential phenotypic markers as requested for taxonomic differentiation. MALDI-TOF represents a universal, fast, and cost-effective alternative to classical phenotypic and genetic identification assays. It is an open system that can constantly be updated with reference data produced in the laboratories themselves depending on their needs.

The MALDI-TOF mass spectrometers designed for microbial identification purpose generally are equipped with databases for the identification of bacteria of primary clinical importance in human medicine and hence lack data for many animal pathogens or opportunists such as species of the family *Pasteurellaceae*. A comprehensive database of MALDI-TOF spectra has recently been developed using a well-characterized strain collection representing type strains and field isolates of a large range of species and also subspecies of *Pasteurellaceae* that are of current relevance in veterinary infectious disease diagnostics [10]. The data obtained revealed that MALDI-TOF is able to discriminate most of *Pasteurellaceae* species tested, while only a few closely related species or subspecies needed additional tests for accurate identification. The current chapter describes the establishment of a MALDI-TOF spectrum database of *Pasteurellaceae* and the method for rapid bacterial identification to be used in diagnostic laboratories. The method is basically adaptable to any other bacterial family, which might be lacking in the commercial databases provided with the MALDI-TOF instruments. Note that MALDI-TOF databases are adapted to the specific mass spectrometers and are not normalized and are applicable to the specific instrument only. Therefore there are currently no online databases for MALDI-TOF-based identification of bacteria available. Spectra are electronically transferable from one instrument to another of the same brand, but adjustments are necessary as there are minor differences from one instrument to another.

2 Materials

Prepare all solutions using ultrapure water and analytical grade reagents. Preparation and storage of reagents is at room temperature unless otherwise indicated.

2.1 Chemicals

1. 0.9 % (w/v) NaCl (=154 mM).
2. Ethanol, absolute.
3. 70 % (v/v) formic acid.
4. Acetonitrile.
5. Organic solvent (OS): 50 % acetonitrile, 2.5 % trifluoroacetic acid (TFA) in H_2O.
6. Matrix solution (10 mg/ml): dissolve 10 mg of α-cyano-4-hydroxycinnamic acid in 1 ml of OS and vortex thoroughly. The matrix solution should be saturated, i.e., some crystals might still be visible even after a few minutes. It can be kept in the dark at room temperature up to 1 week. Aliquots of preweighted powder can be kept at −20 °C and be supplemented with OS just prior to use.
7. Appropriate growth medium for species to be included in database or to be analyzed, e.g., trypticase soy agar supplemented with 5 % sheep erythrocytes or chocolate agar (*see* **Note 1**).

2.2 Equipment

1. MALDI-TOF mass spectrometer for biotyping, such as Bruker Daltonik Microflex LT or Shimadzu AXIMA Microorganism Identification System.
2. General laboratory equipment such as micro-centrifuge.

3 Methods

Procedures can be carried out at room temperature unless otherwise specified. They are given for the Bruker Daltonik Microflex LT (Bruker Daltonik GmbH, Bremen, Germany), using the "Flex control" software, and might vary slightly with other instruments.

3.1 Generation of Reference Spectra for the Establishment of a New or for Upgrading a Database

1. For each species of *Pasteurellaceae* family, grow the type strain and three to four confirmed field strains on appropriate medium, at the appropriate temperature (generally 37 °C) under suitable conditions, such as aerobic, microaerophilic, or capnophilic conditions. Ideally, use field strains for which the species has been confirmed by sequence analysis of the 16S rRNA and housekeeping genes [5, 6].
2. Suspend a few colonies in 300 μl deionized H_2O in an Eppendorf 1.5 ml tube.
3. Add 900 μl of absolute ethanol and mix well.
4. Centrifuge for 2 min in a micro-centrifuge at full speed (15,000 × *g*).
5. Discard liquid and centrifuge again for 2 min at full speed.

6. Remove all liquid with a pipette and air-dry the bacterial pellet for 20–30 min. Suspend the pellet in 50 μl of formic acid 70 % and verify the full suspension of the bacteria.
7. Add 50 μl of acetonitrile and mix well.
8. Centrifuge for 2 min in a micro-centrifuge at full speed.
9. Keep the supernatant for the production of MALDI-TOF spectra.
10. Spot 1 μl aliquots of the supernatant onto the steel target support of the MALDI-TOF mass spectrometer in eight replicas (*see* **Note 2**).
11. Let the samples on steel target support air-dry (2–5 min).
12. Cover each dried sample with 1 μl of α-cyano-4-hydroxycinnamic acid matrix solution (*see* **Notes 2** and **3**).
13. Let the samples on steel target support air-dry (2–5 min).
14. Include a calibration with a bacterial test standard (BTS), which is, in general, a specific strain of *Escherichia coli* provided by the supplier of the MALDI-TOF instrument.
15. Produce reference spectra with the MALDI-TOF mass spectrometer by measuring each spot three times with standard settings resulting in a total of 24 spectra for each strain (Fig. 1). Run one to three BTS calibration spots with each plate read.
16. Import the spectra into the "Flex analysis" software and process it according to the manufacturer's recommendations.
17. Check the quality of the 24 spectra, generate a main spectrum (MSP), and register this as reference for the species in the database of the MALDI-TOF mass spectrometer according to the manufacturer's instructions (*see* **Notes 4** and **5**).
18. Use the MSP (reference spectra) to compile a dendrogram as shown in Fig. 2 using the Biotyper 3.0 software (Bruker) and the correlation distance measure with the average linkage algorithm.

3.2 Diagnostic Identification of Colonies by Direct Transfer

1. Take a single colony from culture medium with a toothpick (*see* **Note 1**).
2. Smear the bacteria on the steel target support (*see* **Note 6**) (Fig. 3).
3. Overlay the bacterial smear with 1 μl of α-cyano-4-hydroxycinnamic acid matrix solution (*see* **Notes 2** and **3**).
4. After air-drying, analyze with the MALDI-TOF mass spectrometer, using standard settings in the "Flex control" software according to the manufacturer's instructions (*see* **Notes 7–12**).
5. Compare the query spectra in the Biotyper 3.0 software against the internal commercial database in combination with the library database generated from additional "in-house" reference spectra.

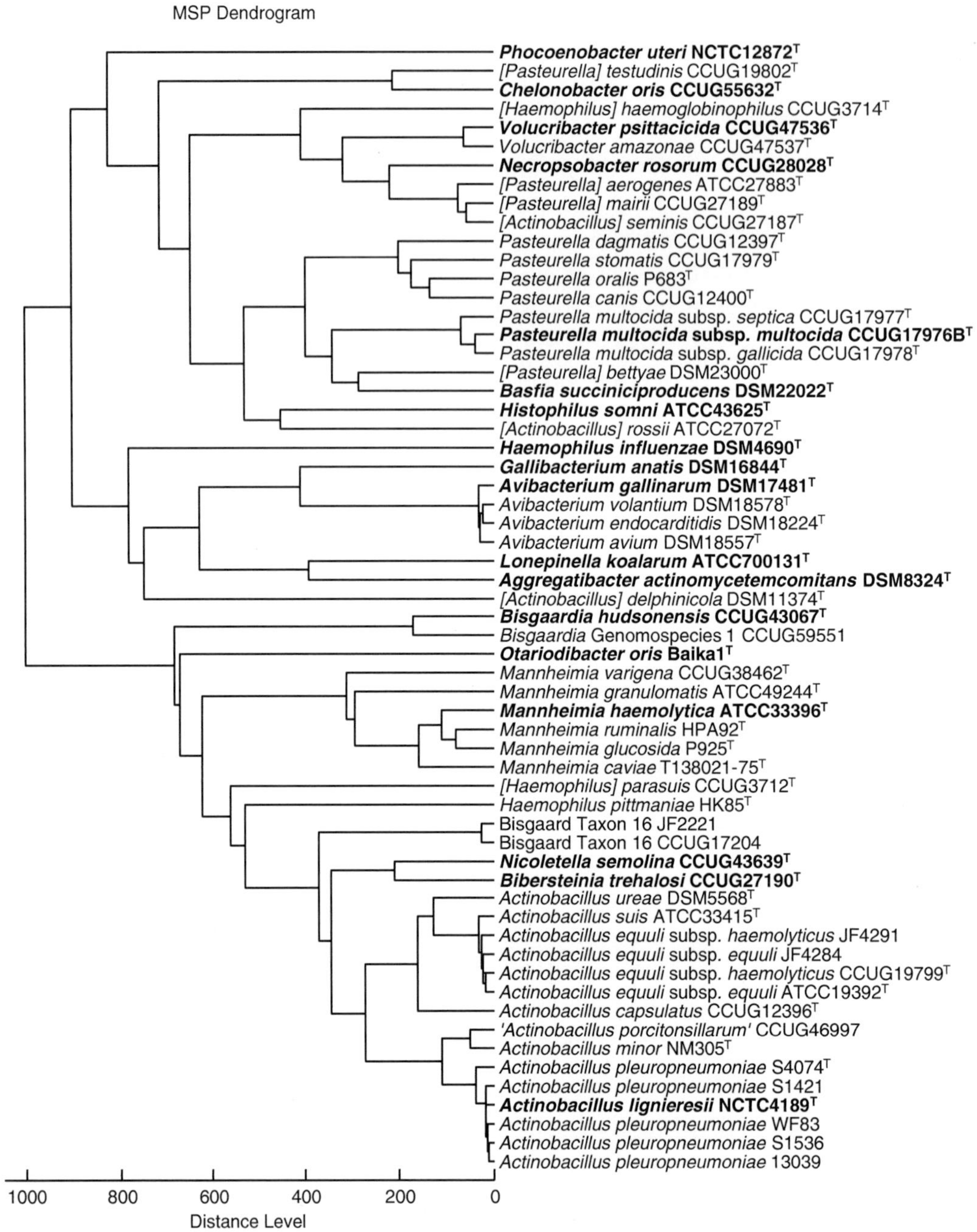

Fig. 2 Dendrogram derived from similarity matrices based on MALDI-TOF MS reference spectra from species of the family *Pasteurellaceae* that are relevant in diagnostics of animal infectious diseases or represent important genera of this family. The distance level is normalized to a maximum value of 1,000. Type species of the currently 18 genera are indicated in *bold*. Species misclassified in the corresponding genus are indicated informally *in brackets* [11]

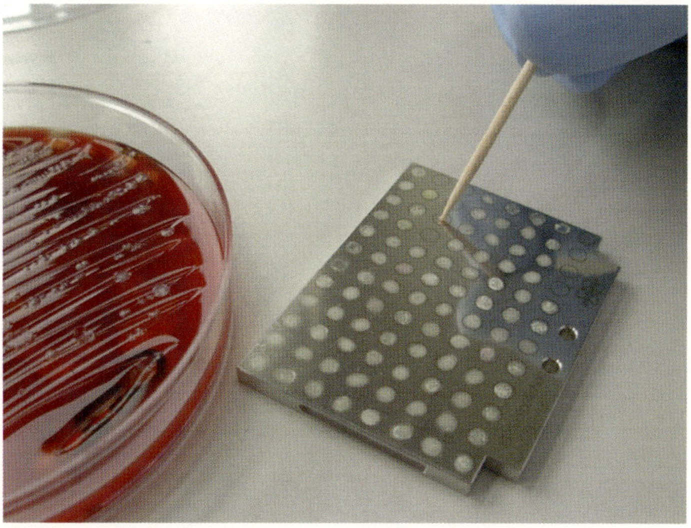

Fig. 3 Simple application of material from individual bacterial colonies onto the steel target support for MALDI-TOF mass spectrometry

4 Notes

1. If using growth liquid media, removal of the media components from the bacterial samples may be important for successful MALDI-TOF analysis. Cell suspension may be centrifuged, and the pellet washed several times with water before performing the analysis.
2. When spotting MALDI-TOF plates, allow the wicking action to pull the sample or matrix solution aliquots off from the pipette rather than touching the surface with the pipette tip, in order to achieve a better homogeneity of the spot.
3. Samples are overlaid with a matrix solution and air-dried. The crystallized organic acid forms the matrix, consisting of laser-absorbing small organic molecules in large excess over the bacterial proteins to be analyzed. Several organic acids are suitable for the matrix solution, but cinnamic acid is adequate for examining proteins (usually α-cyano-4-hydroxycinnamic acid, which enables highly sensitive MALDI-TOF measurement of peptides and proteins from 0.7 to 20 kDa). The solvent acetonitrile leads to co-crystallization of matrix and sample molecules when evaporating.
4. Reference spectra databases can also be transferred from one instrument to another, if the instruments are compatible. However, best results are obtained with reference spectra generated on the proper instrument.
5. For certain bacterial species, reference spectra created on the proper instrument might show differences compared to

reference spectra of the same species or strain present in preset databases. This is due to the fact that preset databases were made on a different instrument.

6. The extraction method with formic acid and acetonitrile results in higher quality and higher similarity indexes compared to the direct transfer method and might exceptionally be necessary for proper identification of certain species, such as *Histophilus somni*.
7. Results of identifications are given by a similarity index starting with the species giving the best match. Good similarity indexes generally are above 2.0. As the MALDI-TOF MS identification is based on the comparative analysis of MS spectra based on ribosomal proteins, the method in general is unable to differentiate subspecies, biotypes, or serotypes, which all were shown to cluster tightly. This is illustrated in Fig. 2 with the reference strains of *A. pleuropneumoniae* serotype 1, S4074^{T}; serotype 2, S1536; serotype 3, 1421; serotype 7, WF83; and serotype 10, 13039, which all form a tight cluster.
8. *Actinobacillus pleuropneumoniae* and *A. lignieresii* are genotypically very closely related. However *A. pleuropneumoniae* is hemolytic and can be readily differentiated from *A. lignieresii* by hemolysis, e.g., on blood-agar medium plates. The species *A. pleuropneumoniae* can be confirmed further by the presence of the *apx*IVA gene using PCR or real-time PCR [11].
9. Some species, e.g., [*Pasteurella*] *testudinis*, [*Actinobacillus*] *rossii*, or [*Haemophilus*] *parasuis*, do not cluster with their corresponding genus (Fig. 2). This is due to their misclassification within this genus, which is therefore given in brackets [5, 12]. However, this does not influence at all the reliable identification of these three species.
10. Subspecies of *Pasteurella multocida* cannot be differentiated as they are phylogenetically very closely related and often only differ by specific virulence attributes.
11. *Actinobacillus suis*, *Actinobacillus equuli* subsp. *haemolyticus*, and *Actinobacillus equuli* subsp. *equuli* represent phylogenetically a tight entity and cannot be separated by MALDI-TOF based on ribosomal protein spectra. *A. equuli* subsp. *equuli* is nonhemolytic, while *A. suis* and *A. equuli* subsp. *haemolyticus* are hemolytic. They differ from each other mainly by the different, hemolytic, RTX toxins of which *A. suis* secretes the porcine-specific toxins ApxI and ApxII and *A. equuli* subsp. *haemolyticus* secretes the equine-specific Aqx toxin. The latter can be differentiated by PCR [13].
12. MALDI-TOF analysis is able to detect and characterize yet unknown or unassigned taxa during research and routine diagnosis. They are evidenced by the fact that their spectra are

clustered and differentiated from those of the known species. The use of reference spectra from new, yet unassigned taxa will help to recognize them for further characterization and finally for the description of new taxa. This is demonstrated by Bisgaard Taxon 16 in Fig. 2.

References

1. Boyce JD, Harper M, Wilkie IW et al (2010) Pasteurella. In: Gyles CL, Prescott JF, Songer JG, Thoen CO (eds) Pathogenesis of bacterial infections in animals. Wiley-Blackwell, Weinheim, pp 325–346
2. Christensen H, Korczak BM, Bojesen AM et al (2011) Classification of organisms previously reported as the SP and Stewart-Letscher groups, with descriptions of *Necropsobacter* gen. nov. and of *Necropsobacter rosorum* sp. nov. for organisms of the SP group. Int J Syst Evol Microbiol 61:1829–1836
3. Foster G, Higgins R, Leclair D et al (2011) Proposal of *Bisgaardia hudsonensis* gen. nov., sp. nov. and an additional genomospecies, isolated from seals, as new members of the family *Pasteurellaceae*. Int J Syst Evol Microbiol 61: 3016–3022
4. Dousse F, Thomann A, Brodard I et al (2008) Routine phenotypic identification of bacterial species of the family *Pasteurellaceae* isolated from animals. J Vet Diagn Invest 20:716–724
5. Korczak BM, Kuhnert P (2008) Phylogeny of *Pasteurellaceae*. In: Kuhnert P, Christensen H (eds) *Pasteurellaceae*: biology, genomics and molecular aspects. Caister Academic Press, Norfolk, UK, pp 27–52
6. Kuhnert P, Korczak BM (2006) Prediction of whole-genome DNA-DNA similarity, determination of G + C content and phylogenetic analysis within the family *Pasteurellaceae* by Multilocus Sequence Analysis (MLSA). Microbiology 152:2537–2548
7. Fenselau C, Demirev PA (2001) Characterization of intact microorganisms by MALDI mass spectrometry. Mass Spectrom Rev 20:157–171
8. Tamura H, Hotta Y, Sato H (2013) Novel accurate bacterial discrimination by MALDI-Time-of-Flight MS based on ribosomal proteins coding in S10-Spc-Alpha operon at strain level S10-GERMS. J Am Soc Mass Spectrom 24:1185–1193
9. Clark AE, Kaleta EJ, Arora A et al (2013) Matrix-assisted laser desorption ionization-time of flight mass spectrometry: a fundamental shift in the routine practice of clinical microbiology. Clin Microbiol Rev 26:547–603
10. Kuhnert P, Bisgaard M, Korczak BM et al (2012) Identification of animal *Pasteurellaceae* by MALDI-TOF mass spectrometry. J Microbiol Methods 89:1–7
11. Schaller A, Djordjevic SP, Eamens GJ et al (2001) Identification and detection of *Actinobacillus pleuropneumoniae* by PCR based on the gene *Apx*IVA. Vet Microbiol 79:47–62
12. Christensen H, Bisgaard M (2008) Taxonomy and biodiversity of members of *Pasteurellaceae*. In: Kuhnert P, Christensen H (eds) *Pasteurellaceae*: biology, genomics and molecular aspects. Caister Academic Press, Norfolk, UK, pp 1–26
13. Kuhnert P, Berthoud H, Straub R et al (2003) Host cell specific activity of RTX toxins from haemolytic *Actinobacillus equuli* and *Actinobacillus suis*. Vet Microbiol 92:161–167

Chapter 19

Gold Nanoparticles as a Potential Tool for Diagnosis of Fish Diseases

Mona Saleh, Hatem Soliman, and Mansour El-Matbouli

Abstract

Infectious diseases are a serious problem and a major contributor to severe economic losses in intensive fish culture. Therefore, rapid and sensitive detection of fish pathogens is extremely important. Although various assays for determination of fish pathogens have been developed, most of these diagnostic methods are time-consuming and laborious. To overcome these limitations, functional nanomaterials have been actively investigated to improve detection ability and rapidity of diagnostic assays. Gold nanoparticles (AuNPs) have been widely studied for their unique optical properties arising from their surface plasmon resonance, which is responsible for their large absorption and scattering properties. These unique properties are four to five orders of magnitude larger than those of conventional dyes and can be controlled by varying their sizes, shapes, and compositions. Moreover, AuNPs can be easily synthesized and functionalized with different biomolecules, including pathogen-specific oligonucleotides or antibodies. Recently, nanoparticle-based assays have been introduced as a tool for laboratory diagnosis. They have been used for the direct detection of unamplified nucleic acids in hybridization assays. Single- and double-stranded oligonucleotides can be adsorbed on AuNPs in colloidal solution under certain conditions. The result of the hybridization process can be visually detected within 1 min after addition of AuNPs, when the color of the reaction mixture changes from red to blue (positive reaction) or remains red (negative). The development of such nanoparticle-based strategies holds the potential to become powerful approaches for diagnosis of fish pathogens.

Key words Diagnosis, Fish pathogens, Gold nanoparticles, Label-free, Colorimetric detection, Unamplified nucleic acids, Nucleic acid probes, Hybridization assay

1 Introduction

Methods conventionally used for the diagnosis of fish diseases mostly require expensive laboratory facilities, preventing their wide-scale use. Additionally, these methods need extensive sample preparation steps and have long readout times, which delay a timely response and hamper effective disease control [1]. Recently, a powerful emerging technology based on the unique properties of nanoscale materials was introduced, which presents a great

Mónica V. Cunha and João Inácio (eds.), *Veterinary Infection Biology: Molecular Diagnostics and High-Throughput Strategies*, Methods in Molecular Biology, vol. 1247, DOI 10.1007/978-1-4939-2004-4_19,

opportunity to develop fast, accurate, and cost-effective diagnostics for the detection of infectious agents [1–3]. The optical transduction by noble metal nanoparticles is based upon the phenomenon of nanoparticle surface plasmon resonance [4–6]. Surface plasmon resonance is the collective oscillations of surface electrons induced by visible light and is responsible for the intense colors exhibited by colloidal solutions of noble metals such as gold and silver [7–11]. Gold nanoparticles (AuNPs) are suitable for a wide range of biological applications due to their unique size-, shape-, and composition-dependent optical, physical, and chemical properties [12].

When in solution, AuNPs are typically stabilized by negatively charged citrate ions adsorbed on their surfaces whose repulsion prevents aggregation due to the strong van der Waals attraction between gold particles [13, 14]. However, on addition of ionic substances such as NaCl, the attraction force becomes stronger than the counteraction, which leads to an aggregation of AuNPs and to the consequent color change of the solution from red to blue [15]. This property, along with the corresponding shift of surface plasmon absorption, has been utilized for the colorimetric detection of DNA and RNA [16–23]. AuNPs-based DNA detection can be generally classified as either being labeled or label-free [22]. In the labeled technique, AuNPs are modified mainly with thiolated single-stranded DNA (ssDNA) and then allowed to hybridize with a complementary target sequence [23]. However, the need for premodification of the AuNPs makes this strategy laborious, complicated, and time-consuming [24].

The label-free method takes advantage of the different electrostatic properties of ssDNA and double-stranded DNA (dsDNA). Since ssDNA is flexible and can partially uncoil, it can be easily adsorbed on AuNPs and enhance the electrostatic repulsion between the nanoparticles. This stabilizes the AuNPs even in the presence of salt. In contrast, because dsDNA cannot easily uncoil and has an exposed negatively charged phosphate backbone, its adsorption to the AuNPs is prevented, and the salt-induced aggregation of the nanoparticles is not blocked [22]. When AuNPs are added to a saline solution containing the target nucleic acid and its complementary unlabeled ssDNA probe, the nanoparticles aggregate, and the solution color changes to blue since the probes are not free to stabilize the AuNPs. On the other hand, in the absence of the target nucleic acid, the probes are free to stabilize the AuNPs, thus preventing its aggregation, and the solution color remains red [22, 23, 25, 26] (Fig. 1). This AuNPs-based label-free strategy has been utilized to develop several colorimetric hybridization assays [25, 27–30]. Gold nanoparticles-based assays have also been used successfully for the detection of fish pathogens [29, 31]. Herein, we describe how these assays can be performed properly to assist rapid, accurate, and affordable diagnosis of fish diseases.

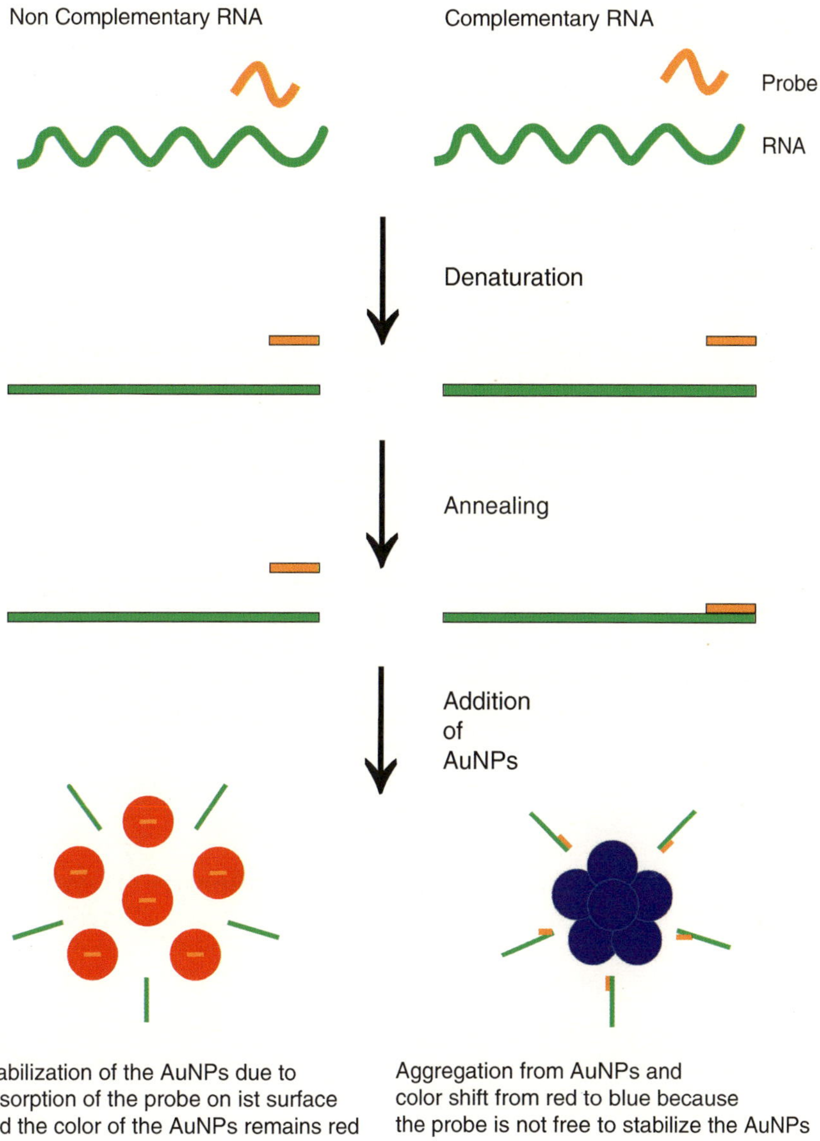

Fig. 1 Schematic diagram of a colorimetric assay based on unmodified AuNPs for detection of unamplified nucleic acids (SVCV RNA). First, the target RNA is denatured and the complementary probe hybridizes to the target forming double strands. Adding AuNPs causes its aggregation since the probe is not free to stabilize the AuNPs, and the solution color changes from *red* to *blue*. In the presence of a noncomplementary target RNA, the probe will be free to adsorb onto and stabilize the AuNPs consequently preventing their aggregation and the solution color remains *red*

2 Materials

2.1 Gold Nanoparticles

1. 38.8 mM sodium citrate solution (Sigma-Aldrich, GmbH, Schnelldorf, Germany).
2. 1 mM aqueous solution of gold (III) chloride trihydrate ($HAuCl_4$) (Sigma-Aldrich, GmbH, Schnelldorf, Germany).

2.2 Oligonucleotide Probes

1. Oligonucleotide probes targeting specific sequences of a particular gene of interest of the pathogen. For example, we have recently described the development of a 26 bp specific probe (5′-GTC TAT CAT CAG CTA CAT CGC ATT CC-3′) designed to target the spring viremia of carp virus (SVCV) glycoprotein gene [29]. Assess the specificity of the probe against other common aquatic pathogens sequences deposited in GenBank.
2. Stock solutions of the probes: order the designed probes commercially and prepare them according to the supplied specification sheet that usually gives instructions needed to rehydrate the probes. For each probe, add the recommended amount of purified, double-distilled, deionized, and autoclaved water (PCR grade water), and mix well to get a stock solution of 100 pmol/μl. Prepare several aliquots from these stock solutions to avoid degradation by repeated freezing and thawing, and keep at −20 °C until required.

2.3 Colorimetric Detection of Nucleic Acids

1. Extracted nucleic acids of the pathogens (DNA or RNA): in this illustrative protocol we use RNA extracted from SVCV grown in epithelioma papulosum cyprinid culture (EPC) [29] (*see* **Note 1**).
2. Hybridization buffer: 10 mM phosphate buffer saline (PBS), pH 7.0, containing 0.4 M of NaCl and 1.8 μM of oligonucleotide probe (*see* **Note 2**).

3 Methods

3.1 Preparation of Gold Nanoparticles

Prepare gold nanoparticles of 13 nm diameter by the citrate reduction method according to Grabar et al. [32] or purchase commercially (e.g., from Strem Chemicals. Newburyport, MA, USA).

1. Add 10 ml of 38.8 mM sodium citrate solution rapidly to 100 ml of vigorously stirred boiling 1 mM $HAuCl_4$ aqueous solution (*see* **Note 3**).
2. The mixture should be boiled for 10 min and stirred for an additional 15 min.

3. Allow the solution to cool to room temperature.
4. Filter and store at 4 °C before use.

3.2 Colorimetric Detection of Nucleic Acids Using Unmodified Gold Nanoparticles

Optimum concentrations of NaCl and oligonucleotide probe (*see* **Note 1**), as well as optimal pH, annealing temperature, and incubation times, need to be determined for each assay. We give an example based on the detection of unamplified SVCV RNA that we recently described [29].

The assay is performed as follows:

1. In a sterile PCR tube place 5 μl of extracted RNA.
2. Add 3 μl of the hybridization buffer.
3. Complete the reaction mixture to 10 μl with sterile distilled water and mix well.
4. Denature the mixture at 95 °C for 30 s, anneal at 58 °C for 30 s, and then cool at room temperature for 10 min.
5. Finally, add 10 μl of colloidal AuNPs to the reaction mixture, and observe the change in the solution color within 1 min (Fig. 2) (*see* **Notes 4–6**).

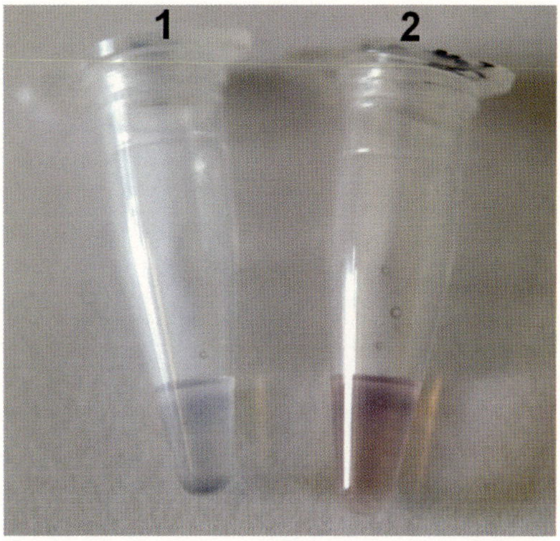

Fig. 2 Colorimetric assay using unmodified AuNPs. Each tube contains 5 μL of sample (SVCV RNA), 1.8 μM of oligonucleotide probe, and 0.1 M of NaCl. The samples were denatured at 95 °C for 30 s and annealed at 58 °C for 30 s and then cooled at room temperature for 10 min. 10 μL of AuNPs solution was added and results were observed within 1 min. Tube 1 contains a positive sample and tube 2 contains a negative sample. In the positive sample, the color changes from *red* to *blue*

4 Notes

1. Inoculate SVCV onto EPC cell line maintained in Eagle's minimal essential medium (EMEM) buffered to pH 7.6 with sodium bicarbonate, supplemented with 2 % of fetal bovine serum (FBS) and standard concentrations of antibiotic. Incubate the inoculated cultures at 15 °C.
2. Optimum concentrations of NaCl and of oligonucleotide probe need to be determined for each assay, allowing the visual detection of the color change of the solutions and, at the same time, an effective annealing of the probe to its complementary target. For the detection of SVCV, the concentration of NaCl sufficient for both aggregation of AuNPs and proper annealing of the probe to its complementary target was 0.4 M. Use different concentrations of the probe to determine the optimum probe concentration sufficient to stabilize the AuNPs in the presence of salt. We found that a final probe concentration of more than 3 μM was too high for any aggregation to occur in the presence of the target, leading to false negative results. In contrast, a probe concentration of less than 0.2 μM did not prevent aggregation of AuNPs in the absence of the target and led to false-positive results.
3. A change in the color of the solution from pale yellow to deep red will be observed.
4. The specificity of the assays should be previously assessed using nucleic acids extracted from closely related organisms as template. Our SVCV-targeted assay showed no false-positive results when tested with nucleic acids extracted from epizootic hematopoietic necrosis virus (EHNV), infectious hematopoietic necrosis virus (IHNV), infectious salmon anemia virus (ISAV), koi herpes virus (KHV), viral hemorrhagic septicemia virus (VHSV), pike fry rhabdovirus (PFRV), zander rhabdovirus (ZRV), and, also, the EPC cells.
5. The lower detection limit of the AuNPs-based assay was determined using a tenfold serial dilution of RNA extracted from SVCV grown in EPC culture with a known titer estimated according to the method described by Reed and Muench [33] (Fig. 3). The detection limit is the lowest RNA concentration able to change the solution color from red to blue upon aggregation of AuNPs.
6. The ability of the AuNPs-based assay to detect SVCV RNA directly from fish specimens can be evaluated by testing RNA samples extracted from SVCV-infected and noninfected fish tissue homogenates. Test outcomes can be compared with those of virus isolation or PCR amplification [34].

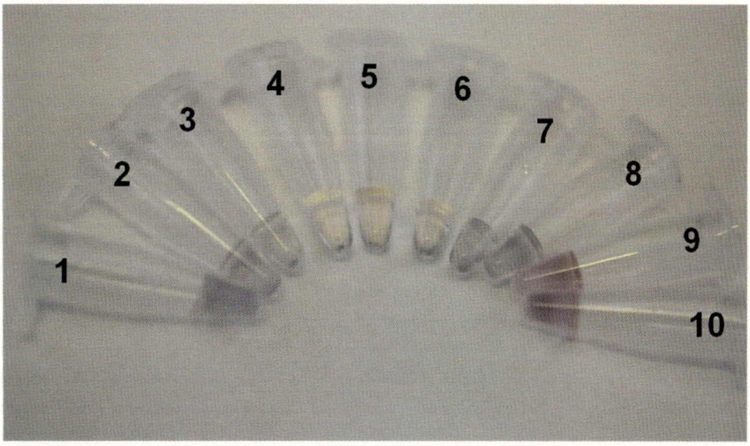

Fig. 3 Lower detection limit of the gold nanoparticle (SVCV-AuNP) assay was estimated in cell culture system using a tenfold dilution series of the nucleic acid tested (SVCV RNA). Tubes 1–10 contain 10^5, 10^4, 10^3, 10^2, 10, 10^{-1}, 10^{-2}, 10^{-3}, 10^{-4}, and 10^{-5} TCID 50 ml^{-1}, respectively. SVC-AuNPs assay detection limit was assessed as about 10^{-3} TCID 50 ml^{-1} (Tube 8; *blue color*)

References

1. Kaittanis C, Santra S, Perez JM (2010) Emerging nanotechnology-based strategies for the identification of microbial pathogenesis. Adv Drug Deliv Rev 62:408–423
2. Jain KK (2005) Nanotechnology in clinical laboratory diagnostics. Clin Chim Acta 358:37–54
3. Rosi NL, Mirkin CA (2005) Nanostructures in biodiagnostics. Chem Rev 105:1547–1562
4. Kreibig U, Genzel L (1985) Optical absorption spectra of pairs of small metal particles. Surf Sci 156:678–700
5. Quinten M, Kreibig U (1986) Optical properties of small metal particles. Surf Sci 172:557–577
6. Link S, El-Sayed MA (2000) Shape and size dependence of radiative, nonradiative, and photothermal properties of gold nanocrystals. Int Rev Phys Chem 19:409–453
7. Nath N, Chilkoti A (2002) A colorimetric gold nanoparticle sensor to interrogate biomolecular interactions in real time on a surface. Anal Chem 74:504–509
8. Nath N, Chilkoti A (2004) Label free colorimetric biosensing using nanoparticles. J Fluoresc 14:4
9. Jain PK, Lee KS, El-Sayed IH, El-Sayed MA (2006) Calculated absorption and scattering properties of gold nanoparticles of different size, shape, and composition: applications in biological imaging and biomedicine. J Phys Chem 110:7238–7248
10. Yguerabide J, Yguerabide EE (1998) Light-scattering submicroscopic particles as highly fluorescent analogs and their use as tracer labels in clinical and biological applications—I. Theory. Anal Biochem 262:137–156
11. Yguerabide J, Yguerabide EE (1998) Light-scattering submicroscopic particles as highly fluorescent analogs and their use as tracer labels in clinical and biological applications—II. Experimental characterization. Anal Biochem 262:157–176
12. Pissuwan D, Cortie CH, Valenzuela SM, Cortie MB (2009) Functionalised gold nanoparticles for controlling pathogenic bacteria. Trends Biotechnol 28:207–213
13. Shaw DJ (1992) Introduction to colloid and surface chemistry, 4th edn. Butterworth–Heinemann, Oxford
14. Hunter RJ (2001) Foundations of colloid science. Oxford University Press, New York
15. Baudhuin P, Van der Smissen P, Beauvios S, Courtoy PJ (1989) Molecular Interactions between Colloidal Gold, Proteins, and Living Cells. In: Hayat MA (ed) Colloidal gold. Academic, San Diego, pp 1–17
16. Peak SH, Seung HL, Joung HC, Young SK (2000) Development of rapid one-step immunochromatographic assay. Methods 22:53–60

17. Huang JT, Hou SY, Fang SB et al (2008) Development of a biochip using antibody-coated gold nanoparticles to detect specific bioparticles. J Ind Microbiol Biotechnol 35: 1377–1385
18. Zhao Y, Zhang G, Lio Q et al (2008) Development of a lateral flow colloidal gold immunoassay strip for the rapid detection of enrofloxacin residues. J Agric Food Chem 56:12138–12142
19. Soo PC, Horng YT, Chang KC et al (2009) A simple gold nanoparticle probes assay for identification of *Mycobacterium tuberculosis* and *Mycobacterium tuberculosis* complex from clinical specimens. Mol Cell Probes 23:240–246
20. Chirathaworn C, Chantaramalai T, Sereemaspun A, Kongthong N, Suwancharoen D (2011) Detection of *Leptospira* in urine using anti-*Leptospira*-coated gold nanoparticles. Comp Immunol Microbiol Infect Dis 34:31–34
21. Saleh M, Soliman H, Haenen O, El-Matbouli M (2011) Antibody-coated gold nanoparticles immunoassay for direct detection of *Aeromonas salmonicida* in fish tissues. J Fish Dis 34:845–852
22. Li H, Rothberg L (2004) Colorimetric detection of DNA sequences based on electrostatic interactions with unmodified gold nanoparticles. Proc Natl Acad Sci U S A 101: 14036–14039
23. Mirkin CA, Letsinger RL, Mucic RC, Storhoff JJ (1996) A DNA-based method for rationally assembling nanoparticles into macroscopic materials. Nature 382:607–609
24. Jung YL, Jung C, Parab H, Li T, Park HG (2010) Direct colorimetric diagnosis of pathogen infections by utilizing thiol-labeled PCR primers and unmodified gold nanoparticles. Biosens Bioelectron 25:1941–1946
25. Elghanian R, Storhoff JJ, Mucic RC, Letsinger RL, Mirkin CA (1997) Selective colorimetric detection of polynucleotides based on the distance-dependent optical properties of gold nanoparticles. Science 277:1078–1081
26. Storhoff JJ, Lucas AD, Garimella V, Bao YP, Müller UR (2004) Homogeneous detection of unamplified genomic DNA sequences based on colorimetric scatter of gold nanoparticle probes. Nat Biotechnol 22:7
27. Li H, Rothberg L (2005) Detection of specific sequences in RNA using differential adsorption of single-stranded oligonucleotides on gold nanoparticles. Anal Chem 77:6229–6233
28. Shawky SM, Bald D, Azzazy HME (2010) Direct detection of unamplified hepatitis C virus RNA using unmodified gold nanoparticles. Clin Biochem 43:1163–1168
29. Saleh M, Soliman H, Schachner O, El-Matbouli M (2012) Direct detection of unamplified spring viraemia of carp virus RNA using unmodified gold nanoparticles. Dis Aquat Organ 100:3–10
30. Saleh M, Soliman H, Sørum H, Fauske AK, El-Matbouli M (2012) A novel gold nanoparticles-based assay for rapid detection of *Melissococcus plutonius*, the causative agent of European foulbrood. Vet Rec 171:400
31. Saleh M, Gotesman M, El-Matbouli M (2013) Going for gold in the detection of Cyprinid herpesvirus-3. In: Diagnostics, Abstract Book, 277 (423) 416–427, 16th international conference on diseases of fish and shellfish, European Association of Fish Pathologists, Sep 2–6, Tampere, Finland
32. Grabar KC, Griffith-Freeman R, Hommer MB, Natan MJ (1995) Preparation and characterization of Au colloid monolayers. Anal Chem 67:735–743
33. Reed LJ, Muench H (1938) A simple method of estimating fifty per cent endpoints. Am J Hyg 27:493–497
34. Koutná M, Vesely T, Psikal I, Hulová J (2003) Identification of spring viraemia of carp virus (SVCV) by combined RT-PCR and nested PCR. Dis Aquat Organ 55:229–235

Chapter 20

Nucleic-Acid Testing, New Platforms and Nanotechnology for Point-of-Decision Diagnosis of Animal Pathogens

Fernando Teles and Luís Fonseca

Abstract

Accurate disease diagnosis in animals is crucial for animal well-being but also for preventing zoonosis transmission to humans. In particular, livestock diseases may constitute severe threats to humans due to the particularly high physical contact and exposure and, also, be the cause of important economic losses, even in non-endemic countries, where they often arise in the form of rapid and devastating epidemics.

Rapid diagnostic tests have been used for a long time in field situations, particularly during outbreaks. However, they mostly rely on serological approaches, which may confirm the exposure to a particular pathogen but may be inappropriate for point-of-decision (point-of-care) settings when emergency responses supported on early and accurate diagnosis are required. Moreover, they often exhibit modest sensitivity and hence significantly depend on later result confirmation in central or reference laboratories. The impressive advances observed in recent years in materials sciences and in nanotechnology, as well as in nucleic-acid synthesis and engineering, have led to an outburst of new in-the-bench and prototype tests for nucleic-acid testing towards point-of-care diagnosis of genetic and infectious diseases. Manufacturing, commercial, regulatory, and technical nature issues for field applicability more likely have hindered their wider entrance into veterinary medicine and practice than have fundamental science gaps. This chapter begins by outlining the current situation, requirements, difficulties, and perspectives of point-of-care tests for diagnosing diseases of veterinary interest. Nucleic-acid testing, particularly for the point of care, is addressed subsequently. A range of valuable signal transduction mechanisms commonly employed in proof-of-concept schemes and techniques born on the analytical chemistry laboratories are also described. As the essential core of this chapter, sections dedicated to the principles and applications of microfluidics, lab-on-a-chip, and nanotechnology for the development of point-of-care tests are presented. Microdevices already applied or under development for application in field diagnosis of animal diseases are reviewed.

Key words Lab-on-a-chip, Microfluidics, Nanotechnology, Nucleic-acid testing, Point of care, Veterinary diagnosis

Abbreviations

AIDS	Acquired immunodeficiency syndrome
BTRP	Biological Threat Reduction Program
CNT	Carbon nanotube
DNA	Deoxyribonucleic acid

Mónica V. Cunha and João Inácio (eds.), *Veterinary Infection Biology: Molecular Diagnostics and High-Throughput Strategies*, Methods in Molecular Biology, vol. 1247, DOI 10.1007/978-1-4939-2004-4_20, © Springer Science+Business Media New York 2015

EIDSS	Electronic Infectious Disease Surveillance System
FIA	Flow-injection analysis
FMD	Foot-and-mouth disease
FMDV	Foot-and-mouth diseases virus
FRET	Fluorescence resonance energy transfer
GNP	Gold nanoparticle
HIV	Human immunodeficiency virus
HPAI	Highly pathogenic avian influenza
LAMP	Loop-mediated isothermal amplification
LATE-PCR	Liner-after-the-exponential PCR
MB	Molecular beacon
MNP	Magnetic NP
MWCNT	Multi-walled CNT
NASBA	Nucleic-acid sequence-based amplification
NP	Nanoparticle
PCR	Polymerase-chain reaction
PDMS	Polydimethylsiloxane
PMMA	Poly(methyl methacrylate)
PNA	Peptide nucleic acid
POC	Point of care
QCM	Quartz-crystal microbalance
QD	Quantum dot
RNA	Ribonucleic acid
rPCR	Real-time PCR
RT-PCR	Reverse-transcription PCR
SARS	Severe acute respiratory syndrome
S/N	Signal-to-noise ratio
S/V	Surface-to-volume ratio
SELEX	Systematic evolution of ligands by exponential enrichment
SPR	Surface plasmon resonance
SWCNT	Single-walled CNT
TADR	Threat Agent Detection and Response

1 The Context of Disease Diagnosis in Veterinary Science, Medicine, and Practice

1.1 Current Situation

As in human medicine, disease diagnosis in veterinary medicine and practice is important for several reasons, including the issues of animal health and welfare, public health (especially in the case of zoonotic agents affecting pets or animals for human consumption), and economy (mainly related to the rules and barriers for the international trade of animals and animal products). In the veterinary field, it is important to consider fauna species other than cattle and farming animals (mainly large terrestrial livestock animals and fishes for aquaculture as well), like pets, captive (e.g., zoo, circus, and aquariums), and wild animals. All of these constitute underestimated sources of many human infectious diseases, especially of viral origin. Animal or human contamination with a veterinary-relevant pathogen may occur through infected animals (live or dead) and infected animal products (e.g., bush meat, unpasteurized milk) or, to a lesser extent, through direct contact with the pathogen itself. In developing countries and regions, the impact of livestock diseases and outbreaks goes far beyond animal welfare and food safety. Too often, farm animals are also the only way of human and cargo transportation and also of income, as feedstock, as a source of manure and draft power, and as raw material for other industries (e.g., leather, shoes, and clothing) [1].

The advent of human immunodeficiency virus (HIV)/acquired immunodeficiency syndrome (AIDS) and other human immune depressing conditions has been a relatively neglected factor of enhanced susceptibility of humans to animal diseases, especially with respect to pets. Immune-depressed individuals or other vulnerable groups, such as children or the elderly, may even become susceptible to subtypes of zoonotic microorganisms that are usually harmless for healthy humans [2]. Interaction between domestic and wild animals may also provide an important via for indirect human contamination [3]. A particularly important group of zoonotic agents is that of enteric pathogens that are transmitted to and between humans and animals through the oral-fecal route, with subsequent dissemination to wastewater effluents. Outbreaks may occur upon contamination of surface waters and groundwater used for recreational and irrigation purposes and insufficient microbial removal of drinking water and/or of treated wastewaters, since many of these enteric pathogens are resilient to classical treatment and disinfection procedures [4]. They often contaminate water supplies in very small concentrations, hence hindering final disinfection and complicating detection as well [5]. Screening of enteric zoonotic agents has been proposed for pets cohabiting with immune-susceptible humans [6]. Very often, the presence of enteric viruses is detected indirectly, through bacterial indicators of fecal contamination, namely, coliforms and enterococci [5]. On the other hand, emerging "wild-type" zoonosis have been transmitted from animals to humans (e.g., SARS and West Nile virus) or after specific mutations that facilitate the "species jump" (e.g., HIV and H5N1 or H1N1 influenza) [7]. Concerning bioterrorism issues and depending on the nature of the infectious pathogen, the detection of potential zoonotic agents in animals should alert for an intentional release act [8]. A successful anti-bioterrorism strategy must not only account for the detection of the known pathogen but also of genetically modified forms. However, only a few potential veterinary pathogens fulfill the criteria for being considered effective bioterrorist agents. The group is composed by the viral agents of rinderpest, classical swine fever, African swine fever, avian influenza, Newcastle disease, Rift Valley fever, and foot-and-mouth disease (FMD) [1]. Among them, FMD and avian influenza are especially important for their high prevalence in the world, zoonotic potential, and ramping spread. FMD is generally considered the most contagious viral disease in animals. Occasional occurrences in non-endemic regions are usually difficult and expensive to control [9]. Avian influenza is a viral disease with pandemic potential; pigs can act as intermediate hosts of influenza viruses between birds and humans. Bidirectional transmission of these viruses between humans and pigs is documented [7].

The diagnosis of air-borne diseases is challenging, with implications in disease control, especially in the case of outbreaks, and in individual case management. For these diseases, timely adoption of quarantine measures and massive antimicrobial therapy administration may be sufficient to contain an emerging outbreak, as long as the first cases are spotted in a short time. However, this may be impracticable in developing countries and regions, where effective routine surveillance flaws. Thus, a successful containment strategy must include rapid diagnosis through inexpensive and easy-to-use portable devices for in-the-field use [10]. As an example, it has been proposed that, within 6 h of the reporting of a suspicious FMD case, definitive detection should be made upon sample transportation to a national or regional laboratory, or else on the farm itself, and that, within 24 h of reporting, definitive identification of the infecting strain/subtype should be accomplished, immediately followed by vaccine production (from stored antigens) and distribution [1].

1.2 The Need for Point-of-Care Testing

Following the trend of human medicine, the diagnosis of animal diseases has also undergone progressive decentralization, from central (reference) laboratories to in-the-field bioanalytical instrumentation, very often in resource-depleted regions and settings, even outside laboratory infrastructures. Essentially, this has been done through adaptation of conventional analytical methods and instrumentation to portable and automated devices, able to be handled by laboratory unskilled personnel (viz., veterinarian practitioners and farmers). Several nomenclatures have been given to these tests. They include the names "field tests", "rapid tests", "biosensors", and "point-of-care (POC) tests"; this last term will be predominantly used throughout this chapter. Improved diagnostic tests are necessary for asymptomatic diseases, for diseases with misleading symptoms, for diseases requiring different treatments, or for diseases that, by their complex or costly treatment, require previous case confirmation. By contrast, these tests will likely have little or no impact for diseases which are easily recognized by their clinical symptoms and for which a syndromic treatment/approach is recommended. There is thus no clinical need to identify the causal agent. However, surveillance and control measures must be maintained for these diseases in order to deal with the risk of major epidemics [11]. It is among livestock animals that disease epidemic outbreaks are more likely to occur, and with higher magnitude, given the physical proximity of many animals under intensive husbandry, the probability of pathogens to contaminate neighboring farms, and the relatively poor biosecurity conditions of most farms, but also in the case of subclinical diseases. As time is crucial when managing the early stages of infectious disease, an immediate preliminary positive result obtained by a POC test strongly argues in favor of precautionary and preventive measures in affected farms and surroundings in order to avoid further transmission, until a definite and more accurate result can be obtained in a reference laboratory [12]. Ideally, POC tests should go towards increased sensitivity, not only for early case identification but also for disease surveillance and epidemiological purposes, as infected animals may suffer and constitute infected reservoirs for disease spreading [11]. During the 2001 FMD outbreak in the United Kingdom, most of the livestock in infected and neighboring farms was targeted for culling during the first 24–48 h, based solely on clinical signs, which may be considerably doubtful, especially in sheep, the main species affected [13]. The time span between animal infection and the onset of clinical symptoms, and hence infection awareness, can take months, usually through rapid and silent spreading within and between herds, which might need to be destroyed [14]. However, indoor controlled studies with experimental infection of cattle with FMD virus (FMDV) showed a smaller-than-expected transmission fraction during the overlapping period between the incubation and the infectious period, suggesting that the importance of common preventive measures taken at endangered farms (viz., preemptive culling of cattle, often with severe economic downturn) has been overestimated [15]. For most viral diseases, since the onset of detectable viremia usually occurs at least 1 day before the onset of infection and/or presentation of clinical signs, efforts should be devoted to the development of new diagnosis methodologies and tools at preclinical stages. Historically, public funds have been used to compensate farmers for massive slaughtering of suspected diseased animals, but it has been argued that this may have generated permissive behaviors and disinterest from livestock industries and owners about transboundary control of cattle diseases [1]. In theory, POC tests are advantageous over laboratory-based tests if they can be used to detect infected animals before they become infectious, especially if this time window is short, as in the case of FMD. This advantage would apply if the time between collection of samples and receipt of results in the laboratory is, at least, 24 h. In the medium term, POC tests for cattle diseases will likely play an increasing role in the screening and triage of biological samples collected on the farm, as a primary support for decision-making during disease outbreaks [16], under a challenging context of permissive biological containment.

In veterinary medicine, POC tests have been largely used, for some decades, for the screening of physiological metabolites in blood and urine. Pathogen detection is a newer application, mainly driven by the increasing number of emerging outbreaks, including those with public health importance. Among these is, for instance, the potentially pandemic H5N1 avian influenza, as well as influenza viruses of putative porcine origin, as the human pandemic strain of 2009 [12]. POC tests have also been developed for important diseases of aquatic animals, using similar technologies to those used for terrestrial animals [17]. The most common layouts of commercially available devices rely on antigen detection in biological samples through affinity binding reactions with immobilized specific antibody probes. Nevertheless, despite the requirement for essentially the same performance features, regulatory approval and introduction of these devices into the market are understandably easier in the veterinary than in the clinical practice [18].

1.3 Difficulties Faced by Point-of-Care Testing

Disease sub-notification remains a major problem for veterinarian health authorities; despite notifiable diseases are of obligatory reporting, too often farmers (and even veterinarians and diagnostic laboratories) ignore or delay the notification process owing to unawareness, minimization, or perceived lack of consequences, which may be aggravated when economic losses are anticipated. It is expected this scenario to worsen as POC tests become more readily available for utilization by farmers, especially in cases of delayed or misleading diagnosis based upon the clinical signs, as a result of disease underestimation or confusion with the signs of non-notifiable endemic diseases [12]. Of course, the interpretation of clinical signs itself and subsequent decision-making processes are compromised by the fact of farmers being unskilled personnel in health and veterinary medicine issues. Reducing the risk of non-reporting depends on tight cooperation and trust between veterinary authorities and livestock farmers and dealers [19]. In the livestock business, especially for important livestock diseases (e.g., classical swine fever), the risk of announcing a false-positive result is particularly worrisome, as it carries detrimental consequences in trade and export. Sanitary requisites on imported livestock for human feeding are very demanding and restrictive in most countries, leading to severe economic losses in cases of insufficient or inaccurate pathogen testing. Therefore, individual animal testing may be one of the main drivers for commercial development of POC tests, because a preliminary positive result with a POC test may prevent further and more expensive testing, while holding the herd being ineligible for export as well [12]. Some animal diseases are particularly contagious and able to spread rapidly. Many of them are considered transboundary diseases, meaning that their detection turns into the prohibition of livestock export and thus in economic losses. The combination of permanent surveillance programs with improved techniques for rapid detection of emerging pathogen subtypes for efficient control of transboundary diseases has been claimed [20]. Unambiguous identification of circulating pathogen subtypes (viz., genotypes and/or serotypes) is frequently a relevant epidemiological feature for the success of disease control programs. For low-prevalence diseases, the proportion of false-positive results is usually higher than for more prevalent ones. In addition, many of the current POC tests are less sensitive and specific than laboratory-based methods. Altogether, this means that, in order to achieve a desired level of performance and confidence in the results, sampling a large number of animals is usually required for POC-based testing of low-prevalent diseases [12]. In pets, the prevalence of many pathogens, particularly of zoonotic parasites, has been probably underestimated as a consequence, among other reasons, of using inadequate and inaccurate diagnostic tests and procedures, including limitations in sample collection and processing, which may directly result in false-negative results [21, 22] and, as such, putting the animals themselves and their owners at greater risk than currently assumed [3].

Intellectual property constraints frequently hamper the passage of these new devices from the proof of principle to the prototype and even commercialization levels. Another bottleneck is the high cost for final development of such devices, the reason why partnerships between research laboratories and biotechnological companies are usually established with such purpose. In this case, of course, the economic leitmotiv is much higher for high-impact diseases, especially those for which control of outbreaks is difficult and expensive. However, even for such diseases (e.g., FMD), the only sporadic and unpredictable character of outbreaks might disincentive investments in individual testing; high demand usually only occurs by the occasion of an outbreak or suspected outbreak. Only a few tests for economically important livestock diseases have been developed and commercialized in developed countries, due to the limited market resulting from only infrequent diseases [12]. It seems that the most promising commercial segment for POC devices for veterinary pathogens concerns multiplexed platforms for a wide range of endemic and non-endemic pathogens [16], taking advantage of the relative simplicity and low cost of incorporating several additional targets in a multiplexed test. Indeed, veterinary health services eagerly lack rapid and simple diagnostic devices designed for in-the-field simultaneous detection, in a single sample, of a broader range of common pathogens [8], thus enabling the rapid gathering of field information on individual animals or whole herds disease status. Currently, simultaneous identification and eventual subtyping of many pathogens in a single test run is a province of central or reference laboratories and only available if the demanding entity (e.g., person, laboratory, or agency) is able to afford to pay for such expensive testing. POC tests have been also used for field differentiation between vaccine and field strains, especially in endemic regions where vaccination is permitted [12]. Suitable application of such differential testing at slaughtering settings to confirm prior livestock vaccination has been argued [1].

1.4 Challenges for Point-of-Care Testing

The ultimate goal of the use of POC portable devices by unskilled and unsupervised practitioners will likely pose enormous challenges for the overall bioanalytical process, from sample acquisition to post-analytical data storage, interpretation, and management. Bearing in mind that most of these devices are to be commonly used in remote and low-resource regions, uncontrolled and irregular reporting of results, in addition to test biosafety, especially when dealing with zoonotic agents, are major issues [23]. For these reasons, a balanced merging between in-the-field testing with remote data analysis and interpretation by competent clinical staff may be desirable. In this regard, telemedicine is an attractive system for healthcare improvement in developing countries, for allowing unskilled persons to provide useful healthcare in remote settings. This can be carried out by using miniaturized analytical devices with integrated hardware for image acquisition and software for storage of results. These results can be downloaded to hard copies or directly transferred online for a remote healthcare central unit for processing and interpretation by expert personal. Processed results can afterwards be returned to the tester, almost in real time [24]. Remote data from POC systems can still be incorporated in national disease surveillance and diagnostic systems, as the Threat Agent Detection and Response (TADR), developed under the Biological Threat Reduction Program (BTRP) of the US Defense Department's Defense Threat Reduction Agency. This system uses real-time polymerase-chain reaction (rPCR) for detection of pathogens. Another surveillance system, the Electronic Infectious Disease Surveillance System (EIDSS), contains a subsystem to report suspicious disease outbreaks in real time. The EIDSS is able to locate disease outbreaks through a geographic positioning device. This system aims to encompassing all available public and animal disease surveillance information. The EIDSS is able to report laboratory results from rPCR up to a few hours, depending on the distance. These systems will eventually enable a shift of paradigm in remote analysis, allowing world reference laboratories to simply handle and manage diagnostic information from pathogens and hosts based on biological samples remotely collected and analyzed, with subsequent reporting of results to the countries and regions of origin [1].

A full evaluation program of POC tests must include performance evaluation (validation), quality assessment (control and assurance), and standardization [25]. The performance of POC tests is highly dependent on the local conditions for their use, on the epidemiology of the pathogen, and on the biology of the host [26]. Thus, the evaluation of such tests sets the particular ranges of in-the-field conditions in which they can be used [27], ideally under multicenter evaluation. Quality control assures correct functioning of the devices with prolonged use; usually, randomly selected units from a given production batch are compared to infer reproducibility. The quality assurance step demonstrates the readiness of the tests to be introduced into the routine diagnostic practice. Standardization is needed in POC diagnostics for veterinary applications, as well as new rules to compare results obtained from the two different methodologies—the POC and the laboratory-based method, respectively—which implicates in the final (accepted) diagnostic result [23, 28]. Proper validation and standardization of many POC tests frequently lack, in part because these often correspond to in-house rather than to well-standardized assays and techniques. It is thus important that national or reference healthcare entities establish quality assurance programs that guarantee the production of reference materials and protocols for effective quality control of rapid diagnostic tests [29]. For the clinics, a set of guidelines for standardization of POC blood-based tests has already been established [30]. Hopefully, in the future, this will also be useful to inspire standardization procedures in new diagnostics for veterinary medicine and practice.

POC tests hold great promise to shift the paradigm of veterinary diagnostics, particularly for field situations, and in cases in which the biological sample is easy to collect and process. However, its advantageous use presumes the availability of sufficient manpower to survey enough animals on high-risk premises, which remains a burdensome challenge. The decision of whether using them or not to manage animal infectious diseases depends on biological and epidemiological factors, on the specific circumstances in which clinical signs arise, on cost-benefit issues (taking into account the costs for deployment, including equipment and reagent storage), and on the relative performance compared to diagnostic tests in reference laboratories. The possibility of sending suspect samples to a central laboratory within 24–48 h has probably discouraged the use of POC tests in some past situations in Western countries, e.g., under medical suspicion of highly pathogenic avian influenza (HPAI); from another point of view, this strengthens the idea of a promising use of these tests in remote regions, far away from laboratory settings. Once POC tests have equivalent analytical sensitivity and specificity to laboratory-based tests, it may be foreseen, on the basis of a POC test alone, to take actions beyond simple restriction/quarantine on suspect premises [12]. Transboundary livestock diseases are probably among the major concerns in veterinary medicine. It has been proposed that an efficient governmental control strategy of these diseases should include legislation enforcing, namely, (a) disease screening in people, conveyances, and goods arriving from other countries, in a reasonable extent, according to previously defined performance benchmarks, including possible use of robotic automated devices; (b) higher extent of screening for people, conveyances, and goods arriving from endemic countries, even reaching exhaustive screening when such countries are recognized as not making acceptable progresses in disease control; and (c) the need to develop tests to certificate animal product's region or country of origin, at the point of importation [1]. These points certainly constitute an immense and valuable fountainhead of opportunities for commercial attraction-driven development of new POC devices in the veterinary field.

2 Nucleic-Acid Testing

2.1 Advantages for Disease Diagnosis

Early disease diagnosis not only prevents or minimizes potential animal suffering but also the risk for infection transmission among susceptible hosts [31]. In contrast, delayed diagnosis carries an increased risk for severe symptoms and complications, ultimately leading to longer suffering, increased toxicity due to accumulated pathogen load and/or virulence effects, and a higher risk for acquisition of drug resistance [12]. Antibody-based detection requires a sufficient level of antibodies to be produced for successful detection, which usually happens only some days after exposure to the pathogen. In this regard, specific detection of pathogen nucleic acids in biological samples by PCR-based methods may be more suitable, since the pathogen genomic material is present in the host from the very beginning of infection and even very little amounts are detectable before the onset of immune response markers or clinical or veterinary signs. Moreover, methods based in nucleic-acid detection are able to detect both live and dead pathogens, an advantage for disease diagnosis [1], especially when time is crucial for disease containment and control. In conventional methods (e.g., cell culturing and serology), pathogen detection strongly depends on the sample quality [13], leading more easily to false-negative or irreproducible results.

Deoxyribonucleic acid (DNA) is a particularly suitable material for biosensing owing to unique characteristics, including the ability for highly specific and mutual recognition between a short immobilized oligonucleotide (probe) and a longer-sized genome and high physicochemical stability. Unlike enzymes and antibodies, DNA forms biological recognition layers easily synthesizable and readily reusable after thermal heating [24]. DNA is also prone to very specific manipulation and processing precision by ligases, nucleases, and other enzymes [32] and is the most easily copyable biomolecule, through PCR and similar techniques of amplification, which is also an enormous advantage for the development of portable and miniaturized diagnostic devices. In addition, DNA micro- and nanoarrays are more suitable than protein counterparts for direct synthesis onto a chip surface, without the need to produce and purify the ligands [33]. Most of these features of DNA are also extensive to ribonucleic acid (RNA). Indeed, nucleic-acid (molecular biology) testing comprises genetic analysis (DNA level) and functional genomics (including mRNA, non-coding RNA, and microRNA). In particular, functional genomics dedicates to the identification and analysis of specific RNA expression patterns (profiles) associated with particular experimental or clinical conditions. DNA (and RNA) microarrays and quantitative PCR have been the most common techniques used with this purpose [34]. DNA microarrays (DNA chips) are usually produced in the form of highly dense arrays printed on a silicon or glass chip, coated with different probes for simultaneous detection of multiple DNA-target sequences [35]. Current microarrays can detect in the order of 10^4 nucleic-acid sequences on a single chip [1]. The Virochip is particularly well succeeded in this regard; it is a panviral DNA microarray platform, able to detect known viruses and new viruses related to known viral families, in a single assay. Its high robustness has been confirmed with viruses of high genetic variability, as the swine virus. This platform is especially useful for detecting viruses for which there are no available reverse transcription-PCR (RT-PCR) assays [7]. Nevertheless, microarrays do not seem promising for the POC use, being too expensive, complex, and bulky [24]. Another peculiarity of DNA-based detection is the superior ability to differentiate strains from the same organism, especially when isolated from different geographical locations. This is useful not only for pathogen identification but also for epidemiological studies. As an example, the significant differences among the nucleic-acid sequences of the different serotypes of FMDV (as in other viruses) and the likelihood for the occurrence of typing errors during viral RNA replication demonstrate how the virus can rapidly evolve in nature [36], which constitutes an enormous challenge for successful viral identification. In influenza viruses, genetic reassortment is able to generate novel subtypes whose cell surface antigens might no longer be recognized by preexisting antibodies (antigenic drift) [37]. The potential for pandemics caused by novel highly pathogenic subtypes strongly stresses the need for specific subtype identification through nucleic-acid testing. Of course, the drifting in influenza viruses, responsible for the sudden onset of dominant subtypes during a yearly season, requires not only rapid development and validation of suitable molecular probes for nucleic-acid tests but also the unobstructed use of such tests. Unraveling the pathogen subtypes circulating in a given region may assist in designing tailored vaccines and disease containment strategies, as well as tracking outbreaks' sources [38].

2.2 Nucleic-Acid Testing in the Point of Care

Most of the current POC tests for human and animal medicine still rely on antigen/antibody bioaffinity reactions, but they are usually handicapped by relatively small sensitivity. Thus, there is a trend for shifting towards more sensitive nucleic-acid detection, usually based on DNA/DNA hybridization schemes. A major challenge for detection of pathogen nucleic acids in host body fluids, apart their scarcity compared to antigenic proteins, is the confinement inside pathogen cells, surrounded by hard biomembranes and cell walls. Consequently, the nucleic-acid levels present in host fluids may be too low for successful diagnosis without prior target amplification by PCR-based techniques. For blood infections in humans, the amount of human genomic DNA can be 10^{14} times higher than that of pathogen DNA [39], an important challenge in terms of sensitivity and selectivity. For POC testing, this constitutes a challenge for the miniaturization of the blood sample preparation step, especially in the case of gram-positive bacteria, whose cell walls are thicker and more rigid than those of gram-negative bacteria. The majority of available POC systems for clinical and veterinary applications require off-device sample preparation (including microorganism concentration and nucleic-acid extraction). This is a traditionally cumbersome and time-consuming step, especially for in-the-field testing, but newer processes, including filter paper capture of nucleic acids and automated extraction procedures and kits, have been developed to simplify such task [40]. In parallel with POC device development, considerable efforts have been spent in the simplification and robustness of sample preparation, in order to minimize manual handling, thus reducing cross-contamination and the effects from potentially interfering substances present during the nucleic-acid amplification assay. Of note are the technical difficulties inherent to the analysis of matrices such as feces, semen, and decomposing tissue or the detection of *Mycobacterium tuberculosis* from saliva [12]. For these cases, it is necessary to incorporate, in POC devices, systems that are able to suppress such interfering substances and that reduce handling prior to the nucleic-acid amplification step.

PCR has been, by far, the most widely employed technique for nucleic-acid amplification in laboratory analysis but also in POC tests. Many similar techniques have been originated from the basic PCR principles, including nucleic-acid sequence-based amplification (NASBA), targeted for direct RNA amplification, thus precluding the need for a previous reverse-transcription step. The development of this panoply of techniques for pathogen detection has been possible due to the increasing availability of whole genomic sequences; a remarkable case in veterinary science is the current possibility of rapidly distinguishing severe acute respiratory syndrome (SARS) from other circulating coronaviruses [41]. Nevertheless, PCR is prone to false-positive results, as a result of unwanted amplification of contaminant nucleic acids. Proper quality management of these issues requires using adequate controls for each stage of the testing process [12]. For RNA analysis through RT-PCR, storing biological samples at very low temperatures is crucial, owing to the high liability of RNA genomes. Innovative lyophilized reagents with enhanced sensitivities have significantly improved the operational conditions for POC disease diagnosis [42]. Moreover, the need for improved stability of RNA used as an internal positive control, especially for real-time RT-PCR assays, has led to the search for new RNA sources. Another approach for improving RNA assays is the use of minor groove-binding probes which, by being short sized, are suitable for multiplexing and for targeting sequences of highly variable genomes [20]. Nevertheless, PCR-based techniques remain challenging for POC pathogen diagnosis in many endemic regions of the world. Even in human medicine, however, RT-PCR, for instance, is only used for clinically important specimens, due to the complexity and time demanding of this technique [43]. Linear-after-the-exponential PCR (LATE-PCR) is another PCR-based technique for detection of RNA. Probably its most known application is in FMDV subtyping, to tackle the difficulty of targeting all field strains with novel sequence mutations, even those in target sequences for which degenerate primers are being used [44]. The amplification process can begin with as few as a single DNA molecule and abundantly generates amplified product over a broad temperature range. The technique employs primers that hybridize to conserved genomic regions and a mismatch-tolerant probe able to target different variable sequences, depending on the temperature. Thus, the technique is especially convenient for detection of RNA viruses [36].

Among the vast diversity of available nucleic-acid amplification schemes and devices, both at the proof-of-concept and commercial levels, the technique of loop-mediated isothermal amplification (LAMP), already widely used in laboratory analysis, seems quite promising for application in POC systems for pathogen detection and identification. In remote PCR-based nucleic-acid testing, power supply is a keystone for device operation, although the use of rechargeable batteries is expected to circumvent this problem, by avoiding the need for an external power source [42]. Advantageously, LAMP does not require thermal cycling for the amplification, rather making use of a simpler power source compared to a PCR thermocycler. Such operation at constant and low temperatures permits LAMP to be incorporated in polymer-based microdevices instead of more traditional and expensive materials, like glass and silicon that, for being temperature-resistant, are required for PCR-based devices. Unlike PCR, LAMP does not require a denatured template for amplification, and given the usual abundance of generated DNA, the amplified product can often be visualized directly [13]. For viral detection, in particular, the technique has shown sensitivity at least equivalent to PCR [45] and even to rPCR [46]. Coupled to easier sample preparation procedures, these features make LAMP inherently simple and hence especially suitable for POC applications [47].

POC tests based on nucleic-acid amplification potentially allow early detection of latently infected animals on targeted high-risk premises, with some examples already being applied in field situations [48]. However, this would require sample collection and testing from many suspect herds, which will require too demanding manpower in the course of an outbreak. This is probably why existing tests have not been adopted in contingency plans in many countries, although the issue remains controversial [12]. During the FMD outbreak in 2007, up to 269 samples were analyzed each day [38], but larger outbreaks would require higher-throughput testing. Of course, from a certain point above, it is admissible that central laboratories would become overloaded and that true POC devices, able to be manipulated by farmers themselves, would be probably the best (or even unique) solution. This, however, by the reasons pointed above, is still far from reality, although the unstoppable technological advances in this field, coupled to new paradigms for decentralized detection, will more and more shorten the present distance to that goal.

3 Methods for Signal Transduction in Biosensors and Point-of-Care Devices

For bioanalysis with prototype biosensors and POC devices, three main types of signal transduction mechanisms have been used: electrochemical, optical, and microgravimetric (mass sensitive). They are well known and have been extensively used in research laboratories for analytical chemistry, holding great promise for new prototype and fully developed bioanalytical and diagnostic microdevices. Among microgravimetric methods, quartz-crystal microbalance (QCM) is the most common; it usually relies on the use of a piezoelectric crystal whose fundamental resonance frequency changes upon successive immobilization of a biorecognition probe and its target. However, the difficulty of miniaturization, the high cost, and the complex influence of multiple interfacial parameters on the sensor response (especially in liquid phase) have hampered wider development of POC devices based on this technique. The applicability of electrochemical methods for nucleic-acid analysis has greatly benefited from the emergence of solid electrodes [24]. Electrochemical-based analytical devices can be relatively simple, rapid, less costly, low-power demanding, and amenable for miniaturization and mass production through standardized microfabrication techniques [49].

Optical detection has been the most widely employed transducing principle in biosensing, partially driven by the unending advances of optic applications in telecommunications and information systems. Furthermore, the very high frequency of optical signals is appropriated for the enormous amount of information that can be carried by optical systems and devices [24]. Conventional optical microscopy has been reliably used for detection and imaging of infectious pathogens (at both cellular and molecular levels), integrated with research and development of new POC diagnostic devices [50]. Within optical detection methods, chemiluminescence and fluorescence have been the most widely used for their versatility of designs and applications. Imaging methods usually require bulky and expensive microscopes and camera-equipped microscopy systems, i.e., in off-device formats. Such equipment is obviously unsuitable for POC diagnostics. The innovative technique of optofluidic seems thus promising in this regard, as this high-throughput and high-resolution on-device technique does not make use of such components [51]. In optofluidic devices, the sample flows through a metal film-etched array with submicron apertures for imaging, onto a plastic platform.

An intrinsic limitation of conventional optical detection is the interference between closely spaced light waves. Understandably, this is especially limiting for the design and performance of miniaturized devices for multi-analyte detection and identification. However, optical transmission through minuscule structures gained a new impulse with the technique of surface plasmon resonance (SPR), in which light waves are directed to the interface between a metal and a dielectric. The technique is label-free and the immobilized probe can be easily reused, although sensitivity must still be improved [24]. Moreover, it faces the challenges of other optical techniques for POC diagnosis, namely, the high cost, instrumental complexity, expensiveness of optical components, and difficulty for miniaturization/portability and mass production. The advent of integrated photodiode detectors is promising for the development of cheap, sensitive, easy-to-use, and easy-to-fabricate fluorescence-based diagnostic microdevices [52]. A remarkable milestone might be the shift from current fluorescent-based detection methods to naked-eye (visual) recognition, which would considerably reduce complexity and costs. These readouts can be recorded as digital images and then transmitted to remote clinicians through trivial and inexpensive telecommunication devices (e.g., digital cameras and scanners); some current examples include the detection of glucose, pH, and proteins [53]. It is expected that future POC diagnostic devices will become connected to wireless communication and information systems through camera-equipped mobile phone networks coupled to web databases, for diagnostic imaging and telemedicine, especially in remote and resource-limited regions and settings [54]. Remote monitoring will not constitute a valuable or even indispensable way for analysis when in-the-field conditions do not allow doing that, but also an approach to improve quality management for tests conducted in the field.

4 New Platforms for Point-of-Care Disease Diagnosis

4.1 Microfluidics

Multiplex PCR and DNA microarrays have been among the most commonly used techniques for the detection and identification of infectious pathogens. Multiplex PCR is frequently limited to the analysis of only a few target genes, owing to interferences between different primer sets in the same reaction vessel. DNA microarrays are usually too expensive, labor intensive, and complex for POC applications; moreover, the microarray assays are usually lengthy due to the slow diffusion-limited hybridization kinetics. On the other hand, lateral-flow devices employed for POC diagnosis usually have relatively low sensitivity; moreover, in the most common format (immunochromatographic format, corresponding to the well-known test strips), they do not provide genetic information, thus hindering the assessment of eventual pathogen subtypes and/or drug resistance markers. In general, the number of targets that can be simultaneously probed in lateral-flow assays is low, thus increasing the cost per assay and limiting the throughput. Also, their degree of multiplexing usually does not reach that of microarrays [55].

The last decade has witnessed tremendous advances in microfluidic sciences and applications for bioanalysis. Microfluidic devices basically consist in a set of microchambers interconnected through microchannels, imprinted onto a suitable solid platform. After injection into the system, the liquid biological sample flows throughout the hydrophilic inner walls of the chambers and channels for final analysis. The flow is usually controlled automatically by mechanical valves. A primary advantage of microfluidics for the development of miniaturized diagnostic devices, especially for POC usage, is the requirement for only very small sample volumes, which permits to save reagents (viz., probes and labels), but also gaining time and sensitivity, as a consequence of the enhanced binding kinetics (unlike in bulky reaction media). It also provides lower power consumption and lower operating costs. Moreover, since the overall analytical process is automated, sample losses and contamination due to human handling can be minimized, in parallel with improved multiplexing capabilities. The confinement and automation of the process also reduces errors due to human manipulation and increases biosafety. In microfluidic devices, the occurrence of nucleic-acid hybridization in solution and the enhanced aqueous mixing allow surpassing the kinetic barriers that slow affinity reactions due to limited diffusion in traditional microarrays [53]. Recent developments in microfluidic technology have pointed towards integrating traditionally off-chip processes into the microdevices. Indeed, significant reduction of bulky, complex, and expensive equipment is mandatory for POC and in-the-field diagnostic applications.

Traditional microfluidic devices usually rely on pressure-driven flow (through a syringe pump or pressure injector) or electroosmotic flow, but these techniques require external bulky and complex equipment, like a power supply. For POC applications, more suitable methods for fluid delivery have been developed, namely, mechanical pumping, capillarity, and light-driven motion [53]. Compared to conventional injection systems, as flow-injection analysis (FIA), microfluidics enables achieving lower detection limits, as a result of enhanced probe/target binding kinetics [56] and of time-dependent target pre-concentration in microchambers. Droplet-based schemes offer a significant improvement in microfluidics, due to the ability to independently control each free droplet containing the target under analysis. In this way, each single droplet functions as a pump, valve, mixer, solid-phase extractor, and thermocycler, thus greatly simplifying the assay design [10].

The first microfluidic devices were manufactured as glass or silicon platforms, but the high cost of these materials led to the widespread use of polydimethylsiloxane (PDMS) for such purpose. However, some properties of PDMS limit its use for biosensing in microfluidic devices, e.g., hydrophobicity and swelling/disintegration in organic solvents. In order to prevent some of the limitations of PDMS, other materials have been used, like paper and thermoplastics. These materials, as well as their fabrication process, are cheaper than PDMS, glass, and silicon, making large-scale fabrication more feasible. This low cost also encourages disposability, an important biosafety asset when dealing with infectious agents, and a way to avoid cross-contamination of biological samples. Moreover, these materials are lightweight and hence easy to transport in the form of portable devices. Finally, their fabrication does not require clean-room settings. Thermoplastics are attractive materials for simple, low-cost, and reproducible fabrication of POC devices by well-known replication molding techniques (e.g., injection molding or hot embossing). An example is poly(methyl methacrylate) (PMMA), which is mechanically stable, is optically transparent, and has an easily modifiable surface. Another example is polycarbonate, whose lower thermic conductivity in comparison with glass or silicon turns it amenable for high-temperature PCR applications [53]. Patterned paper-based microfluidic devices are valuable alternatives to test strips. Advantages of paper include its abundance, easiness to use (e.g., clean rooms or other complex and expensive infrastructures for its manipulation are unnecessary), low cost, disposability, and easily patterned with polymers and other molecules by conventional printing techniques (e.g., photolithography, wax and inkjet printing). Its common white color is particularly suitable for the use of colored substrates in quantitative colorimetric tests. Moreover, unlike in test strips and conventional microfluidics, its porous nature allows capillarity-driven fluid wicking and flow through its structure, without the need for external pumps and pressure source. New three-dimensional structures will enable a vertical flow to be added to the sole lateral flow of two-dimensional devices, in higher complex structures than those presented by plastic frames. In this way, they may exhibit improved abilities for initial purification and concentration as the liquid wicks throughout the inner layers of the device, until final detection [57].

Many current microfluidic devices still rely on complex and bulky laboratorial (off-chip) equipment for fluid delivery and control, making their use impractical in field situations, e.g., by emergency response teams [53]. Other drawbacks faced by microfluidic systems include biomolecule adsorption to microchannel walls, inaccurate control of temperature, liquid evaporation due to heat-generating components, and bubble formation [5]. In addition, future developments in microfluidic platforms may eventually benefit from materials with improved analytical performance [58], as well as simplicity and cost-effectiveness.

4.2 Lab-on-a-Chip

The processes of sample purification and pre-concentration are usually the most complex and cumbersome in biological analysis. In molecular diagnostics, this is particularly true for nucleic-acid isolation procedures, which still remain too complex for in-the-field use. One of commonest requirements is a centrifuge, which obviously hinders the integration of such detection schemes within miniaturized analytical devices. In many diagnostic microdevices, such procedures are carried out off-chip, prior to the detection step itself. Moreover, they strongly depend on the characteristics of the specific biological sample and require relatively high volumes of raw sample for downstream nucleic-acid amplification. In the last years, lab-on-a-chip devices have emerged as second-generation chips, essentially based on the concept of microfluidics. By suitable integration of modules for sample processing and analysis in a single device, they offer enhanced flexibility and discriminatory ability over conventional diagnostic methods and devices. Yet, minimizing and miniaturizing the whole sample preparation procedure towards easiness to use and true POC remains challenging and a relatively underestimated task in the development of POC tests [5]. Compared to conventional detection techniques, lab-on-a-chip devices allow the integration and automation of all (or nearly all) steps for sample processing and analysis; the confinement of the bioelement under measurement in a predefined region of interest facilitates its detection and eventual quantification from very small sample volumes. This, in turn, reduces background noise and hence increases sensitivity [53]. In lab-on-a-chip devices, minimization of the chemical interferences that result from tight spatial confinement is usually envisaged, enabling miniaturization and highly sensitive detection. The high mass transfer rate thus achieved is due to the low diffusional distance and high surface-to-volume ratio (S/V) [59]. Traditional cell analysis and processing, including cell sorting, cell/serum separation (for immunoassays), and cell lysis (for immunoassays or nucleic-acid amplification), can be adapted to POC schemes [53]. Some principles commonly used to separate and concentrate cells within POC devices are cell size, labeling (fluorescent or magnetic), electrophoretic mobility, and cell adhesion [60]. For analysis of real, biological samples, the detection of highly virulent pathogens presumes the ability of detecting very few cells from large sample volumes and, concurrently, washing out sample contaminants (e.g., other cells), in order to prevent, for instance, downstream PCR inhibition and microchannel clogging [61]. In particular, environmental water samples may contain certain substances, like humic acids, that inhibit PCR reactions, able to drastically decrease the resulting signals. The presence of contaminants in biological samples may be particularly troublesome in microfluidic assays for veterinary applications.

A particular advantage of bioanalysis with lab-on-a-chip devices concerns the processing of pathogen RNA. Owing to the confined environment of the purification steps and to the requirement for minimal user handling, the probability for RNA contamination and degradation by ubiquitous RNases is highly decreased [62]. Schemes employing nucleic-acid extraction through detergents rather than high temperature-operating lytic enzymes coupled with isothermal (e.g., LAMP) instead of PCR and RT-PCR amplification processes are also preferred in this regard. In this way, the concept of microfluidics might be able to address a recurrent gap in veterinary literature—the lack of information about RNA quality and integrity, which further complicates the standardization of RT-PCR procedures [34]. Several commercial multiplexed POC tests for diagnosis of influenza and other respiratory viruses are already available, as the FilmArray RP (BioFire Diagnostics, Salt Lake City/UT, United States), the xTAG RVP (Luminex, Toronto, Canada), and the Xpert Flu A Panel (Cepheid, Sunnyvale/CA, United States), consisting in closed systems that include sample preparation and detection by integrated RT-PCR [63, 64]. However, these systems may not be able to detect low viral load specimens, as is the case of the Xpert Flu A Panel with some important avian influenza viruses. In addition, economic constraints still restrict full applicability of some of these tests in POC testing. For the Xpert Flu A panel, it was estimated a cost of 45 euros per test, compared to 15 euros for the antigenic tests [63]. Current lab-on-a-chip devices, despite being simpler than conventional laboratory

Table 1

Illustrative works described in the literature employing nucleic-acid amplification methods for the detection of animal pathogens. POC tests are those claiming, at least, one of the following characteristics: lab-on-a-chip; microfluidics; portability

Target pathogen(s)	POC Yes	POC No	Amplification method	LOD or sensitivity	References
African swine fever virus		×	LAMP	≤330 copies	[67]
Avian influenza virus (H5N1)	×		RT-PCR	–	[10]
Avian influenza virus (H5N1)	×		rRT-PCR	98 %	[42]
Influenza virus	×		LAMP	90.9 %	[43]
Influenza A viruses	×		RT-PCR	400–5,000 viral particles/ml	[63]
Influenza A virus (H1N1)	×		RT-PCR	–	[62]
FMDV	×		rPCR	10^{-9} dilution	[9]
FMDV		×	RT-LAMP	10 copies	[13]
FMDV	[a]		RT-LATE-PCR	10 copies (100 %)	[38]
Respiratory viruses	×		RT-PCR	82.2–100 %	[64]
SARS-CoV		×	RT-LAMP	0.01 PFU (100 %)	[41]
Swine viruses (H1N1 and H2N3); influenza A (flu A; seasonal H1N1; pandemic H1N1)	×		LAMP	<10 copies/μl	[65]
E. coli (O157 and K 12)	×		PCR	0.2 CFU/μl	[61]
S. aureus (MRSA) and FMDV	×		RT-LAMP	17 copies	[40]
E. coli; *B. subtilis*; *E. faecalis*	×		RT-PCR	10^2 to 10^4 CFU/ml	[66]
B. anthracis; *Brucella* spp.; *F. tularensis*; *Y. pestis*	×		rPCR	10–100 fg	[8]
Aquaculture pathogens (*S. agalactiae*; koi herpes virus; Iridovirus; *A. hydrophila*)	×		LAMP	20 copies	[68]

[a]Pilot test adaptable to POC (under development)

analytical apparatus, still require complex and somewhat expensive fabrication procedures onto plastic or glass substrates, thus severely limiting their affordability and availability by poor countries. Table 1 displays some literature references about proof-of-principle schemes and POC devices for detection and identification of some pathogens of veterinary importance.

5 Nanotechnology

An emergent topic in the development of new bioanalytical procedures, structures, and systems is nanotechnology, particularly for the generation of useful nanostructures for diagnostic applications; this is the so-called field of "nanobiotechnology". Novel and improved electronic devices and biosensor platforms have emerged as a consequence of the inherent small size, enlarged surface area, and unusual optical, magnetic, catalytic, and mechanical properties of nanomaterials, unlike those of bulk materials [24]. Depending on their specific nature, for biosensing, nanomaterials may act as labels (including signal amplification), as biomolecule immobilization supports, or even as probes for specific biotarget anchoring. Certain nanomaterials can also be used for pre-concentration of biological targets. Among these applications, labeling has been the most commonly employed. Label-based detection methods are usually more time-consuming and labor intensive than label-free methods due to the labeling steps. Labels have also limited shelf lives and are subjected to leakage from sensing surfaces. However, label-based methods usually provide superior performance, especially in terms of sensitivity, than label-free ones. Moreover, standardized protocols with labeling procedures are already available. Fluorescence labeling has been, by far, the most common approach in this regard, although suffering from pH sensitivity and photobleaching over time [53]. Such handicaps and the advent of nanoengineering have propelled the search and development of new and improved labels.

Nanoparticles (NPs) have been the most widely employed type of nanomaterials for biosensing, especially metallic NPs. Metallic NPs are inorganic NPs that exhibit improved physicochemical characteristics compared to fluorescent labels, including higher sensitivity. In general, they are suitable for construction of high-density bioanalytical devices, taking advantage of their high signal-to-noise ratio (S/N). They are easily synthesizable and functionalized (by simple mixing at room temperature) and have a controlled, self-assembled surface structure [24]. Gold nanoparticles (GNPs), in particular, are already used frequently in molecular diagnosis; some of their advantages include low toxicity and versatility for many specific biorecognition applications and schemes. One common way to enhance the GNP signal even further, and thus the sensitivity of detection, is the inclusion of a final step of silver staining ("silver enhancement"), yielding detection schemes able to preclude the use of a prior PCR amplification step. The high sensitivity exhibited by many NP-based detection layouts, especially in the form of microarrays, has enabled to avoid a prior step of nucleic-acid amplification [69].

Quantum dots (QDs) constitute another class of metallic NPs, able for fluorescence tagging. They are much brighter and more photostable than conventional organic fluorophores. Plus, their color can be directly correlated with size, while exhibiting very broad excitation wavelength windows, very narrow emission wavelength windows, and large Stokes shifts, allowing excitation at wavelengths far removed from their emission peaks [70]. Since QDs of different emission peaks (according to their different sizes) can be excited using a single wavelength excitation source, detection of multiple targets in complex biological systems is a hallmark of these NPs [71]. Another alternative to the overlapping of closely spaced fluorescence emission peaks and consequent limitation of the maximum number of fluorescent dyes that can be discriminated when simultaneously testing multiple pathogens in a single PCR tube is the use of masscode tagging, with a panel of distinct labels with different molecular weights. After an initial step of multiplexed (RT-)PCR using primers labeled with the masscode tags, unincorporated primers are removed, and the photo-cleavable tags of amplifying primers are then released by UV irradiation. Subsequent mass spectrometry analysis assigns each identified tag to its specific pathogen [1]. In principle, the multiplexing ability will only be limited by the highest primer concentration contained by a PCR mix. The method was applied to the identification of respiratory pathogens [72] and hemorrhagic viruses [73]. It offers a rapid, specific, sensitive, and cost-competitive alternative to conventional PCR and RT-PCR for disease diagnosis through POC devices. Nevertheless, some difficulties persist in miniaturizing mass spectrometer devices.

Among metallic NPs are also magnetic NPs (MNPs). Equivalent designations frequently found in the literature include “magnetic nanobeads”, “nanomagnets”, “nanomagnetic beads”, “nanomagnetic spheres”, and “nanospheres”. They have been vastly employed in many biosensor layouts for diagnosis. Despite not matching the nanosize of molecular recognition probes and targets, their microscaled counterparts, magnetic microparticles, are frequently preferred as magnetic labels for biosensing in view of the easiness for detecting the lesser abundant microbeads by routine optical microscopy or by magnetic detection and by the easiness of the purification process, thus allowing more efficient removal of nonspecifically bound labels, with enhancement of the assay performance [74]. However, the higher S/V of nanobeads provides much more binding sites for bioprobe and biotarget anchoring and hence a higher S/N [5]. Very often, magnetic particles are used for target pre-concentration from large initial sample volumes and purification, in parallel with the detection step itself being carried out through another particle that works as the label (e.g., fluorophore or GNP). In this case, there is an initial capture of the target by the probe-functionalized magnetic particle, followed by releasing of the target (“debinding”) for final detection. Through magnetically controlled removal of nonspecifically bound beads (magnetic washing), improved sensitivity can be achieved upon elimination of the time-consuming washing step of nonspecifically bound molecules [75]. This process can, for example, improve significantly the detection specificity of genomic RNA, since RNA enrichment due to magnetic confinement also precludes the effect of common interfering substances and common RNA inhibitors [76]. In addition, the use of magnetic beads permits testing optically opaque samples [29], which is the case of many crude biological samples. Magnetic particles can be manipulated off-chip by a permanent magnet, making easier the design of disposable and inexpensive tests. Moreover, magnetic interactions are not affected by surface charges, pH, ionic strength, or temperature, being thus compatible with most biochemical processes [10].

Unlike inorganic NPs, organic NPs have enhanced structural flexibility and biocompatibility, while being biodegradable. Liposomes constitute an attractive type of organic NPs for efficient DNA-probe labeling and for signal amplification. This is commonly achieved by filling liposome particles with dye and fluorophore molecules, which amplify the response signal and are able to yield quantitative results. Another way of using liposomes in biosensing is in conjunction with resistive techniques. As such, negatively charged liposomes, upon binding to immobilized DNA chains (which are also negative), form giant negatively charged surfaces that repel the target DNA chain, leading to shifts in the electrochemical response [24].

In the last years, chemistry research has rendered a range of new structures based on carbon allotropes. The most promising for biosensing purposes seem to be carbon nanotubes (CNTs), both in the form of single- (SWCNT) or multi-walled CNTs (MWCNTs), depending on the number of cylindrical layers, with unique electronic properties and enlarged surface area for DNA immobilization. They also possess high electrical conductivity (similar to copper and much higher than in polymers), physical robustness, and chemical inertness. Each nanotube may act as an individual nanoelectrode, with sufficient free space between neighboring nanotubes preventing the overlap of their diffusion layers, therefore yielding high S/N values and hence improved detection limits [77]. By providing high sensitivity, they are amenable to PCR-free detection. Their production is sometimes unacceptably irreproducible for ultrasensitive detection, but this has been circumvented by using cheap CNT arrays for multiple biological targets as a way of averaging out between different batches [78].

The recent advances in nucleic-acid synthesis and modification processes and the discovery of nucleic acids with catalytic and regulatory activities have prompted the development of nanoengineered nucleic-acid analogues with new and improved abilities for biorecognition and diagnostic purposes. Among them are aptamers; they are synthetic nucleic acids able to interact with molecular or cellular targets with high specificity and sensitivity for their ability to fold into many tertiary conformations. Aptamers can be generated by "Systematic Evolution of Ligands by Exponential Enrichment" (SELEX), a combinatorial procedure that starts with a pool of candidate nucleic-acid molecules to generate a nucleic-acid library [79]. Compared to antibodies, nucleic-acids can be synthesized in a more reproducible way, have longer shelf lives, and can be reversibly denatured without loss of activity. A remarkable characteristic of these probes for biosensing is that they do not require prior knowledge about the molecular differences between the specific target and nonspecific ones. As shown in cancer diagnosis, the DNA sequences from the DNA library that bind the cell-surface markers of a cancer cell can be determined by comparison with those that bind a healthy (control) cell. In addition, detection occurs before the corresponding antibody against that cancer has been produced [80]. This process is obviously attractive for application to the diagnosis of infectious diseases as well. The high selectivity and sensitivity achieved with aptamers permits eliminating sample pretreatment and is thus promising for POC applications [53]. The inability to distinguish the fluorescent signal from labeled and unlabeled probes is a common problem in microfluidic devices, since labeled probes that did not bind targets cannot be washed out from the microchannels. Different fluorescent labels can be used to tag the probe and the target, with the detection proceeding via fluorescence resonance energy transfer (FRET) upon the occurrence of the bioaffinity reaction. However, this procedure is unpractical in bioanalysis owing to the cumbersome dual labeling procedure [81]. In the case of DNA detection, this can be circumvented with the use of molecular beacons (MBs), which can be considered a particular type of aptamers. MBs are single-stranded oligonucleotides with a hairpin (stem-and-loop) structure, labeled with a fluorophore in one extremity of the chain and a fluorescence quencher in the other extremity. The close proximity between the extremities prevents fluorescence emission, but when a hybridization event occurs with a complimentary chain, the structure becomes linearized and hence fluorescence arises. In this way, target labeling is unnecessary. Another type of synthetic nucleic-acid analogues is constituted by peptide nucleic acids (PNAs), which are in which the sugar-phosphate backbone is replaced by a peptidic structure. When used as probes in nucleic-acid recognition systems, they allow very selective and sensitive hybridization in low ionic-strength media, while having high thermal stability [82]. For being electrically uncharged, PNAs are suitable to promote the occurrence of biochemical events triggered by the formation of the negatively charged PNA/single-stranded DNA hybrid, i.e., a kind of "on/off" processes.

Biosensing schemes reported in the literature employing at least one of the nanotechnology-based structures described above are depicted in Table 2, together with the transduction mechanism employed and performance quantification.

Table 2

Illustrative works described in the literature employing nanostructures for the detection of animal pathogens

Target pathogen(s)	Nanostructures[a]	Transduction mechanism	LOD or sensitivity	References
Canine parvovirus	PNA	Fluorescence	40–2,000 copies/μl (89.8 %)	[105]
Influenza virus (H5)	MB	Fluorescence	0.6 nM	[37]
Influenza virus (H5N1)	GNPs and Ag enhancer	Light scattering	10^3 $TCID_{50}$ units	[69]
Influenza virus (H5N1)	DNA aptamer	SPR	1.28 HAU	[87]
Influenza virus (H1N1)	GNPs	Fluorescence and surface-enhanced Raman scattering	–	[93]
Influenza virus (H5N1)	Complementary oxide semiconductor (CMOS)	Impedance spectroscopy	5 nM (10^{-11} F)	[98]
Influenza virus (H5N1)	DNA aptamer/hydrogel	QCM	0.0128 HAU	[102]
16 avian influenza viruses	Magnetic beads	Colorimetry (HA test and LAT test) and RT-PCR	16–1,024 HAU	[106]
Feline calicivirus	Liposomes	Fluorescence	1.6×10^5 PFU/ml	[5]
Pestiviruses (Classical swine fever virus; Border disease virus; Bovine viral diarrhea virus 1 and 2)	Magnetic beads	Optic (visual; microscopy; chip reader)	–	[55]
Alexandrium sp. complex	PNA and cyanine-derived fluorophore ($DiSC_2(5)$)	Colorimetry	–	[89]
B. anthracis	SWCNT	Raman spectroscopy	–	[97]
B. anthracis	Electrically active magnetic NPs	Cyclic voltammetry	0.01 ng/μl	[94]
B. anthracis	GNPs	QCM	3.5×10^2 CFU/ml	[95]
B. anthracis; *S. enteritidis*	GNPs, magnetic NPs and NP tracers (PbS and CdS)	Square wave anodic stripping voltammetry	50 pg/ml	[90]

(continued)

Table 2
(continued)

Target pathogen(s)	Nanostructures[a]	Transduction mechanism	LOD or sensitivity	References
E. coli	DNA aptamer	Impedance spectroscopy	10^{-7} M	[79]
E. coli	Alginic acid-coated Co magnetic beads	Transmission electron microscopy	10 cells/ml	[86]
E. coli	Fe_2O_3/Au magnetic NP and magnetic NPs	Amperometry	5 CFU/ml	[99]
E. coli O157:H7	Aluminum anodized oxide (AAO) nanopore membrane	Cyclic voltammetry and impedance spectroscopy	0.5 nM	[91]
E. coli O157:H7	Magnetic beads and QDs	Fluorescence	250 zM	[104]
F. tularensis	MB	Fluorescence	–	[84]
M. avium	GNPs	Colorimetry	1.875 ng/µl (87.5–100 %)	[100]
M. tuberculosis; *M. bovis*	GNPs	Colorimetry	5×10^{-8} M	[85]
S. aureus	GNPs/poly-3,4-ethylenedioxythiophene (PEDOT) film	Chronoamperometry	≤150 pM	[96]
S. aureus	GNPs/PANI nanofibers	Cyclic voltammetry	pM range	[101]
S. aureus (MRSA)	PNA	Impedance spectroscopy	10 pM	[103]
Y. enterocolitica	Carbon ionic liquid electrode and V_2O5 nanobelt/MWCNT/chitosan	Differential pulse voltammetry	1.76×10^{-12} M	[92]
C. perfringens; *C. tetani*; *S. pneumoniae*; *P. aeruginosa*; *E. coli*	GNPs	QCM	1.5×10^2 CFU/ml (94.12 %)	[83]
Salmonellae	GNPs and Ag enhancer	Colorimetry	10^4 cells	[88]

[a]Micro-scaled magnetic particle labels are also considered in this table

6 Conclusions

The advances observed on the past decades in proteomics and genomics have led to the discovery of novel diagnostic biomarkers for pathogens relevant in human medicine. In parallel, cutting-edge developments in materials science and in nanotechnology have also been registered. Veterinary science and practice "took the train" and, as such, have been greatly favored from such advances. Microfluidic technologies and nanoengineered structures, especially when coupled together, have led to an unprecedented degree of high-throughput, large-scale genetic analysis, even at whole-genome levels. Ultimately, the high-throughput and multiplexing abilities of in vivo (implanted or swallowed) nanosensor arrays should be able to monitor animals' physiology and health status during their entire lifetime, and even beyond, intended to track and assess the quality of animal products for human feeding. In this way, the current shortcomings related with the limited number of sanitary surveillance resources that can be allocated to guarantee proper product origin, stocking, and shipping could be circumvented. So far, only few POC schemes and devices have reached the exquisite sensitivity thresholds required for detection of nucleic-acid traces in unamplified biological samples, which is the ultimate goal of nucleic-acid testing. As for human diagnostics, the veterinary medicine and practice still lack the commercial availability of more POC devices, more probably as a result of manufacturing and commercial cost-effectiveness constraints than to a shortage of fundamental knowledge. While remaining too expensive for single testing, many tests targeted for POC diagnosis will ultimately prove to be cost-effective when savings with unnecessary laboratory manpower are taken into account. Other major challenges are the need for initial investments that are often prohibitive for small companies and the usual difficulties for obtaining regulatory approvals for testing and commercialization. For effective improvement of human health, more adequate and coordinated actions to face animal diseases are needed, especially concerning livestock. This includes a more effective technology transfer from developed countries to those where diseases are prevalent and where disease preventive measures may be crucial to avoid or contain epidemics. Probably still without meritorious examples in the world, more effective communication and coordination among public health, animal health, and wildlife disease surveillance authorities will be necessary to tackle the problems posed by common and hazardous veterinary diseases, especially in situations of outbreaks endangering animal and human health as well.

References

1. Breeze RG (2006) Technology, public policy and control of transboundary livestock diseases in our lifetimes. Rev Sci Technol 25:271–292
2. Pieniazek NJ, Bornay-Llinares FJ, Slemenda SB et al (1999) New *Cryptosporidium* genotypes in HIV-infected persons. Emerg Infect Dis 5:444–449
3. Robertson ID, Irwin PJ, Lymbery AJ et al (2000) The role of companion animals in the emergence of parasitic zoonoses. Int J Parasitol 30:1369–1377
4. Teles FRR, Prazeres DMF, Lima-Filho JL (2005) Trends in dengue diagnosis. Rev Med Virol 15:287–302
5. Connelly JT, Kondapally S, Skoupi M et al (2012) Micro-total analysis system for virus detection: microfluidic pre-concentration coupled to liposome-based detection. Anal Bioanal Chem 402:315–323

6. Hill SL, Cheney JM, Taton-Allen GF et al (2000) Prevalence of enteric zoonotic organisms in cats. J Am Vet Med Assoc 216: 687–692
7. Nicholson TL, Kukielka D, Vincent AL et al (2011) Utility of a panviral microarray for detection of swine respiratory viruses in clinical samples. J Clin Microbiol 49:1542–1548
8. Matero P, Hemmilä H, Tomaso H et al (2011) Rapid field detection assays for *Bacillus anthracis*, *Brucella* spp., *Francisella tularensis* and *Yersinia pestis*. Clin Microbiol Infect 17:34–43
9. Madi M, Hamilton A, Squirrell D et al (2012) Rapid detection of foot-and-mouth disease virus using a field-portable nucleic acid extraction and real-time PCR amplification platform. Vet J 193:67–72
10. Pipper J, Inoue M, Ng LF-P et al (2007) Catching bird flu in a droplet. Nat Med 13:1259–1263
11. Teles FSRR, Tavira LAPT, Fonseca LJP (2010) Biosensors as rapid diagnostic tests for tropical diseases. Crit Rev Clin Lab Sci 47:139–169
12. Sims L (2012) The use of new technologies for rapid, field-based (point-of-care) testing in the detection of emergency animal diseases. Australian Centre of Excellence for Risk Analysis (ACERA), ACERA Project No. 1004B 2b (final report). http://www.acera.unimelb.edu.au/materials/endorsed/1004B_OID1_Report.pdf. Accessed 28 Aug 2013
13. Dukes JP, King DP, Alexandersen S (2006) Novel reverse transcription loop-mediated isothermal amplification for rapid detection of foot-and-mouth disease virus. Arch Virol 151:1093–1106
14. Scott NR (2007) Nanoscience in veterinary medicine. Vet Res Commun 31(suppl 1):139–144
15. Charleston B, Bankowski BM, Gubbins S et al (2011) Relationship between clinical signs and transmission of an infectious disease and the implications for control. Science 332:726–729
16. King DP (2013) Progress towards the development of simple and rapid diagnostic tests away from centralised laboratories. World Association of Veterinary Laboratory Diagnosticians—16th international symposium, Berlin, Germany, 5–8 June
17. Soliman H, El-Matbouli M (2010) Loop mediated isothermal amplification combined with nucleic acid lateral flow strip for diagnosis of cyprinid herpes virus-3. Mol Cell Probes 24:38–43
18. Niemz A, Ferguson TM, Boyle DS (2011) Point-of-care nucleic acid testing for infectious diseases. Trends Biotechnol 29: 240–250
19. Palmer S, Sully M, Fozdar F (2009) Farmers, animal disease reporting and the effect of trust: a study of West Australian sheep and cattle farmers. Rural Soc 19:32–48
20. Rodriguez-Sanchez B, Sanchez-Vizcaino JM, Uttenthal A et al (2008) Improved diagnosis for nine viral diseases considered as notifiable by the World Organization for Animal Health. Transbound Emerg Dis 55:215–2225
21. Chomel BB (1998) New emerging zoonoses: a challenge and an opportunity for the veterinary profession. Comp Immunol Microbiol Infect Dis 21:1–14
22. Dubey JP (1994) Toxoplasmosis. J Am Vet Med Assoc 205:1593–1598
23. Luppa PB, Müller C, Schlichtiger A et al (2011) Point-of-care testing (POCT): current techniques and future perspectives. Trends Anal Chem 30:887–898
24. Teles FRR, Fonseca LP (2008) Trends in DNA biosensors. Talanta 77:606–623
25. Aguilera-Herrador E, Cruz-Vera M, Valcárcel M (2010) Analytical connotations of point-of-care testing. Analyst 135:2220–2232
26. Banoo S, Bell D, Bossuyt P et al (2006) Evaluation of diagnostic tests for infectious diseases: general principles. Nat Rev Microbiol:S20–S32
27. Special Programme for Research and Training in Tropical Diseases (TDR), Pediatric Dengue Vaccine Initiative (PDVI) (2009) Evaluation of commercially available anti-dengue virus immunoglobulin M tests. Diagnostics Evaluation Series 3, World Health Organization, Geneva, Switzerland
28. Gialamas A, Laurence CO, Yelland LN et al (2010) Assessing agreement between point of care and laboratory results for lipid testing from a clinical perspective. Clin Biochem 43:515–518
29. Special Programme for Research and Training in Tropical Diseases (TDR) (2009) Dengue: guidelines for diagnosis, treatment, prevention and control. World Health Organization, Geneva, Switzerland
30. Briggs C, Carter J, Lee S-H et al (2008) ICSH Guideline for worldwide point-of-care testing in haematology with special reference to the complete blood count. Int J Lab Hematol 30:105–116
31. Bollo E (2007) Nanotechnologies applied to veterinary diagnostics. Vet Res Commun 31(suppl 1):145–147
32. Niemeyer CM (2001) Semi-synthetic nucleic acid-protein conjugates: applications in life sciences and nanobiotechnology. Rev Mol Biotechnol 82:47–66

33. Campbell NF, Evans JA, Fawcett NC et al (1993) Detection of poly (U) hybridization using azido modified poly (A) coated piezoelectric crystals. Biochem Biophys Res Commun 196:858–863
34. Bustin S, Penning LC (2012) Improving the analysis of quantitative PCR data in veterinary research. Vet J 191:279–281
35. Pividori MI, Merkoçi A, Alegret S (2000) Electrochemical genosensor design: immobilisation of oligonucleotides onto transducer surfaces and detection methods. Biosens Bioelectron 14:291–303
36. Pierce KE, Mistry R, Reid SM et al (2010) Design and optimization of a novel reverse transcription linear-after-the-exponential PCR for the detection of foot-and-mouth disease virus. J Appl Microbiol 109:180–189
37. Kerby MB, Freeman S, Prachanronarong K et al (2008) Direct sequence detection of structured H5 influenza viral RNA. J Mol Diagn 10:225–235
38. Reid SM, Pierce KE, Mistry R et al (2010) Pan-serotypic detection of foot-and-mouth disease virus by RT linear-after-the-exponential PCR. Mol Cell Probes 24:250–255
39. Peters RHP, van Agtmael MA, Danner SA et al (2004) New developments in the diagnosis of bloodstream infections. Lancet Infect Dis 4:751–760
40. Bearinger JP, Dugan LC, Baker BR et al (2011) Development and initial results of a low cost, disposable, point-of-care testing device for pathogen detection. IEEE Trans Biomed Eng 58:805–808
41. Thai HTC, Le MQ, Vuong CD et al (2004) Development and evaluation of a novel loop-mediated isothermal amplification method for rapid detection of severe acute respiratory syndrome coronavirus. J Clin Microbiol 42:1956–1961
42. Takekawa JY, Iverson SA, Scultz AK et al (2010) Field detection of avian influenza virus in wild birds: evaluation of a portable rRT-PCR system and freeze-dried reagents. J Virol Methods 166:92–97
43. Abe T, Segawa Y, Watanabe H et al (2011) Point-of-care testing system enabling 30 min detection of influenza genes. Lab Chip 11:1166–1167
44. Hoffmann B, Beer M, Reid SM et al (2009) A review of RT-PCR technologies used in veterinary virology and disease control: sensitive and specific diagnosis of five livestock diseases notifiable to the World Organisation for Animal Health. Vet Microbiol 139:1–23
45. Parida M, Posadas G, Inoue S et al (2004) Real-time reverse transcription loop-mediated isothermal amplification for rapid detection of West Nile virus. J Clin Microbiol 42:257–263
46. Foord A, Boyd V, Heine H (2011) A loop mediated isothermal amplification assay for detection of Hendra virus in the field [Poster]. One health conference, Melbourne, Australia, 14–16 February
47. Mori Y, Notomi T (2009) Loop-mediated isothermal amplification (LAMP): a rapid, accurate, and cost-effective diagnostic method for infectious diseases. J Infect Chemoter 15:62–69
48. Ryan E, Gloster J, Reid SM et al (2008) Clinical and laboratory investigations of the outbreaks of foot-and-mouth disease in southern England in 2007. Vet Rec 163:139–147
49. Kerman K, Kobayashi M, Tamiya E et al (2004) Recent trends in electrochemical DNA biosensor technology. Meas Sci Technol 15:R1–R11
50. Lee WG, Bang H, Yun H et al (2007) On-chip erythrocyte deformability test under optical pressure. Lab Chip 7:516–519
51. Heng X, Erickson D, Baugh LR et al (2006) Optofluidic microscopy—a method for implementing a high resolution optical microscope on a chip. Lab Chip 6:1274–1276
52. Novak L, Neuzil P, Pipper J et al (2007) An integrated fluorescence detection system for lab-on-a-chip applications. Lab Chip 7:27–29
53. Rivet C, Lee H, Hirsch A et al (2011) Microfluidics for medical diagnostics and biosensors. Chem Eng Sci 66:1490–1507
54. Breslauer DN, Maamari RN, Switz NA et al (2009) Mobile phone based clinical microscopy for global health applications. PLoS One 4:e6320(1-7)
55. LeBlanc N, Gantelius J, Schwenk JM et al (2009) Development of a magnetic bead microarray for simultaneous and simple detection of four pestiviruses. J Virol Methods 155:1–9
56. Tai D-F, Lin C-Y, Wu T-Z et al (2006) Artificial receptors in serologic tests for the early diagnosis of dengue virus infection. Clin Chem 5:1486–1491
57. Zimmermann M, Schmid H, Hunziker P et al (2007) Capillary pumps for autonomous capillary systems. Lab Chip 7:119–125
58. Ellerbee AK, Phillips ST, Siegel AC et al (2009) Quantifying colorimetric assays in paper-based microfluidic devices by measuring the transmission of light through paper. Anal Chem 81:8447–8452
59. Ruf HH, Knoll T, Misiakos K et al (2006) Biochip-compatible packaging and micro-

fluidics for a silicon opto-electronic biosensor. Microelectron Eng 83:1677–1680

60. Radisic M, Iyer RK, Murthy SK et al (2006) Micro- and nanotechnology in cell separation. Int J Nanomedicine 1:3–14
61. Beyor N, Yi L, Seo TS et al (2009) Integrated capture, concentration, polymerase chain reaction, and capillary electrophoretic analysis of pathogens on a chip. Anal Chem 81:3523–3528
62. Bhattacharyya A, Klapperich CM et al (2008) Microfluidics-based extraction of viral RNA from infected mammalian cells for disposable molecular diagnostics. Sensor Actuator B 129:693–698
63. Jenny SL, Hu Y, Overduin P et al (2010) Evaluation of the Xpert Flu A Panel nucleic acid amplification-based point-of-care test for influenza A virus detection and pandemic H1 subtyping. J Clin Virol 49:85–89
64. Rand KH, Rampersaud H, Houck HJ (2011) Comparison of two multiplex methods for detection of respiratory viruses: FilmArray RP and xTAG RVP. J Clin Microbiol 49:2449–2453
65. Fang X, Chen H, Yu S et al (2011) Predicting viruses accurately by a multiplex microfluidic loop-mediated isothermal amplification chip. Anal Chem 83:690–695
66. Mahalanabis M, Al-Muayad H, Kulinski MD et al (2009) Cell lysis and DNA extraction of gram-positive and gram-negative bacteria from whole blood in a disposable microfluidic chip. Lab Chip 9:2811–2817
67. James HE, Ebert K, McGonigle R et al (2010) Detection of African swine fever virus by loop-mediated isothermal amplification. J Virol Methods 164:68–74
68. Chang W-H, Yang S-Y, Wang C-H et al (2013) Rapid isolation and detection of aquaculture pathogens in an integrated microfluidic system using loop-mediated isothermal amplification. Sensor Actuator B 180:96–106
69. Zhao J, Tang S, Storhoff J et al (2010) Multiplexed, rapid detection of H5N1 using a PCR-free nanoparticle-based genomic microarray assay. BMC Biotechnol 10:74
70. Hohng S, Ha T (2005) Single-molecule quantum-dot fluorescence resonance energy transfer. Chem Phys Chem 6:956–960
71. Alivisatos AP (2007) Less is more in medicine. Sci Am 23:73–79
72. Briese T, Palacios G, Kokoris M et al (2005) Diagnostic system for rapid and sensitive differential detection of pathogens. Emerg Infect Dis 11:310–313
73. Palacios G, Briese T, Kapoor V et al (2006) MassTag polymerase chain reaction for differential diagnosis of viral hemorrhagic fevers. Emerg Infect Dis 12:692–695
74. Rife JC, Whitman LJ (2004) Fluidic force discrimination. US Patent application publication 2004-0253744
75. Baselt D, Lee GU, Natesan M et al (1998) A biosensor based on magnetoresistance technology. Biosens Bioelectron 13:731–739
76. Lee W-C, Lien K-Y, Lee G-B et al (2008) An integrated microfluidic system using magnetic beads for virus detection. Diagn Microbiol Infect Dis 60:51–58
77. Vaddiraju S, Tomazos I, Burgess DJ et al (2010) Emerging synergy between nanotechnology and implantable biosensors: a review. Biosens Bioelectron 25:1553–1565
78. Gruner G (2007) Carbon nanonets—spark new electronics. Sci Am 17:48–55
79. Queirós RB, de-los-Santos-Álvarez N, Noronha JP et al (2013) A label-free DNA aptamer-based impedance biosensor for the detection of *E. coli* outer membrane proteins. Sensor Actuator B 181:766–772
80. Xu Y, Phillips JA, Yan J et al (2009) Aptamer-based microfluidic device for enrichment, sorting, and detection of multiple cancer cells. Anal Chem 81:7436–7442
81. Jung J, Chen L, Lee S et al (2007) Fast and sensitive DNA analysis using changes in the FRET signals of molecular beacons in a PDMS microfluidic channel. Anal Bioanal Chem 387:2609–2615
82. Wang J, Paleček E, Nielsen PE et al (1996) Peptide nucleic acid probes for sequence-specific DNA biosensors. J Am Chem Soc 118:7667–7670
83. Cai J, Yao C, Xia J et al (2011) Rapid parallelized and quantitative analysis of five pathogenic bacteria by ITS hybridization using QCM biosensor. Sensor Actuator B 155:500–504
84. Ramachandran A, Flinchbaugh J, Ayoubi P et al (2004) Target discrimination by surface-immobilized molecular beacons designed to detect *Francisella tularensis*. Biosens Bioelectron 19:727–736
85. Silva LB, Veigas B, Doria G et al (2011) Portable optoelectronic biosensing platform for identification of mycobacteria from the *Mycobacterium tuberculosis* complex. Biosens Bioelectron 26:2012–2017
86. Geng P, Zhang X, Teng Y et al (2011) A DNA sequence-specific electrochemical biosensor based on alginic acid-coated cobalt magnetic beads for the detection of *E. coli*. Biosens Bioelectron 26:3325–3330
87. Wang R, Zhao J, Jiang T et al (2013) Selection and characterization of DNA aptamers for use

in detection of avian influenza virus H5N1. J Virol Methods 189:362–369
88. Liu C-C, Yeung C-Y, Chen P-H et al (2013) *Salmonella* detection using 16S ribosomal DNA/RNA probe-gold nanoparticles and lateral flow immunoassay. Food Chem 141:2526–2532
89. Duy J, Smith RL, Collins SD et al (2014) A field-deployable colorimetric bioassay for the rapid and specific detection of ribosomal RNA. Biosens Bioelectron 52:433–437
90. Zhang D, Huarng MC, Alocilja EC (2010) A multiplex nanoparticle-based bio-barcoded DNA sensor for the simultaneous detection of multiple pathogens. Biosens Bioelectron 26:1736–1742
91. Wang L, Liu Q, Hu Z et al (2009) A novel electrochemical biosensor based on dynamic polymerase-extending hybridization for *E. coli* O157:H7 DNA detection. Talanta 78:647–652
92. Sun W, Qin P, Gao H et al (2010) Electrochemical DNA biosensor based on chitosan/nano-V_2O_5/MWCNTs composite film modified carbon ionic liquid electrode and its application to the LAMP product of *Yersinia enterocolitica* gene sequence. Biosens Bioelectron 25:1264–1270
93. Ganbold E-O, Kang T, Lee K et al (2012) Aggregation effects of gold nanoparticles for single-base mismatch detection in influenza A (H1N1) DNA sequences using fluorescence and Raman measurements. Colloids Surf B Biointerfaces 93:148–153
94. Pal S, Alocilja EC (2010) Electrically active magnetic nanoparticles as novel concentrator and electrochemical redox transducer in *Bacillus anthracis* DNA detection. Biosens Bioelectron 26:1624–1630
95. Hao R-Z, Song H-B, Zuo G-M et al (2011) DNA probe functionalized QCM biosensor based on gold nanoparticle amplification for *Bacillus anthracis* detection. Biosens Bioelectron 26:3398–3404
96. Spain E, Keyes TE, Forster RJ (2013) DNA sensor based on vapour polymerised pedot films functionalised with gold nanoparticles. Biosens Bioelectron 41:65–70
97. Bansal J, Singh I, Bhatnagar PK et al (2013) DNA sequence detection based on Raman spectroscopy using single walled carbon nanotube. J Biosci Bioeng 115:438–441
98. Lee K-H, Choi S-H, Lee J-O et al (2011) An autonomous CMOS hysteretic sensor for the detection of desorption-free DNA hybridization. Biosens Bioelectron 26: 4591–4595
99. Li K, Lai Y, Zhang W et al (2011) Fe_2O_3@Au core/shell nanoparticle-based electrochemical DNA biosensor for *Escherichia coli* detection. Talanta 84:607–613
100. Liandris E, Gazouli M, Andreadou M et al (2009) Direct detection of unamplified DNA from pathogenic mycobacteria using DNA-derivatized gold nanoparticles. J Microbiol Methods 78:260–264
101. Spain E, Kojima R, Kaner RB et al (2011) High sensitivity DNA detection using gold nanoparticle functionalized polyaniline nanofibres. Biosens Bioelectron 26: 2613–2618
102. Wang R, Li Y (2013) Hydrogel based QCM aptasensor for detection of avian influenza virus. Biosens Bioelectron 42:148–155
103. Corrigan DK, Schulze H, Henihan G et al (2012) Impedimetric detection of single-stranded PCR products derived from methicillin resistant *Staphylococcus aureus* (MRSA) isolates. Biosens Bioelectron 34:178–184
104. Liu Y-J, Yao D-J, Chang H-Y et al (2008) Magnetic bead-based DNA detection with multi-layers quantum-dots labeling for rapid detection of *Escherichia coli* O157:H7. Biosens Bioelectron 24:558–565
105. An D-J, Jeong W, Jeoung H-Y et al (2012) Peptide nucleic acid-based (PNA) array for the antigenic discrimination of canine parvovirus. Res Vet Sci 93:515–519
106. Dhumpa R, Handberg KJ, Jørgensen PH et al (2011) Rapid detection of avian influenza virus in chicken fecal samples by immunomagnetic capture reverse transcriptase-polymerase chain reaction assay. Diagn Microbiol Infect Dis 69:258–265

Part III

Molecular Profiling of Veterinary Relevant Microbial Pathogens

Chapter 21

Molecular Typing Tools: From Pattern Recognition to Genome-Based Algorithms

Konrad Sachse and Petra Moebius

Abstract

In the present chapter, we discuss DNA-based typing methods for microbial pathogens that were frequently used in the past two decades and their essential features, as well as virtues and downsides. We conclude with an outlook on the fundamental changes that can be expected in the era of high-throughput genomics.

Key words Review, RAPD, RFLP, AFLP-PCR, PFGE, VNTR/MLVA, MIRU-VNTR, Spoligotyping, Single-locus sequence typing, MLST, Genomotyping

1 Introduction

Ever since diagnosticians have been trying to identify the origin of disease outbreaks, there was a demand for characterizing and classifying the microbial strain involved. Strain typing can help to reveal important information about the infection, i.e., (1) transmission pathways and patterns, (2) possible association of the strain with clinical manifestations and pathogenicity, (3) specific tissue or organ affinity, and (4) the status of the infection, e.g., new infection, reinfection, or persistent infection.

Historically, the first typing schemes were based on phenotypes, e.g., surface morphology (e.g., gram stain), serotype, biotype, or intrinsic phenotypic properties, such as fermentation of substrates, auxotrophy, or expression of specific antigens. The broad use of DNA amplification and sequencing technology in the past two decades prompted the gradual phasing out of most of these methods and a shift toward genetic typing schemes.

Most of the currently recognized approaches are based on variations in specific genomic loci that are exploited in a direct (i.e., through sequence analysis) or indirect (e.g., through cleavage patterns) fashion. Since the target region for typing is usually selected

Mónica V. Cunha and João Inácio (eds.), *Veterinary Infection Biology: Molecular Diagnostics and High-Throughput Strategies*, Methods in Molecular Biology, vol. 1247, DOI 10.1007/978-1-4939-2004-4_21, © Springer Science+Business Media New York 2015

individually for each microbial agent, the vast majority of the established molecular typing methods were designed for a particular species, group of species, genus, or family. Usually, a single locus or a limited number of loci are targeted. These circumstances imply limitations to the discriminatory capacity of each typing assay. For instance, when restriction fragment length polymorphism analysis (RFLP) and mycobacterial interspersed repetitive unit-variable number tandem repeat (MIRU-VNTR) were used in a comparative study on tuberculosis cases, they produced different clustering of a substantial part of the strains examined [1]. Therefore, a combination of two or more genotyping methods will often be required to improve resolution and ensure accuracy of the findings [2, 3]. Now that high-throughput genome sequencing technology has become more affordable and is within reach for more and more laboratories, it seems certain that typing algorithms for broader use with multiple species will be tomorrow's standards.

An overview of papers on molecular typing methods used for selected microbial agents of veterinary relevance is given in Table 1.

In the present chapter, we discuss DNA-based typing methods that were frequently used in the past two decades, their essential features, as well as virtues and downsides. We conclude with an outlook on the fundamental changes that can be expected in the era of high-throughput genomics.

Some of the typing methods described in the following sections were also used for phylogenetic studies. To justify the latter, more stringent criteria for the choice of target structures have to be applied, namely, stability to evolutionary pressure, which implies a preference for ribosomal RNA and housekeeping genes. In fact, only a minor proportion of the methods are suitable for both epidemiological and phylogenetic purposes.

2 Fingerprint Typing Methods

2.1 RAPD

Random amplified polymorphic DNA (RAPD) analysis represents a special variation of PCR that can be regarded as gross whole-genome characterization. It consists in parallel amplification of an arbitrary set of genomic segments using short oligonucleotide primers of 8–12 nucleotides [4]. The amplification reaction involves one or more primers and is conducted at low-stringency conditions. The low annealing temperature allows primer binding to multiple sites that do not need to be completely complementary, so that the numbers and positions of binding sites are unique for each bacterial strain. Numerous amplicons in the range of 0.1–3 kbp can be produced and subsequently visualized using agarose gel electrophoresis.

Table 1
Selection of published genotyping studies on bacterial pathogens

Agent	Genotyping method	References
Bacillus anthracis	VNTR/MLVA SNP analysis	[91–93] [94, 95]
Borrelia spp.	PCR-RFLP subtyping (*ospA*) MLST	[54, 96] [97]
Brucella spp.	SNP analysis	[98]
B. abortus, *B. suis*, *B. melitensis*, and *B. canis*	VNTR/MLVA MLST	[99–101] [102, 103]
Burkholderia mallei	MLST VNTR/MLVA PFGE	[104–106] [107, 108] [109]
Campylobacter spp.	PFGE MLST PCR-RFLP genotyping (*flaA*) Microarray DNA hybridization assay	[110] [111, 112] [11, 113] [114, 115]
C. fetus subsp. *venerealis* and *C. fetus* subsp. *fetus*	PFGE AFLP MLST	[25, 116] [21, 117] [118, 119]
Chlamydia spp.	MLST	[61, 120]
Chlamydia psittaci	*ompA* genotyping (DNA microarray, RFLP) VNTR/MLVA MLST	[51, 53, 121] [122] [62]
Chlamydia abortus	VNTR/MLVA	[123]
Clostridium botulinum	PFGE VNTR/MLVA	[26, 27] [124]
Clostridium perfringens	PFGE VNTR/MLVA	[125–128] [129, 130]
Clostridium difficile	VNTR/MLVA	[131]
Clostridium septicum	MLST	[132]
Coxiella burnetii	VNTR/MLVA 10-locus multi-spacer sequence typing (MST)	[133–135] [68, 69]
Escherichia coli	Multiplex PCRs for differentiation of *E. coli* pathovars PCR (stx1/stx2 gene) PCR (*eae* gene) PCR-RFLP (*eae* gene) PCRs and PCR-RFLP assay (fedA, K88 gene)	[136–139] [140] [48, 49, 141, 142] [143] [144–146]

(continued)

Table 1 (continued)

Agent	Genotyping method	References
	Microarray genotyping MLST	[147–149] [150]
Francisella tularensis	PFGE AFLP VNTR/MLVA SNP genotyping (RT-PCR, microarray) VNTR+INDELs+SNP	[151] [151] [152, 153] [154] [155, 156]
Mycobacterium avium subsp. *paratuberculosis*	Reviews PFGE IS900-RFLP MIRU-VNTR MLSSR	[157, 158] [159–161] [16, 17] [33] [3, 162–164]
M. avium subsp. *avium*	IS901-RFLP MIRU-VNTR	[165] [33]
M. avium subsp. *hominissuis*	IS*1245*-RFLP, IS1311-RFLP MIRU-VNTR	[166–168] [33]
Mycobacterium tuberculosis complex	IS*6110*-RFLP MIRU-VNTR	[13] [35–38]
M. bovis *M. caprae*	MIRU-VNTR Spoligotyping, microarray spoligotyping	[169] [41, 44]
Mycoplasma mycoides subsp. *mycoides*	VNTR/MLVA MLST	[170] [171–173]
Mycoplasma bovis	RAPD AFLP PFGE VNTR/MLVA MLST	[5] [5] [5] [174, 175] [176]
Salmonella enterica	Reviews PFGE VNTR/MLVA *S.* Typhimurium VNTR/MLVA *S.* Enteritidis VNTR/MLVA *S.* Newport MLST MLST (prophage loci) MLST-seq DNA microarray typing	[177–179] [28, 179, 180] [181] [182–184] [185] [59, 186] (http://mlst.ucc.ie/mlst/dbs/Senterica) [187] [188] [77, 189, 190]
Taylorella equigenitalis	PFGE	[191–194]

RAPD has been used for discriminatory analysis of isolates of many microbial pathogens. For instance, investigating *Mycoplasma bovis* infections in cattle, the number of distinct strains present in a geographical region or a herd was determined based on the obtained banding patterns [5, 6]. This included identification of the strain at the source of the outbreak [7]. Likewise, strains of *Mycobacterium* (*M.*) *avium* were distinguished by their fingerprints using a panel of four or six primers [8, 9]. Differentiation among *M. avium* subsp. *paratuberculosis* strains using RAPD was also attempted [10], but proved more difficult.

The basic asset of the method is its versatility, which allows the use of a theoretically unlimited number of primers and thus offers unlimited capacity for revealing strain-to-strain differences [9]. It also means that the methodology can be adapted individually to any organism. While the method is easy to use, inexpensive, and rapid, its major drawback consists in limited reproducibility. Banding patterns tend to vary considerably from run to run and from laboratory to laboratory. Therefore, it was recommended to conduct RAPD analyses in triplicate [8].

2.2 RFLP

Restriction fragment length polymorphism (RFLP) analysis is based on enzymatic cleavage of genomic DNA of an isolate. The fragments generated by specific restriction endonucleases are separated according to their size using gel electrophoresis. Mutations in the genome can lead to changes in the number of cleavage sites, whereas insertions and deletions can shift their positions and give rise to "fragment length polymorphisms."

A well-known example of RFLP typing refers to *Campylobacter jejuni*, where the tandem flagellin genes *fla*A and *fla*B served as target for subtyping in molecular epidemiological studies [11]. The classical serovars of *Chlamydia psittaci* could be distinguished using PCR-RFLP of the *omp*A gene locus [12].

If an organism's genome carries specific insertion sequences, Southern hybridization with a fluorescent-labeled complementary gene probe can be used to reveal banding patterns that are specific for individual strains. Thus, IS*6110*-RFLP was widely used for genotyping strains of the *Mycobacterium tuberculosis* complex (MTC), e.g., *M. tuberculosis* [13], *M. bovis*, and *M. caprae* [14]. The discriminatory capacity is particularly high for strains with six or more IS*6110* copies [15]. In the case of *M. avium* subsp. *paratuberculosis*, RFLP based on IS*900* and using at least two restriction enzymes can provide high resolution in typing [16, 17]. Ribotyping [18], which was used for years as a versatile typing method for bacterial families, genera, and species, also includes the use of rDNA probes, so that only those bands containing a portion of the ribosomal operon are visualized. The number of reactive bands on Southern blot reflects the multiplicity of rRNA operons in a microbial species. Numerous applications to taxonomic classification, epidemiological tracking, geographical distribution, population biology, and phylogeny were reported [19]. The general use of RFLP-based typing has been in decline for the last few years, not so much for being labor-intensive, time-consuming, and technically demanding, but mainly because more efficient assays have become available (*see* below).

2.3 AFLP-PCR

Amplified fragment length polymorphism (AFLP) analysis is based on selective PCR amplification of restriction endonuclease-digested genomic DNA [20]. The cleavage reaction involving one, (typically) two, or more enzymes is followed by ligation of oligonucleotide adaptors on both termini of the fragments. Subsequent PCR often includes two amplification steps and uses primers complementary to the adaptor sequences to amplify a subset of the restriction fragments. Individual assays can be tailored by using selective bases in the adaptor sequences to keep the number and size of finally generated amplicons in a manageable range, e.g., 50–100 fragments of 50–500 bp. Visualization of the patterns is accomplished through acrylamide gel or capillary electrophoresis.

In a comparative study on *Mycoplasma bovis* isolates from cases of respiratory disease in calves from different regions of the United Kingdom, McAuliffe et al. [5] identified two genetically distinct clusters, whereupon the AFLP-PCR findings largely coincided with those of RAPD. Wagenaar et al. [21] used AFLP-PCR for genotyping of *Campylobacter fetus* strains and were able to differentiate the subspecies *Campylobacter fetus* subsp. *venerealis*. Hu et al. [22] identified phage type-specific markers by using this technique for *Salmonella* Typhimurium strains.

The advantages of AFLP-PCR include its high sensitivity and resolution for genome-wide detection of polymorphisms, as well as relatively good reproducibility. On the other hand, the number of amplified fragments has to be limited in order to keep the performance at high level. All in all, the procedure is relatively elaborate and requires purified and intact double-stranded DNA, as well as specialized equipment and software.

2.4 PFGE

The acronym stands for macro-restriction fragment length polymorphism analysis using pulsed-field gel electrophoresis. The method utilizes specific restriction sites throughout the microbial genome for differentiation below the species level. Bacterial cultures are embedded in agarose blocks, lysed in situ, and digested with rare-cutter restriction endonucleases. The resulting macrorestriction fragments sized up to 10 Mb can only be separated using agarose gel electrophoresis with an alternating electric field [23]. The final fingerprint patterns typically consist of 10–20 fragments. For an update on recent developments in PFGE technology, the reader is referred to an exhaustive review [24].

Due to its high discriminatory power, PFGE analysis evolved as a gold standard for typing of many bacteria, such as *Campylobacter* spp. [25], *Clostridium* spp. [26, 27], and *Salmonella* [28]. There are publicly accessible databases having thousands of individual strain patterns of food-borne pathogens, such as *Salmonella* serovars, *Listeria monocytogenes*, and others (e.g., http://www.pulsenetinternational.org/).

The main reason why the use of the procedure has been confined to a limited circle of specialized laboratories lies in its sophisticated and technically demanding work flow. For instance, the in situ digestion of genomic DNA in the agarose block may prove difficult for certain pathogens. Therefore, it remains a challenge to attain satisfactory interlaboratory reproducibility.

3 Typing Based on Repetitive Elements

3.1 VNTR/MLVA

Variable number tandem repeat (VNTR) analysis is targeting short nucleotide sequences (up to 100 bp) organized as tandem repeats in selected genomic regions [29]. Individual strains may vary in the number of repeat units associated with a certain locus. In the case of mycobacteria and other pathogens, multiple-locus VNTR analysis (MLVA) is an approach characterizing the polymorphism of tandemly repeated sequences in a number of genomic loci. The extensive use of MLVA typing for the characterization of food-borne pathogens, such as *Salmonella enterica*, *Listeria monocytogenes*, *Escherichia coli*, *Brucella* spp., and other bacteria, was reviewed recently by Lindstedt et al. [30]. The reader is also referred to the PulseNet database at http://www.pulsenetinternational.org/.

The practical assay comprises PCR amplification of the respective genomic locus or loci and subsequent electrophoretic separation of the products. The resolution parameters of agarose gel and capillary electrophoresis are comparable [31]. The number of repeats in the loci can be calculated from electrophoresis and combined into the MLVA profile. For instance, in the case of *Coxiella burnetii*, the code 7-6-6-3-5-3-7-3-13 denotes the number of repeats present in loci MS 03, 21, 22, 28, 30, 31, 34, 27, and 36, respectively, which corresponds to the unique profile designated CbNL01 [32]. For *M. avium* subsp. *paratuberculosis*, the panel of tandem repeats denoted 3-2-3-3-2-2-2-8 in the MIRU-VNTR loci 292, X3, 25, 47, 3, 7, 10, and 32, respectively, represents profile INMV2 [33].

VNTR/MLVA can be conducted directly on bacterial cell lysates and is generally well reproducible from laboratory to laboratory. The simple digitized output data format facilitates storage in databases and exchange among collaborators. As the technology allows differentiation below species level and identification of mixed infections, it lends itself for large-scale multilateral epidemiological surveys, as well as phylogenetic studies. However, its use will be confined to those pathogens possessing a sufficient number of highly variable repeat regions.

Table 2
VNTR loci recommended for MLVA typing of *Mycobacterium bovis*, *Mycobacterium caprae*, and other MTC isolates[a]

Locus[b]	Synonym	Specificity
VNTR 424		MTC, *M. bovis*+ *M. caprae*, ***M. caprae***
VNTR 580	ETR D	No diversity in certain geographical regions
VNTR960	MIRU 10	MTC, *M. bovis*+ *M. caprae*
VNTR 1644	MIRU 16	*M. bovis*+ *M. caprae*
VNTR 1955		MTC, *M. bovis*+ *M. caprae*, ***M. bovis***
VNTR 2163a	QUB 11a	MTC, *M. bovis*+ *M. caprae*, ***M. bovis, M. caprae***
VNTR 2163b	QUB 11b	MTC, *M. bovis*+ *M. caprae*, ***M. bovis, M. caprae***
VNTR 2165	ETR A	MTC, *M. bovis*+ *M. caprae*, ***M. bovis, M. caprae***
VNTR 2461	ETR B	***M. bovis***
VNTR 3232	QUB 3232	MTC, *M. bovis*+ *M. caprae*
VNTR 3690		MTC, *M. bovis*+ *M. caprae*
VNTR 4052	QUB 26	MTC, *M. bovis*+ *M. caprae*, ***M. bovis***
VNTR 4156	QUB 4156	MTC, *M. bovis*+ *M. caprae*, ***M. caprae***

Bold print means that the respective loci are particularly suitable for differentiating among *M. bovis* and *M. caprae* strains, respectively

[a]Compiled by the National Reference Laboratory for Bovine Tuberculosis at Friedrich-Loeffler-Institut Jena, Germany (Head: Dr. Irmgard Moser)

[b]All loci have a discriminatory index larger than 0.6 according to Hunter and Gaston [195]

3.2 MIRU-VNTR

MIRU (mycobacterial interspersed repetitive units)-VNTR is a mycobacteria-specific term for an MLVA typing scheme. It is based on 40–100-bp DNA elements arranged as tandem repeats and dispersed in intergenic regions of MTC genomes [34]. MIRU-VNTR typing allows high-throughput discriminatory analysis of clinical MTC isolates. The resolution of a typing assay can be fine-tuned depending on the number of examined loci. Different workers suggested using 24 [35], 12 [36, 37], or 15 [38, 39] loci.

The MTC members of veterinary relevance include *M. bovis*, *M. caprae*, *M. microti*, and *M. pinnipedii*. Their strains can be analyzed based on a variety of VNTR loci as compiled in Table 2. Thus, six loci are recommended for differentiation among *M. bovis* and five for *M. caprae* strains.

3.3 SSR Typing

Short sequence repeat (SSR)-based typing exploits variations in length and distribution of homopolymeric tracts of a single-nucleotide (mononucleotide repeats) or multimeric tracts (di- or trinucleotide repeats) in homogeneous or heterogeneous arrangements. The approach is actually a special case of VNTR analysis.

Genomic regions harboring this kind of repeats are often the most variable targets in a bacterial genome, whereas longer repeats are generally less diverse. SSR typing was suggested for differentiation and subtyping of *Mycoplasma* spp., *Mycobacterium* spp., and other bacteria [29].

The method can be efficient in discriminating between similar strains. However, mononucleotide repeats of more than ten units can give rise to slipped-strand mispairing or replication slippage events affecting the DNA polymerase during the amplification reaction. This leads to inaccurate results as shown in a study on *M. avium* subsp. *paratuberculosis* [40].

3.4 Spoligotyping

As a specialized typing scheme based on repetitive elements, spacer oligonucleotide typing or spoligotyping detects the presence or absence of 43 specific DNA spacer sequences in the direct repeat (DR) genomic region of all currently classified MTC organisms, i.e., *M. tuberculosis*, *M. bovis*, *M. caprae*, *M. africanum*, *M. canettii*, *M. microti*, and *M. pinnipedii*. It was the first PCR-based genotyping method for tuberculosis agents [41] and has become widely accepted for epidemiological tracking [42] and evolutionary studies [43]. To facilitate high-throughput spoligotyping, the conventional membrane-based hybridization protocol may be replaced by a recently developed DNA microarray assay [44]. The resulting hybridization pattern is converted into the generally established binary and octal codes [45], so that the output of this assay can be directly submitted to the international spoligotyping databases SpolDB4.0 [46] and Mbovis.org [47]. The methodology is widely used and well standardized, and the use of databases allows easy interlaboratory comparison of MTC strains. A recent comparative study revealed that spoligotyping is generally less discriminatory for MTC strains than IS*6110* RFLP analysis and MIRU-VNTR using 12 or 15 loci [42].

4 Single-Locus Sequence Typing

Highly variable genomic loci have been used to distinguish among strains of a species. Initially, the relevant genetic polymorphisms were detected using PCR with subsequent restriction enzyme analysis (PCR-RFLP) or Southern hybridization, before direct sequencing became commonly available. In recent years, the tendency toward direct use of nucleotide sequences instead of restriction enzyme digestion has increased. Sequence data have the advantage of being unambiguous, universally applicable and portable. Therefore, they are easily comparable, transferable, and compatible with many different typing approaches.

The first genomic locus used for typing purposes was the ribosomal RNA operon [18]. In the last three decades, ribotyping was used extensively with microorganisms of more than 200 genera for taxonomic classification, epidemiological tracking, and phylogenetic analysis. While comparatively easy to perform and well reproducible, the technique's discriminatory capacity is considered to be limited and less satisfactory in the age of genomics. In a critical review, Bouchet et al. [19] suggested an in silico ribotyping scheme to reflect the complete molecular genetic basis of ribotype polymorphisms. They found out that genetic variation in the housekeeping genes flanking the ribosomal operon was primarily responsible for these polymorphisms and, therefore, had to be taken into account when interpreting ribotyping data.

Strains of enterohemorrhagic *Escherichia coli* produce the outer membrane protein intimin encoded by the *eae* gene. The protein's high variability in the C-terminal region, where the host cell-binding specificity is localized, provided the basis for the *eae* typing scheme [48, 49]. In the area of *Chlamydia* spp., the demonstration of equivalence between traditional serotypes and *omp*A genotypes [50] represented a crucial finding that allowed the replacement of serotyping. To date, at least 15 *omp*A genotypes of *Chlamydia psittaci* have been described, and the original PCR-RFLP procedure has been supplanted by DNA microarray genotyping [51, 52] and real-time PCR [53]. The locus encoding the outer surface protein OspA was shown to differentiate among the species of *Borrelia burgdorferi* sensu lato and within the heterogeneous species of *Borrelia garinii* [54, 55]. Single-locus typing based on nucleotide sequence data can further improve accuracy and repeatability compared to PCR-RFLP. For instance, the modification of *Campylobacter* spp. *flaA* typing to a sequence-based protocol easily allowed inclusion of the *fla*B gene and led to an increase in resolution [56].

While single-locus typing schemes are still widely used, their major caveat is the limited discriminatory potential due to the fact that one locus alone often cannot provide high epidemiological resolution.

5 Multi-locus Sequence Typing (MLST)

Analyzing six to eight genomic loci encoding conserved housekeeping genes has become a widely used approach in epidemiology of microbial infections. Variable segments from each target gene of an average size between 400 and 600 bp are PCR amplified using specific primers and sequenced. The sequence type (ST) or allelic profile of a strain represents a defined set of sequences, each representing a distinct allele within the microbial species. An arbitrary number is assigned to each allele (unique sequence), so that the allelic profile is presented as a combination of numbers.

Since its introduction in 1998 [57], MLST has evolved as the most widely used tool in molecular typing of microbial strains. In a recent review, Pérez-Losada et al. [58] outlined the amazing achievements reached through the use of this typing approach over the past decade. Several publicly accessible MLST databases are available for about 80 microorganisms, mainly bacteria, e.g., http://pubmlst.org and http://www.pasteur.fr. Users can run their sequence data and conduct inquiries for allele sequence identification, allelic profile identification, and matching of isolates. Moreover, there is a number of specialized software programs to process experimental data (for details, *see* ref. 58).

The main areas of application include molecular epidemiology, phylogeny, and taxonomy, as well as population structure and dynamics. An MLST scheme for *Salmonella enterica* comprised seven housekeeping genes, i.e., *aro*C, *dna*N, *hem*D, *his*D, *pur*E, *suc*A, and *thr*A [59]. The scheme revealed a characteristic clustering of serovar Derby isolates from humans and pigs that correlated well with other typing methods, but failed to unambiguously reveal animal-to-human transmission [60].

Korczak et al. [56] introduced an optimized MLST strategy for *Campylobacter jejuni* and *C. coli* that included the *asp*A, *atp*A, *glm*M, *gln*A, *glt*A, *gly*A, and *tkt* loci. This system identified 118 different STs, 34 of which were described for the first time.

In the case of chlamydiae, three different typing schemes have been suggested. Dean et al. [61] selected seven genes on the basis of (1) diverse chromosomal regions where a single recombinational exchange would be unlikely to co-introduce >1 selected gene, (2) regions where several contiguous genes were involved in metabolic or key functions, (3) essential metabolic enzymes (e.g., tRNA synthases), (4) genes without similarity to human genes, and (5) no genes under diversifying selection. The panel includes *gly*A, *mdh*C, *pdh*A, *yhb*G, *pyk*F, *lys*S, and *leu*S loci and is suitable for epidemiological and phenotypic studies.

Pannekoek et al. [62] included seven housekeeping genes (*eno*A, *fum*C, *gat*A, *gid*A, *hem*N, *hlf*X, *opp*A), which allowed the detection of links between individual STs of *Chlamydia psittaci* and *Chlamydia abortus* and their host species. Another approach based on five highly variable but stable genomic loci (*hct*B, CT058, CT144, CT172, and *pbp*B) was intended for short-term clinical epidemiology and outbreak investigations and provided superior resolution [63]. The system was later modified into a DNA microarray assay by Christerson et al. [64] to allow rapid and economical typing at high throughput.

The fact that MLST is strictly sequence based renders it not only unambiguous and highly discriminatory but also portable and repeatable from one laboratory to another. One of the few drawbacks is associated with the selection of the housekeeping loci. The selection criteria applied to the different microorganisms are not always comparable as they depend on current knowledge and certainly also the preferences of individual workers. While the original idea consisted in using only housekeeping genes that were evenly distributed along the chromosome, flanked by genes of known function, and not under diversifying selection [59], later attempts were undertaken to develop alternative typing schemes based on virulence genes, as has been reported for salmonellae [65] and staphylococci [66].

As genetically monomorphic bacterial pathogens, such as mycobacteria, brucellae, and *Bacillus anthracis*, tend to exhibit less DNA sequence diversity in their housekeeping genes, MLST cannot provide the high resolution required for epidemiological studies on these agents [2, 67].

Instead of using functional genes, the genetic variation seen in intergenic spacer regions can also be exploited for typing. Multispacer sequence typing (MST) is a special variant of MLST that was used for *Coxiella burnetii* [68]. The numerical coding is similar to VNTR/MLVA, and the resulting MST genotypes can be identified by visiting a public database at http://ifr48.timone.univ-mrs.fr/MST_Coxiella/mst. MST data are easily comparable between laboratories, but the method is more laborious and less discriminatory than MLVA [69].

Even though there is now a clear tendency toward typing schemes using the entire genome, the MLST approach will certainly retain its importance in the near future, and the extensive data gathered so far will remain important references for comparison.

6 Genome-Wide Typing Approaches

As the demands on epidemiological resolution of typing schemes became ever higher in the last decades, the use of whole-genome sequences (WGS) for intraspecies discrimination and thus the emergence of genomotyping appeared to be only a question of time [70]. Early attempts focused on the utilization of high-density microarray slides covering whole bacterial genomes, similar to those used in transcriptomics. Typically, microarrays carrying 40- to 70-mer oligonucleotide probes to represent each genomic locus were employed [71, 72]. However, this expensive technology was not particularly suitable for routine diagnosis, and the experimental approach proved to have limitations as the accuracy of typing seemed to be satisfactory only among strains of average nucleotide identity (ANI) values higher than 90 % [73]. Another example of microarray-based genomotyping featured *Coxiella burnetii* and was based on the presence or absence of selected genes [74]. In 52 isolates, the authors identified ten genomotypes organized into three groups, of which four types were associated with acute Q fever.

Meanwhile, as more and more WGS have become available, the attractiveness of high-density microarray technology for molecular typing has diminished, because the same information can now be directly extracted from WGS, which is less expensive and strictly sequence based rather than converted into a pattern-like output format. At the same time, more versatile low-density DNA microarray platforms, such as the ArrayStrip™ system, will remain a relevant economical option for specialized typing purposes in diagnostic laboratories. Prominent examples include assays for methicillin-resistant *Staphylococcus aureus* (MRSA) [75], DNA serotyping of *E. coli* [76], as well as identification of antibiotic resistance genes in *Salmonella* [77] and *E. coli* [78].

In an attempt to bridge the gap between PFGE fingerprint typing and genome sequencing, whole-genome mapping (WGM) was used as a strain typing tool in epidemiological surveys. Representing an advanced version of optical mapping introduced in the 1990s [79], the methodology starts with genomic DNA fragments from lysed microbes being immobilized on a glass surface in a microfluidics device. A restriction enzyme specifically cleaves the DNA and leaves the fragments in the original genomic order stretched on a glass slide, where they are subsequently fluorescence stained, analyzed, and assembled to yield a barcode-like map. While the performance of WGM is not yet fully validated to compete with PFGE [80], it has a potential of enhancing differentiation among strains in outbreak situations.

Using a complete genome sequence as the basis of a typing scheme offers a number of advantages: (1) all the genetic information of an organism can be used, (2) standardization of the methodological approach is easier than with most other typing methods, and (3) the universal character of the nucleotide sequence information ensures worldwide comparability and repeatability now and in the future.

The great challenge in designing efficient genome-based typing schemes consists in the necessity to condense the huge amount of sequence data into a handy piece of essential information that will represent a particular genomotype. Currently there are no generally agreed operating procedures, nor criteria or parameters defining such procedures. In a recent review, Sabat et al. [81] singled out three possible strategies that are explained in the following paragraphs.

First, an *extended MLST* (eMLST) approach could be based on all genes of the so-called core genome, i.e., a panel of genes present in all strains of a species. The resulting allelic profile would be composed of hundreds or thousands of different alleles. Larsen et al. [82] used preassembled genome sequences and even short sequence reads to conduct MLST according to the established schemes for about 700 isolates of different bacterial species. This appears to be a realistic option because the costs of high-throughput sequencing have declined, so that the procedure can be cheaper than MLST based on traditional Sanger sequencing.

The use of WGS also allows more sophisticated MLST schemes to be implemented. Strain analysis of a recent outbreak of a multidrug-resistant enterohemorrhagic *E. coli* O104:H4 infection in Germany [83] showed that traditional MLST was unable to reveal distinctions between the outbreak strain and earlier isolates, because it failed to identify the diversity outside the genes covered by MLST. Cody et al. [84] conducted whole-genome MLST on 379 patient isolates of *Campylobacter jejuni* and *Campylobacter coli*. Using the Genome Comparator module of the Bacterial Isolate Genome Sequence Database (BIGSdb) [85] and including a total of 1,595 defined loci, they were able to further discriminate within clonal groups (sequence types) that had been defined by conventional 52-locus MLST.

Second, the *pan-genomic approach* would include the complete sequence information of a given genome, i.e., the core genome, dispensable genes found in a limited number of strains, and unique genes specific to individual strains of a species. Inter-strain relatedness would be defined through the presence or absence of genes. However, the scientific community has yet to agree on a procedure to condense the data into a user-friendly output format.

Third, *comparison of WGS at single-nucleotide resolution* can characterize the distribution of SNPs throughout the genomes, thus enabling high-resolution analysis of sequence variation among related strains and/or along the timeline in epidemiological chains. This was shown in the paper by Roetzer et al. [86], where the number of SNPs emerging in a human-to-human transmission chain was used to calculate the natural mutation rate of *Mycobacterium tuberculosis*. Similarly, Sherry et al. [87] used Ion Torrent sequencing data to conduct SNP analysis, which demonstrated the identity of four outbreak strains of multidrug-resistant *E. coli* in a neonatal intensive care unit.

All in all, WGS-based genotyping is still an emerging field, the number of studies published so far is limited, and its full potential has yet to be explored. The absence of standardization concerning the selection of target loci, the software tools to be used for sequence analysis, and other essential operations is currently the main deficit, and it will certainly take some more time for the research community to agree on these fundamentals. Nevertheless, this area can be expected to develop dynamically in the next few years. One of the most intriguing options opening up refers to the possibility of addressing specific features of a microbial strain, such as virulence, resistance, presence of toxins, or host preference. This means that thematic sequence information can be extracted routinely from WGS to form artificial partial genomes, such as the antibiotic resistome [88, 89], toxome [90], and virulome.

7 Conclusion

The development of microbial typing over the last two decades has significantly contributed to enhanced surveillance and outbreak management [7, 63, 83, 87], as well as to ever more detailed characterization of field strains in terms of virulence properties, antimicrobial resistance, phylogenetic position, etc. As outlined in the previous sections, the evolution of tools shows a clear tendency toward sequence-based methods, with the nascent WGS-based algorithms holding great promise.

Given the diversity in the various methodological approaches and the multitude of typing protocols, it is obvious that there is no single method that would be universally applicable. The choice of the methodology rather depends on the objective of the study, the concrete epidemiological situation, and the budget available.

For instance, in an outbreak scenario, rapid methods are preferable, such as VNTR, partial sequencing, and RAPD. As short-term delivery of relevant strain characteristics is crucial to inform decision makers, it can be more important to use a fast and robust tool rather than aspiring to the highest resolution. In monitoring and surveillance schemes, the overall cost, practical feasibility, and availability of a standardized protocol are likely to be the essential parameters. Therefore, MLST and VNTR schemes are frequently used for this purpose.

Finally, retrospective studies and epidemiological research projects will be demanding ever higher information contents to be obtained on the strains involved, as well as maximum resolution, all of which can be delivered using genome-wide typing methods.

References

1. de Beer JL, van Ingen J, de Vries G et al (2013) Comparative study of IS6110 restriction fragment length polymorphism and variable-number tandem-repeat typing of *Mycobacterium tuberculosis* isolates in the Netherlands, based on a 5-year nationwide survey. J Clin Microbiol 51:1193–1198
2. Pitondo-Silva A, Santos AC, Jolley KA, Leite CQ, Darini AL (2013) Comparison of three molecular typing methods to assess genetic diversity for *Mycobacterium tuberculosis*. J Microbiol Methods 93:42–48
3. Fritsch I, Luyven G, Kohler H, Lutz W, Mobius P (2012) Suspicion of *Mycobacterium avium* subsp. *paratuberculosis* transmission between cattle and wild-living red deer (*Cervus elaphus*) by multitarget genotyping. Appl Environ Microbiol 78:1132–1139
4. Welsh J, McClelland M (1990) Fingerprinting genomes using PCR with arbitrary primers. Nucleic Acids Res 18:7213–7218
5. McAuliffe L, Kokotovic B, Ayling RD, Nicholas RA (2004) Molecular epidemiological analysis of *Mycoplasma bovis* isolates from the United Kingdom shows two genetically distinct clusters. J Clin Microbiol 42: 4556–4565
6. Hotzel H, Schneider B, Sachse K (1998) Investigation of *Mycoplasma bovis* field isolates using PCR fingerprinting. In: Leori G, Santini F, Scanziani E, Frey J (eds) Mycoplasmas of ruminants: pathogenicity, diagnostics, epidemiology and molecular genetics, vol 2. European Commission, Brussels, Belgium, pp 17–19
7. Butler JA, Pinnow CC, Thomson JU, Levisohn S, Rosenbusch RF (2001) Use of arbitrarily primed polymerase chain reaction to investigate *Mycoplasma bovis* outbreaks. Vet Microbiol 78:175–181
8. Schrenzel M, Nicolas M, Witte C et al (2008) Molecular epidemiology of *Mycobacterium*

avium subsp. *avium* and *Mycobacterium intracellulare* in captive birds. Vet Microbiol 126:122–131

9. Kauppinen J, Hintikka E, Iivanainen E, Katila M (2001) PCR-based typing of *Mycobacterium avium* isolates in an epidemic among farmed lesser white-fronted geese (*Anser erythropus*). Vet Microbiol 81:41–50
10. Scheibl P, Gerlach GF (1997) Differentiation of *Mycobacterium paratuberculosis* isolates by rDNA-spacer analysis and random amplified polymorphic DNA patterns. Vet Microbiol 57:151–158
11. Petersen L, Newell DG (2001) The ability of *Fla*-typing schemes to discriminate between strains of *Campylobacter jejuni*. J Appl Microbiol 91:217–224
12. Sayada C, Andersen AA, Storey C et al (1995) Usefulness of *omp1* restriction mapping for avian *Chlamydia psittaci* isolate differentiation. Res Microbiol 146:155–165
13. van Embden JD, Cave MD, Crawford JT et al (1993) Strain identification of *Mycobacterium tuberculosis* by DNA fingerprinting: recommendations for a standardized methodology. J Clin Microbiol 31:406–409
14. Erler W, Martin G, Sachse K et al (2004) Molecular fingerprinting of *Mycobacterium bovis* subsp. *caprae* isolates from central Europe. J Clin Microbiol 42:2234–2238
15. Michel AL, Hlokwe TM, Coetzee ML et al (2008) High *Mycobacterium bovis* genetic diversity in a low prevalence setting. Vet Microbiol 126:151–159
16. Pavlik I, Horvathova A, Dvorska L et al (1999) Standardisation of restriction fragment length polymorphism analysis for *Mycobacterium avium* subspecies *paratuberculosis*. J Microbiol Methods 38:155–167
17. Mobius P, Luyven G, Hotzel H, Kohler H (2008) High genetic diversity among *Mycobacterium avium* subsp. *paratuberculosis* strains from German cattle herds shown by combination of IS900 restriction fragment length polymorphism analysis and mycobacterial interspersed repetitive unit-variable-number tandem-repeat typing. J Clin Microbiol 46: 972–981
18. Grimont F, Grimont PA (1986) Ribosomal ribonucleic acid gene restriction patterns as potential taxonomic tools. Ann Inst Pasteur Microbiol 137B:165–175
19. Bouchet V, Huot H, Goldstein R (2008) Molecular genetic basis of ribotyping. Clin Microbiol Rev 21:262–273
20. Vos P, Hogers R, Bleeker M et al (1995) AFLP: a new technique for DNA fingerprinting. Nucleic Acids Res 23:4407–4414
21. Wagenaar JA, van Bergen MA, Newell DG, Grogono-Thomas R, Duim B (2001) Comparative study using amplified fragment length polymorphism fingerprinting, PCR genotyping, and phenotyping to differentiate *Campylobacter fetus* strains isolated from animals. J Clin Microbiol 39:2283–2286
22. Hu H, Lan R, Reeves PR (2002) Fluorescent amplified fragment length polymorphism analysis of *Salmonella enterica* serovar typhimurium reveals phage-type-specific markers and potential for microarray typing. J Clin Microbiol 40:3406–3415
23. Schwartz DC, Cantor CR (1984) Separation of yeast chromosome-sized DNAs by pulsed field gradient gel electrophoresis. Cell 37: 67–75
24. Herschleb J, Ananiev G, Schwartz DC (2007) Pulsed-field gel electrophoresis. Nat Protoc 2:677–684
25. On SL, Harrington CS (2001) Evaluation of numerical analysis of PFGE-DNA profiles for differentiating *Campylobacter fetus* subspecies by comparison with phenotypic, PCR and 16S rDNA sequencing methods. J Appl Microbiol 90:285–293
26. Nevas M, Lindstrom M, Hielm S et al (2005) Diversity of proteolytic *Clostridium botulinum* strains, determined by a pulsed-field gel electrophoresis approach. Appl Environ Microbiol 71:1311–1317
27. Leclair D, Pagotto F, Farber JM, Cadieux B, Austin JW (2006) Comparison of DNA fingerprinting methods for use in investigation of type E botulism outbreaks in the Canadian Arctic. J Clin Microbiol 44:1635–1644
28. Ribot EM, Fair MA, Gautom R et al (2006) Standardization of pulsed-field gel electrophoresis protocols for the subtyping of *Escherichia coli* O157:H7, *Salmonella*, and *Shigella* for PulseNet. Foodborne Pathog Dis 3:59–67
29. van Belkum A, Scherer S, van Alphen L, Verbrugh H (1998) Short-sequence DNA repeats in prokaryotic genomes. Microbiol Mol Biol Rev 62:275–293
30. Lindstedt BA, Torpdahl M, Vergnaud G et al (2013) Use of multilocus variable-number tandem repeat analysis (MLVA) in eight European countries, 2012. Euro Surveill 18: 20385
31. Jenkins AO, Venter EH, Hutamo K, Godfroid J (2010) Comparison of the capillary and agarose electrophoresis based multiple locus VNTR (variable number of tandem repeats) analysis (MLVA) on *Mycobacterium bovis* isolates. Vet Microbiol 145:172–176
32. Roest HI, Ruuls RC, Tilburg JJ et al (2011) Molecular epidemiology of *Coxiella burnetii*

from ruminants in Q fever outbreak, the Netherlands. Emerg Infect Dis 17:668–675

33. Thibault VC, Grayon M, Boschiroli ML et al (2007) New variable-number tandem-repeat markers for typing *Mycobacterium avium* subsp. *paratuberculosis* and *M. avium* strains: comparison with IS900 and IS1245 restriction fragment length polymorphism typing. J Clin Microbiol 45:2404–2410
34. Supply P, Mazars E, Lesjean S et al (2000) Variable human minisatellite-like regions in the *Mycobacterium tuberculosis* genome. Mol Microbiol 36:762–771
35. Supply P, Allix C, Lesjean S et al (2006) Proposal for standardization of optimized mycobacterial interspersed repetitive unit-variable-number tandem repeat typing of *Mycobacterium tuberculosis*. J Clin Microbiol 44:4498–4510
36. Oelemann MC, Diel R, Vatin V et al (2007) Assessment of an optimized mycobacterial interspersed repetitive-unit-variable-number tandem-repeat typing system combined with spoligotyping for population-based molecular epidemiology studies of tuberculosis. J Clin Microbiol 45:691–697
37. Mazars E, Lesjean S, Banuls AL et al (2001) High-resolution minisatellite-based typing as a portable approach to global analysis of *Mycobacterium tuberculosis* molecular epidemiology. Proc Natl Acad Sci U S A 98: 1901–1906
38. Mandal S, Bradshaw L, Anderson LF et al (2011) Investigating transmission of *Mycobacterium bovis* in the United Kingdom in 2005 to 2008. J Clin Microbiol 49:1943–1950
39. Alonso-Rodriguez N, Martinez-Lirola M, Herranz M et al (2008) Evaluation of the new advanced 15-loci MIRU-VNTR genotyping tool in *Mycobacterium tuberculosis* molecular epidemiology studies. BMC Microbiol 8:34
40. Kasnitz N, Kohler H, Weigoldt M, Gerlach GF, Mobius P (2013) Stability of genotyping target sequences of *Mycobacterium avium* subsp. *paratuberculosis* upon cultivation on different media, in vitro- and in vivo passage, and natural infection. Vet Microbiol 167: 573–583
41. Kamerbeek J, Schouls L, Kolk A et al (1997) Simultaneous detection and strain differentiation of *Mycobacterium tuberculosis* for diagnosis and epidemiology. J Clin Microbiol 35: 907–914
42. Stone MJ, Brown TJ, Drobniewski FA (2012) Human *Mycobacterium bovis* infections in London and Southeast England. J Clin Microbiol 50:164–165
43. Smith NH, Gordon SV, de la Rua-Domenech R, Clifton-Hadley RS, Hewinson RG (2006) Bottlenecks and broomsticks: the molecular evolution of *Mycobacterium bovis*. Nat Rev Microbiol 4:670–681
44. Ruettger A, Nieter J, Skrypnyk A et al (2012) Rapid spoligotyping of *Mycobacterium tuberculosis* complex bacteria by use of a microarray system with automatic data processing and assignment. J Clin Microbiol 50:2492–2495
45. Dale JW, Brittain D, Cataldi AA et al (2001) Spacer oligonucleotide typing of bacteria of the *Mycobacterium tuberculosis* complex: recommendations for standardised nomenclature. Int J Tuberc Lung Dis 5:216–219
46. Brudey K, Driscoll JR, Rigouts L et al (2006) *Mycobacterium tuberculosis* complex genetic diversity: mining the fourth international spoligotyping database (SpolDB4) for classification, population genetics and epidemiology. BMC Microbiol 6:23
47. Smith NH, Upton P (2012) Naming spoligotype patterns for the RD9-deleted lineage of the Mycobacterium tuberculosis complex; www.Mbovis.org. Infect Genet Evol 12: 873–876
48. Oswald E, Schmidt H, Morabito S et al (2000) Typing of intimin genes in human and animal enterohemorrhagic and enteropathogenic *Escherichia coli*: characterization of a new intimin variant. Infect Immun 68:64–71
49. Blanco M, Schumacher S, Tasara T et al (2005) Serotypes, intimin variants and other virulence factors of eae positive *Escherichia coli* strains isolated from healthy cattle in Switzerland. Identification of a new intimin variant gene (eae-eta2). BMC Microbiol 5:23
50. Vanrompay D, Butaye P, Sayada C, Ducatelle R, Haesebrouck F (1997) Characterization of avian *Chlamydia psittaci* strains using *ompl* restriction mapping and serovar-specific monoclonal antibodies. Res Microbiol 148: 327–333
51. Sachse K, Laroucau K, Hotzel H et al (2008) Genotyping of *Chlamydophila psittaci* using a new DNA microarray assay based on sequence analysis of *ompA* genes. BMC Microbiol 8:63
52. Ruettger A, Feige J, Slickers P et al (2011) Genotyping of *Chlamydia trachomatis* strains from culture and clinical samples using an *ompA*-based DNA microarray assay. Mol Cell Probes 25:19–27
53. Geens T, Dewitte A, Boon N, Vanrompay D (2005) Development of a *Chlamydophila psittaci* species-specific and genotype-specific real-time PCR. Vet Res 36:787–797
54. Michel H, Wilske B, Hettche G et al (2004) An ospA-polymerase chain reaction/restriction fragment length polymorphism-based method for sensitive detection and reliable differentiation of all European *Borrelia burgdorferi* sensu

lato species and OspA types. Med Microbiol Immunol 193:219–226

55. Will G, Jauris-Heipke S, Schwab E et al (1995) Sequence analysis of ospA genes shows homogeneity within *Borrelia burgdorferi* sensu stricto and *Borrelia afzelii* strains but reveals major subgroups within the *Borrelia garinii* species. Med Microbiol Immunol 184:73–80
56. Korczak BM, Zurfluh M, Emler S, Kuhn-Oertli J, Kuhnert P (2009) Multiplex strategy for multilocus sequence typing, fla typing, and genetic determination of antimicrobial resistance of *Campylobacter jejuni* and *Campylobacter coli* isolates collected in Switzerland. J Clin Microbiol 47:1996–2007
57. Maiden MC, Bygraves JA, Feil E et al (1998) Multilocus sequence typing: a portable approach to the identification of clones within populations of pathogenic microorganisms. Proc Natl Acad Sci U S A 95:3140–3145
58. Perez-Losada M, Cabezas P, Castro-Nallar E, Crandall KA (2013) Pathogen typing in the genomics era: MLST and the future of molecular epidemiology. Infect Genet Evol 16: 38–53
59. Kidgell C, Reichard U, Wain J et al (2002) *Salmonella typhi*, the causative agent of typhoid fever, is approximately 50,000 years old. Infect Genet Evol 2:39–45
60. Hauser E, Hebner F, Tietze E et al (2011) Diversity of *Salmonella enterica* serovar Derby isolated from pig, pork and humans in Germany. Int J Food Microbiol 151:141–149
61. Dean D, Bruno WJ, Wan R et al (2009) Predicting phenotype and emerging strains among *Chlamydia trachomatis* infections. Emerg Infect Dis 15:1385–1394
62. Pannekoek Y, Dickx V, Beeckman DS et al (2010) Multi locus sequence typing of *Chlamydia* reveals an association between *Chlamydia psittaci* genotypes and host species. PLoS One 5:e14179
63. Klint M, Fuxelius HH, Goldkuhl RR et al (2007) High-resolution genotyping of *Chlamydia trachomatis* strains by multilocus sequence analysis. J Clin Microbiol 45:1410–1414
64. Christerson L, Ruettger A, Gravningen K et al (2011) High-resolution genotyping of *Chlamydia trachomatis* by use of a novel multilocus typing DNA microarray. J Clin Microbiol 49:2838–2843
65. Tankouo-Sandjong B, Sessitsch A, Liebana E et al (2007) MLST-v, multilocus sequence typing based on virulence genes, for molecular typing of *Salmonella enterica* subsp. *enterica* serovars. J Microbiol Methods 69:23–36
66. Verghese B, Schwalm ND 3rd, Dudley EG, Knabel SJ (2012) A combined multi-virulence-locus sequence typing and Staphylococcal Cassette Chromosome mec typing scheme possesses enhanced discriminatory power for genotyping MRSA. Infect Genet Evol 12:1816–1821
67. Scholz HC, Vergnaud G (2013) Molecular characterisation of *Brucella* species. Rev Sci Tech 32:149–162
68. Glazunova O, Roux V, Freylikman O et al (2005) *Coxiella burnetii* genotyping. Emerg Infect Dis 11:1211–1217
69. Santos AS, Tilburg JJ, Botelho A et al (2012) Genotypic diversity of clinical *Coxiella burnetii* isolates from Portugal based on MST and MLVA typing. Int J Med Microbiol 302:253–256
70. Lucchini S, Thompson A, Hinton JC (2001) Microarrays for microbiologists. Microbiology 147:1403–1414
71. Ballerstedt H, Volkers RJ, Mars AE et al (2007) Genomotyping of *Pseudomonas putida* strains using *P. putida* KT2440-based high-density DNA microarrays: implications for transcriptomics studies. Appl Microbiol Biotechnol 75:1133–1142
72. Snyder LA, Davies JK, Saunders NJ (2004) Microarray genomotyping of key experimental strains of *Neisseria gonorrhoeae* reveals gene complement diversity and five new neisserial genes associated with Minimal Mobile Elements. BMC Genomics 5:23
73. Oh S, Yoder-Himes DR, Tiedje J, Park J, Konstantinidis KT (2010) Evaluating the performance of oligonucleotide microarrays for bacterial strains with increasing genetic divergence from the reference strain. Appl Environ Microbiol 76:2980–2988
74. Leroy Q, Armougom F, Barbry P, Raoult D (2011) Genomotyping of *Coxiella burnetii* using microarrays reveals a conserved genomotype for hard tick isolates. PLoS One 6:e25781
75. Monecke S, Coombs G, Shore AC et al (2011) A field guide to pandemic, epidemic and sporadic clones of methicillin-resistant *Staphylococcus aureus*. PLoS One 6:e17936
76. Ballmer K, Korczak BM, Kuhnert P et al (2007) Fast DNA serotyping of *Escherichia coli* by use of an oligonucleotide microarray. J Clin Microbiol 45:370–379
77. Braun SD, Ziegler A, Methner U et al (2012) Fast DNA serotyping and antimicrobial resistance gene determination of salmonella enterica with an oligonucleotide microarray-based assay. PLoS One 7:e46489

78. Perreten V, Vorlet-Fawer L, Slickers P, Ehricht R, Kuhnert P, Frey J (2005) Microarray-based detection of 90 antibiotic resistance genes of gram-positive bacteria. J Clin Microbiol 43: 2291–2302
79. Schwartz DC, Li X, Hernandez LI et al (1993) Ordered restriction maps of *Saccharomyces cerevisiae* chromosomes constructed by optical mapping. Science 262:110–114
80. Miller JM (2013) Whole-genome mapping: a new paradigm in strain-typing technology. J Clin Microbiol 51:1066–1070
81. Sabat AJ, Budimir A, Nashev D et al (2013) Overview of molecular typing methods for outbreak detection and epidemiological surveillance. Euro Surveill 18:20380
82. Larsen MV, Cosentino S, Rasmussen S et al (2012) Multilocus sequence typing of total-genome-sequenced bacteria. J Clin Microbiol 50:1355–1361
83. Mellmann A, Harmsen D, Cummings CA et al (2011) Prospective genomic characterization of the German enterohemorrhagic *Escherichia coli* O104:H4 outbreak by rapid next generation sequencing technology. PLoS One 6:e22751
84. Cody AJ, McCarthy ND, Jansen van Rensburg M, Isinkaye T et al (2013) Real-time genomic epidemiology of human *Campylobacter* isolates using whole genome multilocus sequence typing. J Clin Microbiol 51:2526–2534
85. Jolley KA, Maiden MC (2010) BIGSdb: scalable analysis of bacterial genome variation at the population level. BMC Bioinformatics 11:595
86. Roetzer A, Diel R, Kohl TA et al (2013) Whole genome sequencing versus traditional genotyping for investigation of a *Mycobacterium tuberculosis* outbreak: a longitudinal molecular epidemiological study. PLoS Med 10:e1001387
87. Sherry NL, Porter JL, Seemann T et al (2013) Outbreak investigation using high-throughput genome sequencing within a diagnostic microbiology laboratory. J Clin Microbiol 51: 1396–1401
88. Poirel L, Bonnin RA, Nordmann P (2011) Analysis of the resistome of a multidrug-resistant NDM-1-producing *Escherichia coli* strain by high-throughput genome sequencing. Antimicrob Agents Chemother 55: 4224–4229
89. Forsberg KJ, Reyes A, Wang B et al (2012) The shared antibiotic resistome of soil bacteria and human pathogens. Science 337:1107–1111
90. Koser CU, Holden MT, Ellington MJ et al (2012) Rapid whole-genome sequencing for investigation of a neonatal MRSA outbreak. N Engl J Med 366:2267–2275
91. Keim P, Price LB, Klevytska AM et al (2000) Multiple-locus variable-number tandem repeat analysis reveals genetic relationships within *Bacillus anthracis.* J Bacteriol 182:2928–2936
92. Lista F, Faggioni G, Valjevac S et al (2006) Genotyping of *Bacillus anthracis* strains based on automated capillary 25-loci multiple locus variable-number tandem repeats analysis. BMC Microbiol 6:33
93. Van Ert MN, Easterday WR, Huynh LY et al (2007) Global genetic population structure of *Bacillus anthracis.* PLoS One 2:e461
94. Keim P, Van Ert MN, Pearson T et al (2004) Anthrax molecular epidemiology and forensics: using the appropriate marker for different evolutionary scales. Infect Genet Evol 4:205–213
95. Van Ert MN, Easterday WR, Simonson TS et al (2007) Strain-specific single-nucleotide polymorphism assays for the *Bacillus anthracis* Ames strain. J Clin Microbiol 45:47–53
96. Fingerle V, Michel H, Hettche G, Hizo-Teufel C, Wilske B (2004) *Borrelia burgdorferi* s.l. OspA-types are widespread in Bavaria but show distinct local patterns. Int J Med Microbiol 293(suppl 37):165–166
97. Margos G, Gatewood AG, Aanensen DM et al (2008) MLST of housekeeping genes captures geographic population structure and suggests a European origin of *Borrelia burgdorferi.* Proc Natl Acad Sci U S A 105: 8730–8735
98. Foster JT, Price LB, Beckstrom-Sternberg SM et al (2012) Genotyping of *Brucella* species using clade specific SNPs. BMC Microbiol 12:110
99. Bricker BJ, Ewalt DR, Halling SM (2003) *Brucella* 'HOOF-Prints': strain typing by multi-locus analysis of variable number tandem repeats (VNTRs). BMC Microbiol 3:15
100. Le Fleche P, Jacques I, Grayon M et al (2006) Evaluation and selection of tandem repeat loci for a *Brucella* MLVA typing assay. BMC Microbiol 6:9
101. Whatmore AM, Shankster SJ, Perrett LL et al (2006) Identification and characterization of variable-number tandem-repeat markers for typing of *Brucella* spp. J Clin Microbiol 44: 1982–1993
102. Whatmore AM, Perrett LL, MacMillan AP (2007) Characterisation of the genetic diversity of *Brucella* by multilocus sequencing. BMC Microbiol 7:34
103. Wattiau P, Whatmore AM, Van Hessche M, Godfroid J, Fretin D (2011) Nucleotide

polymorphism-based single-tube test for robust molecular identification of all currently described *Brucella* species. Appl Environ Microbiol 77:6674–6679

104. Godoy D, Randle G, Simpson AJ et al (2003) Multilocus sequence typing and evolutionary relationships among the causative agents of melioidosis and glanders, *Burkholderia pseudomallei* and *Burkholderia mallei*. J Clin Microbiol 41:2068–2079
105. Currie B, Thomas AD, Godoy D, Dance D et al (2007) Australian and Thai isolates of *Burkholderia pseudomallei* are distinct by multilocus sequence typing: revision of a case of mistaken identity. J Clin Microbiol 45: 3828–3829
106. Vesaratchavest M, Tumapa S, Day NP et al (2006) Nonrandom distribution of *Burkholderia pseudomallei* clones in relation to geographical location and virulence. J Clin Microbiol 44:2553–2557
107. Currie BJ, Haslem A, Pearson T et al (2009) Identification of melioidosis outbreak by multilocus variable number tandem repeat analysis. Emerg Infect Dis 15:169–174
108. U'Ren JM, Schupp JM, Pearson T et al (2007) Tandem repeat regions within the *Burkholderia pseudomallei* genome and their application for high resolution genotyping. BMC Microbiol 7:23
109. Chantratita N, Vesaratchavest M, Wuthiekanun V et al (2006) Pulsed-field gel electrophoresis as a discriminatory typing technique for the biothreat agent *Burkholderia mallei*. Am J Trop Med Hyg 74:345–347
110. Ribot EM, Fitzgerald C, Kubota K, Swaminathan B, Barrett TJ (2001) Rapid pulsed-field gel electrophoresis protocol for subtyping of *Campylobacter jejuni*. J Clin Microbiol 39:1889–1894
111. Dingle KE, Colles FM, Wareing DR et al (2001) Multilocus sequence typing system for *Campylobacter jejuni*. J Clin Microbiol 39: 14–23
112. Parsons BN, Cody AJ, Porter CJ et al (2009) Typing of *Campylobacter jejuni* isolates from dogs by use of multilocus sequence typing and pulsed-field gel electrophoresis. J Clin Microbiol 47:3466–3471
113. Nachamkin I, Bohachick K, Patton CM (1993) Flagellin gene typing of *Campylobacter jejuni* by restriction fragment length polymorphism analysis. J Clin Microbiol 31: 1531–1536
114. Buchanan CJ, Yoshida C, Kruczkiewicz P et al (2011) High-resolution comparative genomic fingerprinting of *Campylobacter jejuni* using ArrayTube™ miniaturized diagnostic microarrays. In: Proceedings of 16th international workshop on *Campylobacter*, *Helicobacter* and Related Organisms (CHRO 2011). Vancouver, Canada, p 164
115. El-Adawy H, Hotzel H, Tomaso H et al (2013) Detection of genetic diversity in *Campylobacter jejuni* isolated from a commercial Turkey flock using *flaA* typing, MLST analysis and microarray assay. PLoS One 8:e51582
116. van Bergen MA, van der Graaf-van BL, Visser IJ, van Putten JP, Wagenaar JA (2006) Molecular epidemiology of *Campylobacter fetus* subsp. *fetus* on bovine artificial insemination stations using pulsed field gel electrophoresis. Vet Microbiol 112:65–71
117. van Bergen MA, Simons G, van der Graaf-van BL et al (2005) Amplified fragment length polymorphism based identification of genetic markers and novel PCR assay for differentiation of *Campylobacter fetus* subspecies. J Med Microbiol 54:1217–1224
118. van Bergen MA, Dingle KE, Maiden MC et al (2005) Clonal nature of *Campylobacter fetus* as defined by multilocus sequence typing. J Clin Microbiol 43:5888–5898
119. Miller WG, Chapman MH, Yee E et al (2012) Multilocus sequence typing methods for the emerging *Campylobacter* species *C. hyointestinalis*, *C. lanienae*, *C. sputorum*, *C. concisus*, and *C. curvus*. Front Cell Infect Microbiol 2:45
120. Pannekoek Y, Morelli G, Kusecek B et al (2008) Multi locus sequence typing of Chlamydiales: clonal groupings within the obligate intracellular bacteria *Chlamydia trachomatis*. BMC Microbiol 8:42
121. Geens T, Desplanques A, Van Loock M, Bönner B et al (2005) Sequencing of the *Chlamydophila psittaci ompA* gene reveals a new genotype, E/B, and the need for a rapid discriminatory genotyping method. J Clin Microbiol 43:2456–2461
122. Laroucau K, Thierry S, Vorimore F et al (2008) High resolution typing of *Chlamydophila psittaci* by multilocus VNTR analysis (MLVA). Infect Genet Evol 8:171–181
123. Laroucau K, Vorimore F, Bertin C et al (2009) Genotyping of *Chlamydophila abortus* strains by multilocus VNTR analysis. Vet Microbiol 137:335–344
124. Umeda K, Wada T, Kohda T, Kozaki S (2013) Multi-locus variable number tandem repeat analysis for *Clostridium botulinum* type B isolates in Japan: comparison with other isolates and genotyping methods. Infect Genet Evol 16:298–304

125. Maslanka SE, Kerr JG, Williams G et al (1999) Molecular subtyping of *Clostridium perfringens* by pulsed-field gel electrophoresis to facilitate food-borne-disease outbreak investigations. J Clin Microbiol 37:2209–2214
126. Lukinmaa S, Takkunen E, Siitonen A (2002) Molecular epidemiology of *Clostridium perfringens* related to food-borne outbreaks of disease in Finland from 1984 to 1999. Appl Environ Microbiol 68:3744–3749
127. Johansson A, Aspan A, Bagge E et al (2006) Genetic diversity of *Clostridium perfringens* type A isolates from animals, food poisoning outbreaks and sludge. BMC Microbiol 6:47
128. Ferreira TSP, Moreno AM, de Almeida RR et al (2012) Molecular typing of *Clostridium perfringens* isolated from swine in slaughterhouses from Sao Paulo State, Brazil. Cienc Rural 42:1450–1456
129. Sawires YS, Songer JG (2005) Multiple-locus variable-number tandem repeat analysis for strain typing of *Clostridium perfringens.* Anaerobe 11:262–272
130. Chalmers G, Martin SW, Prescott JF, Boerlin P (2008) Typing of *Clostridium perfringens* by multiple-locus variable number of tandem repeats analysis. Vet Microbiol 128:126–135
131. Knetsch CW, Lawley TD, Hensgens MP et al (2013) Current application and future perspectives of molecular typing methods to study *Clostridium difficile* infections. Euro Surveill 18:20381
132. Neumann AP, Rehberger TG (2009) MLST analysis reveals a highly conserved core genome among poultry isolates of *Clostridium septicum.* Anaerobe 15:99–106
133. Arricau-Bouvery N, Hauck Y, Bejaoui A et al (2006) Molecular characterization of *Coxiella burnetii* isolates by infrequent restriction site-PCR and MLVA typing. BMC Microbiol 6:39
134. Svraka S, Toman R, Skultety L, Slaba K, Homan WL (2006) Establishment of a genotyping scheme for *Coxiella burnetii.* FEMS Microbiol Lett 254:268–274
135. Tilburg JJ, Rossen JW, van Hannen EJ et al (2012) Genotypic diversity of *Coxiella burnetii* in the 2007-2010 Q fever outbreak episodes in The Netherlands. J Clin Microbiol 50:1076–1078
136. Franck SM, Bosworth BT, Moon HW (1998) Multiplex PCR for enterotoxigenic, attaching and effacing, and Shiga toxin-producing *Escherichia coli* strains from calves. J Clin Microbiol 36:1795–1797
137. Nguyen TV, Le Van P, Le Huy C, Gia KN, Weintraub A (2005) Detection and characterization of diarrheagenic *Escherichia coli* from young children in Hanoi, Vietnam. J Clin Microbiol 43:755–760
138. Muller D, Hagedorn P, Brast S, Heusipp G et al (2006) Rapid identification and differentiation of clinical isolates of enteropathogenic *Escherichia coli* (EPEC), atypical EPEC, and Shiga toxin-producing *Escherichia coli* by a one-step multiplex PCR method. J Clin Microbiol 44:2626–2629
139. Casey TA, Bosworth BT (2009) Design and evaluation of a multiplex polymerase chain reaction assay for the simultaneous identification of genes for nine different virulence factors associated with *Escherichia coli* that cause diarrhea and edema disease in swine. J Vet Diagn Invest 21:25–30
140. Scheutz F, Teel LD, Beutin L et al (2012) Multicenter evaluation of a sequence-based protocol for subtyping Shiga toxins and standardizing Stx nomenclature. J Clin Microbiol 50:2951–2963
141. Adu-Bobie J, Frankel G, Bain C et al (1998) Detection of intimins alpha, beta, gamma, and delta, four intimin derivatives expressed by attaching and effacing microbial pathogens. J Clin Microbiol 36:662–668
142. Jores J, Zehmke K, Eichberg J, Rumer L, Wieler LH (2003) Description of a novel intimin variant (type zeta) in the bovine O84:NM verotoxin-producing *Escherichia coli* strain 537/89 and the diagnostic value of intimin typing. Exp Biol Med (Maywood) 228: 370–376
143. Ramachandran V, Brett K, Hornitzky MA et al (2003) Distribution of intimin subtypes among *Escherichia coli* isolates from ruminant and human sources. J Clin Microbiol 41: 5022–5032
144. Barth S, Schwanitz A, Bauerfeind R (2011) Polymerase chain reaction-based method for the typing of F18 fimbriae and distribution of F18 fimbrial subtypes among porcine Shiga toxin-encoding *Escherichia coli* in Germany. J Vet Diagn Invest 23:454–464
145. Franklin MA, Francis DH, Baker D, Mathew AG (1996) A PCR-based method of detection and differentiation of K88+ adhesive *Escherichia coli.* J Vet Diagn Invest 8:460–463
146. Imberechts H, Van Pelt N, De Greve H, Lintermans P (1994) Sequences related to the major subunit gene fedA of F107 fimbriae in porcine *Escherichia coli* strains that express adhesive fimbriae. FEMS Microbiol Lett 119:309–314
147. Schilling AK, Hotzel H, Methner U et al (2012) Zoonotic agents in small ruminants kept on city farms in southern Germany. Appl Environ Microbiol 78:3785–3793

148. Monecke S, Mariani-Kurkdjian P, Bingen E et al (2011) Presence of enterohemorrhagic *Escherichia coli* ST678/O104:H4 in France prior to 2011. Appl Environ Microbiol 77:8784–8786
149. Geue L, Schares S, Mintel B et al (2010) Rapid microarray-based genotyping of enterohemorrhagic *Escherichia coli* serotype O156:H25/H-/Hnt isolates from cattle and clonal relationship analysis. Appl Environ Microbiol 76:5510–5519
150. Wirth T, Falush D, Lan R et al (2006) Sex and virulence in *Escherichia coli*: an evolutionary perspective. Mol Microbiol 60:1136–1151
151. Garcia Del Blanco N, Dobson ME, Vela AI et al (2002) Genotyping of *Francisella tularensis* strains by pulsed-field gel electrophoresis, amplified fragment length polymorphism fingerprinting, and 16S rRNA gene sequencing. J Clin Microbiol 40:2964–2972
152. Johansson A, Farlow J, Larsson P et al (2004) Worldwide genetic relationships among *Francisella tularensis* isolates determined by multiple-locus variable-number tandem repeat analysis. J Bacteriol 186:5808–5818
153. Vogler AJ, Birdsell D, Wagner DM, Keim P (2009) An optimized, multiplexed multilocus variable-number tandem repeat analysis system for genotyping *Francisella tularensis*. Lett Appl Microbiol 48:140–144
154. Vogler AJ, Birdsell D, Price LB et al (2009) Phylogeography of *Francisella tularensis*: global expansion of a highly fit clone. J Bacteriol 191:2474–2484
155. Larsson P, Svensson K, Karlsson L et al (2007) Canonical insertion-deletion markers for rapid DNA typing of *Francisella tularensis*. Emerg Infect Dis 13:1725–1732
156. Svensson K, Back E, Eliasson H et al (2009) Landscape epidemiology of tularemia outbreaks in Sweden. Emerg Infect Dis 15: 1937–1947
157. Castellanos E, de Juan L, Dominguez L, Aranaz A (2012) Progress in molecular typing of *Mycobacterium avium* subspecies *paratuberculosis*. Res Vet Sci 92:169–179
158. Bannantine JP, Li LL, Sreevatsan S, Kapur V (2013) How does a *Mycobacterium* change its spots? Applying molecular tools to track diverse strains of *Mycobacterium avium* subspecies *paratuberculosis*. Lett Appl Microbiol 57:165–173
159. Stevenson K, Hughes VM, de Juan L et al (2002) Molecular characterization of pigmented and nonpigmented isolates of *Mycobacterium avium* subsp. *paratuberculosis*. J Clin Microbiol 40:1798–1804
160. de Juan L, Mateos A, Dominguez L, Sharp JM, Stevenson K (2005) Genetic diversity of *Mycobacterium avium* subspecies *paratuberculosis* isolates from goats detected by pulsed-field gel electrophoresis. Vet Microbiol 106: 249–257
161. Sevilla I, Li LL, Amonsin A et al (2008) Comparative analysis of *Mycobacterium avium* subsp *paratuberculosis* isolates from cattle, sheep and goats by short sequence repeat and pulsed-field gel electrophoresis typing. BMC Microbiol 8:204
162. Amonsin A, Li LL, Zhang Q et al (2004) Multilocus short sequence repeat sequencing approach for differentiating among *Mycobacterium avium* subsp. *paratuberculosis* strains. J Clin Microbiol 42:1694–1702
163. Thibault VC, Grayon M, Boschiroli ML et al (2008) Combined multilocus short-sequence-repeat and mycobacterial interspersed repetitive unit-variable-number tandem-repeat typing of *Mycobacterium avium* subsp *paratuberculosis* isolates. J Clin Microbiol 46:4091–4094
164. Kasnitz N, Kohler H, Weigoldt M, Gerlach GF, Mobius P (2013) Stability of genotyping target sequences of *Mycobacterium avium* subsp. *paratuberculosis* upon cultivation on different media, in vitro- and in vivo passage, and natural infection. Vet Microbiol 167: 573–583
165. Dvorska L, Bull TJ, Bartos M et al (2003) A standardised restriction fragment length polymorphism (RFLP) method for typing *Mycobacterium avium* isolates links IS901 with virulence for birds. J Microbiol Methods 55:11–27
166. van Soolingen D, Bauer J, Ritacco V et al (1998) IS1245 restriction fragment length polymorphism typing of *Mycobacterium avium* isolates: proposal for standardization. J Clin Microbiol 36:3051–3054
167. Johansen TB, Olsen I, Jensen MR et al (2007) New probes used for IS1245 and IS1311 restriction fragment length polymorphism of *Mycobacterium avium* subsp. *avium* and *Mycobacterium avium* subsp. *hominissuis* isolates of human and animal origin in Norway. BMC Microbiol 7:14
168. Johansen TB, Djonne B, Jensen MR, Olsen I (2005) Distribution of IS1311 and IS1245 in *Mycobacterium avium* subspecies revisited. J Clin Microbiol 43:2500–2502
169. McLernon J, Costello E, Flynn O, Madigan G, Ryan F (2010) Evaluation of mycobacterial interspersed repetitive-unit-variable-number tandem-repeat analysis and spoligotyping for genotyping of *Mycobacterium bovis* isolates

and a comparison with restriction fragment length polymorphism typing. J Clin Microbiol 48:4541–4545

170. McAuliffe L, Ayling RD, Nicholas RA (2007) Identification and characterization of variable-number tandem-repeat markers for the molecular epidemiological analysis of *Mycoplasma mycoides* subspecies mycoides SC. FEMS Microbiol Lett 276:181–188
171. Yaya A, Manso-Silvan L, Blanchard A, Thiaucourt F (2008) Genotyping of Mycoplasma mycoides subsp. mycoides SC by multilocus sequence analysis allows molecular epidemiology of contagious bovine pleuropneumonia. Vet Res 39:14
172. Lorenzon S, Arzul I, Peyraud A, Hendrikx P, Thiaucourt F (2003) Molecular epidemiology of contagious bovine pleuropneumonia by multilocus sequence analysis of *Mycoplasma mycoides* subspecies *mycoides* biotype SC strains. Vet Microbiol 93:319–333
173. Churchward CP, Hlusek M, Nicholas RA, Ayling RD, McAuliffe L (2012) A simplified PCR method for genotyping *Mycoplasma mycoides* subspecies *mycoides* small colony: the aetiologic agent of contagious bovine pleuropneumonia. Vet Microbiol 159:257–259
174. Pinho L, Thompson G, Rosenbusch R, Carvalheira J (2012) Genotyping of *Mycoplasma bovis* isolates using multiple-locus variable-number tandem-repeat analysis. J Microbiol Methods 88:377–385
175. Amram E, Freed M, Khateb N et al (2013) Multiple locus variable number tandem repeat analysis of *Mycoplasma bovis* isolated from local and imported cattle. Vet J 197:286–290
176. Manso-Silvan L, Dupuy V, Lysnyansky I, Ozdemir U, Thiaucourt F (2012) Phylogeny and molecular typing of *Mycoplasma agalactiae* and *Mycoplasma bovis* by multilocus sequencing. Vet Microbiol 161:104–112
177. Malorny B, Hauser E, Diekerman R (2011) New approaches in subspecies-level *Salmonella* classification. In: Porwollik S (ed) *Salmonella*, from genome to function. Caister Academic Press, Norfolk, UK, pp 1–24
178. Wain J, Olsen JE (2013) Current and new approaches to typing of *Salmonella*. In: Barrow PA, Methner U (eds) Salmonella in domestic animals. CAB International, Oxfordshire, UK, pp 498–517
179. Wattiau P, Boland C, Bertrand S (2011) Methodologies for *Salmonella enterica* subsp. *enterica* subtyping: gold standards and alternatives. Appl Environ Microbiol 77:7877–7885
180. Peters TM, Maguire C, Threlfall EJ et al (2003) The Salm-gene project—a European collaboration for DNA fingerprinting for food-related salmonellosis. Euro Surveill 8:46–50
181. Torpdahl M, Sorensen G, Lindstedt BA, Nielsen EM (2007) Tandem repeat analysis for surveillance of human *Salmonella* Typhimurium infections. Emerg Infect Dis 13: 388–395
182. Boxrud D, Pederson-Gulrud K, Wotton J et al (2007) Comparison of multiple-locus variable-number tandem repeat analysis, pulsed-field gel electrophoresis, and phage typing for subtype analysis of *Salmonella enterica* serotype Enteritidis. J Clin Microbiol 45:536–543
183. Malorny B, Junker E, Helmuth R (2008) Multi-locus variable-number tandem repeat analysis for outbreak studies of *Salmonella enterica* serotype Enteritidis. BMC Microbiol 8:84
184. Campioni F, Davis M, Medeiros MI, Falcao JP, Shah DH (2013) MLVA typing reveals higher genetic homogeneity among S. Enteritidis strains isolated from food, humans and chickens in Brazil in comparison to the North American strains. Int J Food Microbiol 162: 174–181
185. Davis MA, Baker KN, Call DR et al (2009) Multilocus variable-number tandem-repeat method for typing *Salmonella enterica* serovar Newport. J Clin Microbiol 47:1934–1938
186. Foley SL, White DG, McDermott PF et al (2006) Comparison of subtyping methods for differentiating *Salmonella enterica* serovar Typhimurium isolates obtained from food animal sources. J Clin Microbiol 44:3569–3577
187. Ross IL, Heuzenroeder MW (2005) Discrimination within phenotypically closely related definitive types of *Salmonella enterica* serovar typhimurium by the multiple amplification of phage locus typing technique. J Clin Microbiol 43:1604–1611
188. Singh P, Foley SL, Nayak R, Kwon YM (2013) Massively parallel sequencing of enriched target amplicons for high-resolution genotyping of *Salmonella* serovars. Mol Cell Probes 27:80–85
189. Scaria J, Palaniappan RU, Chiu D et al (2008) Microarray for molecular typing of *Salmonella enterica* serovars. Mol Cell Probes 22: 238–243
190. Huehn S, Malorny B (2009) DNA microarray for molecular epidemiology of *Salmonella*. Methods Mol Biol 551:249–285
191. Matsuda M, Miyazawa T, Moore JE, Buckley TC, Thomas LA (1998) Molecular genotyping by pulsed-field gel electrophoresis of

restricted genomic DNA of strains of *Taylorella equigenitalis* isolated in Ireland and in the United States. Vet Res Commun 22:217–224

192. Kagawa S, Moore JE, Murayama O, Matsuda M (2001) Comparison of the value of pulsed-field gel electrophoresis, random amplified polymorphic DNA and amplified rDNA restriction analysis for subtyping *Taylorella equigenitalis*. Vet Res Commun 25:261–269
193. Kagawa S, Klein F, Corboz L et al (2001) Demonstration of heterogeneous genotypes of *Taylorella equigenitalis* isolated from horses in six European countries by pulsed-field gel electrophoresis. Vet Res Commun 25: 565–575
194. Aalsburg AM, Erdman MM (2011) Pulsed-field gel electrophoresis genotyping of *Taylorella equigenitalis* isolates collected in the United States from 1978 to 2010. J Clin Microbiol 49:829–833
195. Hunter PR, Gaston MA (1988) Numerical index of the discriminatory ability of typing systems: an application of Simpson's index of diversity. J Clin Microbiol 26:2465–2466

Chapter 22

Characterization of *Campylobacter jejuni* and *Campylobacter coli* Genotypes in Poultry Flocks by Restriction Fragment Length Polymorphism (RFLP) Analysis

Ana Cláudia Carreira and Mónica V. Cunha

Abstract

We describe a simple, rapid, and discriminatory methodology that allows the routine molecular characterization of *Campylobacter jejuni* and *Campylobacter coli* isolates. The proposed approach is built on one of the earliest and simplest molecular typing methods ever, consisting on the analysis of the fragments of different lengths generated by digestion of homologous DNA sequences with specific restriction endonucleases, a process known as restriction fragment length polymorphism (RFLP) analysis. The strategy underneath the workflow reported here is meant to explore the polymorphisms of *Campylobacter* spp. *fla*A gene (*fla*A-RFLP) that allows the local investigation of the genetic diversity and distribution of *C. coli* and *C. jejuni* isolates from different sources, namely, chickens' caeca. Although not appropriate for global and long-term epidemiological studies as a single approach, *fla*A-RFLP analysis can be very useful in surveys limited in space and time and, for specific epidemiological settings, an alternative to more modern and resource-demanding techniques.

Key words Genotyping, Restriction fragment length polymorphism, *flaA*-RFLP, *Campylobacter jejuni*, *Campylobacter coli*, Molecular epidemiology

1 Introduction

Campylobacteriosis caused by *Campylobacter* spp. is considered one of the most prevalent zoonotic enteric infections occurring worldwide [1], *Campylobacter jejuni* being associated to the vast majority of human campylobacteriosis cases (about 90 %), followed by *C. coli* (5–10 %) [2, 3]. The main reservoirs of these species are the gastrointestinal tracts of poultry (e.g., chickens, turkeys, ducks, and geese). Handling and consumption of chicken concur as important risk factors in pathogen transmission to humans [4–7].

Isolation, identification, and phenotypic and genetic characterization of pathogens are fundamental to understand the epidemiology of infectious diseases. Using suitable genotyping

Mónica V. Cunha and João Inácio (eds.), *Veterinary Infection Biology: Molecular Diagnostics and High-Throughput Strategies*, Methods in Molecular Biology, vol. 1247, DOI 10.1007/978-1-4939-2004-4_22, © Springer Science+Business Media New York 2015

methodologies, essential information on the sources and routes of pathogen infection may be gathered, which may help to prevent and control infectious diseases and to minimize the occurrence and/or effects of potential outbreaks.

Several methodologies have been developed to genotype *Campylobacter* spp. [8, 9]. However, the procedures applied in different laboratories, both at the national and international levels, lack in standardization. Monitoring prevalence and distribution of different strains at a local, national, and global level is, therefore, hampered [10]. Efforts have been made in this matter, particularly in the United States, through the implementation in 1996 of the PulseNet network (http://www.cdc.gov/pulsenet/). This network is responsible for the standardization of methodologies applied in the subtyping of food-borne pathogens. In the European Union, the Campynet (http://campynet.vetinst.dk/CONTENTS.HTM) network was established in 1998 aiming the uniformization of the methods used in *C. coli* and *C. jejuni* subtyping. Despite these efforts, the progress made in the standardization of *Campylobacter* spp. subtyping has been occurring slowly [10].

In this report, we describe a simple procedure based on the restriction fragment length polymorphism analysis (RFLP) of the *fla*A gene (*fla*A-RFLP). In *Campylobacter* spp., the genetic locus encoding the flagellin is formed by the *fla*A and *fla*B genes arranged in tandem. This locus has both variable and highly conserved regions, which make it suitable for molecular typing [8, 11]. The RFLP methodology exploring the polymorphisms within the flagellin locus is fairly inexpensive, is relatively simple to perform, and is well suited for relatively high-throughput analysis. Still, some limitations have been reported over the years, especially the possibility for genetic recombination in the flagellin locus [12], which hamper molecular tracking in epidemiologically related strains. This method is also not appropriate for global and long-term duration epidemiological studies as a single approach. Over the years, it has been progressively replaced, or complemented, by other methodologies with higher discriminatory power and reproducibility, such as multilocus sequence typing (MLST), based on the nucleotide sequence analysis of housekeeping genes, and the long-standing gold-standard technique, pulsed-field gel electrophoresis (PFGE). On the other hand, *fla*A-RFLP analysis can be very useful in epidemiological studies limited in space and time (e.g., to genotype the isolates from poultry flocks) and, for specific epidemiological scenarios, an alternative to the more resource-demanding techniques mentioned above. Its low cost associated with the quick procedures of the workflow also stands out as major advantage. This method was recently applied with success to the comparative genotypic analysis of *C. jejuni* and *C. coli* isolated from broilers in a nationwide survey in Portugal [13].

Several experimental protocols have been developed for *Campylobacter* spp. typing based on the amplification and restriction of the *fla*A gene, which differ considerably in DNA preparation, the set of primers, the annealing temperature used in PCR, and the restriction enzymes [8]. Various restriction enzymes have been used individually or in combination, in particular, *Alu*I, *Dde*I, *Hinf*I, *Eco*RI, and *Pst*I [14]. The methodology reported in this work is based on the procedure proposed by the Campynet network, which in turn is based on the method originally described by Nachamkin and coworkers [15, 16]. Here, we complement the former protocols with a few adaptations that have been developed to improve the reproducibility and accuracy of the *flaA*-RFLP patterns. From the experimental viewpoint, *fla*A-RFLP analysis can be subdivided into five major procedures: DNA extraction, amplification of a fragment of the *fla*A gene by PCR, amplicon restriction with different endonucleases, electrophoretic separation of generated fragments, and RFLP analysis using suitable software.

2 Materials

2.1 Growth of Campylobacter spp. and Maintenance

1. Growth media: Prepare Columbia blood agar base according to manufacturer's instructions. Sterilize by autoclaving at 121 °C for 15 min. Cool to 50 °C and aseptically add 5 % (v/v) of defibrinated lysed horse or sheep blood.
2. Cryopreservation media: Prepare a mixture of 40 % (v/v) glycerol and 6 % (w/v) Tryptone Soya Broth.
3. Incubation jars of 2.5 L or special incubation bags for the incubation of Petri dishes in an oxygen-depleted and CO_2-enriched atmosphere (*see* **Note 1**).
4. Microaerophilic gas generator systems suitable for incubation bars or for incubation bags.
5. Incubator at 42 °C.

2.2 Isolation of Genomic DNA

Prepare all solutions using ultrapure water. Purify deionized water to reach a resistivity of 18.2 MΩ cm at 25 °C. Keep the reagents/buffers at room temperature, unless otherwise indicated.

1. SET buffer: 150 mM NaCl, 15 mM EDTA, 10 mM Tris–HCl, and pH 8.0.
2. Sodium dodecyl sulfate (SDS) in distilled, deionized water: Prepare a 10 % (w/v) stock solution (*see* **Note 2**).
3. Proteinase K: Prepare a stock solution of 20 mg/mL in distilled water. Keep it at −20 °C.
4. Phenol/chloroform/isoamyl alcohol (25:24:1) solution, saturated with 10 mM Tris (pH 8.0) and 1 mM EDTA. Keep it at 4 °C.

5. 3 M sodium acetate; pH 5.3.
6. Absolute and 75 % (v/v) ethanol.
7. Sterile 1 mL syringes.
8. 1.5 mL sterile tubes.
9. Benchtop centrifuge.
10. DNA vacuum dryer equipment.

2.3 Amplification of flaA Gene by Polymerase Chain Reaction (PCR)

1. Sterile PCR microtubes.
2. Reagents for conventional PCR reactions: *Taq* DNA polymerase and the respective 10× reaction buffer, 25 mM $MgCl_2$, 10 mM deoxynucleoside triphosphate mix (dNTPs), and 0.1 mM of each oligonucleotide primer (primer A1: 5′-GGA TTT CGT ATT AAC ACA AAT GGT GC-3′ and primer A2: 5′-CTG TAG TAA TCT TAA AAC ATT TTG-3′) [15]. Commercially synthetized primers are lyophilized and need to be diluted with nuclease-free water. Stock solutions can be prepared at a standard concentration of 100 pmol/μl and stored at −20 °C. To avoid freeze and thaw, aliquots of 10 pmol/μl working solutions of each primer may be prepared from stock solutions in water and stored also at −20 °C.
3. Sterile PCR-grade nuclease-free water.
4. Reference strains as controls: *C. jejuni* subsp. *jejuni* ATCC 33560 and *C. coli* CCUG 11283.
5. Standard PCR equipment (thermocycler).

2.4 Agarose Gel Preparation and Electrophoresis

1. 5× TBE buffer: 0.89 M Tris Base, 0.89 M boric acid, and 0.5 M EDTA; adjust pH to 8.0. Dilute 200 mL of 5× TBE buffer in 800 mL of purified deionized water to obtain 1 L of 1× TBE buffer. Store at room temperature.
2. Agarose gel: In a glass bottle (*see* **Note 3**), add the appropriate amount of agarose (electrophoresis grade) to 100 mL of 1× TBE buffer [e.g., 1 % (w/v) agarose gel contains 1 g of agarose]. Put the bottle with the cap unscrewed in a microwave (used only for this purpose). Heat until completely liquefied (about 3 min). Let it cool down to 50 °C. Add ethidium bromide at 0.3 μg/mL to the gel (*see* **Note 4**). Ethidium bromide is a known mutagen and should be handled as a hazardous substance. Put the gel into a suitable mold (midi gel dimensions: about 12 cm wide by 10 cm long; pour 100 mL of molten volume). Put one comb inside the mold before the gel polymerizes. After 30/40 min, the gel should be ready to use (*see* **Note 5**). Remove the combs and put the mold with the gel in an electrophoresis tank. Use 1× TBE as running buffer. The gel must be completely covered by the buffer.

3. Molecular weight markers: Select up to three ladders producing regularly spaced 100 bp, 50 bp, and 25 pb fragments.
4. Commercial DNA loading and staining dye or homemade solution (*see* **Note 6**).
5. Standard equipment for performing agarose gel electrophoresis and for detecting nucleic acids under UV light.

2.5 Digestion of Amplified DNA with Restriction Enzymes and Analysis of flaA-RFLP Profiles

1. Restriction enzymes *Dde*I and *Hinf*I.
2. Appropriate 10× restriction buffer for each enzyme.
3. Bovine serum albumin (BSA): 0.1 mg/mL.
4. PCR-grade water.
5. Analysis software: GelCompar II v. 3.50 (Applied Maths).

3 Methods

3.1 Growth of Thermotolerant Campylobacter Strains

1. After detection and identification of *Campylobacter* species, according to ISO 10272-1:2006 standard (E) [17] (*see* **Note 7**), inoculate nonselective Columbia blood agar base plates, supplemented with 5 % (v/v) sheep blood (*see* **Note 8**), with a colony from an agar plate or from a slope, or use a loopful of bacteria from cryotubes.
2. Incubate the plates at 42 °C for 48 h under microaerophilic conditions (5 % O_2, 10 % CO_2), using the appropriate incubation jars/bags (*see* **Note 9**).

3.2 Phenol/Chloroform Extraction of Genomic DNA

1. Collect single colonies (1–3 colonies depending on the size) grown on solid medium using a sterile disposable loop. In a microcentrifuge tube, wash the cells with 1 mL of SET buffer. Then, centrifuge the cell suspension at 7,000 ×*g* at room temperature for 5 min. Discard the supernatant.
2. To lyse the cells, resuspend the pellet in 570 μL SET buffer and add 29 μL of a solution of 10 % (w/v) SDS and 3 μL of proteinase K. Vortex cell suspension briefly and then incubate in a water bath at 50 °C for 1 h without shaking.
3. For the removal of proteins, add 550 μL of phenol/chloroform/isoamyl alcohol solution. Vortex briefly (5–10 min) and centrifuge at 12,000 ×*g* for 8 min to allow organic and aqueous phase separation.
4. Transfer the supernatant (approximately 500 μL) to a new microtube. Add 550 μL of phenol/chloroform/isoamyl alcohol solution. Shake the resulting mixture before proceeding to a new centrifugation under the above conditions. Recover the supernatant into a new tube.

5. In order to precipitate and collect the DNA extracted from the cells, add to the supernatant 40 μL of 3 M sodium acetate and 800 μL of absolute ethanol. Incubate overnight at –20 °C.
6. Perform centrifugation at 12,000 × *g* for 10 min to pellet the DNA in the bottom of the tube. Remove the supernatant carefully with a syringe and wash the pellet with 500 μL of 75 % ethanol (v/v). Repeat the centrifugation under the same conditions.
7. Evaporate ethanol by exposing the open tubes at room temperature for about 1 h and then carry out vacuum drying for 10 min.
8. After drying, resuspend the DNA in 50 μL of autoclaved nuclease-free water. Store at –20 °C until further use (*see* **Note 10**).
9. Other suitable methods may be used to extract *Campylobacter* spp. DNA (*see* **Note 11**).

3.3 Quantitation, Purity, and Integrity of DNA

1. Use disposable plastic cuvettes. Read the optical density of the diluted DNA solutions at 260 and 280 nm. Before reading absorbance of DNA samples, zero the UV spectrophotometer against the control cuvette, containing 1,000 μL of the solvent used for dissolving the DNA samples (e.g., water). Mix 5 μL of the DNA stock solution with 995 μL of the DNA solvent. Rinse the cuvette with deionized water between samples. Alternatively, to spare the DNA solutions, use a nanospectrophotometer.
2. Estimate the purity of DNA solution based on the ratio A_{260nm}/A_{280nm}. Consider that DNA solutions with acceptable purity present reasons comprised between 1.8 and 2.0.
3. To estimate the DNA concentration, consider that each unit of absorbance at 260 nm corresponds to 50 μg/mL for double-stranded DNA. DNA concentration (μg/mL) is given by $A_{260} \times 50 \times$ dilution factor.
4. Add 1 μL of 6× gel loading dye to 5 μL of each DNA solution. Store at 4 °C until electrophoresis is performed.
5. Prepare 1 % (w/v) agarose gel with 1× TBE buffer to verify the integrity of the extracted DNA.
6. Put the DNA samples with the loading dye into the wells using a micropipette. Introduce a molecular weight marker in one of the wells just to check that the gel is appropriately stained. Perform the electrophoresis using the following conditions: 95 V, 60 min (*see* **Note 12**).
7. Examine the gel under UV light (*see* **Note 13**).

3.4 Amplification of flaA Gene by PCR

1. Each PCR reaction should be prepared to a final volume of 50 μL using sterile PCR microtubes. Prepare the master mix containing 1.5 mM $MgCl_2$, 0.2 mM of each dNTP (deoxynucleoside triphosphate mix), 1× *Taq* DNA polymerase reaction buffer, 1 μM of each oligonucleotide primer (primers A1 and A2), and, finally, 0.05 U/μL of reaction mix of *Taq* DNA polymerase (*see* **Note 14**). Add the necessary volume of sterile nuclease-free water to complete the reaction volume. For *N* number of samples, make up sufficient volume for *N*+1 reactions (*see* **Note 15**). Do not forget to prepare reactions for positive (DNA from reference strains) and negative (nuclease-free water) controls.
2. Distribute the reaction mixture by individual 0.2 mL microtubes.
3. Label each tube and, in a different room (if available), add the template DNA (*see* **Note 16**). Each reaction should contain approximately 30 ng/mL of template DNA (*see* **Note 17**).
4. Place the tubes in the thermocycler and start the appropriate program. Use the following amplification conditions: initial denaturation step at 94 °C for 1 min, 35 cycles of denaturation at 94 °C for 15 s, annealing at 50 °C for 45 s, and extension at 72 °C for 105 s; a final step at 72 °C for 5 min is required for extension.
5. Store PCR reactions at 4 °C or −20 °C until ready for analysis by electrophoresis.

3.5 Detection of Amplification Products by Agarose Gel Electrophoresis

1. Prepare 1.5 % (w/v) agarose gel using 1× TBE buffer as previously described.
2. Add 2 μL of 6× gel loading dye to 10 μL of each PCR product.
3. Load the mixture into the wells of the gel. Considering that the amplified *fla*A gene fragment has approximately 1,700 bp, use an appropriate molecular weight marker. It should be placed in the first and last wells and at regular intervals across the gel, ideally after every fifth sample. Use the manufacturer's recommended loading concentration.
4. Electrophoresis conditions: 90 V; 1 h 30 min. Visualize the gel under UV light. An amplicon of ~1,700 bp is expected (*see* **Note 18**).

3.6 Endonuclease Restriction of Amplification Products (flaA-RFLP)

1. Separately, carry out *Dde*I or *Hinf*I restriction reactions of each PCR product corresponding to the amplified *fla*A gene (*see* **Note 19**). Prepare each 30 μL reaction in sterile microtubes by adding the appropriate restriction buffer (1×), BSA in a final concentration of 0.1 mg/mL, 5–10 μL of the PCR product (depending on the concentration, estimated according to the

intensity of the band on agarose gel), and sterile nuclease-free water up to the final reaction volume. Finally, add the restriction enzyme, *Dde*I or *Hinf*I using 0.1 U/μL of reaction mix. Keep the enzymes on ice or in the freezer, until needed.

2. Incubate all the reactions at 37 °C (water bath or oven) during 3 h or overnight (*see* **Note 20**).
3. Visualize the restriction products on 2 % (w/v) agarose gels prepared with 1× TBE buffer (midi gel or a gel with higher dimensions). Perform electrophoresis with the following conditions: 90 V for about 3 h (*see* **Note 21**).
4. Use as standard molecular weight markers 100 bp, 50 bp, and 25 bp fragment DNA ladders in the first and last wells and in regular intervals as previously referred using the final concentration recommended by the manufacturers. Alternate each marker in the gel (*see* **Note 22**).
5. Visualize the gel under UV light under the transilluminator and capture the image of the gel using a digital system for further analysis.
6. Carry out visual analysis of the *fla*A gene restriction profiles (*see* **Note 23**) and complement this analysis with the aid of the GelCompar II software version 3.50, enclosed in the BioNumerics package (Applied Maths, Ghent, Belgium), or with analogous software. Normalize all profiles to the same reference system (e.g., selected DNA ladder) and proceed according to software instructions.
7. To calculate the discriminatory power of the technique, the formula proposed by Hunter [18] can be used. There are also bioinformatic tools available online used to calculate this parameter (e.g., http://insilico.ehu.es/mini_tools/discriminatory_power/).

4 Notes

1. To save on gas generation systems, select an incubation jar or an incubation bag taking into consideration the number of Petri dishes. According to size, incubation bags are normally appropriate for two dishes only.
2. SDS precipitates at 4 °C. Should this occur, warm the solution in a water bath up to 20 °C.
3. The glass bottle should have twice the capacity of the volume of the prepared gel. This prevents spillage of gel upon heating.
4. Staining the gel about 30 min in 1× TBE or in water containing 0.3 μg/mL of ethidium bromide before UV visualization

could be an alternative to the addition of ethidium bromide directly to the gel.

5. The complete polymerization of the agarose gel is essential before loading samples into wells.
6. Alternatively, you can use homemade loading dye: Prepare a solution containing 50 % glycerol (v/v), 0.25 % (w/v) bromophenol blue, and 0.25 % (w/v) cyanol xylene in distilled water. Store at 4 °C.
7. Molecular identification to the species level could also be performed, in addition to the biochemical identification tests (hydrolysis of hippurate and the indoxyl acetate and catalase). For this purpose, use a multiplex PCR assay according to previously established methodologies [19, 20].
8. *Campylobacter* species are unable to metabolize carbohydrates, and their metabolism is dependent on amino acid availability. Supplementation of the culture medium with blood is therefore essential.
9. The strains are generally microaerophilic, which means that, in order to grow, a particular atmospheric environment, comprising approximately 10 % CO_2 and 5 % O_2, is required. The optimum growth temperature ranges from 37 °C to 42 °C. For incubations at 37 °C, extend the incubation period. After growth, the colonies should have typical morphological characteristics—gray and small colonies, with 1–3 mm in diameter.
10. DNA can also be stored in TE buffer.
11. If the phenol/chloroform extraction yield is not satisfactory, try to extract the DNA from cells by the boiling procedure: Depending on size, collect with a sterile 10 μL loop 2 to 4 colonies from the solid media and suspend in 100 μL of TE buffer (prepared with 10 mM Tris base and 1 mM EDTA; pH 8.0) using sterile microtubes. Place the tubes with cell suspensions in a water bath at 100 °C for about 15 min. Centrifuge at 14,000 × *g* for 5 min and transfer the supernatant (with a sterile syringe or 1 mL disposable pipette) to a new sterile tube. Store at −20 °C. This procedure is suitable for the rapid screening of large numbers of isolates, but the long-term storage and reuse of cell lysates could be problematic as the DNA tends to deteriorate.

    For *Campylobacter* spp. DNA extraction using commercial systems, we found that the *High Pure PCR Template Preparation Kit* from Roche is a very effective option.
12. The electrophoresis conditions will vary upon the dimensions and concentration of the agarose gel.
13. Should you verify by gel electrophoresis that the DNA solutions are contaminated with RNA, use RNase for RNA removal.

For this purpose, add 1 μL of RNase (500 μg/mL) to DNA solutions and incubate at 37 °C for 1 h. Let the solutions reach room temperature and then store at −20 °C until further use.

14. Before the DNA, *Taq* DNA polymerase is the last component to be added to the master mix; therefore, keep it on ice or in the freezer until required.
15. Check whether the pipettes are properly calibrated to avoid errors in master mix preparation.
16. The master mix preparation and the DNA addition should be performed in separate rooms in order to avoid DNA carryover.
17. The 1 in 10 dilutions of DNA stock solutions (with sterile deionized water) are frequently of an appropriate concentration to use in PCR reactions. Store the dilutions at −20 °C until needed.
18. If nonspecific products resulting from the PCR reaction are present, the amplified *flaA* gene fragment (with approximately 1.7 kb) needs to be purified. For this purpose, visualize the band of interest in the transilluminator and proceed to its removal from the gel. With protective gloves, use a sterile scalpel and put the excised piece of gel in a microtube. There are many commercial systems available for gel band purification; we found that *illustra GFX PCR DNA and Gel Band Purification Kit* from GE Healthcare is a good option.
19. It is advisable to use more than one restriction enzyme to increase the discriminatory power of the technique.
20. We found that the 3 h duration of the electrophoretic separation of restriction fragments in the referred conditions is an important issue to enable the discrimination of each band and the interpretability and reproducibility among gels.
21. In some restriction profiles, the emergence of very weak bands into a secondary plane could appear. Normally, this situation occurs when the incubation time of the restriction reactions is exceeded. Probably these bands are a result of partial digestion and/or loss of fidelity in relation to enzyme activity (also called "star activity"). Better results may be achieved with less extensive incubation periods (up to 3 h).
22. Bands of high and low molecular weight may be generated in the restriction profiles. It is therefore advisable to switch the two molecular weight markers in the gel in order to facilitate the profile analysis.
23. The restriction profiles should be set based on the bands of greater intensity (foreground) and having in consideration the size of the gene in question.

References

1. FAO/WHO [Food and Agriculture Organization of the United Nations/World Health Organization] (2009) Risk assessment of *Campylobacter* spp. in broiler chickens: Technical Report. Microbiological Risk Assessment Series No 12. Geneva. pp 132
2. Miller WG, Mandrell RE (2005) Prevalence of *Campylobacter* in the food and water supply: incidence, outbreaks, isolation and detection. In: Ketley JM, Konkel M (eds) Campylobacter: molecular and cellular biology. Horizon Bioscience, Norfolk, UK, pp 101–108
3. Wilson DJ, Gabriel E, Leatherbarrow AJH et al (2008) Tracing the source of campylobacteriosis. PLoS Genet. doi:10.1371/journal.pgen.1000203
4. Wingstrand A, Neimann J, Engberg J et al (2006) Fresh chicken as main risk factor for campylobacteriosis, Denmark. Emerg Infect Dis 12:280–285
5. Humphrey T, O'Brien SJ, Madsen M (2007) Campylobacters as zoonotic pathogens: a food production perspective. Int J Food Microbiol 117:237–257
6. Dasti JI, Tareen AM, Raimond L et al (2010) *Campylobacter jejuni*: a brief overview on pathogenicity associated factors and disease-mediating mechanisms. Int J Med Microbiol 300:205–211
7. Silva J, Leite D, Fernandes M et al (2011) *Campylobacter* spp. as a foodborne pathogen: a review. Front Microbiol 2:1–12
8. Wassenaar T, Newell D (2000) Genotyping of *Campylobacter* spp. Appl Environ Microbiol 66:1–9
9. Klena JD, Konkel E (2005) Methods for epidemiological analysis of *Campylobacter jejuni*. In: Ketley JM, Konkel M (eds) *Campylobacter*: molecular and cellular biology. Horizon Bioscience, Norfolk, UK, pp 166–175
10. Fitzgerald C, Sails AD, Fields PI (2005) *Campylobacter jejuni* strain variation. In: Ketley JM, Konkel M (eds) *Campylobacter*: molecular and cellular biology. Horizon Bioscience, Norfolk, UK, pp 59–72
11. Jagannathan A, Penn C (2005) Motility. In: Ketley JM, Konkel M (eds) *Campylobacter*: molecular and cellular biology. Horizon Bioscience, Norfolk, UK, pp 331–344
12. Harrington CS, Thomson-Carter FM, Carter PE (1997) Evidence for recombination in the flagellin locus of *Campylobacter jejuni*; implications for the flagellin gene typing scheme. J Clin Microbiol 35:2836–2892
13. Carreira AC, Clemente L, Rocha T et al (2012) Comparative genotypic and antimicrobial susceptibility analysis of zoonotic *Campylobacter* species isolated from broilers on a nationwide survey, Portugal. J Food Prot 75:2100–2109
14. Ertas HB, Cetinkaya B, Muz A et al (2004) Genotyping of broiler-originated *Campylobacter jejuni* and *Campylobacter coli* isolates using *fla* typing and random amplified polymorphic DNA methods. Int J Food Microbiol 94:203–209
15. Nachamkin I, Bohachick K, Patton CM (1993) Flagellin gene typing of *Campylobacter jejuni* by restriction fragment length polymorphism analysis. J Clin Microbiol 31: 1531–1536
16. Nachamkin I, Ung H, Patton CM (1996) Analysis of HL and O serotypes of *Campylobacter* strains by the flagellin gene typing system. J Clin Microbiol 34:277–281
17. Anonymous (2006) Microbiology of food and animal feeding stuffs—horizontal method for detection and enumeration of *Campylobacter* spp. Part 1. Detection method. ISO10272-1:2006. International Organization for Standardization, Geneva
18. Hunter PR (1990) Reproducibility and indices of discriminatory power of microbial typing methods. J Clin Microbiol 28:1903–1905
19. Denis M, Soumet C, Rival K et al (1999) Development of a m-PCR assay for simultaneous identification of *Campylobacter jejuni* and *Campylobacter coli*. Lett Appl Microbiol 29: 406–410
20. Wang G, Clark C, Taylor T et al (2002) Colony multiplex PCR assay for identification and differentiation of *Campylobacter jejuni*, *C. coli*, *C. upsaliensis*, and *C. fetus* subsp *fetus*. J Clin Microbiol 40:4744–4747

Chapter 23

Pulsed-Field Gel Electrophoresis (PFGE): Application in Population Structure Studies of Bovine Mastitis-Causing Streptococci

Ilda Santos-Sanches, Lélia Chambel, and Rogério Tenreiro

Abstract

Pulsed-field gel electrophoresis (PFGE) separates large DNA molecules by the use of an alternating electrical field, such that greater size resolution can be obtained when compared to normal agarose gel electrophoresis. PFGE is often employed to track pathogens and is a valuable typing scheme to detect and differentiate strains. Particularly, the contour-clamped homogeneous electric field (CHEF) PFGE system is considered to be the gold standard for use in epidemiological studies of many bacterial pathogens. Here we describe a PFGE protocol that was applicable to the study of bovine streptococci, namely, *Streptococcus agalactiae* (group B *Streptococcus*, GBS), *Streptococcus dysgalactiae* subsp. *dysgalactiae* (group C *Streptococcus*, GCS), and *Streptococcus uberis*—which are relevant pathogens causing mastitis, a highly prevalent and costly disease in dairy industry due to antibiotherapy and loss in milk production.

Key words Bovine mastitis, *Streptococcus agalactiae*, *Streptococcus dysgalactiae* subsp. *dysgalactiae*, *Streptococcus uberis*, Molecular typing, Molecular epidemiology, Pulsed-field gel electrophoresis, PFGE, Alternating electrical field, CHEF

1 Introduction

Pulsed-field gel electrophoresis (PFGE) is generally considered the most discriminatory method to infer relationships between strains [1, 2]. Briefly, PFGE is based on enzymatic DNA restriction of bacterial genome (by using rare-cutting restriction endonucleases) to generate DNA fragments, which are subsequently separated on a gel, due to molecular reorientation produced by periodic changes in the electric field, in order to separate the large DNA fragments. The banding pattern obtained from each isolate is then compared with the remaining patterns in order to infer epidemiological relation between the isolates. When two isolates show indistinguishable DNA patterns, it is assumed that they are of the same strain,

Mónica V. Cunha and João Inácio (eds.), *Veterinary Infection Biology: Molecular Diagnostics and High-Throughput Strategies*, Methods in Molecular Biology, vol. 1247, DOI 10.1007/978-1-4939-2004-4_23,

and if the patterns differ, then its epidemiological relation must be evaluated [1, 2]. Different interpretations for analyzing relationships between isolates patterns have been described [2].

1.1 Streptococci Associated with Bovine Mastitis

Bovine mastitis remains the most important disease in the dairy industry because of economic loss due to treatment costs (antibiotherapy) and loss in milk production and quality. *Streptococcus uberis* is traditionally considered an environmental pathogen because it may be found and acquired in the bovine surroundings, such as straw or peat used in bedding materials, in farm soil, and in the nose, vagina, and rumen of the bovines [3]. On the other hand, *S. agalactiae* is considered a contagious pathogen because it is spread from infected to healthy udders, between quarters of the same animal and between animals (e.g., through the milking machine), and is not found in the environment of the bovine [4]. *Streptococcus dysgalactiae* subsp. *dysgalactiae* is considered either an environmental or contagious pathogen [3].

Molecular epidemiology tools offer unique opportunities to advance the study of diseases through the investigation of infectious agents at the molecular level in a veterinary context [5]. We used PFGE as a molecular tool to study the molecular characterization of field *S. agalactiae*, *S. dysgalactiae* subsp. *dysgalactiae*, and *S. uberis* associated with bovine mastitis, which is of utmost importance in order to implement efficient management practices in herds [6–10]. The frequent occurrence of both indistinguishable PFGE profiles and major clonal PFGE groups among *S. agalactiae* isolates collected from the same farm (all farm specific) suggested widespread strain transmission between animals from the same farm and confirmed *S. agalactiae* as a contagious mastitis pathogen. In contrast, the occurrence of identical PFGE patterns (sharing > 82.8 % and 100 % similarity) among *S. dysgalactiae* subsp. *dysgalactiae* isolates collected at different farms suggested an environmental source for this pathogen. Heterogeneity in *S. uberis* PFGE patterns was observed between isolates collected from different farms, while almost half of the isolates were clonal, all farm associated, suggesting direct transmission of *S. uberis* among animals within the same farm. This is indicative that possibly inadequate implementation of management programs for the control of contagious pathogens at farm level may promote the contagious route for *S. uberis* infection within herds, despite it is considered an environmental pathogen.

2 Materials

Prepare all solutions using distilled (or purified) water and analytical grade reagents. Prepare and store all reagents at room temperature (unless indicated otherwise). Sterilize the buffers and solutions by autoclaving at 121 °C for 20 min (or by filtration through a 0.22 μm filter unit, when indicated).

2.1 Solutions for Streptococcal Chromosomal DNA Agarose Discs (for PFGE)

The composition of all the buffers and solutions was previously described by Rato et al. [9] and was based on the original report by Chung et al. [11].

1. 1 M Tris–HCl, pH 8.0: weigh out 121.1 g of Tris base and add 800 ml of distilled water. Adjust to pH 8.0 by adding approximately 42 ml of concentrated HCl and complete volume to 1 L with distilled water.
2. 0.5 M EDTA, pH 8.0: weigh out 186.1 g of EDTA (disodium salt, m.w. = 372.2) and add 800 ml of distilled water. Stir and adjust to pH 8.0 with NaOH (approx. 20 g of NaOH pellets). Add distilled water up to 1 L.
3. TE buffer (1×): 10 mM Tris–HCl, pH 8.0, and 1 mM EDTA. Prepare this solution using a stock solution of TE buffer 10×. Solution is sterilized by filtration (0.22 μm filter unit) and dispensed into vials.
4. PIV: 10 mM Tris–HCl, pH 8.0, and 1 M NaCl. To prepare 500 ml of PIV, add 5 ml of 1 M Tris–HCl, pH 8.0, and 29.2 g of sodium chloride to distilled water up to 500 ml.
5. EC solution: 6 mM Tris–HCl, pH 8.0, 1 M NaCl, 100 mM EDTA, pH 8.0, 0.2 % (w/v) sodium deoxycholate, 0.5 % sodium N-lauroylsarcosinate, and 0.5 % Brij 58. To prepare 500 ml of EC solution, add 3 ml of 1 M Tris–HCl, pH 8.0, 29.2 g of sodium chloride, 100 ml of 0.5 M EDTA, pH 8.0, 1 g of sodiumdeoxycholate, 2.5 g of sodium N-lauroylsarcosinate, and 2.5 g of Brij 58 to distilled water up to 500 ml.
6. EC lysis solution: 1 mg/ml lysozyme, 5 U/ml mutanolysin, and 50 μg/ml RNase in EC solution.

   The enzymes are diluted in EC solution from stock solutions: 10 mg/ml lysozyme in TE buffer; 5 U/μl of mutanolysin in potassium phosphate (0.1 M) buffer; and 10 mg/ml RNase in double-distilled water (*see* **Note 1**).
7. ES buffer: 0.5 M EDTA, pH 9.0, and 1 % sodium N-lauroylsarcosinate. To prepare 500 ml of ES buffer, weigh out 93.1 g of EDTA (disodium salt) and dissolve in 400 ml of distilled water. Adjust the pH to 9.0 by adding NaOH pellets (approximately 10 g). Add 5 g of sodium N-lauroylsarcosinate and complete the volume to 500 ml with distilled water.
8. ESP solution: to prepare 15 ml of ESP solution, add 15 mg of proteinase K (final concentration of 1 mg/ml) to 15 ml of ES buffer (*see* **Note 2**).
9. Pre-SmaI restriction buffer: 6 mM Tris–HCl, pH 8.0, 20 mM KCl, and 6 mM $MgCl_2$.

   To prepare 500 ml, add 3 ml of 1 M Tris–HCl, pH 8.0, 0.75 g of KCl, and 0.61 g of $MgCl_2.6H_2O$ to distilled water up to 500 ml (*see* **Note 3**).

10. SmaI restriction buffer: mix 15 ml of pre-SmaI restriction buffer and 6.3 μl of mercaptoethanol (prepare on the day of use).
11. 10× TBE running buffer: 1 M Tris–HCl, 0.9 M boric acid, and 0.01 M EDTA. Dilute to 0.5× TBE with double-distilled (or ultrapure) water (*see* **Note 4**).
12. Solution of ethidium bromide (1 μg/ml): add 25 μl of a 10 mg/ml stock solution in 300 ml of autoclaved distilled water. The stock solution should be stored away from light at 4 °C.
13. Loading buffer with bromophenol blue (6×): 0.25 % bromophenol blue and 40 % (w/v) sucrose in double-distilled (or ultrapure) water to a final volume of 10 ml. Store at 4 °C.
14. Low melting temperature agarose solution for the DNA discs: weigh out 0.15 g of low melting temperature agarose (we use SeaPlaque™ agarose), add 10 ml of PIV, and heat at the microwave to dissolve completely. Transfer dissolved agarose to a 42 °C water bath where it should stay for at least 10 min before use (prepare just before use).
15. Low melting temperature agarose solution to seal the DNA discs in the gel: to prepare sealing agarose, weigh out 0.075 g of low melting temperature agarose (we use SeaPlaque™ agarose), add 10 ml of 0.5× TBE, and boil on the microwave. Keep at 42 °C until use.
16. SeaKem LE Agarose solution for the gel: 150 ml of 1 % SeaKem LE Agarose. Weigh out 1.5 g of agarose, and add 7.5 ml of 10× TBE and 130 ml of distilled water. Boil in microwave for 1–2 min and mix in between. Adjust the final volume to 150 ml with distilled water. Put a magnetic stirrer bar into agarose; stir slowly at room temperature, until not too hot for hands (about 50 °C); and pour immediately.
17. Running buffer: add 100 ml of 10× TBE in a measuring cylinder and adjust the volume to 2 L with distilled water.

2.2 Other Materials, Equipments, and Software

1. Liquid culture medium Todd–Hewitt (commercially purchased and prepared according to the manufacturer's instructions).
2. Restriction enzyme SmaI (recognizes the nucleotide sequence CCC^GGG and the optimum temperature for the restriction of DNA is 25 °C).
3. Lambda ladder PFG marker (New England Biolabs): successively larger concatemers of lambda DNA embedded in 1 % low melting point (LMP) agarose and supplied in a dispenser (gel syringe type). Size range: 50–1,000 kb. Should be stored at −20 °C.
4. Pulsed-field electrophoresis system for pulsed-field gel electrophoresis (PFGE) (e.g., CHEF-DR®III, BioRad).

5. Digital gel documentation system to capture and image scanning after the pulsed-field gel electrophoresis (PFGE) (e.g., Gel Doc XR system and Quantity One 1-D analysis software, BioRad) or conventional camera photography and a UV-sensitive film.
6. Software for the analysis of DNA banding profiles and construction of dendrograms (e.g., BioNumerics, version 6.6, Applied Maths, Belgium).

3 Methods

Carry out all procedures at room temperature unless otherwise specified. Wear gloves during the protocol to avoid nuclease contamination of the DNA samples from the operator's skin. Use sterile materials throughout (e.g., tubes, tips, etc.).

3.1 Growth of Bacterial Cultures

1. Inoculate 1–2 colonies into a glass tube containing 6 ml of Todd–Hewitt broth.
2. Incubate at 37 °C overnight with aeration without shaking.

3.2 Harvest and Wash of Cells

From this point on, all tubes must be kept on ice.

1. Transfer overnight cultures to 15 ml centrifuge tubes.
2. Centrifuge at 1,800 × *g* (RCF) at 4 °C for 15 min.
3. Discard the supernatants and resuspend cell pellets by adding 1 ml of PIV to each 15 ml centrifuge tube (*see* **Note 5**).
4. Transfer PIV cell suspensions into 1.5 ml centrifuge tubes (which were prechilled on ice).
5. Centrifuge at 11,200 × *g* (RCF) at 4 °C for 5 min.
6. Remove the supernatant with a micropipette (do not touch the pellets; remove carefully the last amounts of supernatant using, e.g., 200 μl volume tips and the correspondent automatic pipette).
7. Resuspend bacterial pellets by adding 200 μl of PIV to each 1.5 ml centrifuge tube (the estimated total volume in each tube is now approx. 210 μl, with the contribution of the pellet volume; resuspend pellets by up and down pipetting with 200 μl volume tips).

3.3 Adjustment of Cell Concentration

1. Label disposable 1 ml plastic spectrophotometer cuvettes.
2. Pipette 1 ml of PIV into each cuvette.
3. Gently vortex cell suspensions (all tubes are on ice) and pipette 5 μl of suspension into the 1 ml PIV containing cuvettes.
4. Cover cuvette with parafilm and mix content by inverting (leave no air bubbles).

5. Discard the parafilm and measure the OD_{620} (which should be between 0.025 and 0.15).
6. Discard cuvettes.
7. To each tube of cell suspension, add PIV to make the $OD_{620} = 5.0$ according to the following formula: $V_{add}\,(\mu l) = (OD_{620} \times 40 \times 210) - 210$ (*see* **Note 6**).

3.4 Preparation of DNA Agarose Discs

1. Prepare glass microscope slides by washing them with 70 % ethanol.
2. Dry the slides by blotting with tissue paper.
3. Take a large piece of glass plate and cover its surface with parafilm completely.
4. Rinse the parafilm surface with 70 % ethanol and dry by gently blotting with tissue paper—it will be onto this large glass plate that the agarose/cell suspensions will be deposited during the preparation of DNA agarose discs (Fig. 1).
5. Pipette 150 μl of the $OD_{620} = 5.0$ cell suspensions into a new set of 1.5 ml centrifuge tubes.
6. Transfer the centrifuge tubes to a 42 °C water bath and incubate for 10 min.
7. Take the first tube and add 150 μl of the low melting agarose (which has been at 42 °C) and vortex briefly.
8. Deposit 20 μl droplets onto the parafilm-coated large glass plate (Fig. 1; use 200 μl pipette tips).
9. Deposit six 20 μl droplets in one row, and in a parallel line deposit a second set of six 20 μl droplets (i.e., a total of 12 droplets for each strain).
10. Cover the two times six droplets with a microscope slide (Fig. 1).
11. When all agarose droplets are lined up on the glass tray covered with the microscope slides, transfer the entire glass tray to the freezer compartment of a refrigerator (−20 °C) for 5 min (do not keep longer than 5 min at −20 °C).
12. Take out the glass tray from the refrigerator and keep it at room temperature for 10 min.
13. Carefully lift off the microscope slides (the agarose droplets are now ready to be used as "agarose DNA discs" for the rest of the PFGE protocol).

3.5 Lysis and Treatment with Proteinase K

1. Remove the agarose discs one by one (from the previous step) into 15 ml plastic tubes containing 1 ml of EC lysis solution in each (use disposable sterile loops to transfer the agarose discs into the tubes; all 12 or more agarose discs containing the same DNA go into the same tube) (*see* **Note 7**).

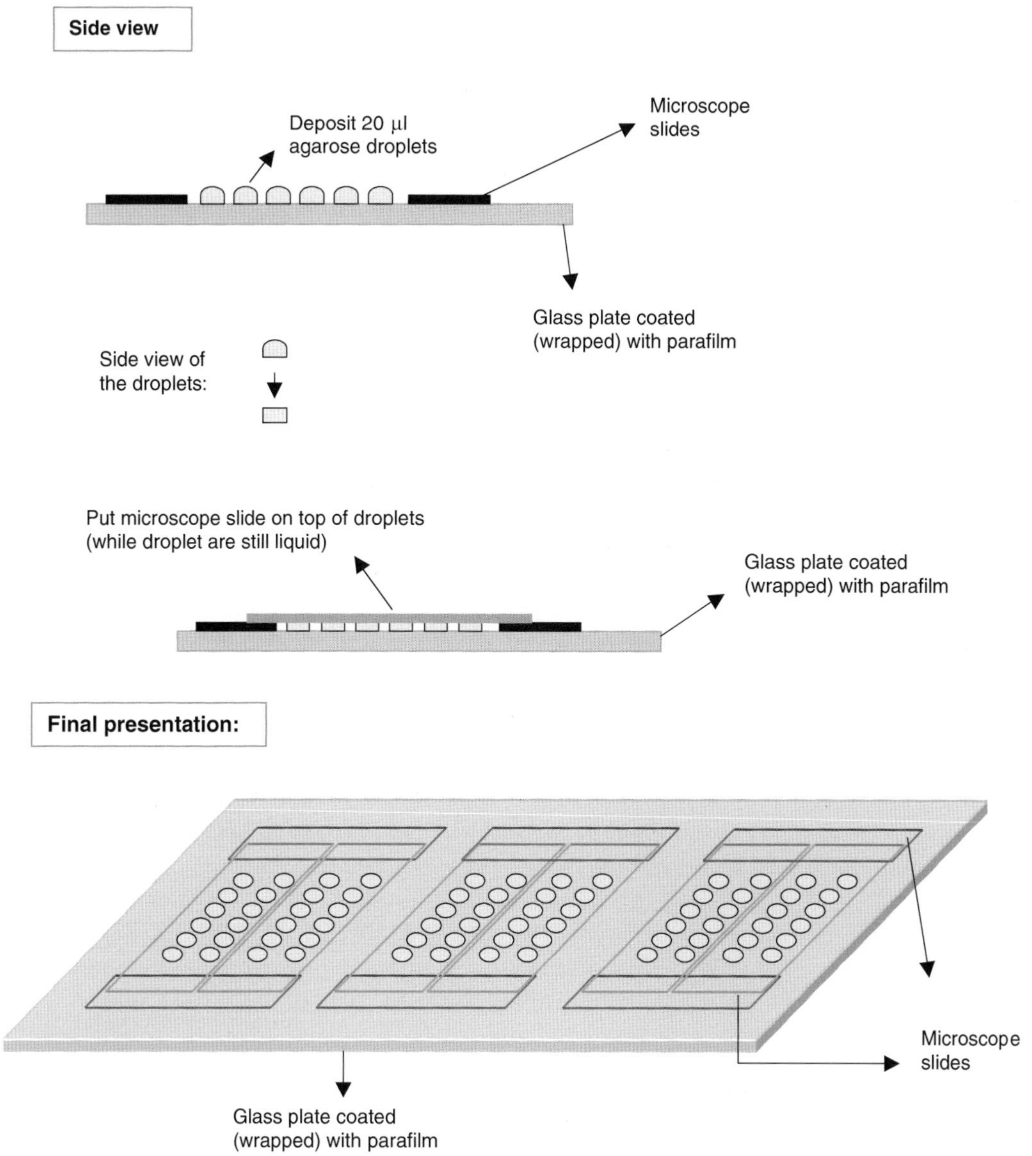

Fig. 1 Schematic drawing of DNA agarose discs preparation (adapted from Chung et al. [11]). Source: H. de Lencastre, ITQB. Portugal)

2. Incubate the agarose discs in EC lysis solution at 37 °C for 3 h (make sure all discs are submerged in the EC lysis solution).
3. Decant carefully the EC lysis solution (use sterilized hydrophilic gauze or muslin cloth) leaving the agarose discs in the 15 ml tube.
4. Remove the last amount of liquid using a 200 µl tip and a pipette.
5. Add 1 ml of ESP solution to each of the 15 ml tubes containing the agarose discs.

6. Incubate at 50 °C overnight (17 h) (no agitation/stirring necessary).
7. Decant the ESP solutions.
8. Add to each tube 13 ml of TE buffer and wash the discs with gentle agitation for at least 30 min at room temperature (during agitation, the 15 ml tubes are in horizontal position, fixed on a shaker).
9. Repeat the washing step for 8 times (at least 30 min each) to remove the proteinase K.
10. After discs have been washed, they can be stored in TE buffer at 4 °C for at least 3–4 months.

3.6 Restriction with SmaI

1. Transfer 1 DNA agarose disc into a 1.5 ml microtube containing 150 μl of pre-SmaI restriction buffer.
2. Incubate at room temperature for 30–40 min and remove the buffer with a pipette.
3. Add 45 μl of SmaI restriction buffer plus 20 units of SmaI enzyme stock per DNA disc (check the equivalent volume in μl) (*see* **Note 3**).
4. Incubate at 25 °C overnight.
5. Add 5 μl of loading buffer (the preparation stays at room temperature while the gel is prepared; if the discs are not immediately used, add 10 μl of ES to the preparation and store the discs at 4 °C for up to 2 days).

3.7 Preparation of the Gel and PFGE Apparatus

1. Prepare agarose, running buffer, and sealing agarose (*see* Subheading 2.1).
2. Clean with distilled water all parts of the casting tray.
3. Assemble apparatus, be sure that it is perfectly horizontal, and add comb.
4. When agarose is ready, pour it in the apparatus slowly to avoid trapping air bubbles (which have to be removed with a pipette tip).
5. Leave the gel to solidify for at least 30 min at room temperature (if the gel is not going to be used within the first hour, wrap it in Saran wrap and keep at 4 °C).
6. Rinse the machine three times with 2 L of autoclaved distilled water. Put the frame into the chamber; add 2 L of running buffer, and turn on the machine, the cooling system, and the variable pump, which should be set at 70. Temperature of cooling system is 11.3 °C. Run parameters: initial time of 5 s, final time of 35 s, running time of 23 h, and voltage of 200 V (6 V/cm).
7. Insert the discs in the gel: take out the agarose disc from the 1.5 ml microtube with a sterile disposable plastic loop, deposit

it on the glass slip, and blot off excess liquid with a soft hand paper towel; with the help of the loop, slide the agarose disc into the first well. Make sure the disc is positioned at the bottom and front part of the well (*see* **Note 8**).

8. Repeat the process for other agarose DNA discs.
9. The PFGE lambda marker is used as a molecular weight standard.
10. At the end, when all the wells are filled, seal them with the sealing agarose (be careful not to leave bubbles inside wells).
11. Put the assembled gel into the PFGE chamber and cover the chamber with the lid.
12. Start running the program.

3.8 Staining and Photography of the Gel

1. Stain the gel by immersing it into 300 ml of 1 μg/ml ethidium bromide solution for 30 min at room temperature.
2. Destain after decanting the ethidium bromide solution and replacing it with 300 ml of distilled water.
3. Place the gel on a shaker for 30–60 min.
4. Images are captured by using the Gel Doc XR system and Quantity One 1-D analysis software or equivalent equipment and software. In alternative, use a conventional camera and a UV-sensitive positive/negative film (keep the negative).
5. Images are usually saved in tagged image file format (TIFF). An example of the typical results produced is shown in Fig. 2. There should be a complete DNA restriction in all lanes (partially restricted DNA produces faint smeared bands between better-defined bands of the profiles).

3.9 Computer-Fingerprinting Analysis

Analysis and interpretation of PFGE profiles is best done using a software program such as BioNumerics software (Applied Maths, Belgium) for computer-assisted cluster analysis. An example is shown in Fig. 3. The PFGE profiles in TIFF images are normalized between all images by using standards (molecular weight standard and duplicated DNAs) included in every gel. Good-quality gel images are essential for the interpretation of PFGE patterns, such as to allow matching PFGE patterns to known PFGE fingerprinting data within a PFGE database. Levels of similarity between fingerprints are calculated by the Dice association coefficient and unweighted pair group method using arithmetic averages (UPGMA) for clustering and produce band-based dendrograms (e.g., with a band position tolerance of 1.5 % and no optimization or 1 % optimization). Groups of patterns with no observed band differences (corresponding to a level of similarity of 100 %) are considered indistinguishable and should be assigned to the same subtype of a PFGE type. Patterns with variation up to six bands are considered related according to previous suggested criteria [1] and are clustered

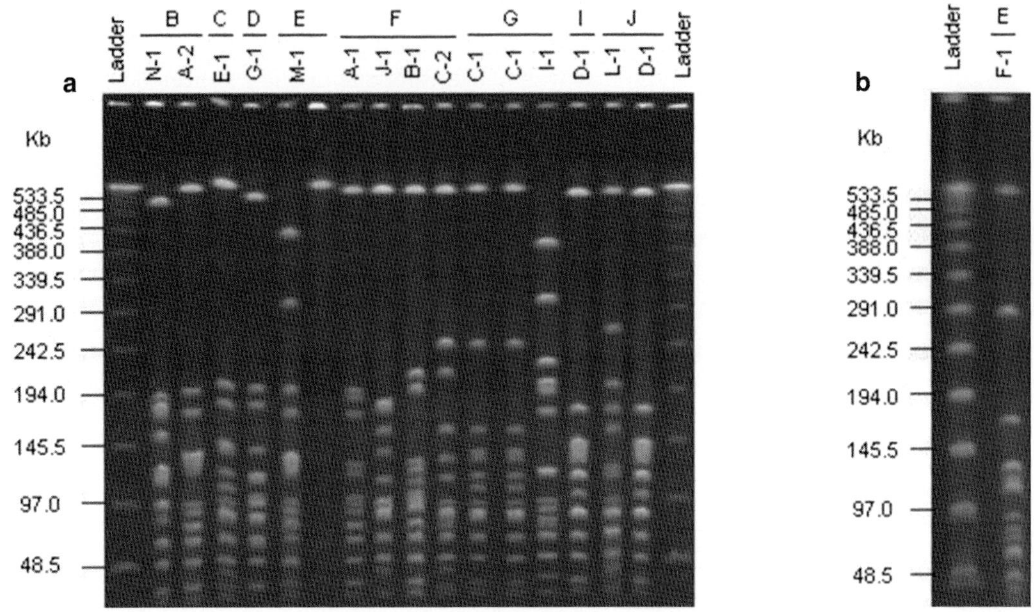

Fig. 2 Representative image of SmaI and Cfr9I PFGE patterns of bovine streptococci (*S. dysgalactiae* subsp. *dysgalactiae*). *Capital letters* B, C, D, E, F, G, I, and J on *top* of PFGE images are farm codes where isolates were collected. *Capital letters and numeral suffix* under farm code represent the PFGE type–subtype patterns. "LADDER" corresponds to lambda ladder PFG marker. (**a**) All PFGE profiles obtained among the 18 bovine isolates using the endonuclease SmaI (one isolate from farm E was resistant to cleavage by endonuclease SmaI). (**b**) PFGE profile of Cfr9I-digested genomic DNA of one isolate (of PFGE F-1) which was resistant to cleavage by SmaI

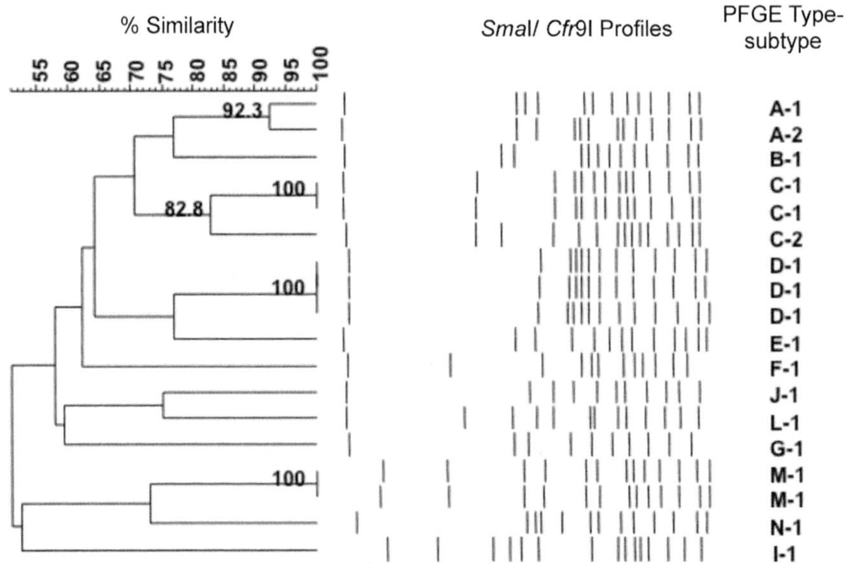

Fig. 3 Representative image of a dendrogram of PFGE patterns of bovine streptococci (*S. dysgalactiae* subsp. *dysgalactiae*) (adapted from Rato et al. (http://wwwnc.cdc.gov/eid/article/16/1/09-0632-f1)) [7]. The dendrogram was produced by using Dice coefficients and an unweighted pair group method using arithmetic averages (UPGMA). Default clustering settings of 0 % optimization (i.e., the relative distance an entire lane is allowed to shift in matching attempts) and 1.5 % band position tolerance were used

in most cases above 80 % similarity. These are assigned to different subtypes of a PFGE type. Patterns with variation of six or more bands (corresponding to levels of similarity of less than 80 %) are considered unrelated and are assigned to distinct PFGE types. PFGE types may be designated with uppercase letters of alphanumeric codes, and each of their subtypes (subclonal variants) may be identified by an additional numeral-or letter-code suffix.

4 Notes

1. Solutions prepared from powdered pancreatic RNase (ribonuclease A from bovine pancreas, Sigma-Aldrich) products can be made free of DNase by boiling. Prepare a 10 mg/ml stock solution in 10 mM sodium acetate buffer, pH 5.2. Heat to 100 °C for 15 min, allow to cool to room temperature, and then adjust to pH 7.4 using 0.1 volumes of 1 M Tris–HCl, pH 7.4. Aliquot and store at −20 °C.
2. The deproteinization solution should be freshly prepared before use.
3. The Cfr9I (*Xma*I) restriction enzyme (C^CCGGG) can be used instead of SmaI (CCC^GGG) when DNAs are uncut by SmaI. If Cfr9I is used, do the equilibration step of the protocol as referred but with pre-Cfr9I restriction buffer (10 mM Tris–HCl, pH 7.2, 5 mM $MgCl_2$, 200 mM sodium glutamate, 100 μg/ml BSA) at 37 °C. For the restriction, add 45 μl of Cfr9I restriction buffer plus 20 units of Cfr9I enzyme stock per DNA disc and incubate at 37 °C overnight.
4. TBE buffer is prone to precipitation over time.
5. Remove supernatants carefully using a 5 ml pipette with an automatic pipette aid.

   Caution: Pellets are easy to lose! Be careful when taking tubes out of centrifuge. Remove the last amounts of supernatant fluid using 1 ml tips and corresponding pipette.
6. The formula is derived as follows:

$$\frac{OD_{620} \times 200}{5.0} = \frac{V_{add} + 210}{210}$$

   where:

   OD_{620}: optical density measured in the cuvette

   200: dilution factor (of 5 μl of cell suspension to 1 ml of PIV in the cuvette)

   $OD_{620} \times 200$: the "true" OD_{620} of the suspension of bacteria (in 210 μl PIV) in the 1.5 ml tubes

   5.0: desired final OD_{620} of the bacterial suspension in the 1.5 ml tubes

V_{add}: volume (μl) to add to the 1.5 ml tubes in order to obtain a final $OD_{620} = 5.0$

210: original volume (μl) of the cell suspension in PIV

$V_{add} + 210$: total volume (μl) in the 1.5 ml tubes, after the addition of the extra volume of PIV

7. Important: the DNA agarose discs are fragile; manipulate them gently.
8. Do not touch agarose disc with hand paper towel.

Acknowledgments

The PFGE data mentioned in this chapter were obtained by Márcia Rato as part of her research leading to Ph.D. thesis. Fundação para a Ciência e a Tecnologia (FCT) is acknowledge for the financial support for the accomplishment of Márcia Rato Doctoral Project (SFRH/BD/32513/2006). The work was supported by the grants Pest-OE/BIA/UI0457/2011-CREM (Centro de Recursos Microbiológicos) and PROC 60839, funded by Fundação para a Ciência e Tecnologia, Portugal and Fundação Calouste Gulbenkian, Portugal (respectively).

References

1. Tenover FC, Arbeit RD, Goering RV et al (1995) Interpreting chromosomal DNA restriction patterns produced by pulsed-field gel electrophoresis: criteria for bacterial strain typing. J Clin Microbiol 33:2233–2239
2. Van Belkum A, Tassios PT, Dijkshoorn L et al (2007) Guidelines for the validation and application of typing methods for the use in bacterial epidemiology. Clin Microbiol Infect 13(suppl 3):1–46
3. Ericsson U, Lindberg A, Persson W et al (2009) Microbial aetiology of acute clinical mastitis and agent-specific risk factors. Vet Microbiol 137:90–97
4. Barkema HW, Green MJ, Bradley AJ, Zadoks RN (2009) Invited review: the role of contagious disease in udder health. J Dairy Sci 92: 4717–4729
5. Muellner P, Zadoks RN, Perez AM et al (2011) The integration of molecular tools into veterinary and spatial epidemiology. Spat Spattemporal Epidemiol 2:159–171
6. Rato MG, Bexiga R, Nunes SF et al (2008) Molecular epidemiology and population structure of bovine *Streptococcus uberis*. J Dairy Sci 91:4542–4551
7. Rato MG, Bexiga R, Nunes SF, Vilela CL, Santos-Sanches I (2010) Human group A streptococci virulence genes in bovine group C streptococci. Emerg Infect Dis 16:116–119
8. Rato MG, Nerlich A, Bergmann R et al (2011) Virulence gene pool detected in bovine group C *Streptococcus dysgalactiae* subsp. *dysgalactiae* using a group A *Streptococcus pyogenes* virulence microarray. J Clin Microbiol 49:2470–2479
9. Rato MG, Bexiga R, Florindo C et al (2013) Antimicrobial resistance and molecular epidemiology of streptococci from bovine mastitis. Vet Microbiol 161:286–294
10. Rato M (2011) Epidemiological characterization, antimicrobial resistance and virulence mechanisms in animal and human streptococci. Ph.D. thesis, Faculdade de Ciências e Tecnologia. Universidade Nova de Lisboa. Portugal. ISBN: 978-989-20-2618-3
11. Chung M, de Lencastre H, Matthews P et al (2000) Molecular typing of methicillin-resistant *Staphylococcus aureus* by pulsed-field gel electrophoresis: comparison of results obtained in a multilaboratory effort using identical protocols and MRSA strains. Microb Drug Resist 6:189–198

Chapter 24

Multiple-Locus Variable-Number Tandem Repeat (VNTR) Analysis (MLVA) Using Multiplex PCR and Multicolor Capillary Electrophoresis: Application to the Genotyping of *Brucella* Species

Giuliano Garofolo

Abstract

The multiple-locus variable-number tandem repeat (VNTR) analysis (MLVA) is a genetic typing method based on the evaluation of the number of repeated sequences in multiple selected loci of microbial DNA. Although several MLVA typing panels have been proposed for brucellae, the 16-loci panel is recognized as the standard genotyping method, also used for the *Brucella* international online database. This chapter describes a high-throughput MLVA-16 protocol using multiplex PCRs and multicolor capillary electrophoresis.

Key words MLVA, Capillary electrophoresis, Multiplex PCR, *Brucella* spp, Genotyping

1 Introduction

Brucellosis is a widespread animal infectious disease and probably the world's most common zoonosis. The *Brucella* genus currently comprises six classical species (*B. abortus*, *B. melitensis*, *B. suis*, *B. ovis*, *B. canis*, and *B. neotomae*) and four novel species (*B. ceti*, *B. pinnipedialis*, *B. inopinata*, and *B. microti*) [1]. New species have been proposed in recent years. The highly monomorphic nature of this genus, presenting few polymorphisms not only within species but between species as well, makes strains particularly difficult to differentiate using most genetic typing techniques. This makes crucial public health tasks, such as diagnosis and strain typing, a challenge for veterinary laboratories testing livestock and wildlife. To date, multiple-locus variable-number tandem repeat (VNTR) analysis (MLVA) [2] is recognized as one of the best genotyping approaches for *Brucella*. Mutation rate variability between loci in *Brucella* allows this method to discriminate closely related strains

Mónica V. Cunha and João Inácio (eds.), *Veterinary Infection Biology: Molecular Diagnostics and High-Throughput Strategies*, Methods in Molecular Biology, vol. 1247, DOI 10.1007/978-1-4939-2004-4_24, © Springer Science+Business Media New York 2015

(through highly mutable loci) as well as yield useful information at the phylogenetic/taxonomic level (through relatively conserved loci). VNTRs are found in both chromosomes and may exhibit several allelic states within a brucellae population. Slipped strand mispairing during DNA replication is the biological reason for such variation. Thus far, MLVA panels of either 21, 16, or 15 loci (MLVA-21, MLVA-16, and MLVA-15, respectively) have been developed [3–5], each with its strengths and weaknesses. A cooperative online public database based on the MLVA-16 panel was established with the aim of promoting the creation of a global epidemiological map of *Brucella* (http://mlva.u-psud.fr/brucella/). The MLVA-16 protocol normally employs singleplex PCRs and agarose gel electrophoresis. We describe an alternative methodology for MLVA-16 *Brucella* genotyping, using multiplex PCRs and capillary electrophoresis performed on an ABI PRISM genetic analyzer. Methods for MLVA data management and analysis, including the submission of queries to international databases, will also be illustrated.

2 Materials

2.1 Laboratory Plasticware

1. 0.5 ml amber-colored tubes (to protect fluorescent dyes from light; in the absence of amber-colored tubes, transparent tubes covered with aluminum foil may be used).
2. 1.5 ml microcentrifuge tubes.
3. 96-well v-bottom PCR plates or blocks for 0.2 ml PCR tubes with caps.
4. Presterile DNase- and RNase-free filter pipette tips (20 μl, 100 μl, 1,000 μl).
5. 1.4 ml noncoded U-bottom bulk tubes (Micronic, Lelystad, The Netherlands).
6. Storage rack for 96 individual tubes (8 × 12)—Comorack-96 (Micronic, Lelystad, The Netherlands).
7. Rubber septa for the 96-well reaction plate.

2.2 Laboratory Reagents

1. Water, Mol Bio grade (i.e., DNase-, RNase-, and protease-free molecular biology grade water).
2. Either TE buffer (i.e., 1× TE: 1 mM Tris–HCl, 0.1 mM EDTA, pH 8.0) or water, Mol Bio grade.
3. Multiplex PCR master mix (we use 2× Type-it microsatellite PCR Master Mix, Qiagen).
4. Q solution, an innovative PCR additive that facilitates amplification of difficult templates (Qiagen).

5. 50 μM primer stock solutions for the following loci: Bruce04, Bruce06, Bruce07, Bruce08, Bruce09, Bruce11, Bruce12, Bruce16, Bruce18, Bruce19, Bruce21, Bruce30, Bruce42, Bruce43, Bruce45, and Bruce55. MLVA primers sequences for the 16 loci and fluorescent dyes used in the capillary electrophoresis are given in Table 1 [6, 7].
6. 10× forward primer mixes (M1fw, M2fw, M3fw, and M4fw mixes) (*see* **Note 1**):
   (a) M1fw: Mix and dilute 4.4 μl of each 50 μM primer stock solutions ["Bruce08 Fw (PET labelled)," "Bruce11 Fw (6FAM labelled)," "Bruce45 Fw (6FAM labelled)," "Bruce30 Fw (PET labelled)," and "Bruce19 Fw (NED labelled)"] in a final volume of 110 μl of TE buffer or Mol Bio grade water to obtain a 2 μM (10×) primer mix working solution (*see* **Note 2**).
   (b) M2fw: Mix and dilute 50 μM primer stock solutions [8.8 μl of "Bruce06 Fw (NED labelled)," 1.1 μl of "Bruce42 Fw (VIC labelled)," and 1.1 μl of "Bruce42 Fw (unlabelled)"] in a final volume of 110 μl of TE buffer or Mol Bio grade water to obtain a 4.0, 0.5, and 0.5 μM (10×) primer mix working solution, respectively (*see* **Note 2**).
   (c) M3fw: Mix and dilute 50 μM primer stock solutions [3.3 μl of "Bruce12 Fw (NED labelled)," 1.1 μl of "Bruce55 Fw (PET labelled)," 1.1 μl of "Bruce55 Fw (unlabelled)," 1.1 μl of "Bruce18 Fw (PET labelled)," 1.1 μl of "Bruce18 Fw (unlabelled)," 4.4 μl of "Bruce21 Fw (6FAM labelled)," and 4.4 μl of "Bruce04 Fw (VIC labelled)"] in a final volume of 110 μl of TE buffer or Mol Bio grade water to obtain a 1.5, 0.5, 0.5, 0.5, 0.5, 2.0, and 2.0 μM (10×) primer mix working solution, respectively (*see* **Note 2**).
   (d) M4fw: Mix and dilute 50 μM primer stock solutions [3.3 μl of "Bruce07 Fw (NED labelled)," 4.4 μl of "Bruce09 Fw (VIC labelled)," 4.4 μl of "Bruce16 Fw (6FAM labelled)," and 3.3 μl of "Bruce43 Fw (6FAM labelled)"] in a final volume of 110 μl of TE buffer or Mol Bio grade water to obtain a 1.5, 2.0, 2.0, and 1.5 μM (10×) primer mix working solution, respectively (*see* **Note 2**).
7. 10× reverse primer mixes (M1rw, M2rw, M3rw, and M4rw mixes) (*see* **Note 1**).
   (a) M1rw: Mix and dilute 4.4 μl of each 50 μM primer stock solutions ["Bruce08 Rw (unlabelled)," "Bruce11 Rw (unlabelled)," "Bruce45 Rw (unlabelled)," "Bruce30 Rw (unlabelled)," and "Bruce19 Rw (unlabelled)"] in a final volume of 110 μl of TE buffer or Mol Bio grade water to obtain a 2 μM (10×) primer mix working solution (*see* **Note 2**).

Table 1
MLVA primers sequences

Multiplex PCR mix[a]	Locus	Primer sequences (5′-3′)[b]	Allele size range (bp)[c]
M1	Bruce30	Fw: PET - TGACCGCAAAACCATATCCTTC Rw: TATGTGCAGAGCTTCATGTTCG	119–199
	Bruce08	Fw: PET - ATTATTCGCAGGCTCGTGATTC Rw: ACAGAAGGTTTTCCAGCTCGTC	312–384
	Bruce11	Fw: 6FAM - CTGTTGATCTGACCTTGCAACC Rw: CCAGACAACAACCTACGTCCTG	257–1076
	Bruce45	Fw: 6FAM - ATCCTTGCCTCTCCCTACCAG Rw: CGGGTAAATATCAATGGCTTGG	133–187
	Bruce19	Fw: NED - GACGACCCGGACCATGTCT Rw: ACTTCACCGTAACGTCGTGGAT	79–205
M2	Bruce06	Fw: NED - GATTGCGGAACGTCTGAACT Rw: TAACCGCCTTCCACATAATCG	312–714
	Bruce42	Fw: VIC - CATCGCCTCAACTATACCGTCA Rw: ACCGCAAAATTTACGCATCG	164–914
M3	Bruce12	Fw: NED - CGGTAAATCAATTGTCCCATGA Rw: GCCCAAGTTCAACAGGAGTTTC	302–452
	Bruce18	Fw: PET - TATGTTAGGGCAATAGGGCAGT Rw: GATGGTTGAGAGCATTGTGAAG	130–186
	Bruce55	Fw: PET - TCAGGCTGTTTCGTCATGTCTT Rw: AATCTGGCGTTCGAGTTGTTCT	193–553
	Bruce21	Fw: 6FAM - CTCATGCGCAACCAAAACA Rw: GTGGATACGCTCATTCTCGTTG	431–463
	Bruce04	Fw: VIC - CTGACGAAGGGAAGGCAATAAG Rw: TGGTTTTCGCCAATATCAACAA	313–473
M4	Bruce07	Fw: NED - GCTGACGGGGAAGAACATCTAT Rw: ACCCTTTTTCAGTCAAGGCAAA	134–246
	Bruce09	Fw: VIC - GCGGATTCGTTCTTCAGTTATC Rw: GGGAGTATGTTTTGGTTGTACATAG	124–292
	Bruce43	Fw: 6FAM - TCTCAAGCCCGATATGGAGAAT Rw: TATTTTCCGCCTGCCCATAAAC	170–194
	Bruce16	Fw: 6FAM - ACGGGAGTTTTTGTTGCTCAAT Rw: GGCCATATCCTTCCGCAATA	227–353

[a]For primer mixes including the forward primers targeting the Bruce18, Bruce42, and Bruce55 loci, equal concentrations of both labelled and unlabelled primers targeting these loci were added to the mix in order to avoid the posterior production of excessive fluorescence during the capillary electrophoresis [6]

[b]Fw, forward primer; Rw, reverse primer

[c]Expected allele size ranges are given in base pairs. The test has been designed so that fragments would differ from one another by either size, fluorescence, or both, to exclude the possibility of overlap in capillary electrophoresis results

(b) M2rw: Mix and dilute 50 μM primer stock solutions [8.8 μl of "Bruce06 Rw (unlabelled)" and 2.2 μl of "Bruce42 Rw (unlabelled)"] in a final volume of 110 μl of TE buffer or Mol Bio grade water to obtain a 4.0 and 1.0 μM (10×) primer mix working solution, respectively (*see* **Note 2**).

(c) M3rw: Mix and dilute 50 μM primer stock solutions [3.3 μl of "Bruce12 Rw (unlabelled)," 2.2 μl of "Bruce55 Rw (unlabelled)," 2.2 μl of "Bruce18 Rw (unlabelled)," 4.4 μl of "Bruce21 Rw (unlabelled)," and 4.4 μl of "Bruce04 Rw (unlabelled)"] in a final volume of 110 μl of TE buffer or Mol Bio grade water to obtain a 1.5, 1.0, 1.0, 2.0, and 2.0 μM (10×) primer mix working solution, respectively (*see* **Note 2**).

(d) M4rw: Mix and dilute 50 μM primer stock solutions [3.3 μl of "Bruce07 Rw (unlabelled)," 4.4 μl of "Bruce09 Rw (unlabelled)," 4.4 μl of "Bruce16 Rw (unlabelled)," and 3.3 μl of "Bruce43 Rw (unlabelled)"] in a final volume of 110 μl of TE buffer or Mol Bio grade water to obtain a 1.5, 2.0, 2.0, and 1.5 μM (10×) primer mix working solution, respectively (*see* **Note 2**).

8. Hi-Di formamide.
9. POP-7 polymer, a separation matrix for performing DNA sequencing and fragment analysis on the Applied Biosystems genetic analyzer instruments (Life Technologies, USA).
10. Anode and cathode buffers, reagents to support electrophoresis on Applied Biosystems genetic analyzer instruments (Life Technologies, USA).
11. GeneScan 1200 LIZ size standard (Life Technologies, USA).
12. DNA samples from one or more reference strains having known MLVA profiles, for comparison (e.g., *B. melitensis* biovar 1 strain 16 M). Be sure to use purified DNAs (A260/A280 ratio ≥1.8).
13. DNA samples to be tested. Be sure to use purified DNAs (A260/A280 ratio ≥1.8).

2.3 Equipment and Instruments

1. PCR plate cooling block or ice.
2. Complete "clean set" (1,000 μl, 200 μl, 100 μl, 20 μl, and 10 μl) of single-channel pipettes for PCR master mix setup.
3. 10 μl single-channel pipettes for DNA solutions.
4. 8-channel pipettes (200 μl and 10 μl) for DNA solutions.
5. Thermocycler with heated lid.
6. Heat block (or thermocycler), capable of operating at 95 °C.

7. Centrifuge and rotors adapted to 0.2 ml PCR tubes, 1.5 ml microcentrifuge tubes, and 96-well v-bottom PCR plates.
8. Mixer.
9. Capillary electrophoresis genetic analyzer (e.g., we use ABI PRISM genetic analyzer, either 3130 or 3500 series) (Life Technologies, USA) (*see* **Note 3**).
10. Capillary arrays, 50 cm.

2.4 Software

1. Data collection software, the operative software to drive the Applied Biosystems genetic analyzer instruments.
2. GeneMapper 4.1 (Life Technologies, USA).

3 Methods

3.1 PCR Setup

1. Defrost all PCR components and keep them on ice during preparation.
2. Briefly vortex and spin down the primer mixes in their amber tubes.
3. Place a 96-well v-bottom PCR plate or the required number of 0.2 ml PCR tubes in a PCR block or on ice.
4. Mark four 1.5 ml microcentrifuge tubes as M1, M2, M3, and M4, respectively, for each of the four multiplex master mixes to be prepared.
5. Prepare each master mix in the correspondent 1.5 ml microcentrifuge tube using the appropriate volumes (*see* Table 2), preferably introducing them in the following order: Mol Bio water, Q solution, 2× Type-it microsatellite PCR Master Mix, and primers.
6. Vortex the master mixes for 1–2 s.
7. Leave the DNA clean room.
8. To optimize the workflow and facilitate the dispensation of DNA samples, it is useful to include 32 samples in each PCR run: 28 DNA samples to be tested, two positive reference DNA samples for positive controls, and two no-template negative controls.
9. Due to differences in the PCR cycling conditions, the M2 PCR should be run separately from M1, M3, and M4 PCRs.
10. In a single 96-well plate or tube rack, dispense M1, M3, and M4 master mixes: 9 μl of each master mix in each well/tube, for each sample to be tested, dedicating distinct columns to each kind of master mix. Using a multichannel pipette, add 1 μl of each DNA sample (1–50 ng) to each master mix, keeping row positions constant across columns.

Table 2
PCR master mixes composition

Component	Volume per reaction (μl)[a]	Final concentration
2× Type-it microsatellite PCR Master Mix	5	1×
Q solution	1	0.5×
10× forward primer mix[b]	1	1×
10× reverse primer mix[b]	1	1×
Mol Bio grade water	1	-
DNA template solution	1	10–50 ng
Final volume (μl)	10	-

[a]The volume of each component to add to the master mix corresponds to the volume per reaction of that component multiplied by the total number of samples (including any positive and negative controls) plus 10 % of the original volume to compensate for eventual pipetting losses (DNA template solutions are not added to master mixes)
[b]Primer mix for the specific multiplex PCR being prepared, primer solutions should be paired as follows: M1fw and M1rw (for multiplex master mix 1—M1), M2fw and M2rw (for multiplex master mix 2—M2), M3fw and M3rw (for multiplex master mix 3—M3), and M4fw and M4rw (for multiplex master mix 4—M4)

11. In a separate 96-well plate or tube rack, dispense 9 μl of M2 master mix in each well/tube for each sample to be tested. Using a multichannel pipette, add 1 μl of each DNA sample (1–50 ng) to the master mix, keeping row positions constant across columns.
12. Keep the plates/racks on ice.
13. Run the PCRs under the following thermocycling conditions: initial activation step at 95 °C for 5 min followed by 30 cycles (for M1, M3, and M4 PCRs) or 26 cycles (for M2 PCR) of denaturation (at 95 °C for 30 s), annealing (at 60 °C for 90 s) and extension (at 72 °C for 30 s) steps, and a final extension step at 60 °C for 45 min and 20 °C for 120 min. Keep the products at 4 °C after the amplification reactions.

3.2 Dilution of PCR Products

1. Prepare as many U-bottom bulk tubes as the wells used in PCR reactions.
2. Insert the tubes in their storage racks.
3. Dispense 450 μl of Mol Bio grade water in each tube (*see* **Note 4**).
4. For each sample, add 2 μl of the PCR product from each reaction (M1, M2, M3, and M4).

3.3 Preparation of the Samples for Capillary Electrophoresis

1. Calculate the volumes of the reagents needed for the formamide/size standard mix by multiplying the volumes required for the injection of a single DNA sample for capillary electrophoresis (i.e., 10.25 μl formamide and 0.3 μl Liz 1200 size standard) by the total number of samples (including any

positive and negative controls). Then, multiply by three, since three capillary electrophoresis injections will be needed to analyze each sample, plus 10 % of the original volumes obtained for each reagent (*see* **Note 5**).

2. Dispense 10.55 μl of the mix into each tube/well of a 96-well PCR plate.
3. Using a multichannel pipette, for each sample, add 2 μl of diluted PCR product; M1 and M2 diluted products should be mixed together in a single well; M3 and M4 should be dispensed separately. Only three capillary electrophoresis injections will therefore be needed to analyze the products of the four multiplex PCRs.
4. Cover the plate with the rubber septa.
5. Denature the sample plate at 95 °C for 3 min, and cool it on ice or ice block for 1 min.
6. Spin down the sample plate to remove any air bubbles.
7. Place the sample plate on a plate base. Snap the plate retainer (cover) onto the plate and plate base. Place the prepared 96-well plate on the autosampler tray of the capillary electrophoresis equipment.

3.4 Capillary Electrophoresis

The following steps are adapted for ABI PRISM genetic analyzer instruments.

1. Power the ABI PRISM genetic analyzer.
2. Run the data collection software.
3. Ensure that consumables (e.g., polymers, buffers) are not expired and that buffer levels are at the fill lines.
4. Set the oven temperature to 60 °C by clicking preheat.
5. Check for and remove any bubbles from the pump assembly.
6. Create a plate record and assign plate contents by entering the following information:
   (a) Sample names: be sure to name the samples in a way that reflects their order in the 96-well plate.
   (b) Assay, set run module parameters as follows: oven temperature (°C) 60, run voltage (kV) 8.5, pre-run voltage (kV) 15, injection voltage (kV) 1.6, run time (sec.) 4900, pre-run time (sec.) 180, injection time (sec.), and data delay (sec.) 480.
   (c) Assign file name convention to each sample: sample name, wells, and capillary number.
   (d) Results group: create a MLVA_*Brucella* folder.
7. Save the plate record.
8. Load the plate onto the instrument, access the plate record created, and link the plate to its plate record.

9. Start run (*see* **Note 6**).
10. After the capillary electrophoresis, an .fsa file containing the results will be generated for each sample.

3.5 GeneMapper Setup

Before starting the first analysis on your .fsa capillary electrophoresis results, prepare GeneMapper by running it on one or more sample files of known *Brucella* reference strains:

1. Create a kit, giving the kit name "MLVA *Brucella*."
2. Create a new bin set with the name "*Brucella*."
3. Create three panels with the names M1–M2, M3, and M4.
4. Add the following new markers for the three panels:
   (a) M1–M2 with Bruce06, Bruce08, Bruce11, Bruce19, Bruce30, Bruce42, and Bruce45.
   (b) M3 with Bruce04, Bruce12, Bruce18, Bruce21, and Bruce55.
   (c) M4 with Bruce07, Bruce09, Bruce16, and Bruce43.
   (d) For each marker, enter the following information (displayed in Table 1): marker name, dye color (6FAM, blue; VIC, green; NED, yellow; and PET, red), and allele size range (minimum and maximum sizes).
5. Create a new project and add all the reference sample files (e.g., *Brucella melitensis* biovar 1 str. 16 M).
6. Set a new analysis method named *Brucella* from the GeneMapper manager. Associate the previously created bin set. Select advanced from the peak detection algorithm drop-down menu. Select partial range for the analysis range. The latter step serves to exclude the primer peak from the analysis range. Under peak quality, set the expected allele number to 1 (for haploid organisms).
7. Set a custom Liz 1200 size standard based on the Liz 1200, but which includes only the values of the partial range.
8. Analyze the samples.
9. Examine the results.
10. Open panel manager and import the reference file.
11. For each of the three panels (corresponding to M1 + M2, M3, and M4), select each marker (locus), add bin, and, on the basis of the observed peak, manually assign it an allelic value (expected VNTR) using Table 3.

3.6 Data Analysis Using GeneMapper

1. After the initial creation of kits, setting of analysis methods and of custom size standard, new samples can be easily analyzed.
2. Open the GeneMapper software.

Table 3
Expected VNTR sizes per locus of *Brucella* sequences currently known and correspondent allelic value[a]

Allelic value	1	2	3	4	5	6	7	8	9	10	11	12	13	14	15	16	17	18	19	20	21	22	23	24	25	26	27	28
Panel 1																												
Bruce06	312	446	**580**	714																								
Bruce08		312	330	**348**	366	384																						
Bruce11		**257**	320	383		509		635	698			887		1013	1076													
Bruce12							302	317	332	347	362	377	**392**	407	422	437	452											
Bruce42	164	289	414	**539**	664	789	914																					
Bruce43	170	**182**	194																									
Bruce45		133	**151**	169	187																							
Bruce55	193	233	**273**	313	353	393	433			553																		
Panel 2A																												
Bruce18			130	138	**146**	154	162	170	178	186																		
Bruce19				79	85	91												**163**	169	175	181	187	193		205			
Bruce21					431	**439**	447	455	463																			
Panel 2B																												
Bruce04	313	**321**	329	337	345	353	361	369	377	385	393	401	409	417	425	433	441	449	457	465	473	481	489					529
Bruce07		134	142	150	**158**	166	174	182	190	198	206	214	222	230		246												
Bruce09			124	132	140	148	156	**164**	172	180	188	196	204	212	220	228	236	244	252	260	268	276	284	292				
Bruce16		227	**235**	243	251	259	267	275	283	291	299	307	315	323	331	337		353										
Bruce30		119	127	135	143	**151**	159	167	175	183	191	199																

[a]Data pertaining to *B. melitensis* biovar 1 str. 16 M is underlined and given in bold; the 16 markers can be split into two groups: one comprises 8 minisatellite loci (panel 1), and the second group contains 8 microsatellite loci (panel 2A and panel 2B). In this approach, the loci are divided into different panels containing increasing levels of genetic resolution: the MLVA-8 (panel 1), MLVA-11 (panels 1 and 2A), and MLVA-16 (panels 1, 2A, and 2B) (for the original source of the table, go to http://mlva.u psud.fr/brucella/IMG/pdf/bru_table_allele_assignement_version3.6.pdf)

Table 4
VNTR size by locus

Locus	VNTR size (bp)
Bruce06	134
Bruce08	18
Bruce11	63
Bruce12	15
Bruce42	125
Bruce43	12
Bruce45	18
Bruce55	40
Bruce18	8
Bruce19	6
Bruce21	8
Bruce04	8
Bruce07	8
Bruce09	8
Bruce16	8
Bruce30	8

3. Import the electrophoresis .fsa files into a new project. Select the previously created analysis method *Brucella* and the panels corresponding to the M1 + M2, M3, and M4 reactions (*see* Subheading 3.5).
4. Analyze the project.
5. Review the sizing quality (SQ).
6. Examine the size standard.
7. View sample information (including raw data).
8. View sample plots.
9. For each marker, check all allele calls against those of the reference strain or strains. Wherever the allele call of the analyzed strain differs from those of your known reference strains, add the new allele to the bin. Putative new alleles will be identified where, in any given locus, the DNA fragment is found to be shorter or longer than expected in light of the VNTR size for that locus and the number of repetitions known to occur in the reference strain or strains (*see* Table 4).

10. Confirm new alleles, whenever possible, through Sanger sequencing.
11. GeneMapper will store all observed and confirmed bins present in the population studied. This information will be used as reference for future analyses.
12. In the GeneMapper, genotype page results are grouped by panel. Export the genotype table of each panel in a .csv file and then merge them together in a single .csv file.
13. Import the data, e.g., into Microsoft Access or Microsoft Excel, and arrange it by loci in the following order: Bruce06, Bruce08, Bruce11, Bruce12, Bruce42, Bruce43, Bruce45, Bruce55, Bruce18, Bruce19, Bruce21, Bruce04, Bruce07, Bruce09, Bruce16, and Bruce30.

3.7 Cluster Analysis

1. Go to the *Brucella* cooperative database (http://mlva.u-psud.fr/mlvav4/genotyping/) using either a Mozilla Firefox or Microsoft Internet Explorer browser (*see* **Note 7**).
2. For each one of tested isolates, submit a query that will compare it to the strains present in the database. From the menu, select the *Brucella* cooperative database, then select the MLVA-16 panel, enter the numeric code for each MLVA marker, and submit the data (for further information, consult the tutorial: http://mlva.u-psud.fr/MLVAnet/IMG/pdf/MlvaBank_tutorial.pdf). The *Brucella* MLVA data efficiently cluster the strains by species. The minimum distance between the isolate submitted and strains previously deposited in the database will determine its species (*see* **Notes 8** and **9**).

4 Notes

1. The preparation of primer mix solutions should be performed in a DNA-free room. Thaw primer stock solutions and place on ice until use. Avoid the exposure of primers to light. In the absence of amber-colored tubes, use aluminum foil to cover the vials.
2. To minimize repetitive freeze-thaw cycles of primer stock solutions, prepare 10 batches of 10× primer mixes (volume 110 μl) every couple of months or if a drop in fluorescence is observed in your old batch. This amount should be sufficient for 1000 PCRs, allowing MLVA on 200–250 strains.
3. Other capillary electrophoresis machines may be used, but it is recommended that fragment analysis be set to 140–1,100 bp and the proper reagents be used, as suggested by the manufacturer.

4. In the first few runs, verify the dilution factor by running one column at a time (M1–M2, M3, and M4 fragments, respectively). If peak fluorescence intensity does not fall between 400 and 6,000 nm, correct the dilution to optimize your electrophoresis. Further PCRs will generate a similar pattern of fluorescence for all samples, provided that equal amounts of purified DNAs are used.
5. For example, for a total of 32 DNA samples: 1082.4 μl of formamide [10.25 μl × 3 injections × 32 (=984 μl) + 10 % of this volume (=98.4 μl)] and 31.6 μl of Liz 1,200 size standard [0.3 μl × 3 injections × 32 (=28.8 μl) + 10 % of this volume (=2.8 μl)].
6. Each injection takes about 1.5 h. The analysis of a single plate involves 12 injections and will thus take about 17 h.
7. A cooperative public online database, based on the MLVA-16 panel, was established with the aim of promoting the creation of a global epidemiological map of *Brucella* and is freely accessible at http://mlva.u-psud.fr/brucella/.
8. MLVA genotypes are considered to be closely related if they share 70 % or more of their VNTR alleles. For MLVA-16, strains having between 11 and 16 alleles in common are said to belong to the same species.
9. Further analysis may be recommended. Both free (e.g., Phyloviz 1.0) and paid (e.g., PAUP 4.0, Bionumerics) software are available for this purpose. UPGMA, neighbor-joining analyses, and minimum spanning trees can be generated to assess fine and broad relationships between the strains analyzed.

References

1. Pappas G (2010) The changing *Brucella* ecology: novel reservoirs, new threats. Int J Antimicrob Agents 36:S8–S11
2. Whatmore AM (2009) Current understanding of the genetic diversity of *Brucella*, an expanding genus of zoonotic pathogens. Infect Genet Evol 9:1168–1184
3. Al Dahouk S, Flèche PL, Nöckler K et al (2007) Evaluation of *Brucella* MLVA typing for human brucellosis. J Microbiol Methods 69:137–145
4. Whatmore AM, Shankster SJ, Perrett LL et al (2006) Identification and characterization of variable-number tandem-repeat markers for typing of *Brucella* spp. J Clin Microbiol 44:1982–1993
5. Bricker BJ, Ewalt DR, Halling SM (2003) *Brucella* 'HOOF-Prints': strain typing by multi-locus analysis of variable number tandem repeats (VNTRs). BMC Microbiol 3:15
6. Garofolo G, Ancora M, Di Giannatale E (2013) MLVA-16 loci panel on *Brucella* spp. using multiplex PCR and multicolor capillary electrophoresis. J Microbiol Methods 92: 103–107
7. Garofolo G, Di Giannatale E, De Massis F et al (2013) Investigating genetic diversity of *Brucella abortus* and *Brucella melitensis* in Italy with MLVA-16. Infect Genet Evol 19: 59–70

Chapter 25

Multilocus Sequence Typing (MLST): Markers for the Traceability of Pathogenic *Leptospira* Strains

Ahmed Ahmed, Ana S. Ferreira, and Rudy A. Hartskeerl

Abstract

Leptospirosis is a major zoonosis with worldwide distribution. Conventional serological typing is arduous and time consuming. Genotyping is increasingly applied for the typing and identification of leptospires and contributes to genetic and virulence divergence and molecular epidemiological characteristics such as host versus leptospires population interactions and dynamics. Presently, multilocus sequence typing (MLST) is the most robust approach. In this chapter, we describe the practical steps of two major multilocus sequence typing methods for leptospires. The first method (denoted as the 6 L scheme) is based on genotyping by phylogeny using concatenated sequences derived from six loci, including genes that encode outer membrane proteins and *rrs* and can be used for typing pathogenic species and strains of intermediate species. The second method (referred to as the 7 L scheme) uses seven loci on housekeeping genes and allows the analysis of seven major *Leptospira* pathogenic species. The 7 L scheme is web based and includes the option to analyze sequence types (STs).

Key words *Leptospira*, Leptospirosis, Genotyping, MLST, Multilocus typing

1 Introduction

Leptospirosis is a hemorrhagic zoonotic disease with a worldwide distribution presenting a major burden for the veterinary and public health. Leptospires, the causative agents, are long (6–20 μm) and thin (0.1–0.2 μm) helically coiled gram-negative bacteria with typically hooked ends from which each of the two endoflagella is extruding. These bacteria belong to the family *Leptospiraceae* and to the genus *Leptospira*. There are free-living saprophytic and pathogenic leptospires, the latter requiring a host for survival. Traditionally, saprophytic and pathogenic leptospires have been denoted as *Leptospira biflexa* and *Leptospira interrogans*, respectively. There is a wide variety of sero- and genotypes of leptospires, which are generally associated with a certain host. Hence, the availability of effective tools to identify infecting leptospires is of utmost importance in both animal and human health fields, not only for

Mónica V. Cunha and João Inácio (eds.), *Veterinary Infection Biology: Molecular Diagnostics and High-Throughput Strategies*, Methods in Molecular Biology, vol. 1247, DOI 10.1007/978-1-4939-2004-4_25, © Springer Science+Business Media New York 2015

the diagnosis of the disease but also for assessing its epidemiology and defining intervention strategies.

Traditionally, the serovar is the basic taxon of leptospires. The serovar is a serological entity determined by the cross agglutinin absorption test (CAAT). To date more than 300 serovars, both saprophytic and pathogenic, have been identified, separated into 26 serogroups on the basis of similarity in serological features. Since the 1990s, speciation of leptospires based on genomic DNA homology has been introduced. This technique, involving heterologous DNA hybridization, allows the speciation of members of *Leptospira* based on the established criterion that >70 % homology under defined stringency conditions corresponds to conspecificity. The method is laborious and tedious, and presently it is only executed at the Centers for Disease Control and Prevention (CDC), Atlanta, USA. Currently, molecular approaches have identified 21 *Leptospira* species, consisting of three clades comprising nine pathogenic, five intermediate, and seven saprophytic species. The molecular and serological classification of leptospires show little correlation.

In the past years, numerous restriction enzyme-generated or PCR-based DNA fingerprinting methods have been described. Among others, pulsed-field gel electrophoresis (PFGE), bacterial endonuclease DNA analysis (BRENDA), and arbitrarily primed PCR (AP-PCR) have been explored to genotype leptospires and, eventually, to achieve molecular speciation, but these methods usually yield complex patterns and lack the ability to directly generate digital data, show low reproducibility, and/or require cultures of viable leptospires. Considering the increasing complexity and associated costs for the international shipment of pathogens, there is a need for typing methods that generate electronically portable data and online databases that can be easily accessed for data insertion and comparison.

Phylogeny-based genotyping has been described for leptospires using sequences of several genes such as *rrs* (16S ribosomal RNA), *secY* (translocase preprotein secY), *gyrB* (DNA gyrase subunit B), *flaB* (flagellar protein B), and *rpoB* (RNA polymerase beta-subunit), some of these presenting a high discriminative power. However, horizontal DNA transfer has been described for *Leptospira*, and thus limitation to one locus holds the risk of misclassification. Therefore, the use of multiple loci for the genotyping of *Leptospira* is imperative. Multilocus sequence genotyping is one of such methods and currently the most robust one. The first *Leptospira* multilocus sequence genotyping system has been developed in the early 2000s [1] and was hampered at that time by a scarcity of available working sequences from public databases. This scheme uses six loci (6 L), including the *rrs* gene and two genes, *lipL32* and *lipL41*, coding for outer membrane proteins. This 6 L scheme for leptospires was followed by additional MLST approaches using seven loci (7 L) [2–4], while a theoretical genotyping scheme based on a super locus comprising four genes was described without information on its practical applicability. The 6 L scheme has the advantage that it can be applied on all pathogenic species of *Leptospira* and seems to enable inclusion of strains of intermediate species. The method uses phylogeny-based approaches on concatenated gene sequences but does not include analysis via sequence types (STs). The other 7 L MLST schemes were originally described for application with *L. interrogans* and, to some extent, the closely related species *L. kirschneri* [2, 3]. One of these schemes was further expanded for the genotyping of additional pathogenic species, namely, *L. borgpetersenii*, *L. noguchii*, *L. santarosai*, *L. weilii*, and *L. alexanderi* [4], and has the advantage that it is web based and includes analysis of STs [2, 4]. Since the availability of gene sequence data from intermediate and saprophytic *Leptospira* species in public databases is limited, both the 7 L and 6 L MLST schemes currently present constraints when analyzing such species. However, a variety of *Leptospira* genomes are being presently sequenced, which will allow the design of novel and more universal primers and the setting of an improved MLST scheme comprising all *Leptospira* clades. A comparison of the 7 L and 6 L MLST schemes showed that both approaches mostly yielded comparable results [5]. It was also demonstrated that the outer membrane encoding genes included in the 6 L scheme did not suffer from unequal evolutionary pressure [5].

This chapter describes the practical application of both the 6 L [1, 5] and the expanded 7 L [4] MLST approaches for the genotyping of pathogenic leptospires.

2 Materials

2.1 DNA Extraction from Cultures

1. 1.0–1.5 ml of fresh fully grown (i.e., approximate optical density at 420 nm is 0.35) purified cultures of the *Leptospira* isolates to genotype, usually in Ellinghausen-McCullough-Johnson-Harris (EMJH) liquid media.
2. Commercial kit for genomic DNA extraction from microbial cultures.
3. Negative (specimen without leptospires) and positive (specimen spiked with 10^4 leptospires/ml) extraction control.
4. Support equipment: centrifuge; thermostatized water bath or heating block (usually adjusted to 56 °C for DNA extraction).

2.2 Multilocus Sequence Typing (6 L and 7 L Schemes)

1. Primer sets for the 6 L (Table 1) [1, 5] and 7 L (Table 2) [4] MLST schemes (*see* **Notes 1** and **2**).
2. Reagents for conventional PCR reactions: DNA polymerase enzyme and respective 10× buffer, $MgCl_2$ (25 mM), dNTPs (25 mM), and distilled PCR grade water.

Table 1
Loci and respective flanking oligonucleotide primers for the *Leptospira* 6 L MLST scheme

Locus/ gene[a]	Primer	Sequence (5′ to 3′)[b]	$MgCl_2$ (mM)[c]	Size of PCR product (bp)	Location of the sequence used to define MLST locus[d, e]	Size of MLST locus (bp)[d]
adk	adkF	GGGCTGGAAAAGGTACACAA *(alternative: ACATTATCTTCATGGGACCTCC)*[f]	1.5	531 557	3458789–3458361	429
	adkR	ACGCAAGCTCCTTTTGAATC *(alternative: TTACACAAGCTCCCTTTGAAT)*[f]				
icdA	icdAF	GGGACGAGATGACCAGGAT	1.5	674	3980926–3980372	555
	icdAR	TTTTTTGAGATCCGCAGCTTT *(alternative: CTTTTTTGAGATCTCCGGCTTT)*[f]		674		
lipL41	LipL41F	TAGGAAATTGCGCAGCTACA	1.5	520	3603644–3604120	477
	LipL41R	GCATCGAGAGGAATTAACATCA				
rrs	rrsF	CATGCAAGTCAAGCGGAGTA	1.5	541	1862535–1862984	450
	rrsR	AGTTGAGCCCGCAGTTTTC				
secY	secYF	ATGCCGATCATTTTTGCTTC	1.5	549	3459402–3458902	501
	secYR	CCGTCCCTTAATTTTAGACTTCTTC *(alternative: CCTTCCTTTAATTTTAGACTTTTTC)*[f]		548		
lipL32	LipL32F	ATCTCCGTTGCACTCTTTGC	1.5	474	1667072–166641	432
	LipL32R	ACCATCATCATCATCGTCCA				

[a] *adk* (adenylate kinase), *icdA* (isocitrate dehydrogenase), *lipL41* (outer membrane lipoprotein LipL41), *rrs* (16S rRNA), *secY* (preprotein translocase SecY protein), and *lipL32* (outer membrane lipoprotein LipL32)

[b] Original primers according to Ahmed et al. [1] and additional alternative primers for some loci according to Ahmed et al. [5]

[c] Concentration of $MgCl_2$ in the PCR mixture as adjusted for each primer pair

[d] The location of the sequence used to define MLST locus and the size of MLST locus (bp) as modified in Ahmed et al. [5]

[e] Nucleotide positions based in the published genome sequence of *L. interrogans* serovar Copenhageni strain Fiocruz L1-130 chromosome I (GenBank Accession Number AE016823)

[f] When using these alternative primers, the annealing temperature should be adjusted to 54 °C in the PCR cycling conditions

Table 2
Loci and respective flanking oligonucleotide primers for the *Leptospira* 7 L MLST scheme

Locus/ gene[a]	Primer	Sequence (5′ to 3′)[b]	$MgCl_2$ (mM)[c]	Size of PCR product (bp)	Location of MLST locus[d]	Size of MLST locus (bp)
glmU	glmU-F_M	AGGATAAGGTCGCTGTGGTA	1.5	650	3784955–3784512	444
	glmU-R_M	AGTTTTTTTCCGGAGTTTCT				
pntA	pntA-FM	TAGGAAARATGAAACCRGGAAC	1.5	621	56347–56871	525
	pntA-RM	AAGAAGCAAGATCCACAAYTAC				
sucA	sucA-FM	TCATTCCACTTYTAGATACGAT	2.5	640	1227474–1227920	447
	sucA-RM	TCTTTTTTGAATTTTTGACG				
tpiA	tpiA-FM	TTGCAGGAAACTGGAAAATGAAT	3.5	639	1694673–1694248	426
	tpiA-RM	GTTTTACRGAACCHCCGTAGAGAAT				
pfkB	pfkB-FM	CGGAGAGTTTTATAARAAGGACAT	1.5	588	1386553–1386984	432
	pfkB-RM	AGAACACCCGCCGCAAAACAAT				
mreA	mreA-FM	GGCTCGCTCTYGACGGAAA	2.0	719	2734550–2734116	435
	mreA-RM	TCCRTAACTCATAAAMGACAAAGG				
caiB	caiB-F	CAACTTGCGGAYATAGGAGGAG	1.5	650	1562845–1563246	402
	caiB-R	ATTATGTTCCCCGTGAYTCG				

[a] *glmU* (UDP-N-acetylglucosamine pyrophosphorylase), *pntA* (NADP transhydrogenase subunit alpha), *sucA* (2-oxoglutarate dehydrogenase decarboxylase component), *tpiA* (triosephosphate isomerase), *pfkB* (ribokinase), *mreA* (rod-shape-determining protein rodA), and *caiB* (carnitine dehydratase)
[b] Primers according to Boonsilp et al. [4]
[c] Concentration of $MgCl_2$ in the PCR mixture as adjusted for each primer pair
[d] Nucleotide positions based in the published genome sequence of *L. interrogans* serovar Lai strain 56601 chromosome I (GenBank Accession Number NC004342)

3. Negative (sample without added DNA from leptospires) and positive (sample spiked with leptospiral DNA approximating 20 ng genomic DNA per reaction) PCR reaction controls.
4. PCR thermocycler.
5. Tris-borate EDTA (TBE) buffer (pH 8.0): 50 mM Tris, 50 mM boric acid, 0.5 mM EDTA.
6. 1.5 % (w/v) agarose gel stained with ethidium bromide: prepare a 1.5 % agarose gel by adding 1.5 g of agarose to 100 mL of TBE buffer. Heat in a microwave and boil for 1–2 min to melt the agarose. Leave it to cool for 3–5 min, add 0.5 μL of a 10 mg/mL stock solution of ethidium bromide, gently mix, and pour the melted gel in the electrophoresis tray with the respective combs.
7. 6× DNA loading dye (blue) containing 0.25 % (W/V) of bromophenol blue, 0.25 % (W/V) of xylene cyanol FF, 40 % (W/V) of sucrose, and 60 mM of EDTA (or orange dye consisting of 0.4 % of orange G, 40 % (W/V) of sucrose) and deionized/milli-Q water.
8. Electrophoresis apparatus and respective power source.
9. Ultraviolet light transilluminator.
10. Sequencing facilities or commercial sequencing services.
11. Informatics programs for nucleic acid sequence processing, alignment, and phylogenetic analysis. We are using SeqMan software (DNASTAR Inc., USA), Chromas Lite (Technelysium Pty Ltd, Australia), Clustal X multiple sequence alignment program [6], Molecular Evolutionary Genetics Analysis (MEGA) [7], and PhyML version 3.0.1 [8].

3 Methods

3.1 6 L MLST Scheme

1. Leptospiral genomic DNA is extracted from cultures as per the manufacturer's commercial kit.
2. Six conventional PCR reactions are performed for each leptospiral isolate, each one containing a pair of forward and reverse primers targeting different loci (according to Table 1) (*see* **Note 1**). The total volume of each reaction is 25 μl and contains 1.5 mM $MgCl_2$ (*see* Table 1), 200 μM dNTPs, 1.25 U of DNA polymerase and the respective 1× buffer, 5 pmol of each forward and reverse primers (*see* Table 1), and approximately 25–50 ng of *Leptospira* DNA (*see* **Note 3**).
3. Run the PCR mixtures with the following program in the thermocycler: one cycle of 95 °C for 5 min; 35 cycles of 94 °C for 30 s, 58 °C (or 54 °C for alternative primers, *see* Table 1) for 30 s, and 72 °C for 1 min; and a final extension step of 72 °C for 7 min (*see* **Note 4**).

4. Run the PCR products in a 1.5 % agarose gel stained with ethidium bromide using standard gel electrophoresis technique (*see* **Notes 5** and **6**).
5. Sequence the PCR products, corresponding to each amplified target locus, for both forward and reverse directions using sequencing "in-house" facilities or commercial services (*see* **Note** 7).
6. After obtaining the nucleotide sequences of all the six loci to be analyzed per *Leptospira* isolate, edit the sequences and trim the same to the correct length spanning each locus, according to the reference lengths and nucleotide positions displayed in Table 1, using appropriate software (e.g., Chromas Lite) (*see* **Notes 8** and **9**).
7. Use appropriate software for the nucleotide sequence analysis (e.g., MEGA), namely, for performing sequence alignments, identifying the polymorphic sites, and the construction of neighbor-joining phylogenetic trees using the concatenated sequences of the six MLST loci (mean pairwise distances are calculated using the Kimura two-parameter nucleotide substitution model) according to the order *adk-icdA-lipL32-lipL41-rrs2-secY* (*see* **Notes 10** and **11**).
8. Construct the likelihood tree from concatenated sequences of MLST loci using an algorithm implemented in PhyML version 3.0.1 (*see* **Notes 10** and **11**).

3.2 7 L MLST Scheme

1. Leptospiral genomic DNA is extracted from cultures as per the manufacturer's commercial kit.
2. Seven conventional PCR reactions are performed for each leptospiral isolate, each one containing a pair of forward and reverse primers targeting different loci (according to Table 2) (*see* **Note 2**). The total volume of each reaction is 25 μl and contains 1.5–3.5 mM $MgCl_2$ (adjusted for each primer pair according to Table 2), 200 μM dNTPs, 1.25 U of DNA polymerase and the respective 1× buffer, 5 pmol of each forward and reverse primers (*see* Table 2), and approximately 25–50 ng of *Leptospira* DNA (*see* **Note 3**).
3. Run the PCR mixtures with the following program in the thermocycler: one cycle of 95 °C for 2 min, 30 cycles of 95 °C for 10 s, 46 °C for 15 s, and 72 °C for 1 min and final extension step of 72 °C for 7 min (*see* **Note 4**).
4. Run the PCR products in a 1.5 % agarose gel stained with ethidium bromide using standard gel electrophoresis technique (*see* **Notes 5** and **6**).
5. Sequence the PCR products, corresponding to each amplified target locus, for both forward and reverse directions using sequencing "in-house" facilities or commercial services (*see* **Note** 7).

6. After obtaining the nucleotide sequences of all the seven loci to be analyzed per *Leptospira* isolate, edit the sequences and trim the same to the correct length spanning each locus, according to the reference lengths and nucleotide positions displayed in Table 2, using appropriate software (e.g., SeqMan or Chromas Lite) (*see* **Notes 8** and **9**).
7. To assign allele numbers and sequence types (STs), access the *Leptospira* MLST database webpage at http://leptospira.mlst.net [2, 4] and use the online software provided for the analysis. Select the Multiple Locus and allelic profile query option, copy the seven trimmed sequences from each isolate into the corresponding query boxes, and submit the search analysis. The allelic profiles of the submitted sequence data will be obtained as well as details of any *Leptospira* isolates presenting identical profiles to the one that has been submitted (*see* **Notes 12–15**).

4 Notes

1. The 6 L MLST scheme was originally developed by Ahmed et al. [1], for genotyping a broad range of pathogenic leptospires. This scheme does not conform to the original concept of MLST as it includes a non-housekeeping gene (*rrs*) and genes that encode cell surface proteins (*LipL32* and *LipL41*). Later, in 2011, Ahmed et al. [5] designed four additional alternative primers for use with the 6 L scheme (*see* Table 1). These primers should be used in a repeat PCR reaction in the event that the original primers fail to generate an amplicon.
2. The 7 L MLST scheme was originally described by Thaipadungpanit et al. [2], in 2007, primarily for genotyping isolates of *L. interrogans*. The scheme followed a conventional strategy for MLST by selecting seven housekeeping genes that were distributed around the genome and were not under positive selection. However, the primers used for this scheme worked variably for other leptospiral species. This scheme was recently further expanded by Boonsilp et al. [4], by updating primers sequences and replacing one of the analyzed locus. Therefore, as presented in this chapter, the modified 7 L MLST scheme can be used to genotype the seven pathogenic species of *Leptospira* linked to the overwhelming majority of disease: *L. interrogans*, *L. kirschneri*, *L. borgpetersenii*, *L. noguchii*, *L. santarosai*, *L. weilii*, and *L. alexanderi*.
3. Defrost the components needed for preparing the PCR mixtures at room temperature but maintain the DNA polymerase at −20 °C (or in ice) and add it to the mixtures in the last. Prepare the required master PCR mixtures (one for each

primer pair targeting distinct loci) containing all components, with the exception of the template DNA, taking into account the total number of reactions to perform and including both positive and negative controls. Distribute the required amount of reaction mixtures by individual microtubes, add the respective DNA template, and proceed for the cycling temperature steps in the thermocycler (can also keep the PCR mixtures at 4 °C if not using immediately). To monitor eventual cross-contaminations, the negative control should be also added in the DNA addition room.

4. Ideally, PCR conditions should be the same for all loci in a MLST scheme. To accomplish this, primers should be designed in order to have comparable melting temperatures and yield amplified DNA fragments of similar lengths.
5. Standard agarose gel electrophoresis can be employed to check that the amplification reactions have been successful and that amplicons of the expected size have been produced. However, when the MLST scheme is fully developed and routinely applied on a large scale, only occasional verification will be necessary.
6. The same primers are used for both the PCR amplification and sequencing reactions. Therefore, it is important that only a single DNA fragment be amplified. The PCR conditions may need to be optimized if more than one fragment is observed in an electrophoresis control gel.
7. Sequence information from both forward and reverse DNA strands of an amplified PCR product should be obtained and used to compile the final accurate consensus sequence. Discrepancies between the forward- and reverse-strand sequences should be resolved by referring to the original electrophoretograms. Only sequencing chromatograms of good quality are acceptable for MLST. The sequencing reactions are easily performed with commercial kits that contain all of the necessary components. A variety of commercial instruments is available for the sequencing of the PCR products. In most cases, they are capillary based and generally operated by "in-house" central sequencing facilities. Commercial companies also offer sequencing services.
8. Although the exact start and stop positions are defined for each locus (Tables 1 and 2), it may be useful to import a known allele for each locus to make trimming easier by comparison
9. Eventually, although it seems to be a rare event, some leptospires may present nonstandard length alleles for some loci. For example, Boonsilp et al. detected two *L. borgpetersenii* isolates with a 78 bp deletion in *caiB* locus [4]. Also, Ahmed et al. detected two *L. interrogans* isolates with a deletion of three nucleotides in the *lipL32* sequence [5].

10. The 6 L MLST scheme is not associated with a public database and website, and therefore the comparative phylogenetic analysis of novel sequences using this scheme requires the download and storage of related sequences from public databases (e.g., NCBI-GenBank) and its offline analysis using dedicated software. Nevertheless, an increasing number of sequences are available for analysis, while an ongoing genome sequencing project will provide additional loci from virtually all serovars. For example, Nalam et al. [9] made available the 6 L loci sequences for a global collection of 271 isolates obtained from a diverse array of hosts and geographic regions.
11. In addition to genotyping of leptospiral isolates, both the 6 L and 7 L MLST scheme can be used to assign genetic species to the same isolates. Isolates of a same pathogenic *Leptospira* species clustered together in the phylogenetic analysis of concatenated loci sequences.
12. A website supporting the sequence analysis of the 7 L MSLT scheme was launched at the time of publication, http://leptospira.mlst.net, which is regularly maintained and updated [2, 4]. Representative isolates of each ST are recorded in a downloadable spreadsheet. This is an easy-to-use online resource, providing tools for comparison of a given strain with all of the other strains in the database. On completion of the 7 L MLST scheme for an isolate, and after submission of the data to the supporting website (http://leptospira.mlst.net), the result is the assignment of an ST to that isolate (e.g., ST50) that is underlain by the allelic profile for the seven loci (i.e., 6, 8, 2, 2, 9, 7, 5 for ST50) (the order of the loci is *glmU-pntA-sucA-tpiA-pfkB-mreA-caiB*). If the allele sequence is novel, all sequences should be checked against the closest alleles in the database, and, if necessary, the original data should be rechecked. If the new allele is confirmed, the novel information should be submitted to the curator for updating the database.
13. The utility of the 7 L MLST scheme, based in ST analysis, was recently demonstrated by providing confirmatory evidence for the role of rodents as major maintenance hosts for *L. interrogans* and bovines as major maintenance hosts for *L. borgpetersenii* and *L. weilii* and was able to identify relatedness between STs in specific geographic regions [4].
14. Leptospires belonging to the same serovar may present unrelated STs, meaning that serovar is a very limited indicator of genetic relatedness. Serovars can vary within a given clone or lineage, which may be most likely due to horizontal gene transfer of genes encoding the surface determinants that confer serovar designation [4].

15. Although the ST assignment to isolates is useful for genotyping, relationships between different STs are not immediately apparent from these notations. One option for showing relationships between STs is to construct phylogenetic trees that show the relationships between isolates. For this, the allele sequences for all seven loci of each strain are compiled in a series, and the resulting concatamers are then compared pairwise and analyzed with appropriate sequence analysis software and algorithms.

References

1. Ahmed N, Devi SM, Valverde Mde L et al (2006) Multilocus sequence typing method for identification and genotypic classification of pathogenic *Leptospira* species. Ann Clin Microbiol Antimicrob 5:28
2. Thaipadungpanit J, Wuthiekanun V, Chierakul W et al (2007) A dominant clone of *Leptospira interrogans* associated with an outbreak of human leptospirosis in Thailand. PLoS Negl Trop Dis 1:e56
3. Leon A, Pronost S, Fortier G et al (2010) Multilocus sequence analysis for typing *Leptospira interrogans* and *Leptospira kirschneri*. J Clin Microbiol 48:581–585
4. Boonsilp S, Thaipadungpanit J, Amornchai P et al (2013) A single multilocus sequence typing (MLST) scheme for seven pathogenic *Leptospira* species. PLoS Negl Trop Dis 7:e1954
5. Ahmed A, Thaipadungpanit J, Boonsilp S et al (2011) Comparison of two multilocus sequence based genotyping schemes for *Leptospira* species. PLoS Negl Trop Dis 5:e1374
6. Jeanmougin F, Thompson JD, Gouy M et al (1998) Multiple sequence alignment with Clustal X. Trends Biochem Sci 23:403–405
7. Tamura K, Peterson D, Peterson N et al (2011) MEGA5: Molecular evolutionary genetics analysis using maximum likelihood, evolutionary distance, and maximum parsimony methods. Mol Biol Evol 28:2731–2739
8. Guindon S, Gascuel O (2003) A simple, fast, and accurate algorithm to estimate large phylogenies by maximum likelihood. Syst Biol 52:696–704
9. Nalam K, Ahmed A, Devi SM et al (2010) Genetic affinities within a large global collection of pathogenic *Leptospira*: Implications for strain identification and molecular epidemiology. PLoS One 5:e12637

Chapter 26

Single-Nucleotide Polymorphism Discrimination Using High-Resolution Melting Analysis for the Genotyping of *Bacillus anthracis*

Sylviane Derzelle

Abstract

High-resolution melting (HRM) is a post-PCR technique that determines with high precision the melt profile of PCR products using a new generation of double-stranded DNA-binding dyes and accurate fluorescence data acquisition over small temperature increments. The method can be used to interrogate small sets of single-nucleotide polymorphisms (SNPs). Here, we describe a simple and cost-effective HRM-based method for the screening of 14 phylogenetically informative SNPs within the genome of *Bacillus anthracis* that subtype the species into 13 major sublineages or subgroups. Fourteen monoplex and seven duplex SNP-discrimination assays have been designed. We detail the parameters most important for the successful application of HRM for *B. anthracis* genotyping.

Key words High-resolution melting (HRM), Single-nucleotide polymorphism (SNP), Genotyping, Phylogeny, Discrimination, Diversity, *Bacillus anthracis*

1 Introduction

Bacillus anthracis, the etiological agent of anthrax, is a spore-forming, Gram-positive bacterium belonging to the *B. cereus* group. Although all mammals are known to be susceptible to anthrax, the bacterium primarily affects wild and domesticated herbivores, causing acute, often fatal disease. Transmission to animals typically occurs through the gastrointestinal tract. Ruminants become infected by ingestion of soil-borne spores while browsing or grazing [1]. Anthrax has been one of the infectious diseases with major mortality among livestock for centuries. It is nowadays considered as a sporadic disease in much of Western Europe, Northern America, and Australia, but anthrax remains endemic in many countries and particularly in Africa [2–4].

B. anthracis is a monomorphic pathogen with extremely low genetic variability [5, 6]. Due to this lack of diversity, only modern molecular characterization techniques with high discrimination

Mónica V. Cunha and João Inácio (eds.), *Veterinary Infection Biology: Molecular Diagnostics and High-Throughput Strategies*, Methods in Molecular Biology, vol. 1247, DOI 10.1007/978-1-4939-2004-4_26, © Springer Science+Business Media New York 2015

power such as multiple-locus variable-number tandem repeat analysis (MLVA) and genome-wide single-nucleotide polymorphism (SNP) analyses are effective to differentiate strains. SNPs are evolutionarily stable markers that make them valuable for broadly defining major phylogenetic divisions [7]. The analysis of a set of 14 diagnostic SNPs (termed canonical SNPs or canSNPs) is currently used to classify *B. anthracis* into three lineages (A, B, and C) and 13 distinct sublineages or groups (e.g., C.Br.A1055, B.Br.001/002, B.Br.KrugerB, B.Br.CNEVA, A.Br.001/002, A.Br.Ames, A.Br.Australia94, A.Br.003/004, A.Br.Vollum, A.Br. 005/006, A.Br.Western North America, and A.Br.008/009 that can be further subdivided into A.Br.008/011 and A.Br.011/009 subgroups) (Fig. 1) [8, 9].

Cost is an important issue for all diagnostic assays. In this respect, high-resolution DNA melting analysis (HRM) has become an attractive real-time technology. HRM techniques can determine with high precision the melt profile of PCR products using a new generation of double-stranded DNA-binding dyes and accurate fluorescence data acquisition over small temperature increments (commonly in 0.2 °C increments) [10]. HRM is an ideal format for scoring a small number of SNPs, with minimal cost and time requirements for new assay development. Two standard primers are used to amplify short segments flanking each SNP. The melt profile of the resulting amplicon is characteristic of its GC content in which a substitution of a G or C to an A or T reduces the melting temperature (*Tm*), while a substitution of an A or T to a G or C increases the *Tm*. The turnaround time for a run and the follow-on data analysis requires less than 2 h. Based on its simplicity, low cost, nondestructive nature, high sensitivity, and specificity, the popularity of HRM analysis has grown considerably in the last few years.

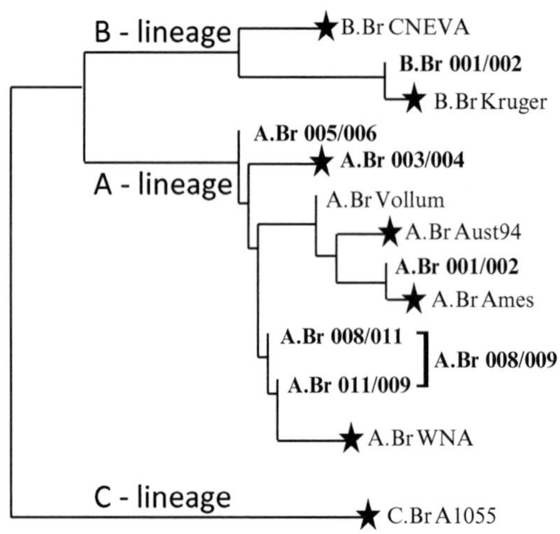

Fig. 1 Phylogeny of the major groups (in *bold*) and sublineages (marked by *stars*) of *B. anthracis* (modified from [8] and [9])

HRM is superior in terms of cost-effectiveness, ease of use, and speed of development compared to alternative SNP-interrogation approaches on real-time technologies, i.e., dual-probe TaqMan PCR assays [11–13] and mismatch amplification mutation assays (MAMA) [14, 15]. TaqMan-minor groove-binding allelic discrimination assays can be cost-prohibitive in studies interested only in small-scale SNP screening, requiring two sequence-specific fluorescently labeled probes. Based on allele-specific (AS) primers, MAMA is another cheap technique. The labeling of AS-forward primers with distinct GC-clamp enables facile differentiation of AS-PCR products through melt curve analysis (Melt-MAMA) [14], agarose gel electrophoresis [15], or capillary electrophoresis [16]. However, MAMA traditionally suffers from high rates of assay design failures and knowledge gaps on assay robustness [15].

Here, we describe 14 monoplex and seven duplex canonical SNP-based discrimination assays that coupled with HRM analysis have the potential to differentiate *Bacillus anthracis* strains into 13 major sublineages or subgroups.

2 Materials

2.1 DNA Preparation

1. Template DNA(s): 5–10 ng genomic DNA. Use template DNA suitable for PCR in terms of purity, concentration, and absence of PCR inhibitors (*see* **Note 1**). Use the same amount of template in each reaction (*see* **Note 2**).
2. Control DNA(s): at least one reference strain of known canSNP genotype has to be used as melt curve standard to ensure that the correct allele is called (*see* **Note 3**).
3. Sterile 0.22 μm filter units (optional). DNA suspensions can be microfiltered on 0.22 μm micro-column for 2 min at 6,000 to 10,000 × g for removal of any live forms of *B. anthracis*.

2.2 PCR–HRM Mix

1. HRM Master Mix: ready-to-use reaction mixes for PCR–HRM are available from various suppliers (*see* **Note 4**). Store at −15 to −25 °C. Keep away from light. Once the kit is opened, avoid repeated freezing and thawing: the Master Mix may be stored up to 4 weeks at +2 to +8 °C. Commercial kits usually include 25 mM $MgCl_2$ stock solution and a Master Mix containing *Taq* DNA polymerase (*see* **Note 5**), reaction buffer, dNTP (*see* **Note 6**), and HRM-compatible saturating fluorescent dye.
2. PCR-grade H_2O: ultrapure water prepared by purifying deionized water, nuclease-free.

Table 1
Set of 14 canonical SNPs and primer sequences

canSNP name		canSNP[a] location	Base change	Forward and reverse primers (5′-3′)	Size (bp)	Duplex concentration	Pair n°
A.Br.001	BA1	182106	T to C	GTGGTAAGGCAAGCGGAAC ACGGTTTCCCTTTATCATCG	76	0.2 µM	1
A.Br.002	BA2	947760	G to A	GCAGAAGGAGCAAGTAATGTTATAGGT CCTAAAATCGATAAAGCGACTGC	62	0.15 µM	2
A.Br.003	BA3	1493157	A to G	AAAGGAATTTAGATTTTCGTGTCG ATAAAAACCTCCTTTTCTACCTCA	58	0.2 µM	3
A.Br.004	BA4	3600659	T to C	ATCGCCGTCATACTTTGGAA GGAATTGGTGGAGCTATGGA	53	0.15 µM	3
A.Br.006	BA5	162509	C to A	GCGTTTTTAAGTTCATCATACCC ATGTTGTTGATCATTCCATCG	54	0.2 µM	4
A.Br.007	BA6	266439	T to C	TTACAAGGTGGTAGTATTCGAGCTG TTGGTAACGAGACGATAAACTGAA	67	0.2 µM	4
A.Br.008	BA7	3947248	T to G	CCAAACGGTGAAAAAGTTACAAA GCAACTACGCTATACGTTTTAGATGG	80	0.2 µM	5
A.Br.009	BA8	2589823	A to G	AATCGGCCACTGTTTTTGAAC AGGTATATTAACTGCGGATGAT	55	0.25 µM	5
B.Br.001	BA9	1455279	T to C	GCACGGTCATAAAAGAAATCG TGTTCAAAAGGTTCGGATATGA	75	0.2 µM	2
B.Br.002	BA10	1056740	G to T	GCACCTTCTGTGTTCGTTGTT TTCACCGAATGGAGGAGAAG	68	0.15 µM	1
B.Br.003	BA11	1494269	G to A	ATTCGCATAGAAGCAGATGAGC TCAAGTTCATAACGAACCATAACG	59	0.2 µM	6
B.Br.004	BA12	69952	T to C	TGCTTGGGTAACCTTCTTTACTT AGAATAAAATGAAGATAATGACAAACG	62	0.3 µM	6
A/B.Br.001	BA13	3697886	A to G	ATTCCAATCGCTGCACTCTT CCCCGATAATTTTCACAAAGC	59	0.2 µM	7
A.Br.011	BA14	2552486	G to A	CGAATTCCCGCTGAAAATAA AAAATCGGAATTGAAGCAGGA	50	0.2 µM	7

[a]Localization on the *Bacillus anthracis* str. Ames Ancestor chromosome (accession no. NC_003997.3)

3. Oligonucleotide primers set (*see* **Note 7**): 100 μM stock solutions diluted in ultrapure water (*see* primer sequences in Table 1). Store at −15 to −25 °C. Primer purification by HPLC is not necessary.

2.3 Equipment

1. A real-time PCR detection system with excellent thermal control and uniformity is important.
2. HRM-dedicated software capable of performing melt profile normalization to discriminate the fine melt profile differences generated from small sequence variations such as SNPs.
3. Standard swing-bucket centrifuge containing a rotor for multiwell plates.

3 Methods

3.1 Preparation of DNA Samples and Biosafety Procedures

Bacillus anthracis is a class 3 pathogen and should be manipulated in a BSL3 laboratory. All security rules and hygiene precautions should be applied during DNA preparation steps (including the elimination of infectious waste).

Viability testing should be systematically performed to assess the complete removal of live forms of *B. anthracis* from DNA samples so that subsequent PCR–HRM analysis could be carried out safely at lower levels of biocontainment (*see* **Note 8**).

3.2 Assay Design

HRM primers have been designed to amplify very small amplicons (50–80 bp) around each SNP to maximize the differences in melting temperature the SNP confers (*see* **Note 9**).

3.3 Real-Time PCR Amplification

1. Using monoplex assays:
   (a) Prepare 14 distinct PCR reaction mixtures for all samples (including template and control DNAs). The total PCR volume is 10 μl per reaction (*see* **Note 10**).
   (b) Mix 0.2 μl of both forward and reverse primers (10 μM work solution) (*see* **Note 11**), 5 μl of Master Mix (2×), 1.2 μl of $MgCl_2$ (3 mM) (*see* **Note 12**), and 2.4 μl of ultrapure water.
2. Using duplex assays:
   (a) Prepare 7 distinct PCR reaction mixtures for all samples.
   (b) Adjust concentration of the two pairs of primers used in each reaction mix as specified in Table 1 (from 0.15 μM to 0.3 μM final) in order to amplify the two coupled canSNP loci with similar efficiency (*see* **Note 13**).
3. Aliquot 9 μl of each monoplex or duplex reaction mix to wells and add 1 μl of template (or control) DNA.
4. Centrifuge the samples prior to the run to remove air bubbles.

5. Run the amplification and HRM steps using the following thermocycling parameters: 95 °C for 10 min, followed by 35 cycles consisting of 10 s at 95 °C, 10 s at 58 °C, and 10 s at 72 °C (*see* **Note 14**). After an additional denaturation (at 95 °C for 1 min) and cooling (to 50 °C for 1 min) steps, melt curves are generated by heating from 65 °C to 90 °C with fluorescence data acquisition at 0.025 °C/s increments (*see* **Note 15**).

3.4 Melt Curve Analysis

The standard workflow to analyze melt curve data and identify changes in the shape of the curve has four basic steps:

1. Check for aberrant amplification plots and eliminate negative samples, i.e., samples with low fluorescence signals or late amplification that lack a prominent melt curve. Results that do not satisfy amplification cutoffs are assigned as no data results (*see* **Note 16**).

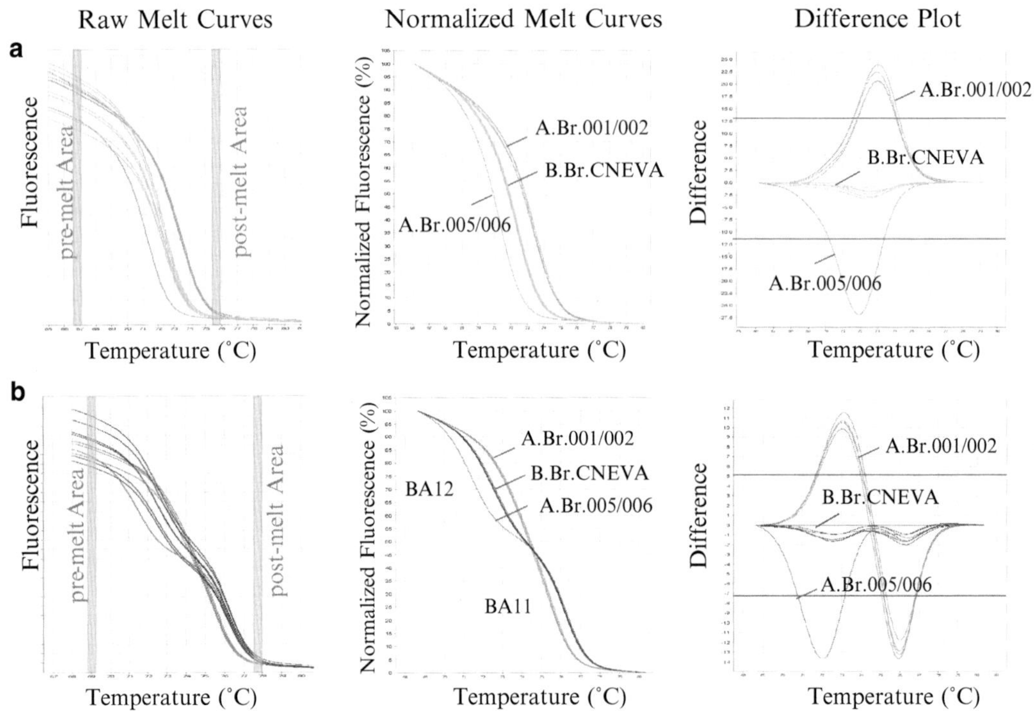

Fig. 2 Representative melt curves and HRM difference plots obtained for three canSNP genotypes (B.Br.CNEVA, A.Br.005/006, and A.Br.001/002) by HRM using the canSNP B.Br.004 (BA12) singleplex assay (**a**) or B.Br.003 and B.Br.004 (pair BA11 and BA12) duplex assays (**b**). Data and plots were produced by the ViiA7 instrument using the ViiA7 v1.2. HRM software (Life Technologies)

2. Normalize the raw melt curve data by setting the pre-melt (initial fluorescence) and post-melt (final fluorescence) signals of all samples to uniform values (*see* Fig. 2). Select manually areas before and after the melt phase on the dissociation curves. Pre-melt fluorescence intensities are then automatically set to a relative value of 100 % by the software, while post-melt signals are set to a relative value of 0 %.
3. Do not perform any temperature (*x*-axis) shifting to avoid superimposition of both alleles. A default temp shift threshold of 5 % to all data is automatically applied by some software. This threshold can be set manually to a different value (zero) (*see* **Note 17**).
4. A difference plot is automatically generated by the software to help clustering samples into groups that have similar melt profiles (*see* Fig. 2). For each temperature point, the average value of a reference curve is calculated and subsequently subtracted from each sample's normalized relative fluorescence unit (RFU) value. The curve used as reference can be modified.

3.5 canSNP Genotype Assignment

1. The cluster detection settings of HRM software include melt curve shape sensitivity (*see* **Note 18**) and *Tm* difference threshold. Adjust empirically the cluster detection settings so that all samples sharing the same allele are called "same" and the remaining ones are denoted as different by the software.
2. On average, differences in *Tm* ranging from 0.7 to about 1 °C are observed between the two allelic states (*see* Table 2). Melt curves are therefore usually considered the same as the defined control if the melting temperature is different by less than 0.5 °C.
3. Alleles can also be determined as same or different by a difference cutoff in the difference graph relative to the sample of interest (*see* Fig. 2). The relative fluorescence unit (RFU) cutoffs in the difference plot have been empirically estimated to 10–15 RFU. But variations among runs may be observed. These variations or errors are sometimes higher than the chosen cutoff for the differential analysis.
4. Use the 14 canSNP profiles (*see* Table 2) to ultimately classify samples into their corresponding canSNP sublineage or subgroup.
5. Any sample with aberrant *Tm* requires further analysis by sequencing. Discrepancies between observed and expected results may suggest unexpected sequence variability at the canSNP locus.

Table 2
canSNP signatures defining *B. anthracis* sublineages and subgroups and representative melting temperatures (*Tm*) for each SNP allele obtained by HRM

canSNP name		Mean *Tm* (°C)		canSNP sublineage													
		A/T allele	C/G allele	C.Br.A1055	B.Br.KrugerB	B.Br.001/002	B.Br.CNEVA	A.Br.Ames	A.Br.001/002	A.Br.Aust94	A.Br.003/004	A.Br.Vollum	A.Br.005/006	A.Br.008/009	A.Br.008/011	A.Br.011/009	A.Br.WNA
A.Br.001	BA1	75.6	76.4	T	T	T	T	**C**	T	T	T	T	T	T	T	T	T
A.Br.002	BA2	77.5	78.3	G	G	G	G	**A**	**A**	G	G	G	G	G	G	G	G
A.Br.003	BA3	72.0	72.9	A	A	A	A	**G**	**G**	**G**	A	A	A	A	A	A	A
A.Br.004	BA4	76.6	77.6	T	T	T	T	**C**	**C**	**C**	**C**	T	T	T	T	T	T
A.Br.006	BA5	76.4	77.3	C	C	C	C	**A**	**A**	**A**	**A**	**A**	**A**	**A**	**A**	**A**	**A**
A.Br.007	BA6	73.9	74.9	T	T	T	T	T	T	T	T	**C**	T	T	T	T	T
A.Br.008	BA7	75.0	75.9	T	T	T	T	T	T	T	T	T	T	**G**	**G**	**G**	**G**
A.Br.009	BA8	78.3	nd	A	A	A	A	A	A	A	A	A	A	A	A	A	**G**
B.Br.001	BA9	74.6	nd	T	**C**	T	T	T	T	T	T	T	T	T	T	T	T
B.Br.002	BA10	77.1	78.3	G	**T**	**T**	G	G	G	G	G	G	G	G	G	G	G
B.Br.003	BA11	75.5	76.2	G	**A**	**A**	**A**	G	G	G	G	G	G	G	G	G	G
B.Br.004	BA12	72.5	73.4	T	T	T	**C**	T	T	T	T	T	tT[a]	T	T	T	T
A/B.Br.001	BA13	74.5	nd	**G**	A	A	A	A	A	A	A	A	A	A	A	A	A
A.Br.011	BA14	76.0	77.0	G	G	G	G	G	G	G	G	G	G	G	G	**A**	**A**

canSNPs that define a particular sublineage or subgroup are underlined and the corresponding allele is indicated in bold. nd: not determined

[a]*Tm* value of 71.5 °C (tT) instead of 72.5 °C (cT) due to a second SNP (C to T) located 5′ to the B.Br.004 canSNP in strains affiliated to the A.Br.005/006 subgroup

4 Notes

1. The following points should be considered when preparing DNA for HRM:
   (a) Use ideally the same extraction procedure to prepare all DNA samples to be analyzed via HRM. This eliminates any subtle differences that might be introduced by the reagent components in the final elution buffers.
   (b) Quantify all DNA samples and adjust to the same concentration.

(c) Target sample purity with A260/280 and A260/230 ratios in the range of 1.8–2.2 and 1.6–2.4, respectively, is recommended. Poor-quality samples may result in high Ct values and noisy HRM results.

(d) The EDTA concentration should be minimized in DNA solution to avoid interference with the activity of some enzymes used in downstream reactions, particularly when at high concentration (>0.5 mM). Optimally, DNA should be in sterile deionized water or 10 mM Tris–HCl (pH 8.0) solution.

2. Standardizing the amount of template DNAs is one means of minimizing reaction-to-reaction variability. The recommended amount is 5–30 nanograms of input template per reaction, which should produce amplification plots with a threshold or quantification cycle value of no more than 30 cycles. Products that amplify late due to limited starting template amount, template degradation, or PCR inhibition may typically produce variable HRM results due to amplification artifacts.

3. HRM assays involve comparing melt profiles from independent PCR reactions. Although the relative temperature calibration is extremely accurate, absolute temperature calibration can vary between runs and instruments (by up to 0.5 °C). A reference sample of known genotype is therefore needed for allele calling in each run.

4. Excellent results have been reported using the LightCycler® 480 High-Resolution Melting Master Mix (Roche Diagnostics).

5. Hot-start *Taq* DNA polymerases are strongly recommended for HRM applications to improve the specificity and sensitivity of PCR. It minimizes the formation of nonspecific amplification products at the beginning of the reaction.

6. dNTP mix with dUTP instead of dTTP can be used for prevention of carry-over contamination in PCR in diagnostic laboratories under quality assurance (optional). Pretreatment of successive PCR mixtures with uracil-DNA glycosylase (UNG) is suitable to avoid preexisting amplicons in PCR mixture. UNG cleaves uracil-glycosidic bonds in DNA, creating alkali-sensitive abasic sites where a deoxyuridylate residue has been incorporated. The resulting abasic sites are next hydrolized by heat treatment during the initial PCR denaturation step and cannot serve as PCR templates. Briefly, add UNG to the PCR mix prior to amplification and incubate the reaction mixture for 2 min at 50 °C (or 10 min at 40 °C) to destroy any contaminating template. The heat-labile UNG is inactivated by performing the 10 min preincubation step (initial denaturation) at 95 °C.

7. Primer pairs have been designed to have annealing temperatures around 60 °C and as little self or cross complementarity as possible (particularly in the 3′ end).

8. Viability testing can be performed by spreading an aliquot of each DNA preparation on blood agar Petri dish and incubation at 37 °C for 18–24 h. In case of growth, perform an additional microfiltration and repeat viability steps.
9. Analyzing short amplicons (50 pb) is preferable since it increases the statistical confidence in calling particular SNPs between samples. The SNP should be in the middle of the amplicon, close to the 3′ end of primers.
10. According to the instrument used, PCR can be performed in reaction volume of less than 10 μl to reduce the cost per analysis. However, it is crucial to minimize reaction-to-reaction variability in HRM assays.
11. Relatively low primer concentrations (less than 300 nM final) are used in the experimental reactions to minimize primer-dimer formation.
12. Salts affect the shape and *Tm* of melt profiles. It is therefore important that the amount of Mg^{2+} in the reaction mix is as uniform as possible for all samples. The optimal $MgCl_2$ concentration that ensures both the specificity and robustness of the PCR depends on the dye used. It may vary from 1.5 to 3.5 mM. As a general rule, lower $MgCl_2$ concentration will give more specific PCR amplification and slightly lower overall *Tm*.
13. In duplex HRM format, input amplicons concentration must be normalized to get consistent SNP genotyping data. Primer concentrations are adjusted so as to yield melting peaks of equivalent height for both amplicons. Correct automatic grouping of both alleles by the software is, however, often problematic and needs empirical adjustments to compensate for variability in PCR efficiency.
14. A number of 35 cycles are suitable for most assays.
15. The melting pre-hold step (50 °C) is optional. It ensures that all PCR products have reassociated and encourages heteroduplex formation. The melt program should start at least 10 °C before and end at least 10 °C after the expected *Tm* values.
16. Successful HRM analysis is highly dependent on the quality of the amplicons being compared. Ensure that only target amplicons of interest are being amplified. Examine amplification data for abnormal amplification curve shapes. A curve with a jagged log-linear phase or one that reaches a low signal plateau compared to other reactions can indicate poor amplification or a fluorescence signal that is too low for analysis. HRM from such samples can cause low resolution and poor or inconsistent classification of samples. Discard these samples [17]. Analyzing real-time PCR amplification data prior to HRM analysis can be extremely useful when troubleshooting HRM experiments.

17. Analyzing the data in temperature-shifted view facilitates detection of heterozygotes. Heterozygotes are typically characterized by a change in melt curve shape (y-axis displacement) generated from base-pairing mismatches resulting from destabilized heteroduplex annealing between some of the wild-type and variant strands. As bacteria are haploid, only homozygote templates are analyzed in this method. Homozygotic SNPs are distinguished by the temperature (x-axis) shift of their melt curves, which is easier to see in the normalized data. Both alleles have similar curve shapes but different *Tm*.

18. The sensitivity parameter, which influences the stringency with which melt profiles are classified into different groups, can be adjusted in some software so that all samples sharing the same allele are called "same" and the remaining ones are denoted as different by the software. A high sensitivity value generally produces more groups than a low value.

References

1. Turnbull PC (2002) Anthrax history, disease and ecology. In: Koehler TM (ed) Anthrax, vol 271, Springer-Verlag. Berlin, Germany, pp 1–19
2. Hugh-Jones M (1999) 1996-97 Global Anthrax Report. J Appl Microbiol 87:189–191
3. Fasanella A, Galante D, Garofolo G et al (2010) Anthrax undervalued zoonosis. Vet Microbiol 140:318–331
4. Derzelle S, Thierry S (2013) Genetic Diversity of *Bacillus anthracis* in Europe: Genotyping Methods in Forensic and Epidemiologic Investigations. Biosecur Bioterror 11:S166–S176
5. Keim P, Gruendike JM, Klevytska AM et al (2009) The genome and variation of *Bacillus anthracis*. Mol Aspects Med 30:397–405
6. Keim P, Price LB, Klevytska AM et al (2000) Multiple-locus variable-number tandem repeat analysis reveals genetic relationships within *Bacillus anthracis*. J Bacteriol 182:2928–2936
7. Pearson T, Busch JD, Ravel J et al (2004) Phylogenetic discovery bias in *Bacillus anthracis* using single-nucleotide polymorphisms from whole-genome sequencing. Proc Natl Acad Sci U S A 101:13536–13541
8. Van Ert MN, Easterday WR, Huynh LY et al (2007) Global genetic population structure of *Bacillus anthracis*. PLoS One 2:e461
9. Marston CK, Allen CA, Beaudry J et al (2011) Molecular epidemiology of anthrax cases associated with recreational use of animal hides and yarn in the United States. PLoS One 6:e28274
10. Erali M, Voelkerding KV, Wittwer CT (2008) High resolution melting applications for clinical laboratory medicine. Exp Mol Pathol 85:50–58
11. Hurtle W, Bode E, Kulesh DA et al (2004) Detection of the *Bacillus anthracis gyrA* gene by using a minor groove binder probe. J Clin Microbiol 42:179–185
12. Easterday WR, Van Ert MN, Simonson TS et al (2005) Use of single nucleotide polymorphisms in the *plcR* gene for specific identification of *Bacillus anthracis*. J Clin Microbiol 43:1995–1997
13. Satterfield BC, Kulesh DA, Norwood DA et al (2007) Tentacle Probes: differentiation of difficult single-nucleotide polymorphisms and deletions by presence or absence of a signal in real-time PCR. Clin Chem 53: 2042–2050
14. Easterday WR, Van Ert MN, Zanecki S et al (2005) Specific detection of *Bacillus anthracis* using a TaqMan mismatch amplification mutation assay. Biotechniques 38:731–735
15. Birdsell DN, Pearson T, Price EP et al (2012) Melt analysis of mismatch amplification mutation assays (Melt-MAMA): a functional study of a cost-effective SNP genotyping assay in bacterial models. PLoS One 7:e32866
16. Price EP, Matthews MA, Beaudry JA et al (2010) Cost-effective interrogation of single nucleotide polymorphisms using the mismatch amplification mutation assay and capillary electrophoresis. Electrophoresis 31:3881–3888
17. Krypuy M, Newnham GM, Thomas DM et al (2006) High resolution melting analysis for the rapid and sensitive detection of mutations in clinical samples: KRAS codon 12 and 13 mutations in non-small cell lung cancer. BMC Cancer 6:295

Chapter 27

Clustered Regularly Interspaced Short Palindromic Repeats (CRISPRs) Analysis of Members of the *Mycobacterium tuberculosis* Complex

Ana Botelho, Ana Canto, Célia Leão, and Mónica V. Cunha

Abstract

Typical CRISPR (*c*lustered, *r*egularly *i*nterspaced, *s*hort *p*alindromic *r*epeat) regions are constituted by short direct repeats (DRs), interspersed with similarly sized non-repetitive spacers, derived from transmissible genetic elements, acquired when the cell is challenged with foreign DNA. The analysis of the structure, in number and nature, of CRISPR spacers is a valuable tool for molecular typing since these *loci* are polymorphic among strains, originating characteristic signatures. The existence of CRISPR structures in the genome of the members of *Mycobacterium tuberculosis* complex (MTBC) enabled the development of a genotyping method, based on the analysis of the presence or absence of 43 oligonucleotide spacers separated by conserved DRs. This method, called spoligotyping, consists on PCR amplification of the DR chromosomal region and recognition after hybridization of the spacers that are present. The workflow beneath this methodology implies that the PCR products are brought onto a membrane containing synthetic oligonucleotides that have complementary sequences to the spacer sequences. Lack of hybridization of the PCR products to a specific oligonucleotide sequence indicates absence of the correspondent spacer sequence in the examined strain. Spoligotyping gained great notoriety as a robust identification and typing tool for members of MTBC, enabling multiple epidemiological studies on human and animal tuberculosis.

Key words Tuberculosis, Bovine tuberculosis, Molecular typing, Direct repeats, Spoligotyping, Epidemiology

1 Introduction

*C*lustered *r*egularly *i*nterspaced *s*hort *p*alindromic *r*epeat (CRISPR) regions are present in the genome of almost all archaea and many bacteria, in association with *cas* (CRISPR-*a*ssociated *s*ystem) genes, which are involved in DNA recombination and repair [1]. The origin of *cas* in prokaryotic genomes is related with the acquisition of heritable immunity against mobile nucleic acid elements, limiting phage infection and horizontal gene transfer of plasmids [2, 3].

Mónica V. Cunha and João Inácio (eds.), *Veterinary Infection Biology: Molecular Diagnostics and High-Throughput Strategies*, Methods in Molecular Biology, vol. 1247, DOI 10.1007/978-1-4939-2004-4_27, © Springer Science+Business Media New York 2015

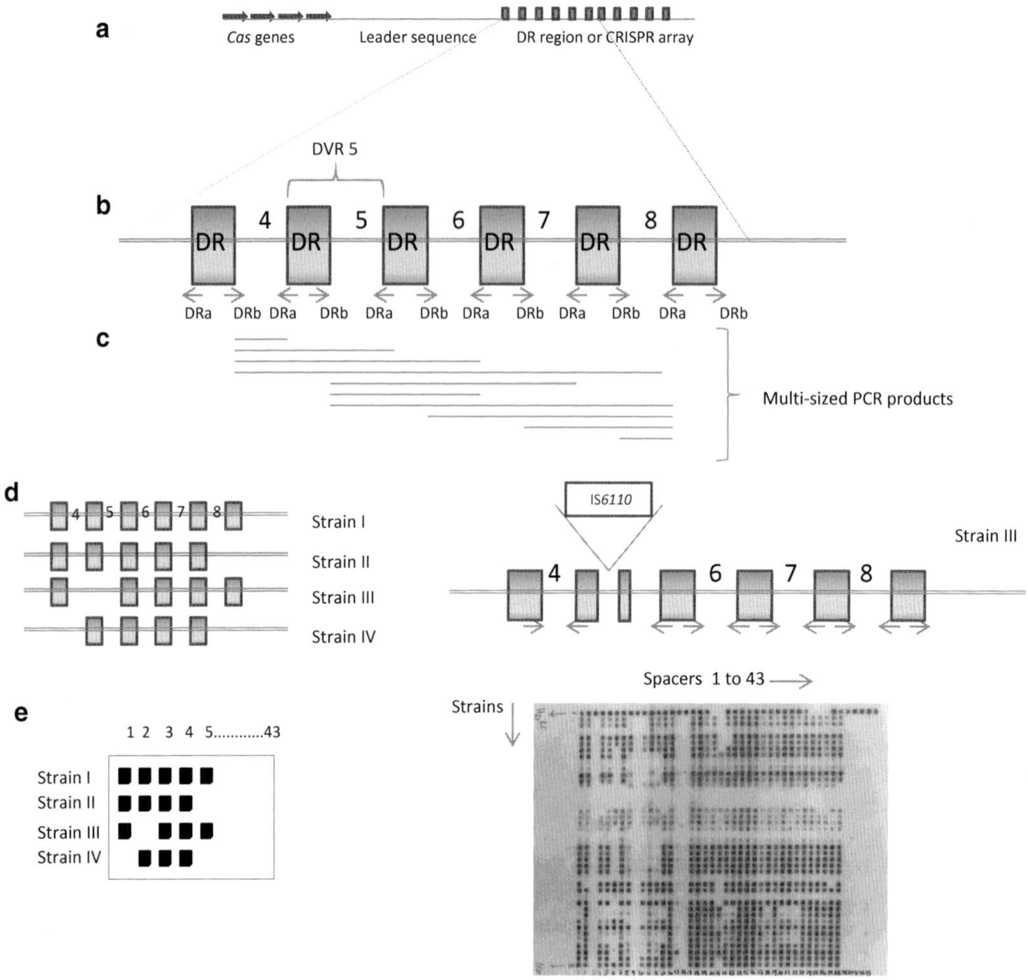

Fig. 1 Schematic structure of a CRISPR/Cas region in MTBC strains and application of the CRISPR array, to the development of the spoligotyping method, using 43 selected spacer sequences. (**a**) General structure of a CRISPR/Cas region; (**b**) structure of DR region: 0–56 copies of 36 bp direct repeats, separated by variable spacer sequences of 36–51 bp, whose order is well conserved in the genome of MTBC. Spacers, here numbered from 4 to 8. The DRs together with the adjacent spacers form the direct variant repeats (DVRs); (**c**) PCR amplification of the DR flanking spacers, using primers DRa and DRb, one of them biotin labeled, complementary to the conserved direct repeats; (**d**) five pretend patterns in the DR region and possible formation of strain III pattern by insertion of IS*6110* sequence in DVR 5, hampering the amplification of spacer 5 by loss of primer DVRb hybridization site. (**e**) Simplified spoligotyping membrane results obtained for the five strains and example of a real spoligotyping membrane. Note that the genome spacer order/number does not correspond to the membrane spacer order/number

A typical CRISPR *locus* is composed of *cas* genes, a leader sequence, and a repeat-spacer array (Fig. 1). These arrays are formed by direct repeat (DR) sequences, of 25–50 base pair (bp) long, interspersed by unique, non-repetitive spacer sequences of similar size. An explanation for the origin of new spacers could be the preferential uptake of bacteriophage DNA, as reported in *Yersinia pestis* [4], or extrachromosomal DNA. CRISPR sequences provide an adaptive, heritable record of past infections and are transcribed into CRISPR RNAs—small RNAs that target invasive nucleic acids [5, 6]. Removal or integration of particular spacers, derived from phage genomic sequences, plasmids, or other recombination event(s), to CRISPR *loci* may modify the phage-resistance phenotype of the cell [2], conferring also a high level of polymorphism to these *loci*, in different strains of the same species. The characteristics of CRISPR *loci* made them useful in biotechnological applications, such as artificial immunization against phage and genomic engineering, and in molecular epidemiology by comparison of CRISPR spacer regions in different bacterial strains, allowing for their discrimination.

The polymorphic property of CRISPR arrays, revealed by the presence or absence of certain spacers, has been used for identification and genotyping of clinical isolates of *Mycobacterium tuberculosis* [7, 8], *Streptococcus pyogenes* [9], and *Campylobacter jejuni* [10] contributing to enlighten the epidemiology of the diseases they cause.

A comprehensive and updated database, containing information about CRISPR systems in several bacterial genomes is available on http://crispr.u-psud.fr/crispr/. Convincing CRISPR structures were found in 1,251 genomes out of 2,630 analyzed so far (as of January 2014).

Within the genus *Mycobacterium*, the presence of CRISPRs structures is exclusive to members of the *Mycobacterium tuberculosis* complex (MTBC). Their number per genome varies from one (in some strains of *Mycobacterium canettii* and of *M. tuberculosis*) to four (in *M. tuberculosis* H37Rv), with an average of two CRISPRs arrays in all *M. bovis* analyzed (http://crispr.u-psud.fr/).

In MTBC strains, a CRISPR array consists of multiple 36 bp tandem DRs, with the consensus sequence TGAGGTGCGGC GTGAGCGCGGGT, interspersed by a total of 94 recognized spacers with 35–41 bp in length [11, 12]. The order and sequence of the spacers is highly conserved between strains of the MTB complex. However, the size of the DR region and, thereby, the presence of spacers differ significantly between strains. Differences have been shown to be due to deletions of spacer sequences in the DR region by transposition of the insertion sequence IS*6110* [11, 13], which is almost invariably present in the DR cluster of MTBC strains, probably driven by homologous recombination between adjacent or distant DRs [7] or by replication slippage.

Based on the nature of the DNA polymorphism in the DR cluster region, two methods of MTBC strain differentiation were developed: direct variable repeat polymerase chain reaction (DVR-PCR) [7], enabling detection and typing of individual *M. tuberculosis* strains in a single PCR, and spoligotyping (spacer oligonucleotide typing) [8]. This last method, also based on PCR coupled with

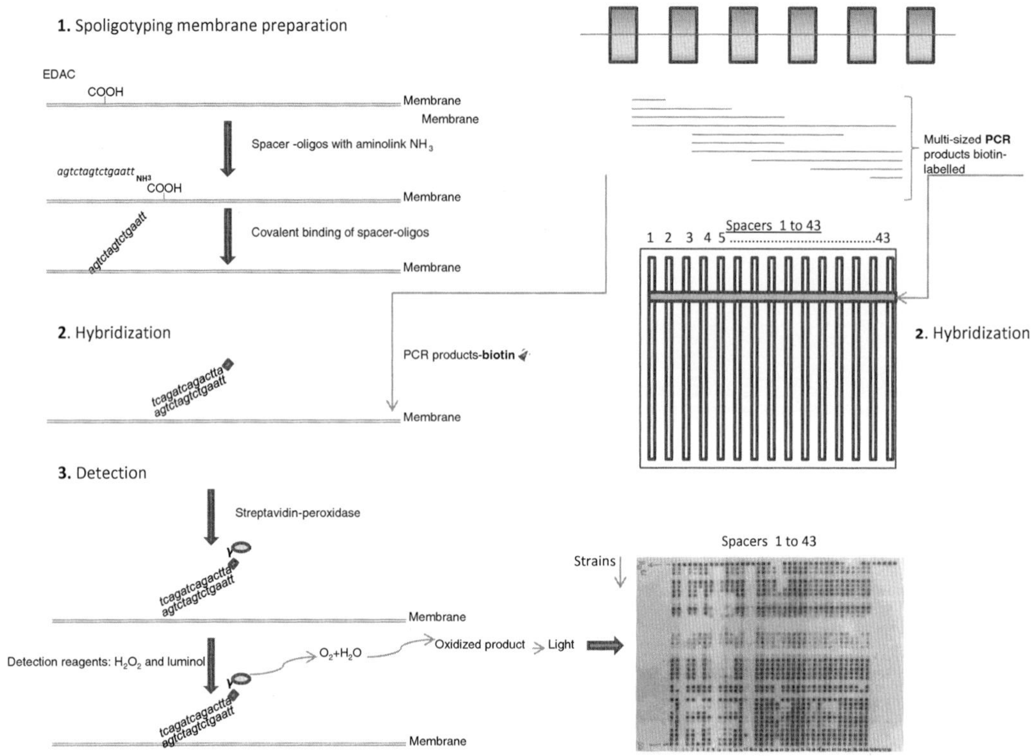

Fig. 2 Schematic basic steps of spoligotyping method. See text for details

reverse line blot hybridization, gained wide diffusion, due to its easy execution and high throughput, to assess global MTBC strain diversity. This technique consists in the amplification of the DR region using two inversely orientated primers, one of them labeled with biotin, complementary to the flanking conserved DR sequence (Figs. 1 and 2). DNA spacer sequences in between adjacent DRs and in between more distantly positioned DRs are amplified [8]. Evaluation of the presence or absence of spacers is done by reverse hybridization of the obtained PCR products with a set of selected 43-spacer oligonucleotides covalently linked to a nylon membrane (Table 1, Fig. 2), designed according to the sequences of *M. tuberculosis* H27Rv and *M. bovis* BCG P3 strains. The PCR products are applied onto the membrane in reverse orientation of the rows with the synthetic oligonucleotides. Since one of the DR primers is labeled with biotin, the detection of hybridization is done by chemiluminescence, through addition of streptavidin-peroxidase conjugate and a substrate (Fig. 2).

Spoligotyping applied to bacterial isolates is simple, robust, and highly reproducible. On the other hand, for MTBC strains containing few copies of the IS*6110* element, such as *M. bovis*, spoligotyping is generally more discriminatory than IS*6110* typing methods, and the DR region is, consequently, also more stable.

Table 1
Sequences and concentrations of the oligonucleotide probes covalently linked to the Biodyne C membrane [8]

Oligonucleotide number order	Sequence (3′-5′ amino)	Concentration (pmol/150 μl)
1	ATAGAGGGTCGCCGGTTCTGGATCA	12.5
2	CCTCATAATTGGGCGACAGCTTTTG	30.0
3	CCGTGCTTCCAGTGATCGCCTTCTA	12.5
4	ACGTCATACGCCGACCAATCATCAG	12.5
5	TTTTCTGACCACTTGTGCGGGATTA	12.5
6	CGTCGTCATTTCCGGCTTCAATTTC	12.5
7	GAGGAGAGCGAGTACTCGGGGCTGC	25.0
8	CGTGAAACCGCCCCCAGCCTCGCCG	50.0
9	ACTCGGAATCCCATGTGCTGACAGC	12.5
10	TCGACACCCGCTCTAGTTGACTTCC	15.0
11	GTGAGCAACGGCGGCGGCAACCTGG	30.0
12	ATATCTGCTGCCCGCCCGGGGAGAT	60.0
13	GACCATCATTGCCATTCCCTCTCCC	12.5
14	GGTGTGATGCGGATGGTCGGCTCGG	30.0
15	CTTGAATAACGCGCAGTGAATTTCG	30.0
16	CGAGTTCCCGTCAGCGTCGTAAATC	12.5
17	GCGCCGGCCCGCGCGGATGACTCCG	100.0
18	CATGGACCCGGGCGAGCTGCAGATG	12.5
19	TAACTGGCTTGGCGCTGATCCTGGT	12.5
20	TTGACCTCGCCAGGAGAGAAGATCA	12.5
21	TCGATGTCGATGTCCCAATCGTCGA	25.0
22	ACCGCAGACGGCACGATTGAGACAA	12.5
23	AGCATCGCTGATGCGGTCCAGCTCG	50.0
24	CCGCCTGCTGGGTGAGACGTGCTCG	50.0
25	GATCAGCGACCACCGCACCCTGTCA	25.0
26	CTTCAGCACCACCATCATCCGGCGC	12.5
27	GGATTCGTGATCTCTTCCCGCGGAT	25.0
28	TGCCCCGGCGTTTAGCGATCACAAC	12.5
29	AAATACAGGCTCCACGACACGACCA	12.5
30	GGTTGCCCCGCGCCCTTTTCCAGCC	12.5

(continued)

Table 1
(continued)

Oligonucleotide number order	Sequence (3′-5′ amino)	Concentration (pmol/150 μl)
31	TCAGACAGGTTCGCGTCGATCAAGT	12.5
32	GACCAAATAGGTATCGGCGTGTTCA	25.0
33	GACATGACGGCGGTGCCGCACTTGA	100.0
34	AAGTCACCTCGCCACACCGTCGAA	25.0
35	TCCGTACGCTCGAAACGCTTCCAAC	12.5
36	CGAAATCCAGCACCACATCCGCAGC	12.5
37	CGCGAACTCGTCCACAGTCCCCCTT	12.5
38	CGTGGATGGCGGATGCGTTGTGCGC	25.0
39	GACGATGGCCAGTAAATCGGCGTGG	25.0
40	CGCCATCTGTGCCTCATACAGGTCC	12.5
41	GGAGCTTTCCGGCTTCTATCAGGTA	12.5
42	ATGGTGGGACATGGACGAGCGCGAC	25.0
43	CGCAGAATCGCACCGGGTGCGGGAG	50.0

A hybridization profile is generated for any MTBC isolate (Fig. 1) allowing, simultaneously, its identification and genotyping, since each species has a specific spoligotype signature [14]. Such is the case of *M. bovis*, *M.canettii*, *M. caprae*, and *M. tuberculosis* (Table 2). The typical signature of most *M. bovis* strains and all *M. bovis* BCG is the absence of spacers 3, 9, 16, and 39–43 [14, 15] (Table 2).

The spoligotyping profile can be expressed as a numerical profile (binary or octal code), which simplifies storing of typing data and facilitates interlaboratory comparison. Most relevant for the global comparison of data is the existence of international spoligotyping databases: SpolDB4 [17] and Mbovis.org [18], the latter specific for *M. bovis* and other non-*M. tuberculosis* isolates, characterized by absence in the genome of RD9 (region of difference). Most spoligotype attribution codes use the international databases calls: ST (for shared types) followed by a number in *M. tuberculosis* databases or SB (for spoligotype bovis) followed by four digits in Mbovis.org database. These databases allow easy interlaboratory comparison of spoligotype patterns and contribute for the definition of the major lineages within *M. tuberculosis* and *M. bovis* strains.

In an attempt to enlarge the discriminatory power of spoligotyping, additional spacers have been evaluated for *M. bovis* [12, 19], *M. africanum* [16], and *M. caprae* [20] strains typing. However, these extended spoligotypes have had few practical applications, since other methods, such as *mycobacterial interspersed*

Table 2
Spoligotyping patterns and signatures of members of the MTBC [14, 21, 22]

MTBC species or strain	Spoligotype pattern[a]	Binary Code[b]	Spoligotype[c]	Species core spoligotype signature[d]
M. bovis BCG	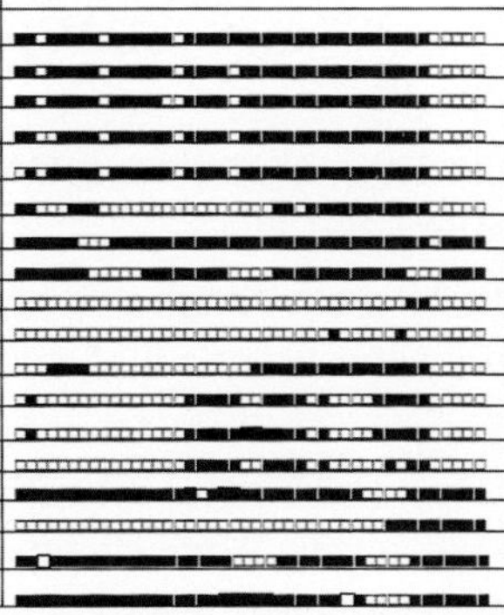	1101111101111110111111111111111111111100000	SB0120	Absence of spacers 3, 9, 16 and 39 to 43
M. bovis		1101111101111110111101111111111111111100000	SB0121	
M. bovis		1101111101111100111101111111111111111100000	SB0119	
M. bovis		1100111101111110111101111111111111111100000	SB1093	
M. bovis		0101111101111110111101111111111111111100000	SB0122	
M. bovis		1100011100000000000000001101111111111100000	SB1175	
M. africanum type 1		1111110001111111111111111111111111111101111	ST181	
M. africanum type 2		1111111000001111111110000111111111110001111	ST331	
M. microti		0000000000000000000000000000000000001100000	ST539	
M. canettii		0000000000000000000000000000010000010000000	ST592	
M. pinnipedii		0001111000000000000000011111111111111100000	ST593	
M. caprae		0100000000000000111110011110100001111100000	SB0157	Absence of spacers 1, 3 to 16 and 39 to 43
M. caprae		0100000000000000111111111110100001111100000	SB0416	
M. caprae		0000000000000000111110011110100000101100000	SB0973	
M. tuberculosis X1		1111111111111111101111111111111100001111111	SB119	
M. tuberculosis W-Beijing		0000000000000000000000000000000000111111111	ST1	
M. tuberculosis LAM1		1111111111111111111100001111111100001111111	ST20	
M. tuberculosis Haarlem 3		1111111111111111111111111111111010000111111	ST50	

[a]Filled square: presence of spacer; open square: absence of spacer

[b]1: Presence of spacer; 0: absence of spacer; underlined numbers mark how spoligotypes SB0121 and SB0119 could have derived from spoligotype SB0120 by deletion of spacers 15 and 21. Other spoligotypes could have evolved from SB0121 by deletion of other spacers: spacers 4 and 1 (double underlined) for, respectively, SB1093 and SB0122. Spacers that make the core signature are indicated in bold. Even for less common spoligotypes, like SB1175, the core spoligotype signature is maintained

[c]Shared type (ST) number or spoligotype bovis (SB) number attributed by, respectively, SpolDB4 and Mbovis.org databases

[d]Based on the consistent absence of certain spacers in all *M. bovis* and *M. caprae* strains analyzed so far

repetitive units variable number of tandem repeats (MIRU-VNTR) in conjunction with spoligotyping, proved to be the most suitable tools to increase the discriminatory power and to further differentiate strains of the MTBC [21, 22].

Provided that suitable quality control measures are adopted, the spoligotyping procedure described below, using 43 spacer analyses, should enable the identification and typing of members of the MTBC. For a self-sufficient procedure and independent from commercial membranes, we describe the in-house preparation of the spoligotyping membrane.

2 Materials

All the solutions should be freshly prepared, with ultrapure water (18.2 MΩ cm at 25 °C) and analytical grade reagents, and stored at room temperature. The stock solutions should be sterilized in autoclave at 121 °C for 15 min. The nylon membrane can be regenerated and reused up to ten times.

2.1 Solutions

2.1.1 Stock Solutions

1. 0.5 M EDTA: For 1,000 ml, weight 186.12 g of ethylenediaminetetraacetic acid (EDTA) and add half the water. Mix until complete dissolution using a magnetic stirrer and adjust to pH 8.0. Complete the volume to 1,000 ml (*see* **Note 1**).
2. 20× SSPE (w/v): Weight 35.6 g of $Na_2HPO_4.2H_2O$, 210.24 g of NaCl, and 7.4 g of EDTA for a final volume of 1,000 ml in water. Mix well and adjust to pH 7.4.

2.1.2 Working Solutions

For Membrane Preparation

1. 500 mM $NaHCO_3$ (pH 8.4): For 250 ml, weight 10.5 g of $NaHCO_3$ and dissolve in water. Mix, adjust to pH 8.4, and add water up to 250 ml.
2. 16 % (w/v) EDAC: For 10 ml, add 1.6 g of 1-ethyl-3-(3-dimethylaminopropyl) carbodiimide (EDAC) and mix with 9.4 ml of water. Store at −20 °C.
3. 100 mM NaOH: Weight 1.0 g of sodium hydroxide (NaOH) and add water up to 250 ml and mix.
4. 10 % SDS (w/v): Weight 10 g of sodium dodecyl sulfate (SDS) to a glass bottle, and add water up to a final volume of 100 ml (*see* **Note 2**).
5. 2× SSPE/0.1 % SDS (w/v): For 250 ml solution, add 25 ml of 20× SSPE to 222.5 ml of water. After stirring, carefully add 2.5 ml of 10 % SDS (w/v) (*see* **Note 3**).
6. 1:100 China ink diluted in 2× SSPE: For 300 μl, add 3 μl of China ink to 297 μl of 2× SSPE.
7. 20 mM EDTA: For 100 ml, add 4 ml of 0.5 M EDTA to 96 ml of water.

For Hybridization

1. 10 % (w/v) SDS: For 130 ml, add 13 g of SDS to 100 ml of water. Stir until complete dissolution using a magnetic stirrer. In a graduated cylinder, add water up to 130 ml final volume (*see* **Note 2**).
2. 2× SSPE (v/v): For 500 ml, add 50 ml of 20× SSPE to 450 ml of water.
3. 2× SSPE/0.1 % SDS: For 300 ml, add 30 ml of 20× SSPE to 267 ml of water. After stirring, carefully add 3 ml of 10 % (w/v) SDS (*see* **Note 3**).
4. 2× SSPE/0.5 % SDS: For 1,000 ml, add 100 ml of 20× SSPE to 850 ml of water. After stirring, carefully add 50 ml of 10 % SDS (*see* **Note 3**).
5. 1 % SDS: For 750 ml, add 75 ml of 10 % SDS to 675 ml of water.
6. 20 mM EDTA: For 1,000 ml, measure 40 ml of 0.5 M EDTA and add water up to 1,000 ml.

2.2 Membrane Preparation

1. Oligonucleotide probes synthesized with a 5′-end amino group (*see* **Note 4**), diluted in 150 μl of 500 mM $NaHCO_3$ pH 8.4.
2. Nylon membrane negatively charged (Biodyne C).
3. 10 ml of 16 % (w/v) EDAC.
4. 300 μl of 1:100 China ink diluted in 2× SSPE.
5. 250 ml of 100 mM NaOH.

6. 250 ml of 2× SSPE/0.1 % SDS.
7. 120 ml of 20 mM EDTA pH 8.0.
8. Ultrapure water.
9. Horizontal platform rocker.
10. Miniblotter (MN45 system).
11. Laboratory trays (about 200 × 300 mm).
12. Vacuum pump.
13. Forceps.

2.3 PCR Amplification

1. Primers DRa: 5′- biotin-GGT TTT GGG TCT GAC GAC- 3′and DRb: 5′- CCG AGA GGG GAC GGA AAC- 3′ (*see* **Note 5**).
2. 50 μl of PCR mix reaction: 1× *Taq* DNA polymerase reaction buffer, 3.5 mM $MgCl_2$, 400 μM dNTPs, 0.4 μM of each primer (DRa and DRb), 1 U of *Taq* DNA polymerase, and 2 μl of genomic DNA.
3. Positive controls: *Mycobacterium tuberculosis* H37Rv (CCUG 37357); *Mycobacterium bovis* BCG (Danish) (CCUG 27863).
4. Negative control: ultrapure water.
5. 2 % (w/v) agarose gel.
6. 1× Tris–Borate–EDTA (TBE) (*see* **Note 6**).
7. 2 % (v/v) GelRed.
8. Horizontal gel electrophoresis system.
9. Power supplies.
10. UV transilluminator.
11. Thermal cycler, 96-well format compatibility.

2.4 DNA Hybridization

1. 20 μl of amplification products diluted in 150 μl of 2× SSPE/0.1 % SDS.
2. Ice.
3. 250 ml of 2× SSPE/0.1 % SDS.
4. 1,000 ml 2× SSPE/0.5 % SDS.
5. 2.5 μl Streptavidin-peroxidase conjugate (500 U/ml).
6. 500 ml of 2× SSPE.
7. Hybridization oven with rolling bottles.
8. Thermal cycler.
9. Forceps.
10. Miniblotter (MN45 system).
11. Nylon membrane Biodyne C.
12. Vacuum pump.
13. Laboratory trays (*see* Subheading 2.2).

2.5 Detection of Hybridizing DNA

1. 10 ml ECL solution 1 from *ECL Direct Labeling and Detection System* (GE Healthcare).
2. 10 ml ECL solution 2 from *ECL Direct Labeling and Detection System* (GE Healthcare).
3. Hyperfilm ECL.
4. Hybridization roller bottles.
5. Autoradiography cassette.
6. Acetate sheet.
7. Blotting paper 3MM.
8. Laboratory trays.
9. Plastic trays.
10. Developer solution.
11. Fixer solution.
12. Red safelight in a dark room.

3 Methods

Always use gloves and forceps to manipulate the membrane.

3.1 Preparation of In-House Membrane with the 43 Oligonucleotides Covalently Linked (See Note 7)

1. Dilute each oligonucleotide probe in the recommended optimized concentrations (*see* Table 1) in 150 μl of 500 mM $NaHCO_3$ (pH 8.3).
2. Incubate the nylon membrane in a laboratory tray containing 10 ml of 16 % (v/v) EDAC solution for 10 min at room temperature to activate the membrane.
3. Discard the EDAC solution and wash the membrane with ultrapure water for 2 min, with orbital shaking.
4. With the forceps, place the membrane on top of the foam cushion of the Miniblotter system and hand-tight the screws.
5. Remove all the residual water of the membrane by aspiration with the vacuum pump (*see* **Note 8**).
6. Fill the slots of the Miniblotter with 150 μl of the 43 diluted oligonucleotide probes, in the order displayed on Table 2, leaving the first and the last slots empty (*see* **Note 9**).
7. Fill the first and the last slots of the Miniblotter with the diluted China ink.
8. Incubate for 2 min at room temperature.
9. Remove all the solutions of the slots of the Miniblotter by aspiration with the vacuum pump, by the same order in which they were filled.

10. Remove the membrane from the Miniblotter using forceps and incubate in a laboratory tray, with 250 ml of 100 mM NaOH for 8 min at room temperature with shaking.
11. Discard the solution and wash the membrane with ultrapure water at room temperature.
12. Wash the membrane with 250 ml of 2× SSPE/0.1 % SDS with gentle shaking for 5 min at 60 °C.
13. The membrane is ready to use or to store.
14. Before storing the membrane, wash it in a laboratory tray, with 100 ml of 20 mM EDTA (pH 8.0), for 15 min at room temperature with gentle shaking.
15. Remove the membrane with forceps and store at 4 °C, in a sealed plastic bag to avoid dehydration, with 10 ml of 20 mM EDTA (pH 8.0) until being used.

3.2 Sample Preparation (In a Biosafety Level 3 Facility)

1. Place 150 μl of ultrapure water in a 2 ml screw-cap tubes.
2. Using a disposable loop, collect sufficient MTBC colonies from culture medium and suspend in the water.
3. In a thermo block, incubate for 30 min at 90 °C to extract the DNA and to kill the bacteria. From this step on, the sample can be manipulated out of the P3 facilities (*see* **Note 10**).

3.3 DR Region Amplification by PCR

1. Prepare PCR reaction mix in a total volume of 50 μl per reaction. *Mycobacterium tuberculosis H37rv* (CCUG 37357) and *Mycobacterium bovis BCG* (CCUG 27863) are used as positive controls and ultrapure water as negative control.
2. Perform the amplification reactions in a thermocycler with an initial step at 96 °C for 3 min, followed by 35 cycles at 96 °C for 1 min, 55 °C for 1 min, and 72 °C for 30 s, ending with a step at 72 °C for 5 min.
3. Analyze the amplified products by electrophoresis in a 2 % (w/v) agarose gel prepared in 1× TBE buffer and stained with 2 % GelRed (*see* **Note 11**). Run the gel at 90 V for 60 min. Visualize the gel under UV light in a transilluminator.

3.4 DNA Hybridization to the Membrane (See Subheading 3.1)

All buffers should be previously warmed to the respective work temperatures, with the exception of 10 ml of 2× SSPE/0.1 % SDS and 2× SSPE that should be at room temperature. Pre-warm the hybridization oven at 60 °C.

1. Dilute 20 μl of the PCR products (maximum of 40 samples, plus two positive controls and one negative control, per membrane) in 150 μl of 2× SSPE/0.1 % SDS buffer.
2. Store the remaining PCR products at 4 °C.
3. Denature the diluted PCR products for 10 min at 99 °C in a thermocycler or in a dry bath, and cool immediately on ice.

4. Place the membrane, with forceps and held by its edges, in a laboratory tray and rinse twice in 250 ml of 2× SSPE/0.1 % SDS for 5 min at 60 °C.
5. Put the foam cushion into the Miniblotter (that acts as a joint) and place the membrane above it, so that the side with the oligonucleotides (spacers) faces the slots and these are perpendicular to the black line of the spacers on the membrane (use the date in the bottom right corner as a marker) (Fig. 2).
6. Tightly fasten the six plastic screws to close the press.
7. Remove the excess of 2× SSPE/0.1 % SDS from each of the slots of the Miniblotter by aspiration with a vacuum pump (*see* **Note 8**).
8. Fill the first slot of the Miniblotter with 150 μl of 2× SSPE/0.1 % SDS to prevent the dehydration of the membrane.
9. Fill the remaining slots, one by one, starting in the second slot, with 150 μl of the diluted PCR products (maximum 43), kept at 4 °C until loading, avoiding air bubbles (*see* **Note 12**). Mark the loading order.
10. Fill the last slot and any empty slots of the Miniblotter with 150 μl of 2× SSPE/0.1 % SDS. The samples must always be surrounded by buffer to prevent leaking.
9. Incubate in a hybridization oven at 60 °C for 1 h without shaking.
10. Remove the samples from the slots of the Miniblotter by aspiration with a vacuum pump, in the same order as they were filled.
11. Disassemble the Miniblotter and, with the forceps, carefully remove the membrane to a laboratory tray, and wash twice with 250 ml of 2× SSPE/0.5 % SDS at 60 °C for 10 min, on the hybridization oven with shaking.
12. Discard the washing buffer and lower the temperature of the hybridization oven to 42 °C (*see* **Note 13**).
13. Add 2.5 μl of streptavidin-peroxidase conjugate (500 U/ml) to 10 ml of 2× SSPE/0.5 % SDS at 42 °C and place the solution in a rolling bottle.
14. Place the membrane and a mesh of the same size in the rolling bottle and incubate at 42 °C during 90 min on the hybridization oven, with rolling movement (*see* **Note 14**).
15. Remove the membrane from the rolling bottle, with the forceps, and wash it twice in a tray with 250 ml of 2× SSPE/0.5 % SDS at 42 °C during 10 min, in the hybridization oven with shaking. Add fresh solution each time.
16. Discard the solution and rinse the membrane twice with 250 ml of 2× SSPE at room temperature for 5 min with shaking. Add fresh solution each time.

3.5 Detection of Hybridized DNA

1. Prepare a light-tight X-ray film holder (autoradiography cassette) placing inside one sheet of blotting paper 3 MM and an acetate sheet (*see* **Note 15**).
2. Immediately before required, prepare 20 ml of solution by mixing 10 ml of each of the solutions supplied in the commercial system ECL (ECL solution 1 and ECL solution 2) in a flask involved in a tinfoil.
3. Place the nylon membrane over one sheet of blotting paper 3 MM to remove the excess of washing buffer.
4. In a complete darkroom, incubate the membrane in 20 ml of the ECL mixture, during 2 min, in a laboratory tray, with gentle manual shaking so that all the membrane is in uniform contact with the liquid (the membranes repel water) (*see* **Note 16**).
5. Remove the excess of ECL mixture from the membrane with a sheet of blotting paper 3 MM. The membrane does not need to be completely dried, but the sharpness of the image is much improved if it is.
6. Place the membrane inside the cassette with the side where the hybridization has occurred up, between the acetate sheet (above) and the blotting paper 3 MM.
7. Place the hyperfilm ECL on top of the acetate sheet and remove the air bubbles. Close the cassette and expose the membrane to the autoradiography film for 10 min (*see* **Note 17**).
8. In the darkroom, remove the hyperfilm ECL as quickly as possible and develop it immediately in an X-ray developer solution during a few seconds (*see* **Note 18**).
9. Wash the autoradiography film with water in a plastic container, for 1 min.
10. Fix the film with a rapid fixer solution in a plastic container, for 5 min.
11. Wash the film with running water for 5 min.
12. Let the film dry and visualize the results.
13. Wash the membrane twice for 15 min with 250 ml of 20 mM EDTA at room temperature, with shaking.
14. Remove the membrane with forceps and store at 4 °C, in a sealed plastic bag to avoid dehydration, with 10 ml of 20 mM EDTA (pH 8.0) until being regenerated in the dehybridization (stripping) step (*see* Subheading 3.7).

3.6 Interpretation of Results

The membrane is analyzed by recording the presence or absence of signals at the sites of DNA/DNA hybridizations, using the binary code (0 for absence, 1 for presence of signal) annotation. The obtained sequence, of 0 and 1, is then checked against the databases (http://www.pasteur-guadaloupe.fr/tb or http://www.mbovis.org) for spoligotype attribution.

Clear sharp signals are easy to interpret, but some weak signals may occur with some spacers, mainly 14, 26, and 33, whose presence or absence is more critical to evaluate. Comparing with well-known control patterns and checking for the presence of the expected spots can clarify some doubts. The negative control should be absolutely clear and with no contamination or leaks. Very faint dots should, in principle, not be considered, unless the positive control gives otherwise information. Obtaining a clear negative control and a correct positive control profile is critical for the assessment of membrane quality and for the interpretation of results.

3.7 Regeneration of the Nylon Membrane for Reuse

The membranes can be reused if the oligonucleotides can be freed from the attached PCR products. As the oligonucleotides (spacers) are covalently fixed to the membrane, the removal method must be highly stringent.

1. Pre-warm the hybridization oven and the 1 % SDS at 85 °C.
2. Place the membrane into a laboratory tray, with the forceps, and wash 3 times for 30 min with 250 ml of 1 % SDS at 85 °C with shaking.
3. Discard the washing solution and wash twice for 15 min with 250 ml of 20 mM EDTA at room temperature, with shaking.
4. Remove the membrane with forceps and store at 4 °C, in a sealed plastic bag to avoid dehydration, with 10 ml of 20 mM EDTA (pH 8.0) until being used.

4 Notes

1. To prepare 1,000 ml of 0.5 M EDTA, weight 186.12 g of EDTA to a glass bottle and add 800 ml of water. It is convenient to dissolve the powder using a magnetic stirrer with maximum speed. Add NaOH pellets to adjust the solution at a pH 8.0. Only a pH 8.0 solution, at 25 °C, completely dissolves the EDTA. Adjust the volume to 1,000 ml with water and mix again. Store at room temperature.
2. To prepare 100 ml of 10 % SDS, weight 10 g of sodium lauryl sulfate to a glass bottle and add 80 ml of water. Dissolve by gentle shaking (to avoid the formation of foam) in a magnetic stirrer with heating up to 68 °C. Adjust the volume to 100 ml with water and mix again. Store at room temperature.
3. Prepare the solutions of 2× SSPE/0.1 % SDS and 2× SSPE/0.5 % SDS firstly mixing the water with the 2× SSPE. After complete homogenization, add the SDS and homogenize again. The addition of the solutions should be as indicated to avoid the formation of a precipitate.

4. All the oligonucleotide probes are synthesized with a 5′-end amino group, to promote the covalent linking to the activated, negatively charged, membrane Biodyne C.
5. The DRa primer is labeled with biotin that binds to streptavidin coupled with peroxidase, making possible to detect any amplification product. The primers are reconstituted in ultrapure water for a stock solution of 100 μM and diluted in water for a working solution of 20 μM. Store the primers in aliquots: the DRa primer at 4 °C, because the repeated freeze-thawing of the biotinylated primer results in a weak reaction, and the DRb primer at –20 °C.
6. To prepare 1,000 ml of 1× TBE, add 200 ml of 5× TBE and mix with 800 ml of water (1,000 ml of 5× TBE is prepared by adding 54 g of Tris base, 27.5 g of boric acid and 800 ml of water to a glass bottle. Mix using a magnetic stirrer. Add 20 ml of 0.5 M EDTA and add water to complete the volume of 1,000 ml).
7. Ready-to-use customized membranes can be obtained from some manufacturers. Also European reference laboratories for tuberculosis can, upon request, supply these membranes.
8. To remove the residual solution from the slots of the Miniblotter, put a 1,000 μl micropipette tip in the top of the tube of the vacuum pump to aspirate the slots. Aspirate the upper slots with the Miniblotter in the horizontal plan and the lower slots with the Miniblotter in a slanting plan.
9. The first and the last slot must be left without oligonucleotide probes because they are going to be used to mark the edges of the membrane with the diluted China ink.
10. The amplification step requires very little DNA concentration. It is therefore better to take fewer bacteria from the agar slopes than to risk taking a large amount of medium. It is important that the bacteria are exactly heated to 90 °C for, at least, 30 min to ensure that they are all killed at this stage. It is also possible to use DNA extracted by phenol–chloroform method or with any commercial DNA extraction kit. Extracted DNA can be stored at –20 °C.
11. The purpose of this step is only to confirm that the amplification of the DR *loci* has occurred. For each sample, it should be observed a smear of bands with different sizes.
12. Fill the slots carefully avoiding air bubbles and using absorbent paper to prevent cross contamination of adjacent slots.
13. The temperature of incubation should be rigorously at 42 °C, since streptavidin-peroxidase conjugate is inactivated above this temperature.

14. Carefully wrap the membrane and the mesh, with the size of the membrane, together and place them inside the rolling bottle. Unroll the membrane and the mesh in the opposite rotation direction to adhere completely at the rolling bottle walls, avoiding bubbles and promoting the contact of the membrane with the streptavidin solution. Place the rolling bottle in the hybridization oven, in the proper rotation direction, in order to prevent the curl of the membrane during the incubation period.
15. To prepare the autoradiography cassette, place a sheet of blotting paper 3 MM and acetate sheet inside the cassette and hold them individually with adhesive tape.
16. Incubate the membrane at room temperature, in the dark room, with the ECL mixture with gentle shaking in order to cover the entire membrane surface.
17. Exposure time can be adjusted according to the results obtained and the intensity of signals. Shorter or longer exposures may vary from 5 to 20 min, depending on the results from the first film.
18. Leave the hyperfilm in the X-ray developer solution the time enough (could be a few seconds) to visualize positive signals, avoiding darkness of the hyperfilm. Once the hyperfilm starts to get dark, wash immediately in water.

Acknowledgments

This work was supported by Fundacão para a Ciência e Tecnologia (FCT) through project PTDC/CVT/117794/2010 and in the framework of Projecto 3599—Promover a Produção Científica e Desenvolvimento Tecnológico e a Constituição de Redes Temáticas.

References

1. Jansen R, van Embden J, Gaastra WL, Schouls M (2002) Identification of genes that are associated with DNA repeats in prokaryotes. Mol Microbiol 43:1565–1575
2. Barrangou R, Fremaux C, Deveau H et al (2007) CRISPR provides acquired resistance against viruses in prokaryotes. Science 31: 1709–1712
3. Deveau H, Garneau JE, Moineau S (2010) CRISPR/Cas system and its role in phage-bacteria interactions. Annu Rev Microbiol 64:475–493
4. Pourcel C, Salvignol G, Vergnaud G (2005) CRISPR elements in *Yersinia pestis* acquire new repeats by preferential uptake of bacteriophage DNA, and provide additional tools for evolutionary studies. Microbiology 151: 653–663
5. Sorek R, Kunin V, Hugenholtz P (2008) CRISPR – a widespread system that provides acquired resistance against phages in bacteria and archaea. Nat Rev Microbiol 6:181–186
6. Marraffini L, Sontheimer EJ (2010) CRISPR interference: RNA-directed adaptive immunity in bacteria and archaea. Nat Rev Genet 11: 181–190
7. Groenen PM, Bunschoten AE, van Soolingen D, van Embden JD (1993) Nature of DNA polymorphism in the direct repeat cluster of *Mycobacterium tuberculosis*; application for strain

differentiation by a novel typing method. Mol Microbiol 10:1057–1065

8. Kamerbeek J, Schouls L et al (1997) Simultaneous detection and strain differentiation of *Mycobacterium tuberculosis* for diagnosis and epidemiology. J Clin Microbiol 35:907–914
9. Hoe N, Nakashima K, Grigsby D et al (1999) Rapid molecular genetic subtyping of serotype M1 group A *Streptococcus* strains. Emerg Infect Dis 5:254–263
10. Schouls LM, Reulen S, Duim B et al (2003) Comparative genotyping of *Campylobacter jejuni* by amplified fragment length polymorphism, multilocus sequence typing, and short repeat sequencing: strain diversity, host range, and recombination. J Clin Microbiol 41:15–26
11. Van Embden JDA, Van Gorkom T, Kremer K, Jansen R et al (2000) Genetic variation and evolutionary origin of the Direct Repeat locus of Mycobacterium tuberculosis complex bacteria. J Bacteriol 182:2393–2401
12. Caimi K, Romano MI, Alito A et al (2001) Sequence analysis of the direct repeat region in *Mycobacterium bovis.* J Clin Microbiol 39: 1067–1072
13. Filliol I, Driscoll JR, Van Soolingen D et al (2003) Snapshot of moving and expanding clones of *Mycobacterium tuberculosis* and their global distribution assessed by spoligotyping in an international study. J Clin Microbiol 41: 1963–1970
14. Streicher EM, Victor TC, van der Spuy G et al (2007) Spoligotype signatures in the *Mycobacterium tuberculosis* complex. J Clin Microbiol 45:237–240
15. Van Soolingen D (2001) Molecular epidemiology of tuberculosis and other mycobacterial infections: main methodologies and achievements. J Intern Med 249:1–26
16. Brudey K, Driscoll JR, Rigouts L et al (2006) *Mycobacterium tuberculosis* complex genetic diversity: mining the fourth international spoligotyping database (SpolDB4) for classification, population genetics and epidemiology. BMC Microbiol 6:23
17. Intitute Pasteur de la Guadeloupe (1993) Tuberculose et Mycobactéries, Abymes Cedex. http://www.pasteur-guadeloupe.fr/tb/bd_myco.html. Accessed 10 Jan 2014
18. *Mycobacterium bovis* spoligotyping Database. http://www.Mbovis.org. Accessed 10 Jan 2014
19. van der Zanden AGM, Kremer K, Schouls LJ et al (2002) Improvement of differentiation and interpretability of spoligotyping for *Mycobacterium tuberculosis* complex isolates by introduction of new spacer oligonucleotides. J Clin Microbiol 40:4628–4639
20. Javed MT, Aranaz A, de Juan L et al (2007) Improvement of spoligotyping with additional spacer sequences for characterization of *Mycobacterium bovis* and *M. caprae* isolates from Spain. Tuberculosis 87:437–445
21. Duarte EL, Domingos M, Amado A, Botelho A (2008) Spoligotype diversity of *Mycobacterium bovis* and *Mycobacterium caprae* animal isolates. Vet Microbiol 130:415–421
22. Rodríguez S, Bezos J, Romero B, de Juan L et al (2011) *Mycobacterium caprae* infection in livestock and wildlife, Spain. Emerg Infect Dis 17:532–535

Chapter 28

Rapid Microarray-Based Genotyping of *Chlamydia* spp. Strains from Clinical Tissue Samples

Konrad Sachse and Anke Ruettger

Abstract

Pathogenic *Chlamydia (C.) psittaci* and *C. trachomatis* strains can be genotyped based on variations in the *omp*A genomic locus. In the present chapter, we describe rapid genotyping assays for both chlamydial agents using the ArrayStrip™ (AS) microarray platform. The test is targeting multiple discriminatory sites in the variable domains of the *omp*A gene by using 35 (*C. psittaci*) and 61 (*C. trachomatis*) oligonucleotide probes representing genotype-specific polymorphisms. In addition to discrimination among the established genotypes, this approach allows identification of atypical strains that were not accessible to typing using previously established techniques, such as PCR-RFLP or serotyping.

The present DNA microarray assay can be conducted directly on clinical tissue samples and is suitable for tracing epidemiological chains and exploring the dissemination of particular genotypes. The procedure is easy to handle and economically affordable, and it allows genotyping of up to 32 clinical samples per day, thus lending itself for routine diagnosis as well.

Key words *Chlamydia psittaci*, *Chlamydia trachomatis*, *omp*A genotyping, Diagnostic DNA microarray test, Direct testing of clinical samples

1 Introduction

1.1 History of Typing

Members of the family *Chlamydiaceae* represent obligate intracellular bacteria that are distinguished by a characteristic biphasic developmental cycle. There are several well-established pathogens among them. For instance, *Chlamydia (C.) psittaci*, the causative agent of psittacosis in birds and humans, is responsible for outbreaks in psittacine birds and domestic poultry [1], as well as cases of atypical pneumonia in exposed individuals [2, 3]. The fact that *C. psittaci* is a heterogeneous taxon in terms of host range and virulence entailed the development of a serotyping scheme in the 1990s [4]. Strains of the agent were assigned to serovars A, B, C, D, E, and F on the basis of their immune reaction with a panel of monoclonal antibodies (MAbs) recognizing specific epitopes of the major outer membrane protein (MOMP). Later on, Sayada

Mónica V. Cunha and João Inácio (eds.), *Veterinary Infection Biology: Molecular Diagnostics and High-Throughput Strategies*, Methods in Molecular Biology, vol. 1247, DOI 10.1007/978-1-4939-2004-4_28, © Springer Science+Business Media New York 2015

et al. [5] suggested restriction fragment length polymorphism (RFLP), i.e., PCR amplification of the *omp*A gene with subsequent restriction enzyme analysis, for differentiation among *C. psittaci* isolates. The finding by Vanrompay et al. [6] that serotypes and RFLP genotypes were generally equivalent rendered strain typing accessible to all laboratories without access to the specific MAbs. However, there were obvious limitations to PCR-RFLP typing. To obtain distinctive and reproducible RFLP patterns on ethidium bromide-stained agarose gels, substantial amounts of target DNA and PCR amplicon were required. Some of the related genotypes gave quite similar patterns and were difficult to distinguish, and different enzymes could produce ambiguous or even contradictory patterns (e.g., *Alu*I vs. *Mbo*II). Finally, atypical strains were not amenable to this genotyping procedure.

The use of real-time PCR [7] helped to further increase sensitivity but also failed to cover the entire spectrum of natural sequence diversity at the target locus.

Historically, nine genotypes (former serotypes) were postulated, and a certain degree of host preference was assigned to them [4, 8–10], i.e., genotype A occurring in psittacine birds, B in pigeons, C in ducks and geese, D in turkeys, E in pigeons, ducks, and others, E/B in ducks, F in parakeets, WC in cattle, and M56 in rodents. In reality, the host specificity of most of these types is limited (*see* Table 1).

Based on the original serotyping scheme [11], an analogous *omp*A-based genotyping system has also been in use for strains of the human pathogen *C. trachomatis* The agent can also be found occasionally in animals [12, 13]. There are 17 generally recognized genotypes, i.e., A, B, Ba, C (associated with trachoma), D, Da, E, F, G, H, I, Ia, J, K (urogenital infections), L1, L2, and L3 (lymphogranuloma venereum). Like in the case of *C. psittaci*, they are equivalent to the previously defined serotypes.

1.2 Genotyping Using DNA Microarrays

In principle, sequencing of the *omp*A gene can also be used to identify the genotype of *C. psittaci*, as well as *C. trachomatis*. However, there are no generally agreed criteria in terms of sequence similarity, so that the assignment remains somewhat arbitrary. Detailed analysis of *omp*A sequence data deposited at the GenBank database led Sachse et al. [14] to the conclusion that at least 15 *omp*A genotypes of *C. psittaci* are occurring in nature. A summary of this classification in Table 1 shows that the more heterogeneous types A, D, and E/B can be further divided into subtypes. The host range of the proposed new genotypes 1V, 6N, Mat116, R54, YP84, and CPX0308 is not yet fully known, but they seem to occur predominantly in wildlife birds.

The fact that genotype-specific sites of *C. psittaci* are located in *omp*A's variable domains (VD) 2 and 4 allows a molecular definition of individual genotypes at the nucleotide level.

Table 1
***ompA* genotypes and subtypes of *Chlamydia psittaci* [Adapted from reference [14]]**

Genotype	Known hosts	Subtypes	Type strain (representative strain of subtype)	GenBank acc. no.
A	Psittacine, pigeon, canary, turkey	A-VS1	VS1, MN Zhang	AF269281
	pheasant, chicken, duck, cattle	A-6BC	**6BC**	X56980
	swine, sheep, horse, human	A-8455	84-55	Y16561
B	Pigeon, canary, budgerigar, chicken, pheasant, turkey		**CP3**	AF269265
C	Duck, goose, swan, sheep, human		**GR9**, avian type C	L25436
D	Turkey, human	D-NJ1	**NJ1**	AF269266
		D-9 N	9 N	EF375557
E	Pigeon, duck, turkey, ostrich, human		**CPMN**, EAE A22/M	X12647
EB	Duck, human	EB-E30	**WS/RT/E30**	AY762613
		EB-859	06-859/1	EU159263
		EB-KKCP	KKCP-1	AB284062
F	Psittacine		**VS225**	AF269259
M56	Muskrat, snowshoe hare		**M56**	AF269268
WC	Cattle		**WC**	AF269269
1 V[a]	Crow		1 V	EF028916
6 N[a]	Crow		6 N	EF197820
Mat116[a]	Psittacine, budgerigar		Mat116	AB284058
R54[a]	Antarctic skua		R54	AJ243525
YP84[a]	Psittacine		Daruma-1981	AB284065
CPX0308[a]	Stork		CPX0308	AB284064

[a]Additional genotypes proposed by Sachse and colleagues [14]

In this situation, the use of DNA microarray technology can provide added value because of its potential to simultaneously exploit minor sequence differences at multiple target sites. In the present chapter, we describe a rapid genotyping assay using the ArrayStrip™ (AS) platform that was shown to work with clinical samples under the conditions of routine diagnosis [14, 15]. The AS platform is open and flexible, so that iterative adaptation of probes and extension beyond the currently covered genotypes will always be possible, for instance, in the case of newly emerging types. Comments on the platform's major performance parameters and comparison with PCR-RFLP and *omp*A sequencing are given in **Note 1**. While both sensitivity and specificity of the microarray assay are high, its main assets include rapidity, ease of operation, and the possibility of mixed genotype identification, as well as high-throughput and moderate costs. An AS unit consists of eight connected plastic vessels in microtiter format, each of which carrying a microarray chip on the bottom.

The present genotyping procedure is based on target DNA being amplified using duplex PCR with 5′-biotinylated primers to generate a 418-bp product encompassing VD1 and VD2, as well as a 570-bp fragment covering VD3 and VD4. Subsequently, the amplification products are subjected to hybridization on the microarray. Based on the analysis of *omp*A sequences described above, 35 hybridization probes derived from the discriminatory sites of VD2 and VD4 were selected. They had an average size of 26 nt (22–30), average melting temperature of 60.3 °C (59.7–61.2), and G+C contents of 46.0 mol % (37.0–59.0).

Similarly, an *omp*A genotyping microarray assay was developed for *C. trachomatis* [16]. Variable domains 1, 2, and 4 of the *omp*A locus were amplified using a multiplex PCR with biotinylated primers. A total of 61 oligonucleotide probes representing genotype-specific polymorphisms in the same variable domains were included.

2 Materials

2.1 DNA Extraction

Commercially available DNA extraction kit for PCR template preparation. We use the High Pure PCR Template Preparation Kit (Roche Diagnostics, Mannheim, Germany) for cultured strains and nearly all kinds of tissue samples, e.g., nasal, vaginal, and conjunctival swabs, mucus, bronchoalveolar lavage, organs, feces, and milk.

2.2 Biotinylation PCR and Agarose Gel Electrophoresis

1. Water. Deionized water must be used throughout.
2. PCR reagents. We use the QIAGEN Multiplex PCR Kit (QIAGEN, Hilden, Germany) according to the instructions of the manufacturer (*see* **Note 2**).
3. Primers. Sequences, primer concentrations, and other parameters are given in Table 2. The oligonucleotides are stored at −20 °C in 100 μM stock solutions. The concentration of primer working solutions is 10 μM.
4. Agarose, molecular biology grade: 1.5 % (w/v) gels for the PCR products mentioned in Table 2.
5. Tris–borate EDTA electrophoresis buffer (TBE): 0.09 M Tris–borate, 0.002 M EDTA, pH 8.0. For 1 L of 10× TBE, mix 108 g of Tris-base, 55 g of boric acid, and 80 mL of 0.25 M EDTA, make up with water. Dilute 1:10 before use.

Table 2
Primers for *ompA* genotyping of *C. psittaci and C. trachomatis*

Designation	Nucleotide sequence (5′-3′)[a]	Amount per reaction (μL)[b]	Amplicon size (bp)
C. psittaci			
VD1-fw	5′-ACT ACG GAG ATT ATG TTT TCG ATC GTG T-3′	1	418 bp
VD2-rev	5′-Bio-CGT GCA CCY ACG CTC CAA GA-3′	1	
201CHOMP	5′-GGI GCW GMI TTC CAA TAY GCI CAR TC-3′	2	570 bp
ompA-rev	5′-Bio-TCC TTA GAA TCT GAA TTG AGC-3′	2	
C. trachomatis			
Trach-VD1-fw	5′-Bio-ACC AAG CCT TAT GAT CGA C-3′	3	326 bp
Trach-VD1-rev	5′-Bio-AGA ATA CAT CAA AAC GAT CCC A-3′	1	
Trach-VD2-rev	5′-Bio-TTG AGC ATA TTG GAA AGA AGC-3′	2	572 bp (with Trach-VD1-fw)
Trach-VD4-fw	5′- Bio-CTT ACA TTG GAG TTA AAT GGT CT-3′	1	231 bp
Trach-VD4-rev	5′-Bio-CTA CTG CAA TAC CGC AAG A-3′	1	

[a]Bio: oligonucleotide biotinylated at 5′-end
[b]The concentration of primer working solutions is 10 pmol/μL (10 μM)

6. Gel loading buffer (GLB): 20 % (v/v) glycerol, 0.2 M EDTA, 0.01 % (w/v) bromophenol blue, 0.2 % (w/v) Ficoll 400.
7. Ethidium bromide stock solution: 1 % (10 mg/mL) solution in water. CAUTION: The substance is presumed to be mutagenic. Avoid direct contact with skin. Wear gloves when preparing solutions and handling gels.
8. DNA size marker. We mostly use the O'Range Ruler ("100-bp ladder") (Fermentas, St. Leon-Rot, Germany).

2.3 DNA Microarray Hybridization

The Identibac™ Hybridisation Kit (Alere Technologies, Jena, Germany) contains all necessary reagents and is the most efficient and convenient option (*see* **Note 3**): hybridization buffer (C1), washing buffers (C2, C5), streptavidin-peroxidase conjugate (C3 + C4), and TMB-substrate (D1).

2.4 General Equipment and Consumables

1. ArrayMate transmission reader (Alere Technologies, Jena, Germany).
2. Iconoclust software, version 2.3 or higher (Alere Technologies, Jena, Germany).

3. *Chlamydia* ArrayStrips, version 4 or higher (layout "Chlam_gesamt_4_AS") (Alere Technologies, Jena, Germany). These arrays are commercially available from Alere. The company also has a service for ordering customized arrays. The sequences of the oligonucleotide probes immobilized on these arrays were previously published in Sachse et al. [14] (*C. psittaci* assay) and Ruettger et al. [16] (*C. trachomatis* assay).
4. Heatable horizontal tube shaker. We recommend the Bioshake iQ (Quantifoil Instruments, Jena, Germany; *see* **Note 4**).
5. Thermal cycler. We use the Mastercycler personal (Eppendorf, Hamburg, Germany).
6. Vortex shaker, e.g., Vortex 1 (IKA Labortechnik, Staufen, Germany).
7. Benchtop centrifuge with rotor for 0.2 mL or 0.5 mL plastic tubes, e.g., Centrifuge 5415R (Eppendorf, Hamburg, Germany).
8. Apparatus for horizontal gel electrophoresis.
9. UV transilluminator, 254 nm and/or 312 nm.
10. Video documentation or photographic equipment.
11. Set of pipettes covering the whole volume range from 0.1 to 1,000 μL. We use the Eppendorf Research series (Eppendorf, Hamburg, Germany).
12. Aerosol-resistant pipette tips (filter tips).
13. Plastic tubes 0.2 mL or 0.5 mL, sterile, thin-walled, DNase- and RNase-free for PCR.
14. Plastic tubes 1.7 mL and 2.0 mL for pre-PCR operations.

3 Methods

3.1 DNA Extraction

Follow the protocol given by the commercial supplier of the DNA extraction kit.

3.2 Biotinylation PCR

1. The reaction volume is 20 μL. For each amplification, pipette 10 μL of Master Mix solution of the QIAGEN Multiplex PCR Kit and the amount of primers as given in Table 2, and make up with water to 19 μL.
2. Add template to each reaction vessel: 1 μL of DNA extract from your sample. If the DNA contents of the extract is low, up to 4 μL of sample DNA can be used and the amount of water be reduced accordingly.
3. Include external amplification controls: DNA of a chlamydial reference strain (positive control) and water (reagent control) instead of sample extract.

4. Run PCR according to the following temperature-time profile: Initial denaturation at 95 °C for 15 min, 40 cycles of denaturation (94 °C for 30 s), primer annealing (50 °C for 90 s) and primer extension (72 °C for 90 s), final extension at 72 °C for 10 min.
5. Run agarose gel electrophoresis. Correct amplification leads to the formation of two products in the case of *C. psittaci* and three products in the case of *C. trachomatis*. Amplicon sizes are given in Table 2.

3.3 DNA Microarray Hybridization

1. Transfer 1 μL of the PCR product from Subheading 3.2 into a 1.7-mL plastic tube and add 99 μL of hybridization buffer (Buffer C1).
2. Denature DNA by heating at 95 °C for 5 min. Cool down immediately by putting the tube on ice for 1 min. Spin down the liquid by short centrifugation.
3. Condition the ArrayStrip by adding 100 μL of water to each well. Rinse by pipetting the liquid up and down four times, and then discard it.
4. Add 100 μL of buffer C1 to each well, and shake on Bioshake iQ at 48 °C and 550 RPM for 5 min. Remove liquid.
5. Hybridization. Add the hybridization mix (100 μL each) from **step 2** to AS wells. Incubate on Bioshake iQ at 48 °C and 550 rpm for 60 min. Remove supernatant and discard it.
6. Add 200 μL of washing buffer C2 to each well, and wash at 48 °C and 550 rpm for 10 min. Remove liquid and discard it.
7. Repeat **step 6**.
8. Combine 792 μL of C4 and 8 μL of C3 solutions (horseradish peroxidase conjugated with streptavidin) in a plastic tube, vortex, and spin down. The amount is for a single AS unit, i.e., 8 wells. Add 100 μL of this mix to each well. Incubate at 30 °C and 550 rpm for 10 min. Remove supernatant.
9. Wash wells by adding 200 μL of washing buffer C5 and 4 times up-and-down pipetting at room temperature. Remove all the liquid thoroughly and completely.
10. Add 100 μL of D1 solution (peroxidase substrate) to each well, and incubate at room temperature for 5 min.
11. Remove liquid and put AS into the ArrayMate reader.

3.4 Data Processing

1. Conduct the reading process according to the instructions for the ArrayMate equipment.
2. Transfer the image files (bmp format) to your computer and process the data using the Iconoclust software.
3. Determine the genotype using the PatternMatch algorithm of the software (*see* **Note 5**).

4 Notes

1. Genotyping analysis using the AS assay can be accomplished within a working day (6–8 h). This renders the procedure faster than PCR-RFLP and *ompA* sequencing. Furthermore, AS genotyping is easy to handle as it mainly involves standard laboratory equipment and requires less hands-on time than PCR-RFLP and less experience than sequencing. The expenses for consumables are moderate, and the equipment costs considerably less (about 25 %) than that for DNA sequencing. The microarray technology is manageable in a high-throughput environment, with up to 32 samples per day and technician.
2. Amplification can also be accomplished using standard PCR reagents and preparing the reaction mixes in the usual way. The main arguments in favor of using the present kit are that it is convenient to use as it contains all reagents and that the commercial mix is optimized for high yield.
3. Alternatively, buffers can be prepared manually according to the protocols published previously [14, 15].
4. For the sake of high specificity and stringency of the hybridization reaction, it is extremely important to ensure that the prescribed temperatures are actually attained in the AS vessel itself. This requires heat transfer from the heatable shaker to the liquid contents of the AS vessel to be very rapid and efficient. Most of the commercially available shakers are too slow, so that too much time (and, consequently, specificity) is lost until the necessary in-tube temperature has been reached. In our hands, the Bioshake iQ fulfills the criteria to be used in the hybridization process.
5. The PatternMatch algorithm compares the experimentally obtained signal pattern with those of reference strains representing the genotypes of *C. psittaci* or *C. trachomatis*, respectively. It provides combined bar diagrams of sample and reference (*see* an example in Fig. 1), as well as two numerical parameters to assess the similarity of two patterns and the accuracy of identification. The matching score (MS) represents the sum of numerical differences between corresponding signal intensities of sample and theoretical and/or practical reference hybridization patterns. Thus, the MS value is a measure of the overall dissimilarity between two hybridization patterns. An ideal match of two patterns based on the same set of oligonucleotide probes would yield MS = 0, but practical values can be in the order of 100. Prior to the examination of field samples, the user should run a series of samples of known genotypes in order to determine the practical MS range and set the upper threshold, above which the best match is no more valid for genotyping.

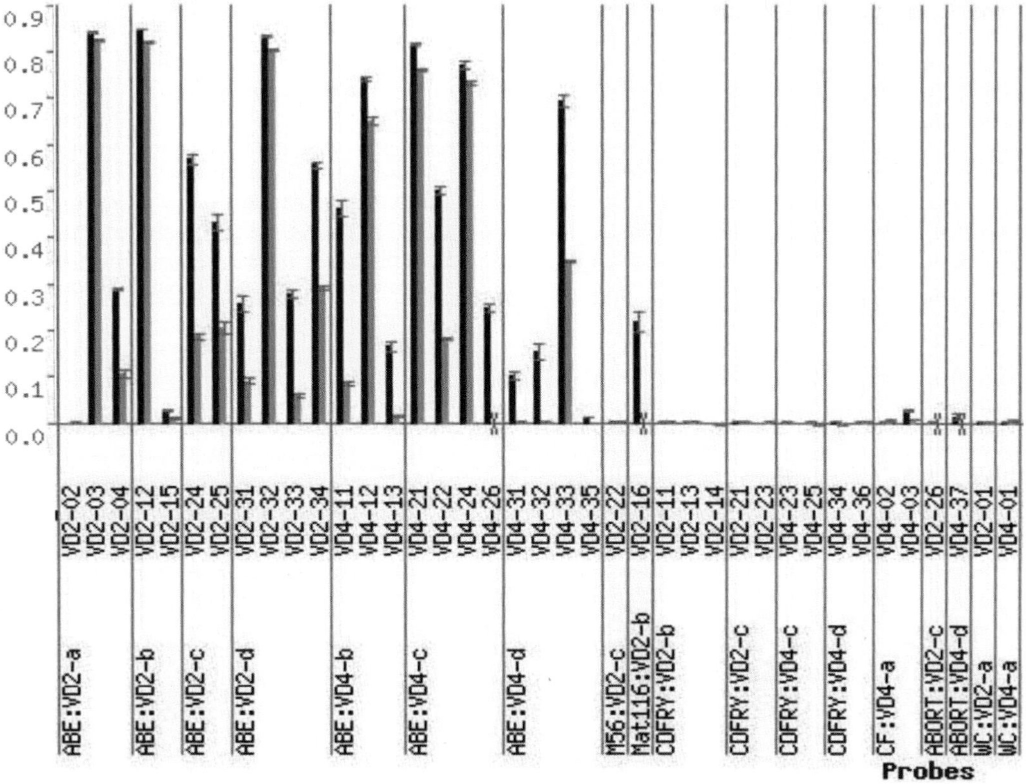

Fig. 1 Identification of the *omp*A genotype of the *C. psittaci* strain from the feces sample of a diseased pigeon (sample ID 11G1376). Using the PatternMatch function of the software, the experimentally obtained hybridization pattern of the sample (*black bars*) is compared to the closest match of a panel of reference strains, i.e., type strain CP3 of genotype B (*gray bars*). The matching score (MS) of 154.12 is a measure of dissimilarity between sample and reference, and the Delta MS value of 1.2 represents the numerical difference between best and second best match. These values confirm that the assignment of the present sample to genotype B is valid

The second parameter is the arithmetic difference between best and second best match, termed Delta MS, and indicates the reliability of a given genotyping result. Values of Delta MS ≥ 0.5 are regarded as representing a sufficient degree of distinction between best and second best matches.

References

1. Harkinezhad T, Geens T, Vanrompay D (2009) *Chlamydophila psittaci* infections in birds: a review with emphasis on zoonotic consequences. Vet Microbiol 135:68–77
2. Gaede W, Reckling K-F, Dresenkamp B et al (2008) *Chlamydophila psittaci* infections in humans during an outbreak of psittacosis from poultry in Germany. Zoonoses Public Health 55:184–188
3. Laroucau K, de Barbeyrac B, Vorimore F et al (2009) Chlamydial infections in duck farms associated with human cases of psittacosis in France. Vet Microbiol 135:82–89
4. Andersen AA (1991) Serotyping of *Chlamydia psittaci* isolates using serovar-specific monoclonal antibodies with the microimmunofluorescence test. J Clin Microbiol 29:707–711

5. Sayada C, Andersen AA, Storey C et al (1995) Usefulness of *omp1* restriction mapping for avian *Chlamydia psittaci* isolate differentiation. Res Microbiol 146:155–165
6. Vanrompay D, Butaye P, Sayada C, Ducatelle R, Haesebrouck F (1997) Characterization of avian *Chlamydia psittaci* strains using *omp1* restriction mapping and serovar-specific monoclonal antibodies. Res Microbiol 148:327–333
7. Geens T, Dewitte A, Boon N, Vanrompay D (2005) Development of a *Chlamydophila psittaci* species-specific and genotype-specific real-time PCR. Vet Res 36:787–797
8. Andersen AA (1997) Two new serovars of *Chlamydia psittaci* from North American birds. J Vet Diagn Invest 9:159–164
9. Vanrompay D, Andersen AA, Ducatelle R, Haesebrouck F (1993) Serotyping of European isolates of *Chlamydia psittaci* from poultry and other birds. J Clin Microbiol 31:134–137
10. Geens T, Desplanques A, Van Loock M et al (2005) Sequencing of the *Chlamydophila psittaci ompA* gene reveals a new genotype, E/B, and the need for a rapid discriminatory genotyping method. J Clin Microbiol 43:2456–2461
11. Wang SP, Grayston JT (1991) Serotyping of *Chlamydia trachomatis* by indirect fluorescent-antibody staining of inclusions in cell culture with monoclonal antibodies. J Clin Microbiol 29:1295–1298
12. Kauffold J, Melzer F, Berndt A et al (2006) Chlamydiae in oviducts and uteri of repeat breeder pigs. Theriogenology 66:1816–1823
13. Sachse K, Kuehlewind S, Ruettger A, Schubert E, Rohde G (2012) More than classical *Chlamydia psittaci* in urban pigeons. Vet Microbiol 157:476–480
14. Sachse K, Laroucau K, Hotzel H et al (2008) Genotyping of *Chlamydophila psittaci* using a new DNA microarray assay based on sequence analysis of *ompA* genes. BMC Microbiol 8:63
15. Sachse K, Laroucau K, Vorimore F et al (2009) DNA microarray-based genotyping of *Chlamydophila psittaci* strains from culture and clinical samples. Vet Microbiol 135:22–30
16. Ruettger A, Feige J, Slickers P et al (2011) Genotyping of *Chlamydia trachomatis* strains from culture and clinical samples using an *ompA*-based DNA microarray assay. Mol Cell Probes 25:19–27

Chapter 29

Multiplexed Genotyping of *Bacillus anthracis* by Luminex xMap Suspension Array

Simon Thierry and Sylviane Derzelle

Abstract

The Luminex® xTAG technology is a medium to high throughput, open methodology able to test many single nucleotide polymorphisms (SNPs) in a single reaction and a minimum time. Multiplex SNPs interrogation are conducted on the Luminex xMAP system, which uses lasers to read universal tag, color-coded microspheres that attach to specific nucleic acid sequences. The present method describes a Multiplex Oligonucleotide Ligation-PCR procedure (MOL-PCR) for the simultaneous interrogation of 13 phylogenetically informative SNPs within the genome of *Bacillus anthracis*. The reported 13-plex assay enables efficient *B. anthracis* genotyping into major sublineages and groups. While cost-effective compared to other monoplex methods, the present MOL-PCR method also offers a high degree of flexibility and scalability. It can easily accommodate newly identified SNPs to increase resolving power to the canSNP typing of *B. anthracis*.

Key words *Bacillus anthracis*, Genotyping, SNP, MOL-PCR, Suspension microarray, Luminex

1 Introduction

Single nucleotide polymorphisms (SNPs) represent a major source of genetic variation in *Bacillus anthracis*. Recently, a set of 14 representative SNPs that define major clades within the *B. anthracis* species have been selected and used for assigning an isolate to one sublineages or subgroups [1–3]. These canonical SNPs (canSNPs) subdivided all *B. anthracis* isolates into three major lineages (A, B, and C), with further subdivisions into seven distinct sublineages (C.Br.A1055, B.Br.KrugerB, B.Br.CNEVA, A.Br.Ames, A.Br.Australia94, A.Br.Vollum, A.Br.Western North America) and six subgroups (B.Br.001/002, A.Br.001/002, A.Br.003/004, A.Br.005/006, A.Br.008/011, A.Br.011/009). CanSNP analysis is currently considered the reference method in *B. anthracis* genotyping.

Several platforms and methods exist for SNP-based genotyping [4, 5], including ultra-high-throughput array-based technologies, such as those offered by Illumina [6] and Affymetrix [7]. But only few of them are at the same time flexible, rapid (<1 day), cost-effective,

Mónica V. Cunha and João Inácio (eds.), *Veterinary Infection Biology: Molecular Diagnostics and High-Throughput Strategies*, Methods in Molecular Biology, vol. 1247, DOI 10.1007/978-1-4939-2004-4_29,

and capable of detecting multiplexed signals simultaneously with medium to high throughput [8–10]. The xMAP system's unique "liquid array" technology is one of these platforms. This suspension array format implies the use of a set of up to 100 universal tag-coupled, color-coded microspheres that allow the simultaneous capture and detection of many specific nucleic acid targets from a sample. Once bound, the target DNA molecules are fluorescently tagged with streptavidin-R-phycoerythrin, and the beads are individually analyzed by flow cytometry on the Luminex® platform. A red laser recognizes the microsphere set, and a green laser provides a quantitative readout of the reporter dye captured during the assay [11]. Unlike with flat arrays, xMAP arrays give tight inter-assay reproducibility. The microarray format exhibits rapid hybridization kinetics and flexibility in assay design and is cost-effective [10]. In addition, suspension microarrays can be compiled as desired by adding or replacing beads and probes without having to reformat and print new arrays [12]. This represents a clear advantage, knowing that new diagnostic SNPs that further resolve *B. anthracis* population substructure are continuously published following the completion of a growing number of new genome sequences [13–17].

Conceptually related to multiplex ligation-dependent probe amplification (MLPA) technique [18], the Multiplex Oligonucleotide Ligation-PCR (MOL-PCR) is a smart method adapted to the Luminex® platform to carry out SNP multilocus genotyping/SNP interrogation [19, 20]. In MOL-PCR, detection probes (MOLigoP) consist of modular components that enable target detection, probe amplification, and subsequent capture onto microsphere arrays. MOL-PCR uses allele-specific ligation for allele discrimination, monoplex PCR for signal amplification, and hybridization to fluorescent microspheres (beads) for signal detection on a flow cytometer (*see* in Fig. 1). The assay consists of three main steps: (a) annealing of competitive MOLigo pairs P1 and MOLigoP2 adjacent to each other on target canSNPs sequences and ligation of the MOLigos by a thermostable DNA ligase if complementary to the target SNP, (b) amplification of the ligation products (all ligated oligonucleotides) using universal primers, and (c) hybridization of the amplicons to microspheres using xTAG sequences complementary to anti-tag probes and signal detection on the Luminex flow cytometer. In the 13-plex assay designed for the simultaneous interrogation of 13 out of the 14 reported *B. anthracis* lineage-specific canSNPs, a Dual Priming Oligonucleotide (DPO) system [21] was also coupled to the MOL-PCR procedure to increase assays specificity [22].

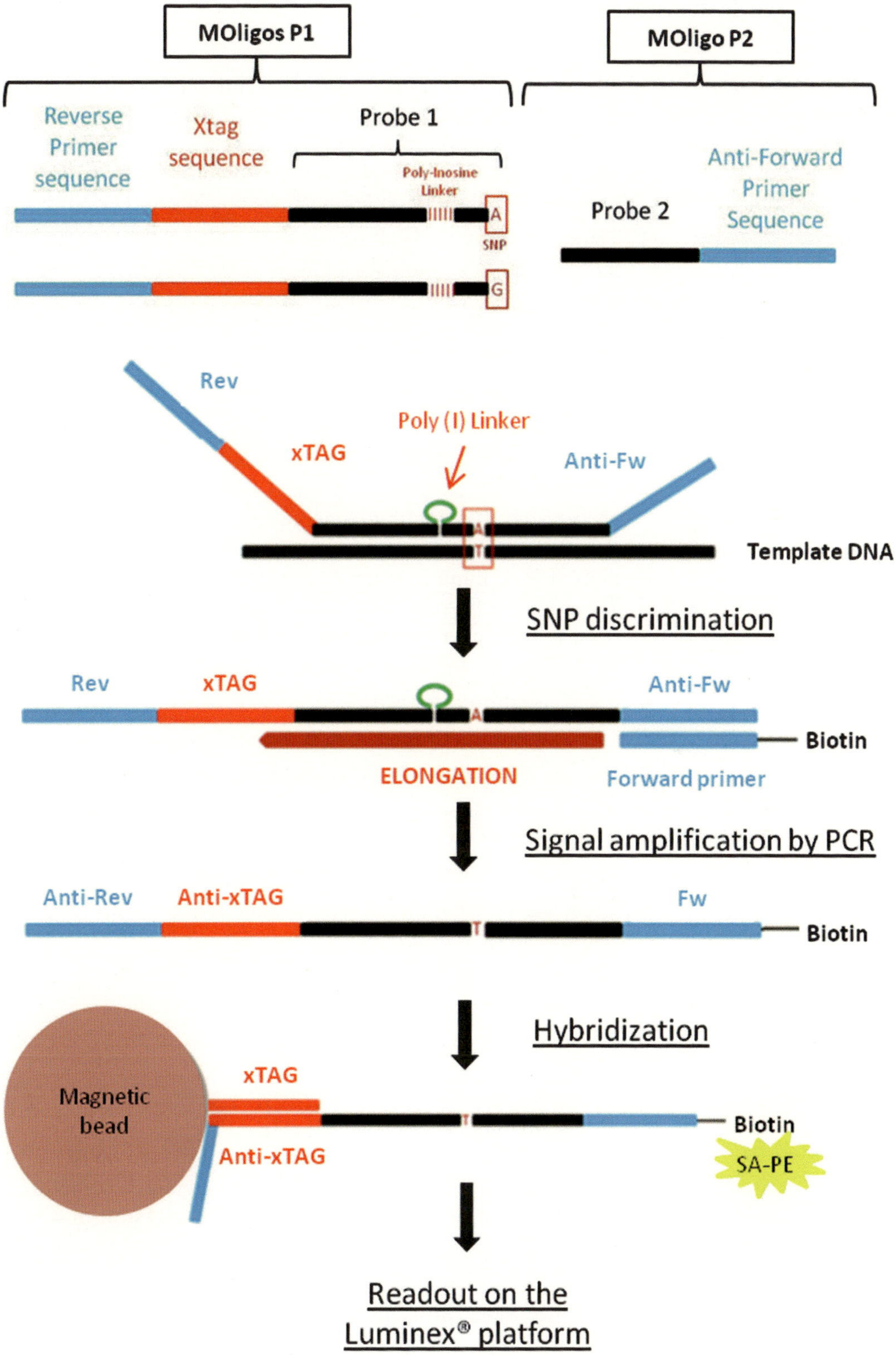

Fig. 1 MOL-PCR general scheme

2 Materials

2.1 DNA Preparation and Biosafety Procedures

1. *Bacillus anthracis* is a class 3 pathogen and should be manipulated in a BSL3 laboratory. Viability testing should be systematically performed to assess the complete removal of live forms of *B. anthracis* from DNA samples so that subsequent analysis could be carried out safely at lower levels of biocontainment (*see* **Note 1**).
2. Template DNA(s): 5–10 ng genomic DNA (*see* **Note 2**). Use template DNA suitable for PCR in terms of purity, concentration, and absence of PCR inhibitors.

2.2 MOL-PCR

1. 10× Ampligase DNA Ligase Buffer (Epicentre, Madison, USA).
2. Ampligase DNA Ligase, 5 U/μL (Epicentre, Madison, USA) (*see* **Note 3**).
3. A set of 39 modular single-stranded DNA oligonucleotides (termed MOLigo probes): a pair of competing allele-specific probes (MOLigoP1) and one common probe (MOLigoP2) per canSNP (*see* **Notes 4** and **5**). 100 μM stock solutions diluted in ultrapure water (*see* oligonucleotide sequences in Table 1). The 5′-end of each MOLigoP2 probe is phosphorylated to enable covalent linkage to MOLigoP1 in the presence of DNA ligase and target DNA.
4. dNTP solution (100 μM).
5. 10× *Taq* Buffer (Qiagen, Courtaboeuf, France).
6. Hot Start *Taq*, 5 U/μL (Qiagen, Courtaboeuf, France).
7. Biotinylated Universal Forward primer (*see* primer sequence in Table 1): 100 μM stock solutions. The primer is tagged with three biotin moieties to guarantee sensitivity at the readout step.
8. Universal Reverse primer (*see* primer sequence in Table 1): 100 μM stock solutions.
9. PCR-grade H_2O: ultrapure water prepared by purifying deionized water, nuclease-free.
10. Thermocycler.

2.3 Luminex Equipment and Reagents

1. *Tm* Hybridization Buffer 1.1× (THB 1.1×): for a final volume of 250 mL, add 27.5 mL of 1 M Tris–HCl, pH 8.0; 11 mL of 5 M NaCl; 0.22 mL Triton® X-100; to 211.28 mL of ultrapure water (*see* **Note 6**). Mix until Triton is completely solubilized. Filter the solution on a 0.22 μm membrane and store at 4 °C.
2. TE pH 8: for a final volume of 1 L, add 10 mL of 1 M Tris-HCl, pH 8.0; 2 mL of 0.5 M EDTA, pH 8.0; to 988 mL of ultrapure water. Mix, autoclave, and store at 4 °C.

Table 1
Oligonucleotide sequences of all probes and primers used

canSNP	xTAG	Allele	MOLigo	Sequence (5'-3')[a]
BA1 A.Br.001	B007	C	P1	5'-ACTCGTAGGGAATAAACCGT AAATTGTGAAAGATTGTTTGTGTA CAAATTTAATCTTTAAAGGAAAIIIIIACCGAAAC-3'
	A014	T	P1	5'-ACTCGTAGGGAATAAACCGT ATTGTGAAAGAAAGAGAAGAAATT CAAATTTAATCTTTAAAGGAAAIIIIIACCGAAAT-3'
	–	–	P2	5'P-TTGAAGTCGATGATAAAGGGAAACCGTATTATA TCTCACTTCTTACTACCGCG-3'
BA2 A.Br.002	A021	C	P1	5'-ACTCGTAGGGAATAAACCGT ATTAAGTAAGAATTGAGAGTTTGA AGAAGGAGCAAGTAATGTTATAGIIIIIGTTTAGGC-3'
	A022	T	P1	5'-ACTCGTAGGGAATAAACCGT GATTGATATTTGAATGTTTGTTTG AGAAGGAGCAAGTAATGTTATAGIIIIIGTTTAGGT-3'
	–	–	P2	5'P-TGGGCGGCAGTCGCTTTATC TCTCACTTCTTACTACCGCG-3'
BA3 A.Br.003	A025	G	P1	5'-ACTCGTAGGGAATAAACCGT GTATGTTGTAATGTATTAAGAAAG TGTATAAAAACCTCCTTTTTCTIIIIIACCTCAAG-3'
	A026	A	P1	5'-ACTCGTAGGGAATAAACCGT TTTGATTTAAGAGTGTTGAATGTA TGTATAAAAACCTCCTTTTTCTIIIIIACCTCAAA-3'
	–	–	P2	5'P-TTGAGGTAGAAAAAGGAGGTTTTTATACAATGACA TCTCACTTCTTACTACCGCG-3'
BA4 A.Br.004	A027	T	P1	5'-ACTCGTAGGGAATAAACCGT AAGATGATAGTTAAGTGTAAGTTA GACATCGCCGTCATACTTIIIIITGGAATGT-3'
	A028	C	P1	5'-ACTCGTAGGGAATAAACCGT GATAGATTTAGAATGAATTAAGTG GACATCGCCGTCATACTTIIIIITGGAATGC-3'
	–	–	P2	5'P-CCCTAATCCTTCCATAGCTCCACCA TCTCACTTCTTACTACCGCG-3'
BA5 A.Br.006	B008	T	P1	5'-ACTCGTAGGGAATAAACCGT TGTAAGTGAAATAGTGAGTTATTT CGTTTTTAAGTTCATCATACCIIIIICATGCACT-3'
	A015	G	P1	5'-ACTCGTAGGGAATAAACCGT GTTGTAAATTGTAGTAAAGAAGTA CGTTTTTAAGTTCATCATACCIIIIICATGCACG-3'
	–	–	P2	5'P-AGGCGATGGAATGATCAACAACATATTGA TCTCACTTCTTACTACCGCG-3'

(continued)

Table 1
(continued)

canSNP	xTAG	Allele	MOLigo	Sequence (5'-3')[a]
BA6 A.Br.007	A029	T	P1	5'-ACTCGTAGGGAATAAACCGT TTTAAGTGAGTTATAGAAGTAGTA AGACGATAAACTGAATAATACCIIIIIATCCTTAT-3'
	A030	C	P1	5'-ACTCGTAGGGAATAAACCGT GTGTTATAGAAGTTAAATGTTAAG AGACGATAAACTGAATAATACCIIIIIATCCTTAC-3'
	–	–	P2	5'P-ATTCAGCTCGAATACTACCACCTTGTAATTC TCTCACTTCTTACTACCGCG-3'
BA7 A.Br.008	B009	T	P1	5'-ACTCGTAGGGAATAAACCGT GAATTGTATAAAGTATTAGATGTG TATACGTTTTAGATGGAGATAIIIIIATTCTTCT-3'
	A018	G	P1	5'-ACTCGTAGGGAATAAACCGT GTAATTGAATTGAAAGATAAGTGT TATACGTTTTAGATGGAGATAIIIIIATTCTTCG-3'
	–	–	P2	5'P-CCGCTTGTTAAACGTATATTTGTAACTTTTTCAC TCTCACTTCTTACTACCGCG-3'
BA8 A.Br.009	A033	C	P1	5'-ACTCGTAGGGAATAAACCGT TATTAGAGTTTGAGAATAAGTAGT AGGTATATTAACTGCGGATGIIIIIATGCAAGC-3'
	A034	T	P1	5'-ACTCGTAGGGAATAAACCGT TGATATAGTAGTGAAGAAATAAGT AGGTATATTAACTGCGGATGIIIIIATGCAAGT-3'
	–	–	P2	5'P-AAAGCCGTTCAAAAACAGTGGCC TCTCACTTCTTACTACCGCG-3'
BA9 B.Br.001	A035	G	P1	5'-ACTCGTAGGGAATAAACCGT AATAAGAGAATTGATATGAAGATG CGGATATGATACCGATACCTIIIIITCTTATCC-3'
	A036	T	P1	5'-ACTCGTAGGGAATAAACCGT TTGTGTAGTTAAGAGTTGTTTAAT CGGATATGATACCGATACCTIIIIITCTTATCT-3'
	–	–	P2	5'P-TCTTCTATTGTACCGATTTCTTTTATGACCG TCTCACTTCTTACTACCGCG-3'
BA10 B.Br.002	A037	T	P1	5'-ACTCGTAGGGAATAAACCGT TGTATATGTTAATGAGATGTTGTA ACCTTCTGTGTTCGTTGTTAAIIIIICGTTACTT-3'
	A038	G	P1	5'-ACTCGTAGGGAATAAACCGT AGTAAGTGTTAGATAGTATTGAAT ACCTTCTGTGTTCGTTGTTAAIIIIICGTTACTG-3'

	–	–	P2	5'P-CTGTTCCTTTTGCAACTTCTCCTCCA <u>TCTCACTTCTTACTACCGCG</u>-3'
BA11 B.Br.003	A012	G	P1	5'-<u>ACTCGTAGGGAATAAACCGT</u> AGTAGAAAGTTGAAATTGATTATG GCATAGAAGCAGATGAGCTTAIIIIICATATCCG-3'
	A019	A	P1	5'-<u>ACTCGTAGGGAATAAACCGT</u> GTGTGTTATTTGTTTGTAAAGTAT GCATAGAAGCAGATGAGCTTAIIIIICATATCCA-3'
	–	–	P2	5'P-CTTCACGTTATGGTTCGTTATGAACTTGAG <u>TCTCACTTCTTACTACCGCG</u>-3'
BA12 B.Br.004	A013	A	P1	5'-<u>ACTCGTAGGGAATAAACCGT</u> AGTGAATGTAAGATTATGTATTTG TAAAATGAAGATAATGACAAAIIIIICGGGATGA-3'
	A020	G	P1	5'-<u>ACTCGTAGGGAATAAACCGT</u> AAATTAGTTGAAAGTATGAGAAAG TAAAATGAAGATAATGACAAAIIIIICGGGATGG-3'
	–	–	P2	5'P-TAGAAGTAAAGAAGGTTACCCAAGCACTTG <u>TCTCACTTCTTACTACCGCG</u>-3'
BA14 A.Br.011	A039	T	P1	5'-<u>ACTCGTAGGGAATAAACCGT</u> TTGTGATAGTAGTTAGATATTTGT TTGAAGCAGGAIIIIIGCGCCCCT-3'
	A042	C	P1	5'-<u>ACTCGTAGGGAATAAACCGT</u> ATTTGTTATGATAAATGTGTAGTG TTGAAGCAGGAIIIIIGCGCCCCC-3'
	–	–	P2	5'-P-ATTATTTTCAGCGGGAATTCGTTTCTTTTTAG <u>TCTCACTTCTTACTACCGCG</u>-3'
Forward	–	–	–	5'**<u>BIOT</u>**-CGCGG**<u>T</u>**AGTAAGAAG**<u>T</u>**GAGA-3'
Reverse	–	–	–	5'-ACTCGTAGGGAATAAACCGT-3'

[a]Primer, xTAG, and DNA target sequences of MOLigos are indicated, respectively, by underlined, italic and bold, and light gray sequences. The forward primer is biotinylated at its 5′ end and at two internal T nucleotides (positions are underlined and indicated in bold). The 5′-end of each MOLigoP2 probe is phosphorylated

3. 26 MagPlex beads (Luminex, Austin, USA) with a unique spectral signature (*see* region names and tag-coated sequences in Table 1). Store at 2–8 °C.
4. Streptavidin-phycoerythrin (SA-PE) 100× (Bio-Rad, Hercules, USA) (*see* **Note 3**). Store at 2–8 °C. Keep away from light.
5. Luminex 200 (Luminex, Austin, USA) or BioPlex 200 platform (Bio-Rad, Hercules, USA).

3 Methods

Carry out all procedures at room temperature.

Each experiment must include two controls for the calculation of signal-to-noise ratio: a bead-only control that reports background fluorescence obtained from the microspheres alone and a no template PCR control (H_2O) that reports cross reactivity between MOLigo pairs in the absence of any DNA template.

3.1 MOL-PCR Method

1. Prepare ligation and amplification mixes for all samples, including two, no template, PCR controls (*see* **Notes 7** and **8**), as follows:
2. The ligation mix includes 5 U of Ampligase® DNA ligase, 0.1 nmol of each MOLigo probe (*see* Table 1) and 1× Ampligase® DNA Ligase Buffer. Make up to 8 µl per reaction with TE buffer.
3. The amplification mix includes 2.5 U of Hot Start *Taq* polymerase, 2.5 µM of each dNTP, 1× *Taq* Buffer, 100 pmol of biotin-labeled Universal Forward primer, and 2 pmol of Universal Reverse primer. The total PCR volume is 12 µl per reaction.
4. Aliquot 8 µL of ligation mix to wells or PCR microtubes and store the amplification mix at 4 °C until use.
5. Add 2 µL of template DNA (sample) to each ligation mix reaction or 2 µL of ultrapure water to PCR negative controls wells.
6. Run the ligation step using the following thermocycling parameters: DNA denaturation at 95 °C for 5 min, followed by 10 ligation cycles of 60 °C for 5 min and 95 °C for 2 min, and a final ligase denaturation step at 98 °C for 5 min.
7. Aliquot 12 µL of amplification mix to new PCR microtubes or multiwell plate.
8. Add 8 µL of the ligation products.
9. Run the amplification step as follows: 95 °C for 15 min, 45 cycles of 95 °C for 30 s, 55 °C for 30 s, and 72 °C for 30 s. Reactions are then cooled to 4 °C and either used immediately in the bead hybridization step or stored at −20 °C before proceeding with the hybridization step.

3.2 Hybridization on Beads and SA-PE Incubation

1. Equilibrate the MagPlex beads and the THB 1.1× at room temperature (*see* **Note 9**).
2. Prepare enough mix of 26 MagPlex beads to perform all analyses in duplicate, including the two no template PCR controls and an additional bead-only control that reports background fluorescence obtained from the microspheres alone. Dilute 1,250 magnetic beads of each region (*see* **Note 10**) in 32 μL of THB 1.1× solution per reaction. A final volume of 45 μL is obtained. Turn on the Luminex platform and equilibrate the calibration beads at room temperature (*see* **Note 11**).
3. When the lasers are warmed up, perform a calibration of the system as recommended by the manufacturer (*see* **Note 12**) and set the platform heater to 52 °C.
4. Vortex, then sonicate the MagPlex beads, and mix briefly (about 20 s each step).
5. Aliquot 45 μL of this mix into a multiwell plate. The no template PCR and only-bead controls (in duplicate) have to be clearly separated from the other samples to avoid cross contamination.
6. Add 5 μL of amplicons (or water for the only-beads controls) to each well. Seal and vortex briefly.
7. Run the bead hybridization thermocycling program: 95 °C for 2 min followed by array hybridization at 52 °C for 30 min.
8. Separate the beads from the supernatant (*see* **Note 13**).
9. Prepare a SA-PE mix at a final concentration of 3× by dilution in THB 1.1×. The final volume is 75 μL per reaction (*see* **Note 14**).
10. Resuspend the pelleted MagPlex-TAG microspheres in 75 μL SA-PE mix.
11. Briefly vortex the plate until the pellet is totally resuspended.
12. Incubate at 52 °C for 15 min in the Luminex platform.

3.3 Luminex Readout

1. Run the protocol on the Luminex platform, using the reading of 100 beads per region setting (*see* **Notes 11** and **15**).
2. When the run is over, export the results in Excel file for data analysis.
3. Rinse and shut down the system according to manufacturer recommendations.

3.4 Data Analysis

The standard workflow to analyze Luminex output data has four basic steps:

1. Correct raw Mean Fluorescence Intensity (MFI) values by subtracting the MFI values of the bead-only control. All resulting negative MFI values are set to 1.

2. Determine the absolute minimal threshold value of the run by calculating the median values of all no template PCR controls (MFI_{H2O}). No template PCR control values (MFI_{H2O_allele}) below that threshold are replaced by the threshold value in Eq. 1. This step avoids SNP calling failure linked to excessive variations observed between no template PCR controls values.
3. Calculate an allelic ratio (AR) for each biallelic canSNP and sample to genotype according to Eq. 1 [20]:

$$AR = \left(MFI_{allele1} / MFI_{H2O\_allele1}\right) / \left(\begin{array}{l} \left(MFI_{allele1} / MFI_{H2O\_allele1}\right) \\ +\left(MFI_{allele2} / MFI_{H2O\_allele2}\right) \end{array} \right) \quad (1)$$

4. Assign allele calling using the following general rules: SNP is called "allele 2" if the AR is less than 0.4 ($AR < 0.4$) and "allele 1" if it is greater than 0.6 ($AR > 0.6$). Between both AR values, manual inspection of raw data is used for allele calling.

4 Notes

1. Viability testing can be performed by spreading an aliquot of each DNA preparation on blood agar Petri Dish and incubation at 37 °C for 18–24 h. In case of growth, perform microfiltration and repeat viability step.
2. Assay limit of detection was determined to be 2 ng of genomic DNA per ligation reaction.
3. The supplier of DNA ligase (Epicentre) and streptavidin-phycoerythrin (Bio-Rad) is critical for the method. Use the specified products.
4. MOLigoP1 probes contains three functional components that allow (a) detection of target sequences, (b) universal amplification of successfully ligated probes, and (c) capture of amplified products onto a microsphere array. Each pair contains a 5′-end universal PCR Reverse primer sequence common for all the different MOLigoP1, an internal 24 bp xTAG sequence unique for each MOLigoP1 probe for capture to conjugated xTAG microsphere, and a 3′-end sequence complementary to the specific target DNA including the allele-specific nucleotide (SNP) at its 3′ end. To improve allele specificity, the 3′ specific target sequence is separated into two distinct priming regions by a polydeoxyinosine (Poly(I)) linker, according to the DPO principle [21]. The longer 5′ segment initiates stable priming. The shorter 3′ segment determines target-specific extension and SNP discrimination).

5. MoLigoP2 probes consist of two sequences: the 5′-end reverse complement of a Universal Forward primer and a 3′-end locus-specific portion complementary to the specific target sequence located just after the SNP.
6. Use the reagent at room temperature to facilitate Triton® X-100 mixing.
7. Prepare $n+1$ ligation and amplification mixes to ensure sufficient volume for all samples (n = number of strains to genotype + 2 no template controls).
8. Vortex both mixtures thoroughly; it has to be homogenous as much as possible.
9. Keep the MagPlex beads away from light as much as possible during all the processes.
10. The canSNP genotyping assay implies 26 different bead regions. Two unique anti-xTAG bead regions are associated with each biallelic-specific canSNP and the corresponding competitive MOLigoP1 pair (*see* Table 1).
11. The Luminex system needs 30 min to warm up the lasers; this also applies to the calibration beads.
12. We recommend calibrating the system once per day of use.
13. Three different methods of separation are recommended by the manufacturer: using a magnetic plate separator, an automatic plate washer, or centrifugation. In the last case, pellet the MagPlex-TAG microspheres by centrifugation at $\geq 2{,}250 \times g$ for 3 min and remove the supernatant.
14. The SA-PE mix is very sensitive to light, so use a dark tube or keep it in the dark as much as possible.
15. To enhance the signal, use the option "Run at High RP1 Target" in the software (if available).

Acknowledgments

This research was supported by/executed in the framework of the EU-project AniBioThreat (Grant Agreement: Home/2009/ISEC/AG/191) with the financial support from the Prevention of and Fight against Crime Programme of the European Union, European Commission–Directorate General Home Affairs. This publication reflects the views only of the author, and the European Commission cannot be held responsible for any use which may be made of the information contained therein.

References

1. Pearson T, Busch JD, Ravel J et al (2004) Phylogenetic discovery bias in *Bacillus anthracis* using single-nucleotide polymorphisms from whole-genome sequencing. Proc Natl Acad Sci U S A 101:13536–13541
2. Marston CK, Allen CA, Beaudry J et al (2011) Molecular epidemiology of anthrax cases associated with recreational use of animal hides and yarn in the United States. PLoS One 6:e28274
3. Van Ert MN, Easterday WR, Huynh LY et al (2007) Global genetic population structure of *Bacillus anthracis*. PLoS One 2:e461
4. Kim S, Misra A (2007) SNP genotyping: technologies and biomedical applications. Annu Rev Biomed Eng 9:289–320
5. Kwok PY (2001) Methods for genotyping single nucleotide polymorphisms. Annu Rev Genomics Hum Genet 2:235–258
6. Gunderson KL, Steemers FJ, Ren H et al (2006) Whole-genome genotyping. Methods Enzymol 410:359–376
7. Kennedy GC, Matsuzaki H, Dong S et al (2003) Large-scale genotyping of complex DNA. Nat Biotechnol 21:1233–1237
8. Price EP, Matthews MA, Beaudry JA et al (2010) Cost-effective interrogation of single nucleotide polymorphisms using the mismatch amplification mutation assay and capillary electrophoresis. Electrophoresis 31:3881–3888
9. Bruse S, Moreau M, Azaro M, Zimmerman R, Brzustowicz L (2008) Improvements to bead-based oligonucleotide ligation SNP genotyping assays. Biotechniques 45:559–571
10. Dunbar SA (2006) Applications of Luminex xMAP technology for rapid, high-throughput multiplexed nucleic acid detection. Clin Chim Acta 363:71–82
11. Dunbar SA, Vander Zee CA, Oliver KG, Karem KL, Jacobson JW (2003) Quantitative, multiplexed detection of bacterial pathogens: DNA and protein applications of the Luminex LabMAP system. J Microbiol Methods 53:245–252
12. Janse I, Bok JM, Hamidjaja RA, Hodemaekers HM, van Rotterdam BJ (2012) Development and comparison of two assay formats for parallel detection of four biothreat pathogens by using suspension microarrays. PLoS One 7:e31958
13. Kenefic LJ, Pearson T, Okinaka RT et al (2009) Pre-Columbian origins for North American anthrax. PLoS One 4:e4813
14. Kuroda M, Serizawa M, Okutani A, Sekizuka T, Banno S, Inoue S (2010) Genome-wide single nucleotide polymorphism typing method for identification of *Bacillus anthracis* species and strains among *B. cereus* group species. J Clin Microbiol 48:2821–2829
15. Birdsell DN, Pearson T, Price EP et al (2012) Melt analysis of mismatch amplification mutation assays (Melt-MAMA): a functional study of a cost-effective SNP genotyping assay in bacterial models. PLoS One 7:e32866
16. Van Ert MN, Easterday WR, Simonson TS et al (2007) Strain-specific single-nucleotide polymorphism assays for the *Bacillus anthracis* Ames strain. J Clin Microbiol 45:47–53
17. Girault G, Madani N, Derzelle S (2013) Anthrax in France: a pangenomic study. In: *Bacillus ACT* 2013, Victoria, Canada
18. Schouten JP, McElgunn CJ, Waaijer R et al (2002) Relative quantification of 40 nucleic acid sequences by multiplex ligation-dependent probe amplification. Nucleic Acids Res 30:e57
19. Deshpande A, Gans J, Graves SW et al (2010) A rapid multiplex assay for nucleic acid-based diagnostics. J Microbiol Methods 80:155–163
20. Stucki D, Malla B, Hostettler S et al (2012) Two new rapid SNP-typing methods for classifying *Mycobacterium tuberculosis* complex into the main phylogenetic lineages. PLoS One 7:e41253
21. Chun JY, Kim KJ, Hwang IT et al (2007) Dual priming oligonucleotide system for the multiplex detection of respiratory viruses and SNP genotyping of CYP2C19 gene. Nucleic Acids Res 35:e40
22. Thierry S, Hamidjaja RA, Girault G et al (2013) A Multiplex bead-based suspension array assay for interrogation of phylogenetically informative single nucleotide polymorphisms for *Bacillus anthracis*. J Microbiol Methods 95(3):357–365

Part IV

Integrative Omics and High-Throughput Platforms to Unravel the Biology of Pathogens and Their Interaction with the Host

Chapter 30

Next-Generation Sequencing in Veterinary Medicine: How Can the Massive Amount of Information Arising from High-Throughput Technologies Improve Diagnosis, Control, and Management of Infectious Diseases?

Steven Van Borm, Sándor Belák, Graham Freimanis, Alice Fusaro, Fredrik Granberg, Dirk Höper, Donald P. King, Isabella Monne, Richard Orton, and Toon Rosseel

Abstract

The development of high-throughput molecular technologies and associated bioinformatics has dramatically changed the capacities of scientists to produce, handle, and analyze large amounts of genomic, transcriptomic, and proteomic data. A clear example of this step-change is represented by the amount of DNA sequence data that can be now produced using next-generation sequencing (NGS) platforms. Similarly, recent improvements in protein and peptide separation efficiencies and highly accurate mass spectrometry have promoted the identification and quantification of proteins in a given sample. These advancements in biotechnology have increasingly been applied to the study of animal infectious diseases and are beginning to revolutionize the way that biological and evolutionary processes can be studied at the molecular level. Studies have demonstrated the value of NGS technologies for molecular characterization, ranging from metagenomic characterization of unknown pathogens or microbial communities to molecular epidemiology and evolution of viral quasispecies. Moreover, high-throughput technologies now allow detailed studies of host-pathogen interactions at the level of their genomes (genomics), transcriptomes (transcriptomics), or proteomes (proteomics). Ultimately, the interaction between pathogen and host biological networks can be questioned by analytically integrating these levels (integrative OMICS and systems biology). The application of high-throughput biotechnology platforms in these fields and their typical low-cost per information content has revolutionized the resolution with which these processes can now be studied.

The aim of this chapter is to provide a current and prospective view on the opportunities and challenges associated with the application of massive parallel sequencing technologies to veterinary medicine, with particular focus on applications that have a potential impact on disease control and management.

Key words Next-generation sequencing, Animal infectious disease management, OMICS

The Epi-SEQ consortium (www.epi-seq.eu)

Mónica V. Cunha and João Inácio (eds.), *Veterinary Infection Biology: Molecular Diagnostics and High-Throughput Strategies*, Methods in Molecular Biology, vol. 1247, DOI 10.1007/978-1-4939-2004-4_30,

1 Introduction

Genetic characterization of infectious agents plays a central role in the diagnosis, monitoring, and control of infectious diseases. The development of rapid DNA sequencing methods based on the selective incorporation of chain-terminating dideoxynucleotides ([1]; later termed "first-generation sequencing technologies") and the polymerase chain reaction (PCR) DNA amplification technologies ([2]; reviewed in [3]) has paved the way for the study of biological and evolutionary processes at the molecular level. Such technologies have been extensively applied to the diagnosis and molecular epidemiology of infectious diseases of livestock and become important tools for targeted research on host-pathogen interactions. The most recent versions of these first-generation sequencing technologies are widely accessible and provide high-quality data. However, their application to projects such as whole genome sequencing is expensive and time-consuming, often requiring prior knowledge of the target genome for specific template amplification. These limitations have been particularly problematic for large sequencing projects and have motivated the development of alternative, post-Sanger sequencing technologies ("next-generation sequencing" or NGS).

Next-generation sequencing platforms provide unprecedented throughput, generating hundreds of gigabases of data in a single experiment. Although the initial capital investment and cost per experiment remain high, the price per information unit (nucleotide) has been dramatically reduced in comparison with first-generation sequencing. Moreover, these technologies allow unbiased sequencing without prior knowledge of the complete DNA content in a sample while retaining the flexibility to allow for targeted sequencing.

This paradigm shift in the scale of DNA sequence data has revolutionized the way biological and evolutionary processes can be studied at the molecular level, enabling genome projects previously restricted to high profile model organisms and human pathogens to target pathogens of lesser economic and medical significance.

Such advancements are now being increasingly applied to veterinary medicine. As a result, the increasing availability of these technologies combined with the rapid development of applied tools and protocols has provided a diverse array of applications for use in genomics and transcriptomics and even routine diagnostics.

In this chapter, we review recent advances in NGS technologies that are becoming commonplace in many laboratories, with an emphasis on the applications that have the potential to significantly impact on diagnosis, prevention, and control of infectious diseases in animals.

2 Massive Parallel Sequencing

2.1 Technologies

A number of different NGS platforms are currently available, with each utilizing different sequencing chemistries and detection strategies. This has led to individual systems having their own strengths and limitations (reviewed in [4–6]). *Second-generation sequencing platforms* vary in technology and chemistry used but have the following properties in common:

- A DNA library is made from the sample. This library is either representing all DNA in sample without prior knowledge or a targeted library using PCR amplification or alternative enrichment methods. Adapter sequences are joined to the DNA molecules (by ligation or amplification) and can include a barcode sequence that allows multiplexing of several samples in an experiment.
- Individual DNA molecules in each library are clonally amplified.
- Clonal DNAs are sequenced by massive parallel sequencing.
- Hundreds of thousands of DNA sequence reads result and need to be processed.

The second-generation sequencing platforms first emerged on the market with an emphasis on extreme high-throughput sequencing applications and initially were restricted to genome sequencing centers or core facilities. These technologies use different detection principles including pyrosequencing (454 Life Sciences, acquired by Roche, available since 2005, but planned to be discontinued by mid-2016), Illumina's sequencing by synthesis (previously Solexa, available since 2007), SOLiD ligation-based sequencing (Life Technologies, available since 2006), and, more recently, the Ion Torrent semiconductor sequencing technology. Over the last 5–7 years, all of the major platforms have made significant improvements, with notable advancements made in terms of protocol complexity, overall performance (including read length, fidelity, lower input DNA), and cost efficiency. More recently, smaller benchtop sequencers [7] have become available, making the technology more accessible for use in routine microbiology laboratories, while academic core facilities and commercial service providers focused increasingly upon providing users with access to a wider diversity of the sequencing technologies available. These developments will bring NGS technologies within the reach of many more research groups and diagnostic laboratories where NGS analysis of a single isolate will generate significant quantities of data, many orders of magnitude greater than that generated by other typing methods.

In addition to the continuous improvement of existing platforms, newer methodologies are being developed. *Third-generation sequencing technologies* are defined as single-molecule sequencers (reviewed in [6, 8]). These approaches promise additional advantages such as scalability, simplicity, long read length, and low operational costs and do not require clonal amplification of template DNA molecules, thereby removing potential errors associated with clonal amplification. A single third-generation platform is currently available on the market since 2011 (PacBio, Pacific Biosciences) that sequences long single DNA molecules in real time, known as SMRT sequencing. Other technologies are still under development (e.g., [4]) such as DNA sequencing in nanopores that offer the potential of simple, inexpensive, single-molecule sequencing in miniaturized or highly scalable devices [9]. Although substantial validation data is still required, these technologies have the potential to make NGS even more widely available in diagnostic labs.

2.2 Challenges

While the advantages of NGS are numerous (unprecedented scale of genomic information, scalability, low-cost per information content, and high throughput), several challenges remain to be addressed.

Several processes in the NGS workflow, from sample selection to data interpretation, are potentially vulnerable to bias and/or error introduction (Fig. 1). This includes the *error rates* of the

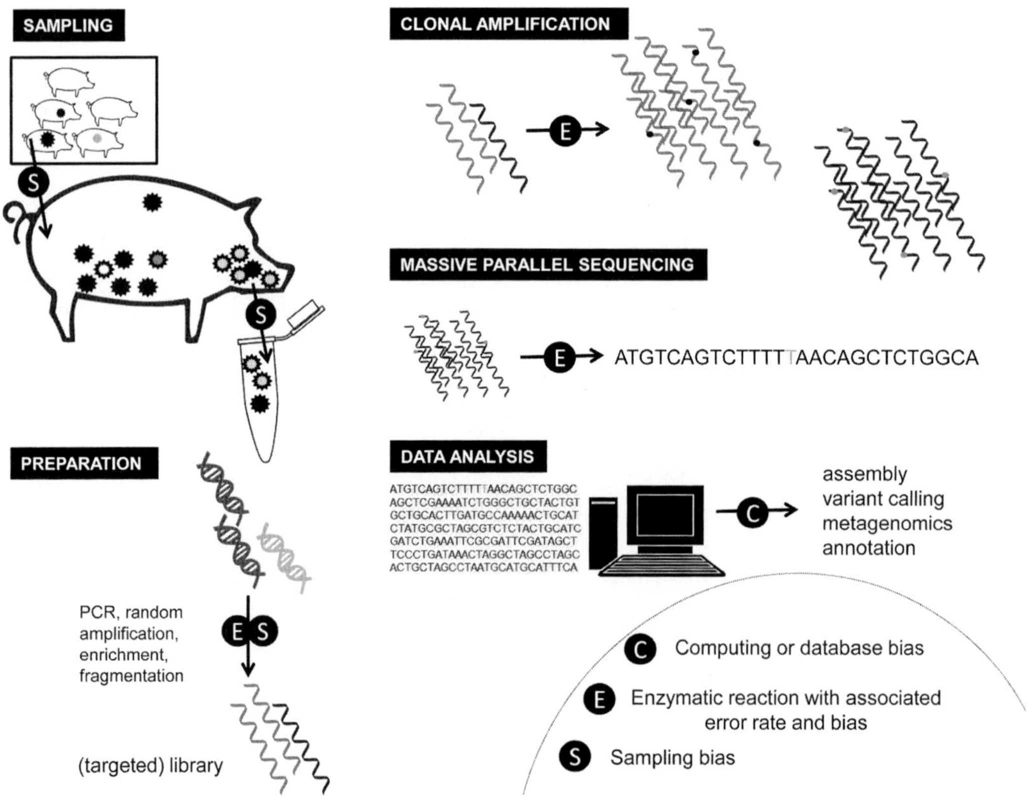

Fig. 1 Steps in next-generation sequencing and data analysis workflows where error and bias introduction may occur

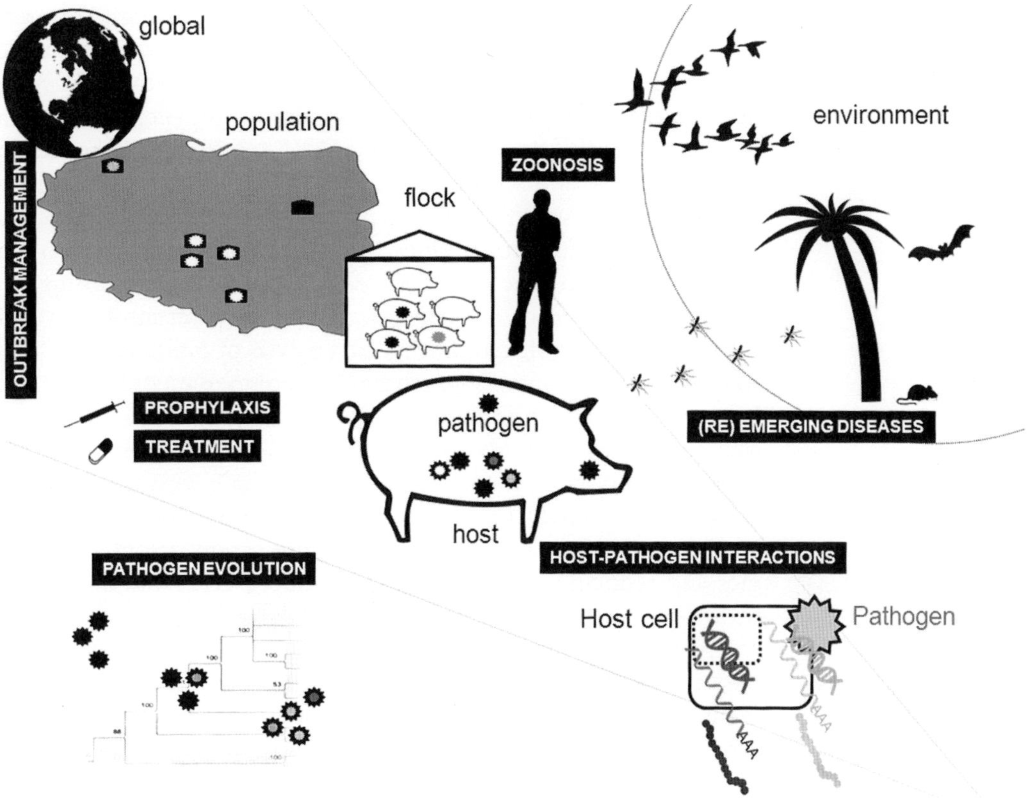

Fig. 2 High-throughput technologies can be applied to numerous aspects of animal infectious diseases

sequencing chemistry and library construction, as well as point mutations and insertions/deletions that may arise during reverse transcription and PCR amplification. The amplification of DNA by PCR to obtain clonal template sequences is subject to error introduction [8] and may result in an amplification bias impacting the relative frequency of sequence variants present in the sample. *Sampling bias* can be introduced when a relatively small number of samples are analyzed per epidemiological unit (e.g., single animal or herd) due to financial constraints restricting the thorough use of NGS. When only a small proportion of the nucleic acids in a single sample are subjected to sequence analysis, technical sampling bias occurs. While NGS data provides a high resolution of an individual sample, the resolution of higher epidemiological scales (Fig. 2) may thus be compromised due to insufficient sampling. Moreover, as a minimum amount of genetic material is needed as input for NGS workflows, this can result in bias towards samples with the highest pathogen titers. Errors and bias may also be introduced by methods to increase the sensitivity of the workflow, such as targeted pathogen genome amplification [10–12] or enrichment (e.g., [13]).

Furthermore, reagent contamination has been reported to interfere with metagenomic analyses [14, 15]. Errors can also be made during the sequencing process itself via base miscalls by NGS machines. For example, the loss of synchronicity (dephasing) in a percentage of the clonally amplified DNA template [16] results in increased noise and sequencing errors [17, 8]. Each of the different NGS platforms available has its own distinct characteristics in terms of read and error profiles, with the Illumina platform often regarded as having the lowest error rate, while other platforms can produce longer reads [7, 18, 19]. In addition, certain biases and errors can be introduced during the analysis of NGS datasets, due to the limitations of the algorithms or reference data used [20, 21]. For example, genomic repeat regions are a well-known problem for sequence assembly algorithms [22]. However, software advancements combined with platform and chemistry developments are expected to further reduce operational costs, error rates, and input DNA quantities, allowing more careful sampling strategies and reducing experimentally introduced error and bias in the future.

As a result of errors and bias introductions, NGS data needs to be "cleaned". This includes sequence filtering (removing low-quality sequences) and alignment followed by variant calling and error correction. Discriminating true biological variants from those due to experimental noise is an important issue when trying to identify low-frequency variants in a population, for example, in viral quasispecies or metagenomic analyses, and there are currently a number of bioinformatics tools to aid in this (e.g., [23–26, 19]). Currently, a multitude of software has been developed to address different aspects of NGS analyses [27, 28]. However, the available algorithms for both genome assembly and amplicon analysis can present some limitations [29], meaning that custom-made scripting and in-house resolution of bioinformatic problems are often needed to investigate novel datasets and specific hypotheses. In this context, researchers are frequently faced with the need to acquire computer skills and bioinformatics expertise. To evaluate the potential of NGS for a wider group of scientists and diagnosticians, there is a real need to develop flexible and practical bioinformatics workflows that can provide user-friendly tools for the analysis of massive datasets and that become publicly available. Although some software with a menu-driven approach is available (e.g., Geneious, CLC Workbench, Galaxy), most applications are optimized on UNIX-based operating systems and require some bioinformatics expertise. Although less user-friendly, UNIX-based pipelines are typically freely available to the NGS user community and are equipped with algorithms that track the high pace of innovation in the NGS field.

A further issue is the scale of genetic data produced by NGS technologies which presents a physical constraint in terms of data storage and analysis. Although limited datasets (e.g., resulting from the desktop-range 2nd-generation sequencers) can be managed using modest computing resources, like high-end desktop computers running virtual Linux machines [4], larger datasets typically require high-performance computational clusters, which present a considerable investment and require sufficient information technology (IT) support. Cloud computational resources (i.e., renting time from commercial high-performance computational clusters) may be a solution [30] although further developments are needed, given the data transfer issues resulting from huge file sizes [4]. Another issue for diagnostic laboratories is protection of data from unauthorized access, which cannot be guaranteed in the cloud, as data from diagnostic examinations need to be kept confidential. For labs frequently producing NGS data, data storage and backup costs can be substantial. Ideally, these huge genetic datasets should be made publicly available to the scientific community as they provide a source of information applicable to better understanding disease, design of targeted assays, systems biology, and integrated OMICS analysis approaches. To this end, online repositories such as the Sequence Read Archive (SRA; [31]) have been created to store both raw NGS and intermediate analysis files.

It will also be important to consider how results from complex and massive NGS datasets will be communicated to policy groups and the public and become a decision-supporting tool. To this end, it is necessary that scientists and diagnosticians develop and agree on data formats for the communication of NGS results for analyses that go beyond simple genome sequences, for instance, for reporting quasispecies compositions.

3 Application of NGS to Animal Infectious Disease

NGS technology is now being increasingly applied to study the etiology, genomics, evolution, and epidemiology of animal infectious diseases as well as host-pathogen interactions (Fig. 2). These applications have provided novel insights and illustrate the potential of this new technology to directly impact on our understanding and control strategies for animal infectious disease.

NGS platforms have been instrumental in the completion of large *animal genomes* and the documentation of genomic variation (reviewed in [32]). Available livestock genomes now include bovine, pig, sheep, equine, and avian [32] which provide an important source of knowledge for understanding food production and animal interaction with infectious pathogens. Additional livestock genome sequencing efforts have documented genomic variation providing information for the development of genetic markers applicable to animal breeding genetics [33–35], including traits related to pathogen resistance and interaction with microbial communities in poultry [36]. Others have used novel sequencing technologies for the targeted study of specific gene families occupying key roles in host immunology (e.g., Toll-like receptor (TLR) gene family [37]).

The high variability and large size of the mitochondrial genome (mtDNA) of *eukaryotic parasites* have been recently explored using NGS (reviewed by [38]). mtDNA sequences proved very informative in epidemiological studies [38] but also include comparative mtDNA sequencing of parasites with low and high zoonotic potential [39]. Targeting specific polymorphic genes in the *Cryptosporidium parvum* genome using NGS, extensive intra-host genetic diversity was documented [40]. Studies of the *transcriptome* (all mRNA transcripts in an organism, tissue, or cell; also called *RNA-Seq*) of different parasite species and/or developmental stages provide insights into aspects of gene expression, regulation, and function, which are major steps to understanding their biology (reviewed in [41]). Examples include the characterization of the transcriptome from *Eimeria* sp. from chicken [42] and *Taenia* sp. from sheep [43]. In addition, RNA-Seq data have been used to predict potential drug targets [44] and to identify key genes involved in anthelmintic resistance [45].

Over the last five years, NGS has been used as an extremely important tool in the tracing of transmission, genome characterization, and outbreak management of both viral and bacterial diseases. The sequencing of these two pathogen types poses very different sets of challenges and issues, where the large data output expressed typically in the Mb (megabase) to Gb (gigabase) range [4] is particularly suited for the sequencing of larger bacterial genomes. The high plasticity of some microbial genomes, with large mobile elements, gene-coding plasmids, chromosomal genes, and regions of extensive genetic variability, can frequently complicate genome assembly [46]. While most viral genomes are significantly smaller than their bacterial counterparts, the viral replication biology (particularly that of RNA viruses) poses its own unique problems. These involve the inherent variability of many viral genomes due to replication machinery lacking efficient proofreading mechanisms. This, combined with a short generation time and high replication rate, results in a complex mix of differing genomes (a "swarm" of closely related viruses) within a single host that are often termed as "*quasispecies*," reviewed in [47]. In addition, recombination and reassortment of segmented viral genomes frequently occur. NGS techniques offer an unprecedented "step-change" increase in the amount of sequence data that can be generated from both types of these samples.

Figure 3 (different scales of sequence analysis) highlights where genetic analyses can target different biological scales and whether these are within an individual host, or between hosts,

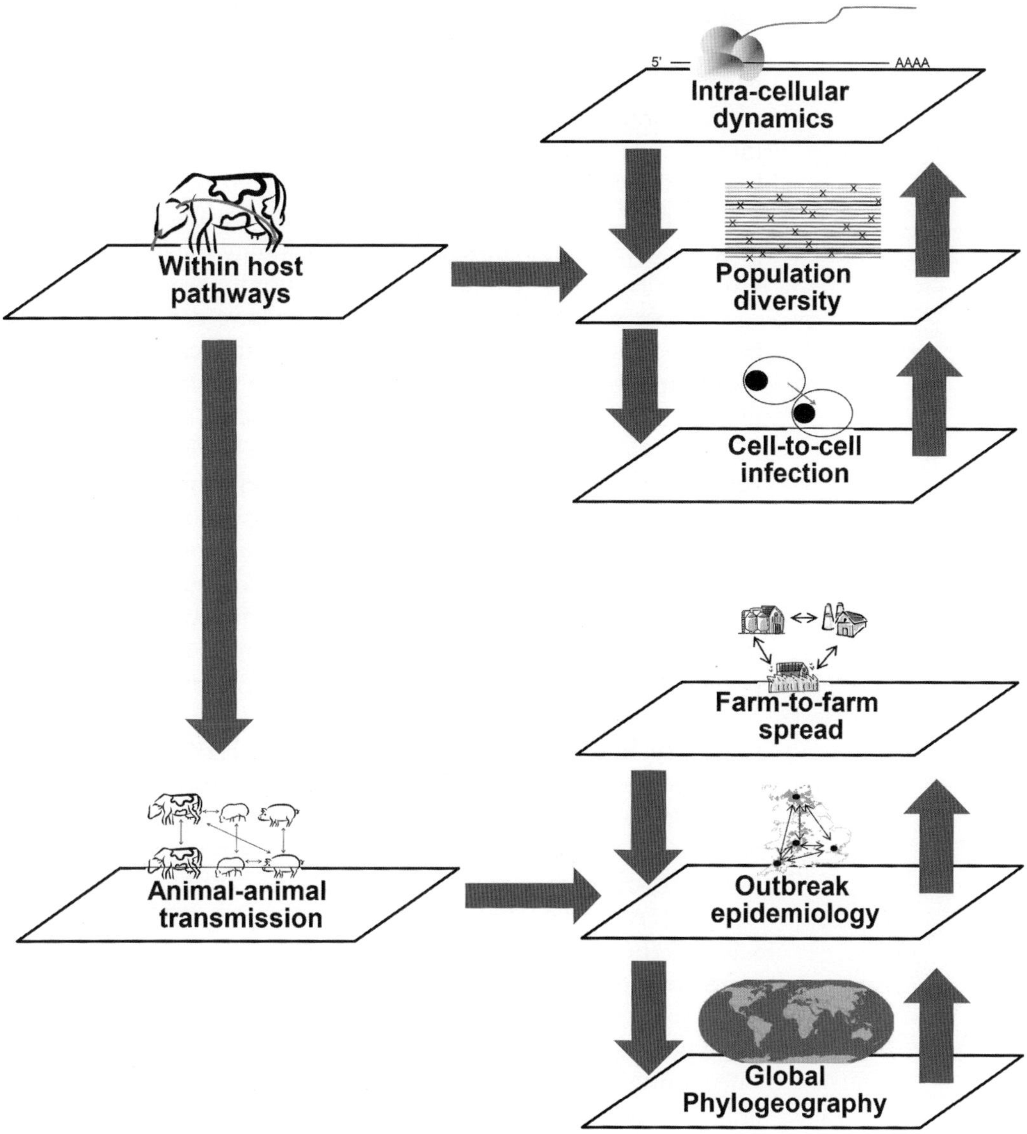

Fig. 3 The differing levels of intra- and inter-host variation that can be explored using NGS technologies range from intracellular dynamics to epidemiological applications

resulting in either host variation or inter-herd diversity/outbreak transmission.

At the level of the quasispecies, NGS technologies can now determine complete viral genomes to a fine-point resolution, allowing the quantification of viral diversity within samples [48] and making the sequencing of large numbers of samples economically feasible. The technology will allow the comparison of genetically diverse populations from different replication sites within a host [49, 50]. Wright and colleagues investigated the genetic diversity and resulting quasispecies population after inoculation of foot-and-mouth disease virus (FMDV) into a single animal and identified genetically distinct populations originating from different lesions [50]. Morelli and colleagues [51] studied the evolution of FMDV intra-sample sequence diversity during serial transmission in bovine hosts, providing novel insights into the fine-scale evolution of an RNA virus. NGS can also provide insights on microevolutionary processes of viruses at different scales, including the fine-point resolution molecular epidemiology analysis of outbreaks [52].

Recent studies on influenza A viruses have demonstrated that minority variants present in the donor population can be successfully transmitted to the recipient host and become prevalent with unpredictable impact on the virus biological properties [53, 54]. These findings suggest that the use of NGS approaches in RNA virus surveillance will be strategic to promptly detect biologically relevant viral quasispecies and will help in expanding our understanding of viral dynamics and emergence and the possible implications of mutation emergence for studies done using isolated viruses [55, 56].

The study of the viral swarm within individual hosts also has implications for understanding the evolutionary dynamics of viral populations under selection pressures, e.g., antiviral drugs. This has been a particularly active field in human medicine, e.g., with regard to human immunodeficiency virus (HIV) antiviral drugs response, drug resistance, and viral tropism (reviewed in [57–59]) and human influenza A (e.g., [60]) studies. The technologies' application to personalize antiviral treatment as a function of genetic marker makeup in human medicine is just around the corner [61]. Although at present only an emerging field in veterinary science, the development of antiviral drugs has the potential to translate into efficient animal infectious disease control strategies (e.g., [62, 63]).

The majority of the papers using NGS to investigate animal infectious disease focus specifically upon the level of animal-to-animal transmission and the characterization of pathogens within a single host, as this yields the most useful data in terms of outbreak management and identifying mechanisms/sources of disease transmission. For example, Lefébure and colleagues [64] used NGS to study genome complexity and horizontal gene transfer in foodborne *Campylobacter* spp. Biek et al. [65] studied local transmission patterns of *Mycobacterium bovis* in cattle and wildlife reservoirs using whole genome sequences from 31 samples originating on five farms. These demonstrated enough diversity between individual outbreaks to determine evolutionary variation down to herd level. The identification of novel antimicrobial resistance genes in the foodborne pathogen *Campylobacter coli* [66] was possible using NGS, and the application of NGS technologies during a recent crisis involving foodborne enterohemorrhagic *Escherichia coli* O104:H4 allowed a swift genomic identification [67] that was key to the management of this crisis. Finally, the technology also proved very informative to study the molecular epidemiology and evolutionary history of extremely monomorphic *Mycoplasma mycoides* subsp. *mycoides* SC [68] in addition to studies tracing medically significant pathogens [69–71]. Samples from the US 2006–2007 West Nile virus (WNV) outbreak in birds were characterized using Illumina sequencing, resulting in the identification of a new genetic variant containing a 13-nucleotide indel [72]. A survey of Chinese domestic fowl using RNA-Seq on an Ion Torrent identified a novel Coronavirus, providing insights into the diversity and distribution of avian coronaviruses [73]. A further study has also investigated the role of Usutu virus in causing epizootic infection in blackbirds in Germany [74].

The advent of NGS has also led to the cost-efficient sequencing of complete viral genomes including avian influenza virus [75–78], classical swine fever virus [79], and bluetongue viruses [80]. An optimized method incorporating 454 sequencing for universal nonspecific RNA viral genomes from brain and cell culture material was applied to Lyssaviruses [81]. Other groups have reported the characterization of Louping ill virus in lambs [82], porcine reproductive and respiratory syndrome virus [83], and herpesviruses from Asian elephants [84]. Furthermore, studies using random amplification techniques have identified mixed infections of paramyxoviruses and avian influenza in bird populations [77, 85, 78]. Efficient influenza A-specific resequencing strategies [86, 87] have allowed the study of quasispecies-scale genetic variability with implications for immune response [88, 89], host cell line adaptation [90, 91], antiviral drug resistance [92], and pathogenicity [53]. Likewise, efficient targeted CSFV genome sequencing using NGS has led to insights in classical swine fever virus (CSFV) epidemiology based on isolates from an outbreak in wild boar from Germany [79] and in the role of quasispecies diversity in CSFV pathogenicity [93].

NGS technology has also allowed the characterization of complete microbial communities without prior knowledge. For instance, the unbiased characterization of conserved bacterial ribosomal RNA-encoding sequences (rRNA profiling) has been applicable to whole microbial community characterization (e.g., [94, 95]) and to molecular characterization of (uncultured) bacteria [96]. *Metagenomics* is the determination of the sequence content of a complete microbial community (reviewed in [97]). The analysis of the resulting data can be taxonomy oriented (identification and quantification of species diversity; [98]) or function based (identification of coding gene diversity, e.g., [99]). The latter has significant potential, e.g., in the screening for virulence-associated, antibiotic resistance genes, and vitamin production-associated genes in microbial communities [100]. NGS also offers the potential of unbiased sequencing of the nucleic acid content of a sample and has been applied to the characterization of the *viral metagenome* in samples [101] or the identification of unknown or unexpected viruses in diseased animals or insect vectors. Furthermore, metagenomic NGS workflows allow the study of the interaction of treatment with an animal's microbiome [102]. In the microbiology lab, NGS has the potential for greater diagnostic resolution than any other typing method, and clinical microbiology labs are currently investigating its potential for routine diagnosis [103, 104].

Using NGS-based metagenomic approaches, multiple potential disease agents have been identified in a wide range of both domestic and wild animals (reviewed in [105–109]). Although the common goal is to identify potential pathogens, the studies can roughly be divided into three categories: (1) investigations of outbreaks of unknown etiology, (2) investigations of well-known disorders presumed to be of multifactorial etiology, and (3) metagenomic studies of reservoir species and vectors. Examples of the first category include the identification of a novel Orthobunyavirus affecting cattle (described in more detail below), an astrovirus in the brain of farmed minks suffering from encephalomyelitis [110], and a novel picornavirus as candidate etiologic agent for turkey viral hepatitis [111], among others. The second category encompasses investigations aimed at finding contributing infectious agents to complex diseases, such as colony collapse disorder of honey bees [112, 113] and postweaning multisystemic wasting syndrome in pigs [114]. Studies in the third category have been performed on diverse animal species suspected to be important reservoirs, such as bats [115, 116], African bush pigs [117], and red fox [118], as well as typical vector organisms, such as ticks [119].

Although it is an important first step, the identification and genetic characterization of candidate pathogens are not enough to establish causal relationships or understand how they may be associated with disease. It is therefore necessary to use a synergistic approach combining molecular diagnostic tools, such as NGS-based metagenomics and follow-up PCR-based assays targeting detected pathogen sequences, with more conventional diagnostic methods, including isolation and characterization. This is crucially important in situations where metagenomic data indicate the potential presence of multiple pathogens. While PCR-based prevalence studies in matching disease cases and healthy controls can provide further evidence for disease association, isolation of candidate pathogens is required to assign causality by addressing Koch's postulates [120]. The assembled data from such a multidisciplinary (pathology, epidemiology, metagenomic data, PCR prevalence studies, isolation, characterization, etc.) should be used to identify the most likely candidate etiologic agent and to make informed intervention decisions. The synergetic and parallel use of molecular and classical methods not only results in detection of infectious agents and development of targeted diagnostic tests but also has the potential to make isolates or strains available shortly after the occurrence of outbreaks. The availability of isolates or strains is of special importance to allow the design of effective vaccines or antimicrobial drugs.

The power of NGS to boost the veterinary laboratory community's responsiveness to emerging diseases was demonstrated through the discovery of a novel Orthobunyavirus in 2011 associated with fever, decreased milk production, and diarrhea in dairy cattle. Metagenomics, using 454 technology, allowed the identification of a novel virus, subsequently named Schmallenberg virus (SBV), in an epidemiological cluster of diseased cattle in Germany [121]. These viral sequences were used to rapidly design targeted molecular tests that were used to confirm a clear association between the presence of the virus and affected animals [110]. International adoption of these molecular tests identified a widespread occurrence of SBV in European countries (http://www.efsa.europa.eu/en/supporting/pub/429e.htm) and its detection in stillborn and malformed lambs [122, 123], as well in insect vectors [124, 125]. The molecular tests were also helpful in targeting samples for isolation of the virus, which ultimately led to the development of a prototype vaccine currently under evaluation [126].

Metagenomic NGS workflows also have the potential use for quality control of biological products [127] and vaccines [128–132] and provide a powerful approach for the identification and characterization of unexpected of highly divergent pathogen variants [133, 85] that may remain undetected using targeted diagnostic tests.

The technological possibility to study both the host and the pathogen with high resolution on the level of their genome, transcriptome, or proteome opens opportunities to study *host/pathogen interactions* at several levels ((genomics, transcriptomics, *microRNAs* (miRNA)) and ultimately to analytically integrate these levels (integrative omics or systems biology) aiming to study the interaction of pathogen, microbiome, and host biological networks with many examples in veterinary science. Nordentoft and colleagues [134] used NGS metagenomics to study the influence of livestock management parameters and infection with *Salmonella enteritidis* on the microbial community in the chicken intestinal tract. Another study [135] documented the effect of *Campylobacter jejuni* infection on the chicken fecal microbiome. The application of metagenomic techniques in poultry production could lead to the development of novel alternatives to antibiotic growth promoters and better understanding of the colonization of food production animals by foodborne pathogens such as *Salmonella enterica* and *Campylobacter* spp. [36]. Other studies investigated the host response to pathogen infection. Glass and colleagues [136] used NGS transcriptomics to document bovine resistance and tolerance traits to parasitic infection. The technology was also used to study the ferret transcriptome response to influenza infection [137], the chicken transcriptome response to Marek's disease [138], the swine response to porcine reproductive and respiratory syndrome virus infection [139], and the changes in the mouse transcriptome after *Brucella* sp. infection [140].

microRNAs are considered to be a key mechanism of gene regulation in both parasites and viruses. Their characterization contributes to better understanding the complex biology of pathogens. Wang and coworkers [141] characterized microRNA sequences from *Orientobilharzia turkestanicum*, a fluke with zoonotic potential infecting sheep, and identified key target miRNAs for parasite energy metabolism, transcription initiation factors, signal transduction, and growth factor receptors. Virus-encoded microRNAs (vmiRNA) regulating viral or cellular transcripts can be targeted for virus discovery [142, 143]. miRNAs also play important roles in regulating host-pathogen interactions. NGS has been applied to investigate whether infection can modulate miRNA biogenesis and has also been used to identify miRNAs that influence pathogen replication, tropism, and pathogenic potential [144–149]. In particular, cellular miRNAs have been shown to interact with the viral genomic RNA or mRNA, facilitating or inhibiting the virus life cycle. These molecules have demonstrated immense potential as a source of antiviral therapeutics effective against a number of viruses (adenovirus, rabies, Venezuelan equine encephalitis, porcine reproductive and syndrome virus [150–153]) or for the design of live-attenuated virus vaccine based on miRNA-mediated gene silencing [154, 155, 147].

4 Conclusions

Next-generation sequencing technologies have the potential to revolutionize our understanding of the complex dimensions of animal infectious disease and infection biology (Fig. 2), ranging from the intracellular interactions to disease epidemiology. The application of high-throughput biotechnology platforms in these fields and their typical low-cost per information content has increased the resolution with which these processes can now be studied.

We now have high-resolution tools that provide veterinary diagnostic laboratories with the ability to undertake swift and flexible responses to emerging infectious diseases and unexpected pathogen variants. Moreover, these tools provide an increased resolution for the characterization of pathogens and provide important assets to improve our understanding. Fundamental research on pathogen evolution, adaptation, and virulence determinants can now be studied on a scale allowing within and between host dissections of genetic variability. Moreover, high-throughput tools open new perspectives to study the complex interaction between pathogen, host, and microbiome with very high resolution and to deepen our understanding of the key biological processes leading to protective immunity.

Not only will our increased understanding of pathogens and their interaction with livestock impact on future disease prevention, control, and management strategies, but the technologies may themselves become part of the intervention strategies, providing high-resolution data for molecular epidemiology to rapidly trace the origin and spread of outbreaks, for molecular typing, for predicting, and for optimizing the outcome of targeted treatment with antibiotics, antivirals, and anthelmintic.

The ready availability of high-resolution genomic and transcriptomic data will impact upon the targeted development of novel vaccines and drugs [156, 157], while NGS has the potential to become a powerful tool for the control of vaccines and other biological products.

As with any new technology, challenges remain. In the case of NGS, these include the requirement for expertise in both the laboratory and in the analysis of huge datasets and the current need for high investment in laboratory and data analysis hardware. As the technology is ever evolving towards lower cost, user-friendliness, and accessibility for smaller research and diagnostic labs, efforts are needed to make the data analysis more accessible to nonexpert users. This includes proper modeling of the sources of error introduction, solutions for public data storage, development of user-friendly but high standard analysis pipelines for routine applications, etc. Both the industry and the NGS user community can play a role in this evolution.

Similarly, recent improvements in protein and peptide separation efficiencies and highly accurate mass spectrometry have promoted the identification and quantification of proteins in a given sample [158]. Directly targeting peptide and protein content in a sample, proteomic approaches provide important additional information taking known issues, such as the quantitative discrepancy between mRNA transcript levels and final protein levels and posttranslational modification, into account [159].

Novel proteomic approaches have been applied to animal infectious disease research, including the study of *E. coli* response to chicken sera [160], proteomic profiling of porcine sera after FMDV infection [161], host-pathogen interaction during bovine mastitis [159], and metaproteomic studies characterizing the collective proteome of microbial communities [162].

This section contains excellent contributions exploring the application of high-throughput technologies to animal infectious diseases, including functional genomics of tick vectors infected with eukaryotic parasites, metagenomic approaches to detect bee viral pathogens, proteomics of vector-host-pathogen interactions, and NGS applications exploring parasites and intervention strategies.

Acknowledgments

The collaboration between the authors was supported by Epi-SEQ: a research project supported under the 2nd joint call for transnational research projects by EMIDA ERA-NET (FP7 project nr 219235). Additional support for this work in the United Kingdom was obtained from the Department of Environment, Food and Rural Affairs (Defra project SE2940) and BBSRC (BB/I014314/1).

References

1. Sanger F, Nicklen S, Coulson AR (1977) DNA sequencing with chain-terminating inhibitors. Proc Natl Acad Sci U S A 74:5463–5467
2. Mullis K, Faloona F, Scharf S et al (1986) Specific enzymatic amplification of DNA in vitro: the polymerase chain reaction. Cold Spring Harb Symp Quant Biol 51:263–273
3. Bartlett JM, Stirling D (2003) A short history of the polymerase chain reaction. Methods Mol Biol 226:3–6
4. Glenn TC (2011) Field guide to next-generation DNA sequencers. Mol Ecol Resour 11:759–769
5. Radford AD, Chapman D, Dixon L et al (2012) Application of next-generation sequencing technologies in virology. J Gen Virol 93: 1853–1868
6. Pareek CS, Smoczynski R, Tretyn A (2011) Sequencing technologies and genome sequencing. J Appl Genet 52:413–435
7. Loman NJ, Misra RV, Dallman TJ et al (2012) Performance comparison of benchtop high-throughput sequencing platforms. Nat Biotechnol 30:434–439
8. Schadt EE, Turner S, Kasarskis A (2010) A window into third-generation sequencing. Hum Mol Genet 19(R2):R227–240
9. Eisenstein M (2012) Oxford Nanopore announcement sets sequencing sector abuzz. Nat Biotechnol 30:295–296
10. Brodin J, Mild M, Hedskog C et al (2013) PCR-induced transitions are the major source of error in cleaned ultra-deep pyrosequencing data. PLoS One 8:e70388
11. Kim KH, Bae JW (2011) Amplification methods bias metagenomic libraries of uncultured single-stranded and double-stranded DNA viruses. Appl Environ Microbiol 77:7663–7668
12. Rosseel T, Van Borm S, Vandenbussche F et al (2013) The origin of biased sequence depth in sequence-independent nucleic Acid amplification and optimization for efficient massive parallel sequencing. PLoS One 8:e76144
13. Pettengill JB, McAvoy E, White JR et al (2012) Using metagenomic analyses to estimate the consequences of enrichment bias for pathogen detection. BMC Res Notes 5:378
14. Lysholm F, Wetterbom A, Lindau C et al (2012) Characterization of the viral microbiome in patients with severe lower respiratory tract infections, using metagenomic sequencing. PLoS One 7:e30875
15. Naccache SN, Greninger AL, Lee D et al (2013) The perils of pathogen discovery: origin of a novel parvovirus-like hybrid genome traced to nucleic acid extraction spin columns. J Virol 87:11966–11977
16. Whiteford N, Skelly T, Curtis C et al (2009) Swift: primary data analysis for the Illumina Solexa sequencing platform. Bioinformatics 25:2194–2199
17. Metzker ML (2010) Sequencing technologies—the next generation. Nat Rev Genet 11:31–46
18. Quail MA, Smith M, Coupland P et al (2012) A tale of three next generation sequencing platforms: comparison of Ion Torrent, Pacific Biosciences and Illumina MiSeq sequencers. BMC Genomics 13:341
19. Zagordi O, Klein R, Daumer M, Beerenwinkel N (2010) Error correction of next-generation sequencing data and reliable estimation of HIV quasispecies. Nucleic Acids Res 38:7400–7409
20. Archer J, Rambaut A, Taillon BE et al (2010) The evolutionary analysis of emerging low frequency HIV-1 CXCR4 using variants through time—an ultra-deep approach. PLoS Comput Biol 6:e1001022
21. Degner JF, Marioni JC, Pai AA et al (2009) Effect of read-mapping biases on detecting

allele-specific expression from RNA-sequencing data. Bioinformatics 25:3207–3212

22. Treangen TJ, Salzberg SL (2012) Repetitive DNA and next-generation sequencing: computational challenges and solutions. Nat Rev Genet 13:36–46
23. Archer J, Baillie G, Watson SJ et al (2012) Analysis of high-depth sequence data for studying viral diversity: a comparison of next generation sequencing platforms using Segminator II. BMC Bioinformatics 13:47
24. Macalalad AR, Zody MC, Charlebois P et al (2012) Highly sensitive and specific detection of rare variants in mixed viral populations from massively parallel sequence data. PLoS Comput Biol 8:e1002417
25. Quince C, Lanzen A, Davenport RJ, Turnbaugh PJ (2011) Removing noise from pyrosequenced amplicons. BMC Bioinformatics 12:38
26. Yang X, Chockalingam SP, Aluru S (2013) A survey of error-correction methods for next-generation sequencing. Brief Bioinform 14: 56–66
27. Flicek P, Birney E (2009) Sense from sequence reads: methods for alignment and assembly. Nat Methods 6(11 Suppl):S6–S12
28. Horner DS, Pavesi G, Castrignano T et al (2010) Bioinformatics approaches for genomics and post genomics applications of next-generation sequencing. Brief Bioinform 11: 181–197
29. Finotello F, Lavezzo E, Fontana P et al (2012) Comparative analysis of algorithms for whole-genome assembly of pyrosequencing data. Brief Bioinform 13:269–280
30. Angiuoli SV, White JR, Matalka M, White O, Fricke WF (2011) Resources and costs for microbial sequence analysis evaluated using virtual machines and cloud computing. PLoS One 6:e26624
31. Leinonen R, Sugawara H, Shumway M (2011) The sequence read archive. Nucleic Acids Res 39(Database issue):D19–21
32. Bai Y, Sartor M, Cavalcoli J (2012) Current status and future perspectives for sequencing livestock genomes. J Anim Sci Biotechnol 3:8
33. Aslam ML, Bastiaansen JW, Elferink MG et al (2012) Whole genome SNP discovery and analysis of genetic diversity in Turkey (*Meleagris gallopavo*). BMC Genomics 13:391
34. Ramos AM, Crooijmans RP, Affara NA et al (2009) Design of a high density SNP genotyping assay in the pig using SNPs identified and characterized by next generation sequencing technology. PLoS One 4:e6524
35. Rubin CJ, Zody MC, Eriksson J et al (2010) Whole-genome resequencing reveals loci under selection during chicken domestication. Nature 464:587–591
36. Diaz-Sanchez S, Hanning I, Pendleton S, D'Souza D (2013) Next-generation sequencing: the future of molecular genetics in poultry production and food safety. Poult Sci 92:562–572
37. Fisher CA, Bhattarai EK, Osterstock JB et al (2011) Evolution of the bovine TLR gene family and member associations with *Mycobacterium avium* subspecies *paratuberculosis* infection. PLoS One 6:e27744
38. Jex AR, Littlewood DT, Gasser RB (2010) Toward next-generation sequencing of mitochondrial genomes-focus on parasitic worms of animals and biotechnological implications. Biotechnol Adv 28:151–159
39. Webb KM, Rosenthal BM (2011) Next-generation sequencing of the *Trichinella murrelli* mitochondrial genome allows comprehensive comparison of its divergence from the principal agent of human trichinellosis, *Trichinella spiralis*. Infect Genet Evol 11: 116–123
40. Grinberg A, Biggs PJ, Dukkipati VS, George TT (2013) Extensive intra-host genetic diversity uncovered in *Cryptosporidium parvum* using Next Generation Sequencing. Infect Genet Evol 15:18–24
41. Cantacessi C, Campbell BE, Gasser RB (2012) Key strongylid nematodes of animals—Impact of next-generation transcriptomics on systems biology and biotechnology. Biotechnol Adv 30:469–488
42. Matsubayashi M, Hatta T, Miyoshi T et al (2013) High-throughput RNA sequencing profiles and transcriptional evidence of aerobic respiratory enzymes in sporulating oocysts and sporozoites of *Eimeria tenella*. Infect Genet Evol 18:269–276
43. Wu X, Fu Y, Yang D et al (2012) Detailed transcriptome description of the neglected cestode *Taenia multiceps*. PLoS One 7:e45830
44. Romine NM, Martin RJ, Beetham JK (2013) Computational cloning of drug target genes of a parasitic nematode, *Oesophagostomum dentatum*. BMC Genet 14:55
45. Cwiklinski K, Merga JY, Lake SL et al (2013) Transcriptome analysis of a parasitic clade V nematode: comparative analysis of potential molecular anthelmintic targets in *Cylicostephanus goldi*. Int J Parasitol 43:917–927
46. Tritt A, Eisen JA, Facciotti MT, Darling AE (2012) An integrated pipeline for de novo

assembly of microbial genomes. PLoS One 7:e42304

47. Lauring AS, Andino R (2010) Quasispecies theory and the behavior of RNA viruses. PLoS Pathog 6:e1001005
48. Watson SJ, Welkers MR, Depledge DP et al (2013) Viral population analysis and minority-variant detection using short read next-generation sequencing. Philos Trans R Soc Lond B Biol Sci 368:20120205
49. Stack JC, Murcia PR, Grenfell BT, Wood JL, Holmes EC (2013) Inferring the inter-host transmission of influenza A virus using patterns of intra-host genetic variation. Proc Biol Sci 280:20122173
50. Wright CF, Morelli MJ, Thebaud G et al (2011) Beyond the consensus: dissecting within-host viral population diversity of foot-and-mouth disease virus by using next-generation genome sequencing. J Virol 85: 2266–2275
51. Morelli MJ, Wright CF, Knowles NJ et al (2013) Evolution of foot-and-mouth disease virus intra-sample sequence diversity during serial transmission in bovine hosts. Vet Res 44:12
52. Orton RJ, Wright CF, Morelli MJ et al (2013) Observing micro-evolutionary processes of viral populations at multiple scales. Philos Trans R Soc Lond B Biol Sci 368:20120203
53. Fusaro A, Monne I, Hughes J, et al. (2013) Evolution of H7 viruses in poultry: convergent and divergent mutations. Paper presented at the Options for the Control of Influenza VIII, Cape Town, South Africa
54. Wilker PR, Dinis JM, Starrett G et al (2013) Selection on haemagglutinin imposes a bottleneck during mammalian transmission of reassortant H5N1 influenza viruses. Nat Commun 4:2636
55. Szpara ML, Parsons L, Enquist LW (2010) Sequence variability in clinical and laboratory isolates of herpes simplex virus 1 reveals new mutations. J Virol 84:5303–5313
56. Wellehan JF Jr, Yu F, Venn-Watson SK et al (2010) Characterization of San Miguel sea lion virus populations using pyrosequencing-based methods. Infect Genet Evol 10: 254–260
57. Vrancken B, Lequime S, Theys K, Lemey P (2010) Covering all bases in HIV research: unveiling a hidden world of viral evolution. AIDS Rev 12:89–102
58. Swenson LC, Daumer M, Paredes R (2012) Next-generation sequencing to assess HIV tropism. Curr Opin HIV AIDS 7:478–485
59. Swenson LC, Mo T, Dong WW et al (2011) Deep sequencing to infer HIV-1 co-receptor usage: application to three clinical trials of maraviroc in treatment-experienced patients. J Infect Dis 203:237–245
60. Ghedin E, Laplante J, DePasse J et al (2011) Deep sequencing reveals mixed infection with 2009 pandemic influenza A (H1N1) virus strains and the emergence of oseltamivir resistance. J Infect Dis 203:168–174
61. Capobianchi MR, Giombini E, Rozera G (2013) Next-generation sequencing technology in clinical virology. Clin Microbiol Infect 19:15–22
62. Backer JA, Vrancken R, Neyts J, Goris N (2013) The potential of antiviral agents to control classical swine fever: a modelling study. Antiviral Res 99:245–250
63. Lefebvre DJ, De Vleeschauwer AR, Goris N et al (2013) Proof of Concept for the Inhibition of Foot-and-Mouth Disease Virus Replication by the Anti-Viral Drug 2′-C-Methylcytidine in Severe Combined Immunodeficient Mice. Transbound Emerg Dis. doi:10.1111/tbed.12069
64. Lefebure T, Bitar PD, Suzuki H, Stanhope MJ (2010) Evolutionary dynamics of complete *Campylobacter* pan-genomes and the bacterial species concept. Genome Biol Evol 2:646–655
65. Biek R, O'Hare A, Wright D et al (2012) Whole genome sequencing reveals local transmission patterns of *Mycobacterium bovis* in sympatric cattle and badger populations. PLoS Pathog 8:e1003008
66. Chen Y, Mukherjee S, Hoffmann M et al (2013) Whole-Genome Sequencing of Gentamicin-Resistant *Campylobacter coli* Isolated from U.S. Retail Meats Reveals Novel Plasmid-Mediated Aminoglycoside Resistance Genes. Antimicrob Agents Chemother 57:5398–5405
67. Mellmann A, Harmsen D, Cummings CA et al (2011) Prospective genomic characterization of the German enterohemorrhagic *Escherichia coli* O104:H4 outbreak by rapid next generation sequencing technology. PLoS One 6:e22751
68. Dupuy V, Manso-Silvan L, Barbe V et al (2012) Evolutionary history of contagious bovine pleuropneumonia using next generation sequencing of *Mycoplasma mycoides* subsp. *mycoides* "Small Colony". PLoS One 7:e46821
69. Das S, Roychowdhury T, Kumar P et al (2013) Genetic heterogeneity revealed by sequence analysis of *Mycobacterium tuberculosis* isolates from extra-pulmonary tuberculosis patients. BMC Genomics 14:404
70. Eyre DW, Golubchik T, Gordon NC, et al. (2012) A pilot study of rapid benchtop

sequencing of Staphylococcus aureus and Clostridium difficile for outbreak detection and surveillance. BMJ Open 2 (doi: 10.1136/bmjopen-2012-001124)
71. Koser CU, Holden MT, Ellington MJ et al (2012) Rapid whole-genome sequencing for investigation of a neonatal MRSA outbreak. N Engl J Med 366:2267–2275
72. Grinev A, Chancey C, Anez G et al (2013) Genetic analysis of West Nile virus isolates from an outbreak in Idaho, United States, 2006-2007. Int J Environ Res Public Health 10:4486–4506
73. Chen GQ, Zhuang QY, Wang KC et al (2013) Identification and survey of a novel avian coronavirus in ducks. PLoS One 8:e72918
74. Becker N, Jost H, Ziegler U et al (2012) Epizootic emergence of Usutu virus in wild and captive birds in Germany. PLoS One 7:e32604
75. Croville G, Soubies SM, Barbieri J et al (2012) Field monitoring of avian influenza viruses: whole-genome sequencing and tracking of neuraminidase evolution using 454 pyrosequencing. J Clin Microbiol 50: 2881–2887
76. Dugan VG, Dunham EJ, Jin G et al (2011) Phylogenetic analysis of low pathogenicity H5N1 and H7N3 influenza A virus isolates recovered from sentinel, free flying, wild mallards at one study site during 2006. Virology 417:98–105
77. Ramakrishnan MA, Tu ZJ, Singh S et al (2009) The feasibility of using high resolution genome sequencing of influenza A viruses to detect mixed infections and quasispecies. PLoS One 4:e7105
78. Van Borm S, Rosseel T, Vangeluwe D, Vandenbussche F, van den Berg T, Lambrecht B (2012) Phylogeographic analysis of avian influenza viruses isolated from Charadriiformes in Belgium confirms intercontinental reassortment in gulls. Arch Virol 157:1509–1522
79. Leifer I, Ruggli N, Blome S (2013) Approaches to define the viral genetic basis of classical swine fever virus virulence. Virology 438:51–55
80. Rao PP, Reddy YN, Ganesh K, Nair SG, Niranjan V, Hegde NR (2013) Deep sequencing as a method of typing bluetongue virus isolates. J Virol Methods 193:314–319
81. Marston DA, McElhinney LM, Ellis RJ et al (2013) Next generation sequencing of viral RNA genomes. BMC Genomics 14:444
82. Marston DA, Mansfield KL, Mearns R, Ellis RJ, Fooks AR, Johnson N (2013) Louping ill virus genome sequence derived from the spinal cord of an infected lamb. Genome Announc 1 (doi:10.1128/genomeA.00454-13)
83. Kvisgaard LK, Hjulsager CK, Fahnoe U, Breum SO, Ait-Ali T, Larsen LE (2013) A fast and robust method for full genome sequencing of Porcine Reproductive and Respiratory Syndrome Virus (PRRSV) Type 1 and Type 2. J Virol Methods 193:697–705
84. Wilkie GS, Davison AJ, Watson M et al (2013) Complete genome sequences of elephant endotheliotropic herpesviruses 1A and 1B determined directly from fatal cases. J Virol 87:6700–6712
85. Rosseel T, Lambrecht B, Vandenbussche F, van den Berg T, Van Borm S (2011) Identification and complete genome sequencing of paramyxoviruses in mallard ducks (*Anas platyrhynchos*) using random access amplification and next generation sequencing technologies. Virol J 8:463
86. Hoper D, Hoffmann B, Beer M (2011) A comprehensive deep sequencing strategy for full-length genomes of influenza A. PLoS One 6:e19075
87. Kampmann ML, Fordyce SL, Avila-Arcos MC et al (2011) A simple method for the parallel deep sequencing of full influenza A genomes. J Virol Methods 178:243–248
88. Hoper D, Kalthoff D, Hoffmann B, Beer M (2012) Highly pathogenic avian influenza virus subtype H5N1 escaping neutralization: more than HA variation. J Virol 86:1394–1404
89. Hutter J, Rodig JV, Hoper D et al (2013) Toward animal cell culture-based influenza vaccine design: viral hemagglutinin N-glycosylation markedly impacts immunogenicity. J Immunol 190:220–230
90. Bourret V, Croville G, Mariette J et al (2013) Whole-genome, deep pyrosequencing analysis of a duck influenza A virus evolution in swine cells. Infect Genet Evol 18:31–41
91. Roedig JV, Rapp E, Hoper D, Genzel Y, Reichl U (2011) Impact of host cell line adaptation on quasispecies composition and glycosylation of influenza A virus hemagglutinin. PLoS One 6:e27989
92. Wu NC, Young AP, Dandekar SW et al (2013) Systematic identification of H274Y compensatory mutations in influenza A virus neuraminidase by high-throughput screening. J Virol 87:1193–1199
93. Topfer A, Hoper D, Blome S et al (2013) Sequencing approach to analyze the role of quasispecies for classical swine fever. Virology 438:14–19
94. Fouts DE, Szpakowski S, Purushe J et al (2012) Next generation sequencing to define

prokaryotic and fungal diversity in the bovine rumen. PLoS One 7:e48289

95. Oikonomou G, Machado VS, Santisteban C, Schukken YH, Bicalho RC (2012) Microbial diversity of bovine mastitic milk as described by pyrosequencing of metagenomic 16 s rDNA. PLoS One 7:e47671
96. Kolbert CP, Rys PN, Hopkins M et al (2004) 16S ribosomal DNA sequence analysis for identification of bacteria in a clinical microbiology laboratory. In: Persing DH, Tenover FD, Versalovic J et al (eds) Molecular microbiology: diagnostic principles and practice. ASM Press, Washington, DC, pp 361–377
97. Thomas T, Gilbert J, Meyer F (2012) Metagenomics—a guide from sampling to data analysis. Microb Inform Exp 2:3
98. Petrosino JF, Highlander S, Luna RA, Gibbs RA, Versalovic J (2009) Metagenomic pyrosequencing and microbial identification. Clin Chem 55:856–866
99. Ferrer M, Ghazi A, Beloqui AV et al (2012) Functional metagenomics unveils a multifunctional glycosyl hydrolase from the family 43 catalysing the breakdown of plant polymers in the calf rumen. PLoS One 7:e38134
100. Singh KM, Jakhesara SJ, Koringa PG, Rank DN, Joshi CG (2012) Metagenomic analysis of virulence-associated and antibiotic resistance genes of microbes in rumen of Indian buffalo (*Bubalus bubalis*). Gene 507:146–151
101. Day JM, Ballard LL, Duke MV, Scheffler BE, Zsak L (2010) Metagenomic analysis of the turkey gut RNA virus community. Virol J 7:313
102. Danzeisen JL, Kim HB, Isaacson RE, Tu ZJ, Johnson TJ (2011) Modulations of the chicken cecal microbiome and metagenome in response to anticoccidial and growth promoter treatment. PLoS One 6:e27949
103. Long SW, Williams D, Valson C et al (2013) A genomic day in the life of a clinical microbiology laboratory. J Clin Microbiol 51: 1272–1277
104. Sherry NL, Porter JL, Seemann T et al (2013) Outbreak investigation using high-throughput genome sequencing within a diagnostic microbiology laboratory. J Clin Microbiol 51:1396–1401
105. Barzon L, Lavezzo E, Militello V, Toppo S, Palu G (2011) Applications of next-generation sequencing technologies to diagnostic virology. Int J Mol Sci 12:7861–7884
106. Belak S, Karlsson OE, Blomstrom AL, Berg M, Granberg F (2013) New viruses in veterinary medicine, detected by metagenomic approaches. Vet Microbiol 165:95–101
107. Bexfield N, Kellam P (2011) Metagenomics and the molecular identification of novel viruses. Vet J 190:191–198
108. Bishop-Lilly KA, Turell MJ, Willner KM et al (2010) Arbovirus detection in insect vectors by rapid, high-throughput pyrosequencing. PLoS Negl Trop Dis 4:e878
109. Blomstrom AL (2011) Viral metagenomics as an emerging and powerful tool in veterinary medicine. Vet Q 31:107–114
110. Blomstrom AL, Widen F, Hammer AS, Belak S, Berg M (2010) Detection of a novel astrovirus in brain tissue of mink suffering from shaking mink syndrome by use of viral metagenomics. J Clin Microbiol 48:4392–4396
111. Honkavuori KS, Shivaprasad HL, Briese T et al (2011) Novel picornavirus in Turkey poults with hepatitis, California, USA. Emerg Infect Dis 17:480–487
112. Cox-Foster DL, Conlan S, Holmes EC et al (2007) A metagenomic survey of microbes in honey bee colony collapse disorder. Science 318:283–287
113. Granberg F, Vicente-Rubiano M, Rubio-Guerri C et al (2013) Metagenomic detection of viral pathogens in Spanish honeybees: co-infection by Aphid Lethal Paralysis, Israel Acute Paralysis and Lake Sinai Viruses. PLoS One 8:e57459
114. Blomstrom AL, Belak S, Fossum C et al (2009) Detection of a novel porcine boca-like virus in the background of porcine circovirus type 2 induced postweaning multisystemic wasting syndrome. Virus Res 146:125–129
115. Ge X, Li Y, Yang X et al (2012) Metagenomic analysis of viruses from bat fecal samples reveals many novel viruses in insectivorous bats in China. J Virol 86:4620–4630
116. Li L, Victoria JG, Wang C et al (2010) Bat guano virome: predominance of dietary viruses from insects and plants plus novel mammalian viruses. J Virol 84:6955–6965
117. Blomstrom AL, Stahl K, Masembe C et al (2012) Viral metagenomic analysis of bushpigs (*Potamochoerus larvatus*) in Uganda identifies novel variants of Porcine parvovirus 4 and Torque teno sus virus 1 and 2. Virol J 9:192
118. Bodewes R, van der Giessen J, Haagmans BL, Osterhaus AD, Smits SL (2013) Identification of multiple novel viruses, including a parvovirus and a hepevirus, in feces of red foxes. J Virol 87:7758–7764
119. Carpi G, Cagnacci F, Wittekindt NE et al (2011) Metagenomic profile of the bacterial communities associated with *Ixodes ricinus* ticks. PLoS One 6:e25604

120. Fredericks DN, Relman DA (1996) Sequence-based identification of microbial pathogens: a reconsideration of Koch's postulates. Clin Microbiol Rev 9:18–33
121. Hoffmann B, Scheuch M, Hoper D et al (2012) Novel orthobunyavirus in Cattle, Europe, 2011. Emerg Infect Dis 18:469–472
122. De Regge N, van den Berg T, Georges L, Cay B (2013) Diagnosis of Schmallenberg virus infection in malformed lambs and calves and first indications for virus clearance in the fetus. Vet Microbiol 162:595–600
123. van den Brom R, Luttikholt SJ, Lievaart-Peterson K et al (2012) Epizootic of ovine congenital malformations associated with Schmallenberg virus infection. Tijdschr Diergeneeskd 137:106–111
124. De Regge N, Deblauwe I, De Deken R et al (2012) Detection of Schmallenberg virus in different *Culicoides* spp. by real-time RT-PCR. Transbound Emerg Dis 59:471–475
125. Elbers AR, Meiswinkel R, van Weezep E, van Oldruitenborgh-Oosterbaan MM, Kooi EA (2013) Schmallenberg virus in *Culicoides* spp. biting midges, the Netherlands, 2011. Emerg Infect Dis 19:106–109
126. Wernike K, Nikolin VM, Hechinger S, Hoffmann B, Beer M (2013) Inactivated Schmallenberg virus prototype vaccines. Vaccine 31:3558–3563
127. Van Borm S, Rosseel T, Steensels M, van den Berg T, Lambrecht B (2013) What's in a strain? Viral metagenomics identifies genetic variation and contaminating circoviruses in laboratory isolates of pigeon paramyxovirus type 1. Virus Res 171:186–193
128. Baylis SA, Finsterbusch T, Bannert N, Blumel J, Mankertz A (2011) Analysis of porcine circovirus type 1 detected in Rotarix vaccine. Vaccine 29:690–697
129. Farsang A, Kulcsar G (2012) Extraneous agent detection in vaccines-a review of technical aspects. Biologicals 40:225–230
130. Neverov A, Chumakov K (2010) Massively parallel sequencing for monitoring genetic consistency and quality control of live viral vaccines. Proc Natl Acad Sci U S A 107(46): 20063–8
131. Onions D, Kolman J (2010) Massively parallel sequencing, a new method for detecting adventitious agents. Biologicals 38:377–380
132. Victoria JG, Wang C, Jones MS et al (2010) Viral nucleic acids in live-attenuated vaccines: detection of minority variants and an adventitious virus. J Virol 84:6033–6040
133. Miller PJ, Afonso CL, Spackman E et al (2010) Evidence for a new avian paramyxovirus serotype 10 detected in rockhopper penguins from the Falkland Islands. J Virol 84:11496–11504
134. Nordentoft S, Molbak L, Bjerrum L et al (2011) The influence of the cage system and colonisation of *Salmonella* Enteritidis on the microbial gut flora of laying hens studied by T-RFLP and 454 pyrosequencing. BMC Microbiol 11:187
135. Qu A, Brulc JM, Wilson MK et al (2008) Comparative metagenomics reveals host specific metavirulomes and horizontal gene transfer elements in the chicken cecum microbiome. PLoS One 3:e2945
136. Glass EJ, Crutchley S, Jensen K (2012) Living with the enemy or uninvited guests: functional genomics approaches to investigating host resistance or tolerance traits to a protozoan parasite, *Theileria annulata*, in cattle. Vet Immunol Immunopathol 148:178–189
137. Leon AJ, Banner D, Xu L et al (2013) Sequencing, annotation, and characterization of the influenza ferret infectome. J Virol 87:1957–1966
138. Maceachern S, Muir WM, Crosby S, Cheng HH (2011) Genome-wide identification of allele-specific expression (ASE) in response to Marek's disease virus infection using next generation sequencing. BMC Proc 5(Suppl 4):S14
139. Miller LC, Fleming D, Arbogast A et al (2012) Analysis of the swine tracheobronchial lymph node transcriptomic response to infection with a Chinese highly pathogenic strain of porcine reproductive and respiratory syndrome virus. BMC Vet Res 8:208
140. Wang F, Hu S, Liu W et al (2011) Deep-sequencing analysis of the mouse transcriptome response to infection with *Brucella melitensis* strains of differing virulence. PLoS One 6:e28485
141. Wang CR, Xu MJ, Fu JH et al (2012) Characterization of microRNAs from *Orientobilharzia turkestanicum*, a neglected blood fluke of human and animal health significance. PLoS One 7:e47001
142. Kong BW (2011) Identification of virus encoding microRNAs using 454 FLX sequencing platform. Methods Mol Biol 733:81–91
143. Ma M, Huang Y, Gong Z et al (2011) Discovery of DNA viruses in wild-caught mosquitoes using small RNA high throughput sequencing. PLoS One 6:e24758
144. Cullen BR (2006) Viruses and microRNAs. Nat Genet 38(Suppl):S25–30
145. Eulalio A, Schulte L, Vogel J (2012) The mammalian microRNA response to bacterial infections. RNA Biol 9:742–750

146. Gottwein E, Cullen BR (2008) Viral and cellular microRNAs as determinants of viral pathogenesis and immunity. Cell Host Microbe 3:375–387
147. Perez JT, Pham AM, Lorini MH et al (2009) MicroRNA-mediated species-specific attenuation of influenza A virus. Nat Biotechnol 27:572–576
148. Wang Y, Brahmakshatriya V, Lupiani B et al (2012) Integrated analysis of microRNA expression and mRNA transcriptome in lungs of avian influenza virus infected broilers. BMC Genomics 13:278
149. Wang Y, Brahmakshatriya V, Zhu H et al (2009) Identification of differentially expressed miRNAs in chicken lung and trachea with avian influenza virus infection by a deep sequencing approach. BMC Genomics 10:512
150. Bhomia M, Sharma A, Gayen M, Gupta P, Maheshwari RK (2013) Artificial microRNAs can effectively inhibit replication of Venezuelan equine encephalitis virus. Antiviral Res 100:429–434
151. Ibrisimovic M, Kneidinger D, Lion T, Klein R (2013) An adenoviral vector-based expression and delivery system for the inhibition of wild-type adenovirus replication by artificial microRNAs. Antiviral Res 97:10–23
152. Israsena N, Supavonwong P, Ratanasetyuth N, Khawplod P, Hemachudha T (2009) Inhibition of rabies virus replication by multiple artificial microRNAs. Antiviral Res 84:76–83
153. Xia B, Song H, Chen Y et al (2013) Efficient inhibition of porcine reproductive and respiratory syndrome virus replication by artificial microRNAs targeting the untranslated regions. Arch Virol 158:55–61
154. Barnes D, Kunitomi M, Vignuzzi M, Saksela K, Andino R (2008) Harnessing endogenous miRNAs to control virus tissue tropism as a strategy for developing attenuated virus vaccines. Cell Host Microbe 4:239–248
155. Kelly EJ, Hadac EM, Greiner S, Russell SJ (2008) Engineering microRNA responsiveness to decrease virus pathogenicity. Nat Med 14:1278–1283
156. Luciani F, Bull RA, Lloyd AR (2012) Next generation deep sequencing and vaccine design: today and tomorrow. Trends Biotechnol 30:443–452
157. Woollard PM, Mehta NA, Vamathevan JJ et al (2011) The application of next-generation sequencing technologies to drug discovery and development. Drug Discov Today 16:512–519
158. Mann M, Hendrickson R, Pandey A (2001) Analysis of proteins and proteomes by mass spectrometry. Annu Rev Biochem 70:437–473
159. Boehmer JL (2011) Proteomic analyses of host and pathogen responses during bovine mastitis. J Mammary Gland Biol Neoplasia 16:323–338
160. Li G, Cai W, Hussein A et al (2012) Proteome response of an extraintestinal pathogenic *Escherichia coli* strain with zoonotic potential to human and chicken sera. J Proteomics 75:4853–4862
161. Liu Y, Zhang K, Zheng H et al (2011) Proteomics analysis of porcine serum proteins by LC-MS/MS after foot-and-mouth disease virus (FMDV) infection. J Vet Med Sci 73:1569–1572
162. Kolmeder CA, de Vos WM (2013) Metaproteomics of our microbiome—Developing insight in function and activity in man and model systems. J Proteomics 97:3–16

Chapter 31

Impact of Next-Generation Technologies on Exploring Socioeconomically Important Parasites and Developing New Interventions

Cinzia Cantacessi, Andreas Hofmann, Bronwyn E. Campbell, and Robin B. Gasser

Abstract

High-throughput molecular and computer technologies have become instrumental for systems biological explorations of pathogens, including parasites. For instance, investigations of the transcriptomes of different developmental stages of parasitic nematodes give insights into gene expression, regulation and function in a parasite, which is a significant step to understanding their biology, as well as interactions with their host(s) and disease. This chapter (1) gives a background on some key parasitic nematodes of socioeconomic importance, (2) describes sequencing and bioinformatic technologies for large-scale studies of the transcriptomes and genomes of these parasites, (3) provides some recent examples of applications and (4) emphasizes the prospects of fundamental biological explorations of parasites using these technologies for the development of new interventions to combat parasitic diseases.

Key words Parasitic nematodes, Genomics, Transcriptomics, Bioinformatics, Next-generation sequencing, Post-genomics, Anthelmintic resistance, Drug targets, Diagnostic markers

1 Introduction

Parasitic nematodes (roundworms) of humans and other animals are of particular significance as pathogens [1–5]. For example, the soil-transmitted helminths (STHs) *Ascaris* spp. (large roundworm), *Ancylostoma duodenale*, *Necator americanus* (hookworms) and *Trichuris trichiura* (whipworm) are estimated to infect almost one sixth of all humans [6, 7], and parasitic nematodes of livestock, including species of *Haemonchus*, *Ostertagia*, and *Trichostrongylus*, cause substantial losses estimated at billions of dollars per annum, due to poor productivity, failure to thrive, the costs of anthelmintic treatment and deaths [8–10]. In addition to their socioeconomic impact, anthelmintic resistance in nematodes of livestock [11–13] has stimulated research towards developing alternative intervention and control

Mónica V. Cunha and João Inácio (eds.), *Veterinary Infection Biology: Molecular Diagnostics and High-Throughput Strategies*, Methods in Molecular Biology, vol. 1247, DOI 10.1007/978-1-4939-2004-4_31,

strategies against these parasites. In spite of some knowledge of parasites and the diseases that they cause [14, 15], little is known about essential molecular processes and mechanisms in parasitic nematodes. Gaining an improved understanding of the molecular biology of these organisms offers a possible pathway for discovering new methods of diagnosis, treatment and control of parasitic diseases.

Advances in genomic and bioinformatic technologies provide exciting opportunities to explore, for example, basic developmental and reproductive processes in nematodes. In particular, studies of the transcriptomes of parasites have become instrumental in various areas, such as gene discovery and characterization, and for gaining insights into aspects of gene expression, regulation and function [16–19]. The purpose of this chapter is to (1) give a background on some socioeconomically important parasitic nematodes of animals, (2) describe sequencing and bioinformatic technologies for large-scale studies of the transcriptomes and genomes of these parasites, (3) provide some recent examples of applications, and (4) emphasize the prospects of fundamental biological explorations of parasites using these technologies for the development of new interventions to combat parasitic diseases.

2 Brief Background on Parasitic Nematodes

As one of the most diverse phyla in the animal kingdom, the phylum Nematoda includes > 28,000 species, of which >16,000 are parasites of animals or plants [14, 20]. This phylum consists of two main classes, the Adenophorea and the Secernentea [21]. Within the Secernentea, species within the orders Ascaridida, Oxyurida, Spirurida and Strongylida are parasites of humans and other vertebrates [14]. Within the latter order, the superfamily Strongyloidea includes, among others, some intestinal parasites of pigs, ruminants (Chabertiidae) and equids (family Strongylidae) [14]. Members of this superfamily are characterized by complex buccal capsules, often with a series of leaflike structures on the border of the labial region (*corona radiata*) [22]. In contrast, the buccal capsule, lips, and *corona radiata* of species of parasitic nematodes of the superfamily Trichostrongyloidea are greatly reduced or absent [23–25]. Members of this latter superfamily (commonly known as "trichostrongyles") are key parasites of some mammals, particularly ruminants [14, 26]. The superfamily Ancylostomatoidea ("hookworms") includes blood-feeding nematodes, characterized by large, globular buccal capsules, which enable them to attach to the intestinal wall to feed on blood [14]. According to a molecular classification proposed by Blaxter et al. [27], members of the Strongylida, such as trichostrongyles and hookworms, as well as the free-living nematodes of the suborder Rhabditina (e.g., *Caenorhabditis elegans*) and order Diplogasterida (e.g., *Pristionchus pacificus*), belong to "clade V" of the Nematoda.

2.1 Selected Examples of Nematodes (Order Strongylida) of Major Socioeconomic Importance

2.1.1 Trichostrongyles

Within the superfamily Trichostrongyloidea, *Haemonchus contortus* (barber's pole worm) and *Trichostrongylus* spp., for example, are responsible for substantial production losses in the livestock industries worldwide [10, 28]. *H. contortus* is the most important nematode of small ruminants in subtropical and tropical (summer rainfall) areas, whereas some *Trichostrongylus* spp. are often dominant in winter rainfall areas due to their ability to develop and survive at lower temperatures than *H. contortus* does [29]. The life cycles of *H. contortus* and *T. colubriformis* are similar and direct, with eggs being laid by females in the abomasum (*H. contortus*) or small intestine (*Trichostrongylus*) of the host [26, 30, 31]. Under suitable environmental conditions [30, 32], first-stage larvae (L1s) hatch from eggs to develop, via the second-stage larvae (L2s), to infective, third-stage larvae (L3s). The cuticle of the L2 is retained as a sheath around the L3 and protects it from desiccation [14, 30, 32]. Small ruminants acquire the infection by ingesting L3s from contaminated pastures. The L3s pass through the forestomachs and undergo an exsheathment process to then establish, via the parasitic fourth-stage larvae (L4s), as adult males and females in the abomasum (*H. contortus*) or small intestine (*Trichostrongylus* spp.) within ~3 weeks [14, 26, 30, 32]. The exsheathment process is triggered by stimuli within the host and may include (depending on the species of nematode) dissolved gaseous CO_2 and undissociated carbonic acid (*H. contortus*) or hydrochloric acid and pepsin (*T. colubriformis*) in the abomasum. L3s respond to these stimuli by producing an exsheathment fluid which determines the detachment of the sheath from the bodies of the larvae [5, 33–35].

The adults of *H. contortus* feed on blood from vessels in the gastric wall. Consequently, the main clinical signs of acute haemonchosis are anemia, variable degrees of edema, as well as lethargy, decreased live-weight gain, impaired wool/milk production, and decreased reproductive performance, often leading to death in severely affected animals [36, 37]. Trichostrongylosis is triggered by the presence of adult parasites in mucus-covered tunnels in the epithelial surface of the small intestine [38], usually associated with extensive villous atrophy, combined with hyperplasia of the submucosal glands, mucosal thickening, and erosion as well as infiltration of lymphocytes and neutrophils into affected areas [38–42]. Clinical signs of trichostrongylosis include malabsorption, weight loss, progressive emaciation, and diarrhea (scouring or "black scour").

2.1.2 Hookworms

The hookworms *N. americanus* and *A. duodenale* of humans are estimated to infect ~1 billion people in rural regions of the subtropics and tropics [1], with the highest prevalence (~17 %) recorded in areas of sub-Saharan Africa and China [1, 43, 44], and cause an estimated disease burden of 22 million disability-adjusted life years (DALYs) [45]. Although *N. americanus* is the most widely distributed hookworm of humans globally [1], a related species, *A. caninum*, is a cosmopolitan hookworm of the small intestine of dogs and other canids [14, 26]. The life cycle of these nematodes is direct, with female hookworms excreting thin-shelled eggs, which are passed in the feces of the host [26, 46]. Under suitable environmental conditions (i.e., 23–33 °C), the L1s hatch from the eggs [26, 46], feed on microbes, and, within 2 days, molt to L2s and then to L3s within 4–5 days. The L3 stage retains the cuticle of the L2 (i.e., sheath) and is called a "filariform" larva [46]. Infection occurs when the L3s penetrate the skin of the vertebrate host following cuticular shedding [47]; then, the larvae enter the subcutaneous tissues and migrate via the circulatory system to the heart and lungs, where they molt to fourth-stage larvae (L4s). From the lungs, the larvae migrate (via the airways and pharynx) to the small intestine, where they develop to adult males and females within 2–7 weeks, depending on species [14, 26, 48, 49]. The adult stages attach by their buccal capsule to the intestinal mucosa, rupture capillaries and feed on blood [50, 51]. Although skin penetration is considered the main route, ingestion of L3s might also lead to infection [52]. L3s of *Ancylostoma* spp. can undergo hypobiosis (developmental arrest) in the somatic tissues of the vertebrate host and, following activation during pregnancy, undergo transmammary transmission to the offspring [53–55].

Hookworm disease relates mainly to the blood-feeding activity by the adult worms within the host [50]. Focal lesions caused by the attachment of the worms are characterized by local hemorrhage, tissue cytolysis and a neutrophilic immune response [50]. The clinical expression of disease relates mainly to iron-deficiency anemia, which can cause physical and mental retardation and sometimes deaths in children as well as maternal mortality, impaired lactation, prematurity and low birth rates [3, 56, 57].

2.2 Host Immune Responses

Various studies have described molecules and cells implicated in host immune responses against parasitic nematodes [2, 58–70]. The primary immunological responses induced by nematodes are dependent on the processes and mechanisms of invasion of and establishment in the host [2]. For example, migrating hookworm L3s stimulate a marked peripheral blood eosinophilia in the mammalian host, both systemic and in the lungs [71, 72]. Conversely, nematodes that do not undergo extensive tissue migration stimulate a mucosal immune response at the site of infection [73]. For instance, the invasion of the abomasa of small ruminants by the larvae of *H. contortus* and *Trichostrongylus axei* leads to a localized IgE-mediated immune response [73]. However, it has been observed that the infection of pigs with L3s of *Oesophagostomum dentatum* is associated with a systemic production of IgG antibodies [74–76], followed by the formation of eosinophilic cysts containing the larvae (nodules) within the intestinal mucosa [77].

In spite of variation in immune responses induced by larvae of strongylid nematodes, adult stages appear to stimulate similar immunological responses in their mammalian host(s). These responses include (1) increased production of mucus by the gastrointestinal epithelium of the host, (2) eosinophilia and increased presence of mast cells and leucocytes at the infection site and (3) production of specific antibodies [2, 60]. Responses against primary infections by gastrointestinal parasitic nematodes are reported to be linked to a T helper (Th) 2-type immune response which, in turn, relates to the secretion of multiple types of cytokines, including IL-4, IL-5, IL-9 and IL-13 [2, 62, 68, 78–80]. In contrast, immunological responses in hosts with chronic infections appear to be regulated mainly by a Th1-type immune response, characterized by a production of IL-2, IL-18 and interferon-γ [65, 66, 70]. In particular, individuals infected chronically by hookworms show a significant alteration of the immune response to helminth infections, characterized by a dysfunction of the antigen-presenting ability of dendritic cells, which results in a "hyporesponsiveness" of the antigen-induced proliferation of T lymphocytes [79].

2.3 Drugs and Vaccine Research

The control of gastrointestinal nematodes relies heavily on the use of anthelmintic drugs [81]. Such drugs include imidazothiazoles/tetrahydropyrimidines (e.g., levamisole and pyrantel), benzimidazoles (e.g., albendazole and mebendazole) and macrocyclic lactones (e.g., ivermectin and moxidectin) [81]. Levamisole and pyrantel act by binding to a subgroup of nematode acetylcholine receptor ion channels in parasite nerves and muscles of parasitic nematodes, resulting in an overstimulation, spastic muscle contraction [82] and paralysis of the worms; the parasites are unable to move in the intestinal tract and are removed by peristalsis. Benzimidazoles are active against a range of species of nematodes [83]; they block microtubular matrix formation by binding to tubulin (cytoskeletal protein), which is essential for various biological processes in the cell, including chromosome movement and cell division [11, 81, 84]. Macrocyclic lactones act by opening glutamate-gated chloride channels, thus increasing the flow of chloride ions and subsequently leading to defects in neurotransmission and flaccid paralysis [84]. Recently, new classes of anthelmintics, including cyclooctadepsipeptides (e.g., emodepside), amino acetonitrile derivatives (e.g., monepantel) and 2-deoxy-paraherquamides (e.g., derquantel) have become available commercially [85]. These compounds act by binding to presynaptic latrophilin-like receptors (emodepside), some acetylcholine receptors (monepantel) or B-subtype nicotinic acetylcholine receptors (derquantel) and cause spastic (monepantel) or flaccid (emodepside and derquantel) paralysis of some parasitic nematodes and subsequent death [85].

The relatively low cost, ease of administration and efficacy of anthelmintic drugs against various gastrointestinal parasitic nematodes of humans and animals have led to their extensive use and, consequently, to the emergence of resistance [11]. Indeed, resistance in nematodes of livestock to imidazothiazoles/tetrahydropyrimidines, benzimidazoles and macrocyclic lactones has been reported, particularly in Africa, Australia, New Zealand, Asia and South America [11, 12, 37, 84, 86]. Three mutations in the gene encoding the beta-tubulin isotype 1 in *H. contortus* were proposed to be involved in the mechanism of benzimidazole resistance [87]. Although it was suggested that a less frequent use of anthelmintics in humans (compared with their extensive use in livestock) should reduce the emergence of resistance in parasitic nematodes [88–91], some studies [92–97] have reported a reduction in efficacy of mebendazole and pyrantel in *N. americanus* and *A. duodenale* in areas of Mali, Zanzibar and North Western Australia, proposed to be attributed to resistance. Given the incomplete knowledge of the molecular mechanisms associated with resistance in parasitic nematodes [11], much attention is now directed towards the identification of new drug targets and the development of new, effective, and safe anthelmintics [98, 99] and effective strategies to prevent drug resistance [100–102].

Over the years, considerable research has focused on developing vaccines against selected parasitic nematodes [8, 9, 57, 80, 103–108]. For instance, irradiated larvae were used as the basis for a vaccine against *H. contortus* and *A. caninum* infection in sheep and dogs, respectively [109–112]. More recently, various proteins of the epithelial cell-surface membrane of the digestive tract of some gastrointestinal nematodes have been evaluated as vaccine candidates in experimental murine models or in livestock [9, 106, 107, 113]. For example, a 110 kDa integral membrane aminopeptidase of *H. contortus*, which is heavily glycosylated and localized in the brush border of the epithelial cells of the gut of the adult worm, was shown to be effective in reducing the intensity of *H. contortus* infection in different breeds and ages of sheep [114–117]. However, protection is limited to native proteins, administered multiple times, usually in Freund's adjuvant [118]. Another peptidase complex (P1), separated from the membrane aminopeptidase H11 by ion-exchange chromatography, was identified and shown to represent a ubiquitous component of the microvillar membrane of the intestinal cells of *H. contortus* [119]. Although vaccination with this protein complex resulted in a significant reduction (69 %) in the number of *H. contortus* eggs in the feces of vaccinated sheep following *H. contortus* challenge infection, P1 led only to an ~22–38 % reduction of infection intensity (parasite burden) [115]. On the other hand, vaccination with the glucose-binding glycoprotein complex (H-gal-GP), separated by lectin affinity chromatography from other integral membrane proteins from the gut of adult *H. contortus*, achieved ~53–72 % protection and a >90 % reduction in the number of eggs in the feces of vaccinated sheep [120]. However, the vaccination of lambs (9 months of age) with prokaryotically expressed recombinant H-gal-GP failed to induce protective immunity against challenge infection with *H. contortus* L3s [121].

Other vaccine candidates have been derived from the excretory/secretory products (ES) from worms [57, 80, 106, 122]. For example, proteases in ES from parasitic nematodes have been a major focus for vaccine development, given their inferred roles in the digestion of nutrients acquired from the host and/or during the penetration and migration through host tissues [122]. Metalloproteases, aspartic proteases and cysteine proteases have received considerable attention for blood-feeding nematodes, such as *H. contortus*, *A. caninum*, and *N. americanus* [57, 106, 123–128]. For instance, vaccination with a cysteine protease-enriched fraction from membrane extracts from the microvillar surface of intestinal cells from adult *H. contortus* [129] was demonstrated to reduce infection intensity by 47 % and the number of eggs in feces by 77 % in sheep following a single challenge infection [130]. Similarly, the vaccination of dogs with recombinant forms of a cysteine or aspartic protease from *A. caninum* (designated *Ac*-CP-2 and *Ac*-APR-1, respectively) resulted in partial protection against this hookworm, characterized by an absence of clinical signs and a reduced fecundity of the adult worms in dogs [126, 131]. In addition, vaccination of hamsters with the *N. americanus* homologue of *Ac*-CP-2 (i.e., *Na*-CP-2) was shown to induce partial protection, achieving an ~30–46 % reduction of infection intensity, following challenge infection with L3s [132].

Proteases from larval stages have also been the focus of vaccine research, because of their proposed role(s) in host invasion [80, 133]. In ES from hookworm larvae, for example, an astacin-like zinc metalloprotease from *A. caninum*, called *Ac*-MTP-1, has been demonstrated to degrade fibronectin, laminin, and collagen [134, 135]. Based on the results of a vaccine trial in hamsters, this protein was proposed as a potential candidate for the development of a multi-epitope vaccine [132]. In addition, two cysteine-rich secretory proteins, known as "*Ancylostoma*-secreted proteins" (ASPs) [136–139], major components of ES of hookworm L3s, can represent vaccine candidates [140]. However, the development of ASP-based vaccines has been impaired by evidence that such molecules can cause allergic reactions in humans previously infected with *N. americanus* hookworms [141, 142].

Collectively, the results of studies focusing on the identification of suitable immunogens and the development of effective vaccines against gastrointestinal parasitic nematodes show that progress has been made over the years. However, there is still limited information on parasite-host interactions at the molecular level. Clearly, advanced molecular technologies provide unique opportunities to explore the molecular biology of parasitic nematodes, parasite-host interactions and diseases on a global scale and should thus underpin the discovery of new intervention strategies. Indeed, high-throughput technologies are revolutionizing the way biology is done, allowing systems biological investigations of parasites and other pathogens. This statement applies to many areas, including genomics, proteomics and metabolomics, but also the detailed explorations of transcriptomes and associated molecular processes.

3 Some Key Techniques for Transcriptomic Investigations of Parasitic Nematodes

3.1 Conventional Methods

The genome of any living organism includes coding regions that are transcribed into mRNAs, which are subsequently translated into proteins. Techniques, such as Northern blot [143], quantitative real-time, reverse transcription PCR (qRT-PCR; 144) and differential display (DD; 145), have been used to define patterns of transcription for single genes or small numbers of molecules in parasitic nematodes, such as species of *Trichostrongylus*, *Haemonchus*, *Oesophagostomum*, and *Ostertagia* [146–153]. Another approach is the serial analysis of gene expression (SAGE) [154], which is based on the generation of a short specific tag (14 bp) from each mRNA present in the sample; these tags are used for the construction of a SAGE library. The sequencing of these tags allows a relatively high-throughput determination of their frequencies in the library, which are correlated with relative amounts of the corresponding mRNAs. Despite its demonstrated utility in studies of yeast [155] and humans [156, 157], the application of SAGE for investigations of transcription in parasitic nematodes has remained limited [158]. A single study [159] used SAGE to sequence and analyze ~3,000 transcripts from adult *H. contortus*, of which ~60 % had homologues in public databases.

The analysis of conventional expressed sequence tag (EST) datasets has been a widely used approach for investigations of the transcriptomes of parasitic nematodes. In vitro, mRNAs are reverse-transcribed, resulting in stable complementary DNAs (cDNAs); ESTs usually represent single-pass DNA sequence reads derived from cloned cDNAs [160, 161]. Traditional sequencing [162, 163] involves the use of a DNA polymerase, an oligonucleotide primer and four deoxyribonucleotide triphosphates (dNTPs) to synthesize the complementary strand to the template sequence [162–164]. The advent of EST sequencing marked a revolution in the field of parasitology and has been used in a range of studies aimed at investigating fundamental molecular processes in parasitic nematodes as well as drug and vaccine target discovery (e.g., 17, 165–172). For nematodes of animals, applications range from the analyses of stage- and gender-enriched molecules (e.g., 149, 153, 167, 173, 174) to global analyses of gene transcription (e.g., 166, 170, 175–177).

The cDNA microarray technology [178] was a significant advance for large-scale studies of the transcriptomes of parasitic nematodes [179]. In microarrays, thousands of oligonucleotides, usually cDNAs, EST clones or fragments of PCR products (which correspond to previously characterized genes/transcripts), are "spotted" ("arrayed") on to glass slides or chips in precise positions. The mRNAs from different stages or tissues are labeled with different fluorescent or radioactive markers and hybridized to the spots on the array. The relative abundance of hybridization for each mRNA population is then determined by comparing the relative signal intensity of each marker [178]. Supported by the increasing amount of sequence data available in public databases, microarray technology has allowed comparisons of levels of transcription of large numbers of mRNAs in, for instance, different tissues, developmental stages, and sexes of these nematodes to be performed, ultimately providing researchers with the opportunity to identify molecules considered to play essential roles in fundamental biological pathways of survival, development, and reproduction [9, 179, 180]. The use of microarray technology has resulted in an expanded knowledge of the transcriptomes of socioeconomically important strongylids, including *H. contortus*, *T. vitrinus*, *O. dentatum*, *Teladorsagia circumcincta* and *A. caninum* [153, 174, 181–185]. In addition, the combined application of suppressive-subtractive hybridization (SSH) and microarray analysis has been useful in enabling rapid comparisons of transcriptional profiles between/among life cycle stages, genders and/or species of parasitic nematodes [153, 183, 184, 186–188].

Knowledge of the complement of molecules transcribed in the larval stages of strongylid nematodes should also aid the elucidation of pathways associated with infectivity and interactions with the vertebrate host. The molecular mechanisms that regulate the transition from the free-living stage to the parasitic stage of nematodes may allow the development of novel strategies to disrupt this transition. Previous studies have analyzed differences in transcription between the ensheathed, free-living L3 and exsheathed L3 of *H. contortus* [152, 167, 189] and the related strongylid, *A. caninum* [182, 183]. The results of a cDNA microarray analysis, complemented by qRT-PCR of differentially transcribed molecules, showed that, among others, most transcripts encoding ASPs were upregulated in free-living L3s compared with parasitic, serum-stimulated larvae of *A. caninum* [182]. However, a study using

SSH-based microarray analysis [183] showed a substantial "upregulation" in the numbers and levels of transcripts encoding ASPs in serum-activated L3s [183].

To date, molecular studies of hookworms have mainly involved *A. caninum*, because of its use as a model for species infecting humans [182, 183, 190–192]. Clearly, detailed knowledge and understanding of the molecules transcribed in all stages of different species of hookworms, including *N. americanus* and *A. duodenale* of humans, should facilitate the identification of conserved pathways linked to development, survival, reproduction, parasite interactions and disease, and could assist in the discovery of new intervention strategies.

3.2 High-Throughput Sequencing Techniques

Recent advances in sequencing technologies [193–196]; Table 1) now provide the unique opportunity to perform de novo analyses of the whole transcriptomes of different species, sexes and/or developmental stages of nematodes of socioeconomic importance. Currently available massively parallel sequencing platforms include the 454/Roche [193]; www.454.com), Illumina/Solexa [194]; www.illumina.com), and SOLiD (Supported Oligonucleotide Ligation and Detection) [195]; http://www.invitrogen.com/site/us/en/home/Products-and-Services/Applications/Sequencing/Next-Generation-Sequencing.html) platforms (Table 1). Due to their capacity of generating millions or hundreds of millions of

Table 1
Technical features of next-generation sequencing platforms (i.e., 454/Roche, Illumina/Solexa, and SOLiD)[a]

Description	454/Roche	Illumina/Solexa	SOLiD
Platform	Genome Sequencer FLX	Genome Analyzer IIx	SOLiD 3 Plus System
Sequencing method	Emulsion PCR of bead-bound oligos	Isothermal bridge amplification on flow cell	Emulsion PCR of bead-bound oligos
Sequencing chemistry	Pyrosequencing using polymerase	Ligation ("dual-base encoding" octamers)	Reversible terminator using polymerase
Reads per run	~1 million	Up to 3 billion	1.2 to 1.4 billion
Read length	1,000 bp	50–250 bp	100 bp
Run time	~12 h	~2–9 days	~3 days
Peer-reviewed manuscripts	++++	+++	++
Examples of applications	De novo sequencing, metagenomics, targeted sequencing	Resequencing, RNA-Seq, DNA methylation studies	Resequencing, RNA-Seq

[a]Based on information available on July 2012

sequences simultaneously, these platforms have been at the forefront of the genomic and transcriptomic research [197–199] and are powerful tools for investigating the transcriptomes of parasitic nematodes on an unprecedented scale.

The 454/Roche platform [193] uses a sequencing-by-synthesis approach. For transcriptomic studies, cDNA is randomly fragmented (by "nebulization") into sections of variable size; adaptors are ligated to each end of these fragments, which are then mixed with a population of agarose beads whose surfaces anchor oligonucleotides complementary to the 454-specific adapter sequence, such that each bead is associated with a single fragment. Each of these complexes is transferred into individual oil–water micelles containing amplification reagents and is then subjected to an emulsion PCR (emPCR) step, during which ~10 million copies of each cDNA are produced and bound to individual beads. Subsequently, in the sequencing phase, the beads anchoring the cDNAs are deposited on a picotiter plate, together with other enzymes required for the pyrophosphate sequencing reaction (i.e., ATP sulfurylase and luciferase), and sequencing is carried out by flowing the reagents (nucleotides and buffers) over a plate [200].

Following the introduction of the 454 technology, the first Illumina (formerly Solexa) sequencer became available [194]. This technology involves fragmentation of cDNA sample into a shotgun library, followed by the in vitro ligation of Illumina-specific adaptors to each cDNA template; the termini of the template are covalently attached to the surface of a glass slide (or flow cell). Attached to the flow cell are primers complementary to the other end of the template, which bend the cDNAs to form bridge-like structures. During the amplification step (bridge-PCR), clonal clusters, each consisting of ~1,000 amplicons, are generated; subsequently, the cDNAs are linearized, and the sequencing reagents are directly added to the flow cell, with four types of fluorescently labeled nucleotides. After the incorporation of a fluorescent base, the flow cell is interrogated with a laser in several locations, which results in several image acquisitions at the end of a single synthesis cycle [200]. This technology is considered ideal for both de novo and resequencing projects, targeted sequencing, single-nucleotide polymorphism (SNP) analyses and gene transcription studies.

The sequencing process of the SOLiD platform [195] employs the enzyme DNA ligase, instead of a polymerase [200]. Briefly, after an emPCR step, the adaptor sequences of the cDNA templates bind to complementary primers that are covalently anchored to a glass slide. Subsequently, a set of four fluorescently labeled di-probes (octamers of random sequence, except known dinucleotides at the 3′-terminus) are added to the sequencing reaction. In case an octamer is complementary to the template, it will be ligated, and the two specific nucleotides can be called; subsequently, an image is acquired and the fluorescent dye is removed, so that other octamers can be ligated. After multiple ligations (e.g., seven ligations for a 35 bp read), the newly synthesized cDNA is removed and the primer is inactivated. This process is repeated multiple times from different starting points of the cDNA templates, so that each position is sequenced at least twice. This technique, known as "two-base calling," allows the correction of sequencing errors, thus providing accurate base calling [200]. Because of the short read length, the range of applications of the SOLiD system is considered similar to that of the Illumina technology and includes (targeted) resequencing projects, SNP detection and gene transcription studies.

In the past few years, numerous studies have demonstrated the utility of high-throughput sequencing for investigating, for example, aspects of the systematics, population genetics and molecular biology of helminths [192, 201–211]. For instance, Illumina technology alone has been used to sequence the entire genomes of *Ascaris suum* [202] and the human blood fluke, *Schistosoma haematobium* [211], whereas the 454 technology has been instrumental for de novo sequencing of the transcriptomes of important parasitic worms, such as *N. americanus, Clonorchis sinensis, Opisthorchis viverrini, Fasciola hepatica* and *F. gigantica* of humans and other animals [205, 208–210]. Several thousands of unique and novel sequences were characterized for each of these parasites, demonstrating the capacity of this technology to generate large and informative datasets. The development of suitable bioinformatic tools has become crucial for the detailed analyses of such datasets.

3.3 Bioinformatics

The increasing number of high-throughput sequence datasets in public databases has been accompanied by an expansion of bioinformatic tools for the analysis of such datasets, at the cDNA, genomic DNA and protein levels. This expansion has resulted in the development of a number of web-based programs and/or integrated pipelines [16, 206, 212–218]. In brief, following the acquisition of sequence data, these are firstly screened for sequence repeats, contaminants and/or adaptor sequences [215, 219]. Following the preprocessing, sequences are "clustered" (assembled) into contiguous sequences (of maximum length) based on sequence similarity.

3.3.1 Assembly

The main goal of sequence assembly is to determine, with confidence, the sequence of a target transcript/gene. This process involves the alignment and merging of fragments of nucleic acids to form long, contiguous sequences (i.e., contigs) [18, 215]. Long (e.g., generated by Sanger sequencing or 454 technology) and short reads (e.g., Illumina or SOLiD platform) are assembled using algorithms for "overlap-layout consensus" [220] and "de Bruijn graph" [221, 222], respectively.

For the former algorithm [220], all pairwise overlaps among reads are computed and stored in a graph; all graphs are used to compute a layout of reads and then a consensus sequence of contigs [223, 224]. Some of the assemblers designed to support long-read assembly include PHRAP [225], the *c*ontig *a*ssembly *p*rogram v.3 (CAP3; 212), the TIGR assembler [226], the *p*arallel *c*ontig *a*ssembly *p*rogram (PCAP; 227) and the *m*imicking *i*ntelligent *r*ead *a*ssembly program (MIRA; 228).

For the "de Bruijn graph" [221, 222], reads are fragmented into short segments, called "k-mers," where "k" represents the number of nucleotides in each segment. Overlaps between or among k-mers are captured and stored in graphs, which are subsequently used to generate the consensus sequences [223, 224]. Examples of programs specifically designed for the assembly of short reads include the *s*hort *s*equence *a*ssembly by *k*-mer search and 3′-read *e*xtension (SSAKE; 229), Velvet [222], Oases [230], the *e*xact de novo *a*ssembler (EDENA; 231), Euler-SR [232], the *a*ssembly *by* *s*hort *s*equencing (ABYSS; 233), the *s*hort *o*ligonucleotide *a*nalysis *p*ackage (SOAP; 234) and Trinity [235].

3.3.2 Annotation and Analyses

Following assembly, the contigs and single reads (or singletons) are compared with known sequence data available in public databases, in order to assign a predicted identity to each query sequence if significant matches are found [206, 215]. In addition, assembled nucleotide sequences are usually conceptually translated into predicted proteins using algorithms that identify protein-coding regions (open reading frames, ORFs) from individual contigs. Examples of such algorithms are OrfPredictor [236], ESTScan [213], DECODER [237] and ORFcor [238]. Once peptide sequences are predicted, they are compared with amino acid sequence data available in public databases to identify protein domains [206, 215]. For instance, the software InterProScan [216] provides an integrated tool for the characterization of a protein family or an individual protein sequence, domain and/or functional site by comparing sequences with information available in the databases PROSITE [239], PRINTS [240], Pfam [241], ProDom [242], SMART [243] and/or Gene Ontology (GO; 244). In addition, other programs are available for the prediction of transmembrane domains (e.g., TMHMM; 245) and/or signal peptide motifs (e.g., SignalP; 246).

Different types of the Basic Local Alignment Software Tool (BLAST; 247) are used for comparing the nucleotide sequence data with DNA or cDNA (BLASTn) or amino acid (BLASTx) sequences or conceptually translated peptides with protein sequences (BLASTp), available in databases [206, 215]. Public databases represent comprehensive collections of nucleotide and amino acid sequences. Due to the rapid progress in the discovery and characterization of novel genes and proteins, online public databases have become primary sources for sequence data storage, analysis and annotation. For example, the International Nucleotide Sequence Database Collaboration includes three "sister" databases, namely GenBank [248], the Enterprise Management Technology Transfer nucleotide database curated by the European Molecular Biology Laboratory (EMBL; 249) and the DNA Data Bank of Japan (DDBJ; 250). In these databases, all publicly available nucleotide sequences are stored and curated; in addition, each sequence is stored as a separate record and linked to information, such as primary source references and predicted and/or experimentally verified biological features. For high-throughput sequencing projects, raw sequence data are often stored in subdivisions of these nucleotide databases, such as UniGene [251] and the Sequence Read Archive [252]. Various databases, which exclusively store known amino acid sequence data, are also available. For instance, the Protein Data Bank (PDB; 253), maintained by the Research Collaboratory for Structural Bioinformatics, represents the primary source for protein structures, whereas the SWISS-PROT database [254] is a protein sequence database for a number of prokaryotes and eukaryotes. The TrEMBL [255] division of SWISS-PROT contains a non-redundant set of translations for all coding sequences in the EMBL nucleotide sequence database that do not correspond to existing SWISS-PROT entries. In addition to these comprehensive general databases, there is a number of specialized collections of gene and protein information on particular organisms. Examples include the databases for *Saccharomyces cerevisiae* (yeast) (www.yeastgenome.org; 256), *Drosophila melanogaster* (vinegar fly) (http://flybase.org; 257), *Mus musculus* (mouse) (www.informatics.jax.org; 258) and *C. elegans* (free-living nematode) (WormBase at www.wormbase.org; 259). WormBase is a comprehensive repository of information on *C. elegans* and related nematodes, such as *C. briggsae* [259]. Here, essentially all information and data on classical genetics, cellular biology, and structural and functional genomics of these free-living nematodes are stored and continually curated [259–262].

The functional annotation of sequence data for parasitic nematodes has often relied on pairwise homology-based comparative analyses with already annotated and curated sequence datasets for a range of organisms [203, 204]. However, many genes, transcripts and gene products of these worms (often ≥50 %) cannot be functionally annotated using this approach, because closely related, homologous molecules do not exist in transcriptomic and/or genomic datasets available in public databases and/or because sequence datasets are incomplete. In addition, as functional genomic tools are not yet practical or established for most parasitic helminths, improved bioinformatic approaches need to be established and continually enhanced to achieve enhanced functional annotation of genes and gene products. Recently, Mangiola et al. [263] tackled this issue and compiled transcriptomic datasets of key, socioeconomically important parasitic helminths, constructed and validated a curated database (HelmDB; www.helmdb.org), and showed how data integration and clustering can achieve improved functional annotations. HelmDB provides a practical and user-friendly toolkit for sequence browsing and comparative analyses among divergent helminth groups (including nematodes and trematodes) and should be readily adaptable and applicable to a wide range of parasites.

4 *Caenorhabditis elegans* as Major Resource for Comparative Studies

The annotation and analysis of sequence data derived from many parasitic nematodes, particularly Strongylida, relies on information available for *C. elegans* (in WormBase). The latter nematode is simple in its anatomy (959 somatic cells in the hermaphrodite and 1,031 in the male), has a short life cycle (~3 days) and is easy to culture in vitro [264]. The genome of *C. elegans* is ~100 Mb in size [265]. Currently, WormBase contains detailed and curated information on ~20,000 *C. elegans* genes and associated data on, for instance, transcription/expression profiles in different developmental stages, tissues and cells, mutants and their phenotypes, genetic and physical maps, SNPs, information on gene-gene and protein-protein interactions, as well as all peer-reviewed literature pertaining to *C. elegans.*

The advent of double-stranded RNA interference (RNAi; 266) has revolutionized the study of gene function in metazoan organisms and led to detailed information on the functions of ~96 % genes in *C. elegans* [267–271]. The principle of RNAi relies on the introduction of double-stranded RNA (dsRNA) into the cells of a living organism, which induces the degradation of the homologous (target) mRNA [266]. The dsRNA can be introduced directly into *C. elegans* by injection [266], by soaking worms in solution [272] or by feeding worms *Escherichia coli* expressing a dsRNA fragment of a target gene [273]; it can also be introduced using a transgene expressing dsRNA [274, 275]. This gene silencing approach opened up avenues for large-scale studies of molecular function in *C. elegans* [267–270, 274, 276, 277] as well as for comparative studies (e.g., comparison with parasitic nematodes or humans) [278–282].

Transgenesis of *C. elegans* has also been widely used for assessing gene function [283, 284]. This technique can involve the microinjection of expression constructs, which usually comprise plasmid or cosmid DNA, often incorporating green fluorescent protein (GFP; 285) into the syncytium (mitotically active) region of the adult hermaphrodite gonad ("gonadal microinjection");

alternatively, the DNA constructs can be transferred directly into target cells via high-density microparticles of gold or tungsten ("biolistics" or "particle bombardment") [286]. Introduced DNA does not usually integrate into the chromosome, but rather it forms a multi-copy extrachromosomal array which can be inherited. Labeling with GFP allows the study of a number of (temporal and spatial) biological processes, including gene expression, protein localization and dynamics, protein-protein interactions, cell division, chromosome replication and organization, intracellular transport pathways, organelle inheritance and biogenesis [287].

In addition to investigations of gene expression and localization, patterns of gene transcription during key developmental and reproductive processes have also been studied in *C. elegans*, employing microarray technology [288–290]. In an early study [288], various groups of molecules were demonstrated to have high expression levels in the germ-line tissues of *C. elegans*, i.e., the "germ-line-intrinsic" molecules (expressed in the germ line of hermaphrodites producing either sperm or oocytes and proposed to play key roles in biological processes linked to meiosis, stem cell recombination and germ-line development), and molecules highly expressed either in oocyte-producing or sperm-producing hermaphrodites [288]. The latter group included a large number of molecules, such as protein kinases and phosphatases, associated with spermatogenesis, in accordance with other studies investigating gender-enriched transcriptional patterns in parasitic nematodes (e.g., 153, 174, 181). Previously, genetic studies had indicated that ~50–70 % of genes in parasitic nematodes have orthologues in *C. elegans* [27, 171], which supported the grouping of this free-living nematodes into "clade V" of the phylum Nematoda, together with parasitic nematodes of the order Strongylida [27, 291]. These results, together with similarities in various characteristics (such as body plan and molting) between *C. elegans* and some parasitic nematodes (e.g., 5, 292), indicate that this free-living nematode provides a useful system for comparative investigations of many conserved biochemical and molecular pathways linked to development in related nematodes.

5 Understanding Nematodes of Socioeconomic Importance Through Genomics and Transcriptomics: Examples

High-throughput sequencing technologies (Table 1) and improved bioinformatic tools are providing unparalleled opportunities for global analyses of the genomes and transcriptomes of key nematodes, such as *A. suum* [202] and *Trichinella spiralis* (trichina; 293). Recent studies have utilized such technologies to explore the transcriptomes of different developmental stages and both sexes of key strongylid nematodes, including *N. americanus*, *H. contortus*, *T. colubriformis* and *O. dentatum* [203–206].

Although human hookworms are of major socioeconomic importance [1, 3, 6, 7], genomic and molecular studies have mostly involved *A. caninum* (e.g., 182, 183, 190–192). Recently, 454 sequencing and bioinformatic analyses were conducted to investigate, for the first time on a large scale, the transcriptome of the adult stage of *N. americanus* [205]. The results showed that transcripts encoding proteases and Kunitz-type protease inhibitors were most abundantly represented in the transcriptome of this nematode, supporting the fundamental roles that these molecules play in multi-enzyme cascades to digest hemoglobin and other serum proteins [294, 295], and in preventing homeostasis and inhibiting host proteases [296, 297]. Using a combination of orthology-mapping and functional data available for *C. elegans*, Cantacessi et al. [205] predicted 18 potential drug targets in the transcriptome of the adult stage of *N. americanus*, which included, for instance, mitochondria-associated proteins known to be essential in *C. elegans* [298].

In *H. contortus*, high-throughput sequencing and bioinformatic analyses were used to explore differences in gene transcription between the free-living (L3) and the parasitic (xL3) third larval stages and to predict the roles that key transcripts play in the metabolic pathways linked to larval development [204]. These analyses revealed that transthyretin-like proteins (TTLs) and calcium-binding proteins were highly represented in the transcriptome of both *H. contortus* L3 and xL3, whereas selected transcripts encoding collagens and neuropeptides were present exclusively in L3 and proteases in xL3 [204]. In nematodes, the synthesis of collagens has been observed to increase significantly prior to a molt [299], whereas proteins involved in the development of the nervous system are essential in the cascade of events that lead to the growth and development of the larval stages [300]. Therefore, increased transcription of neuropeptides in L3s of *H. contortus* might relate to axon guidance and synapse formation during the L3's transition to parasitism [204]. This statement is supported by the fact that, in *H. contortus*, the transition from the free-living L3 to the parasitic L3 is triggered by gaseous CO_2, detected by chemosensory neurons of amphids, which are located in the anterior end of the L3 stage, ultimately leading to the secretion of the neurotransmitter noradrenaline [5]. Conversely, the largest number of *C. elegans* orthologues of *H. contortus* xL3-specific transcripts encoded peptidases and other enzymes involved in amino acid catabolism, supporting previous evidence that cysteine proteases play a crucial role in the catabolism of globin, as is the case for *A. caninum* and *N. americanus* [146, 294, 295, 301]. A similar spectrum of proteases and other molecules linked to catalytic activity had been shown also to be highly represented in the transcriptomes of activated xL3 stages of both *H. contortus* and *A. caninum* in comparison with their L3s [183, 204]. This finding, for two hematophagous bursate nematodes with differing life histories, is likely to reflect the key roles that these molecules play in host tissue invasion, degradation and/or digestion.

In the transcriptome of *T. colubriformis*, molecules encoding peptides which are predicted to be associated with the nervous system (i.e., "transthyretin-like" and "neuropeptide-like" proteins (TTLs and NLPs, respectively)), digestion of host proteins, or inhibition of host proteases (i.e., proteases and protease inhibitors, respectively) were highly represented [203], with serine and metalloproteases and "Kunitz-type" protease inhibitors being the vast majority of molecules characterized [203]. In strongylid nematodes, these molecules play fundamental roles in the invasion of the vertebrate host by mediating, for example, tissue penetration, feeding and/or immune evasion by (1) digesting antibodies, (2) cleaving cell-surface receptors for cytokines and/or (3) causing the direct lysis of immune cells [302–306].

In an effort to predict and prioritize molecules that could represent novel drug targets and are expressed across different stages of development, Cantacessi et al. [206] employed high-throughput sequencing and predictive algorithms to explore similarities and differences in the transcriptomes of the L3, L4, and adult male and female of *O. dentatum* [206]. Most of the molecules unique to the adult male and female of *O. dentatum* could be linked to pathways associated with reproductive processes. For instance, a large number of *O. dentatum* male-specific molecules encoded major sperm proteins (MSPs), in accordance with previous studies of male-enriched datasets of other species of trichostrongylid nematodes, including *T. vitrinus* and *H. contortus* [174, 181]. Based on the observation that MSPs from various nematodes, including *C. elegans*, are characterized by significant amino acid sequence conservation (~67 %; 307), a similar role has been proposed for these proteins in processes linked to the maturation of oocytes in the uterus of female nematodes [308, 309]. In addition, a large proportion (17 %) of molecules unique to the larval stages of *O. dentatum* represented proteases that, in this species, have been reported to evoke immunological and/or inflammatory reactions (including infiltrations of neutrophils and eosinophils) surrounding the encapsulated larvae [77, 180]. In addition, somatic extracts of and supernatants from in vitro maintenance cultures of *O. dentatum* L4s have been shown to induce the proliferation of porcine mononuclear cells in vitro [310], which supports the hypothesis that L4-specific proteases play an active role in the modulation of the host's immune response [302–304]. The results from a recent study showed also that a high proportion (27–32 %) of transcripts encoding protein kinases and phosphatases were common among all developmental stages of *O. dentatum* investigated [206]. Supported by investigations of the free-living nematode *C. elegans*, other studies have predicted, for instance, that some kinases and phosphatases could represent targets for novel nematocidal drugs [99, 311]. Some cantharidin/norcantharidin analogues [312–314] are known to display exquisite and specific inhibitory activity against PP1 and PP2A phosphatases, which indicated that some of them could be designed to selectively inhibit essential serine/threonine phosphatase (STPs) of nematodes [311] (*see* Subheading 6). In addition to phosphatases, other molecules, such as chitin-binding proteins or proteases, might be interesting drug target candidates, given that they are proposed to have crucial roles in pathways linked to developmental and reproductive processes in some nematodes [180, 206, 315].

Highly represented in the transcriptomes of a number of strongylid nematodes [203–206] are proteins containing a "sperm-coating protein (SCP)-like extracellular domain" (InterPro: IPR014044), also called SCP/Tpx-1/Ag5/PR-1/Sc7 (SCP/TAPS, Pfam accession number no. PF00188), or ASPs [139]. Due to their abundance in the excretory/secretory products from serum-activated L3s (aL3s) of *A. caninum* and high transcriptional levels of mRNAs encoding ASPs in activated L3s compared with non-activated, ensheathed L3s, these molecules have been hypothesized to play a major role in the transition from the free-living to the parasitic stages of this hookworm [137, 183]. Other ASP homologues have been characterized for the adult stage of hookworms and are proposed to play a role in the initiation, establishment and/or maintenance of the host-parasite relationship [183, 316, 317]. Due to the immunogenic properties of ASPs, one member of this protein group (i.e., *Na*-ASP-2) has been under investigation as a vaccine candidate against necatoriasis in humans [57, 132, 318–320]. Whether SCP/TAPS proteins or their genes represent drug target candidates still remains to be determined. For ASPs, a focus of future research could be on studying their structure and function in parasitic helminths, to pave the way for applied outcomes, such the development of vaccines and/or drugs [321].

6 Opportunities for Drug Discovery Using Global Datasets

For parasitic nematodes, the prediction of drug target candidates from global genomic and transcriptomic datasets can be assisted by using extensive information on the functionality and essentiality of homologues in *C. elegans*, *D. melanogaster*, *M. musculus* and/or *S. cerevisiae* (accessible via public databases www.wormbase.org, http://flybase.org, www.informatics.jax.org, and www.yeastgenome.org) [202–206, 211]. Since most effective drugs achieve their activity by competing with endogenous small molecules for a binding site on a target protein [322], the amino acid sequences produced from essential genes can be screened for the presence of conserved ligand-binding domains [322, 323] and lists of prioritized inhibitors compiled [323]. The comparison of various studies shows consistently that some proteases, G protein-coupled receptors (GPCRs), guanosine triphosphatases (GTPases), kinases and phosphatases are salient among essential molecules and, thus, represent potential targets for nematocides [202–206].

Protein kinases (PTKs) have shown considerable promise as drug targets in protozoa, such as *Plasmodium* and *Giardia* [324–326] and in helminths, including *Schistosoma mansoni* and *Echinococcus multilocularis* [327]. In the latter two species, for example, PTK inhibitors (i.e., tyrphostins AG1024 and AG538) have been shown to affect the survival and development of the parasite through the inhibition of glucose uptake [327]. In another study, the inactivation of *S. mansoni* PTKs with herbimycin A (an Src kinase inhibitor) was shown to disrupt mitosis, thus reducing the expression of proteins essential for egg production, including the formation of the eggshell, in adult females [328]. Although crystal structures of PTKs from parasitic nematodes have not yet been determined, some advances have been made in the identification and design of effective inhibitors based on homology models for protein kinases from humans [327]. There is evidence that the active sites of parasite PTKs display a variable degree of structural divergence compared with their human counterparts [326, 327], which seems promising for designing selective kinase inhibitors for helminths.

Recent work has also shown potential for atypical protein kinases (aPKs; 324) as targets for the development of novel intervention strategies. Among these aPKs, the RIO kinases (RIOKs: RIOK-1, RIOK-2 and RIOK-3) are considered essential for life [329]. RIOKs of parasitic strongylid nematodes have close homologues in *C. elegans* [329, 330]; however, almost nothing is known about the function or biology of RIOKs in parasitic nematodes and in most other metazoans. Although there are some conserved elements in each of the three RIOKs of different organisms, these aPKs from nematodes cluster, with high statistical support, to the exclusion of those of other eukaryotic organisms, including mammals [329], indicating prospects for the design of a new class of nematode-specific inhibitors of these aPKs. Using in silico screening of the SPECS database (www.specs.net), Campbell et al. [329] identified compounds that bind in silico to RIOK-1 of *H. contortus* (*Hc*-RIOK-1). For some of these compounds, multiple, highly scored binding modes were observed, indicating an increased likelihood that these aPKs would display productive interactions in an in vitro assay [329]. In addition, the hydrogen-bond interactions between the compounds identified and the *Hc-RIOK-1* model involved multiple conserved side chains in the active site (including the P-loops, catalytic loops, and metal-binding loops); however, all compounds identified were also involved in interactions with residues that are not conserved and specific to *Hc*-RIOK-1 [329] and are thus considered important for the design of selective inhibitors of *Hc*-RIOK-1. A screen of the BRENDA database (www.brenda-enzymes.org; 322) for compounds with similar chemical structures to known kinase effectors identified two molecules with significant similarity to the protein kinase inhibitor emodol (an anthraquinone found in several plants), providing a useful starting point for drug development [329]. Also identified were molecules with some structural similarity to known kinase effectors, such as the flavonoids apigenin and kaempferol (known to possess cancer-protective effects; 331–333) and prunitrin, a naturally occurring isoflavonoid in species of *Trifolium* (clover) and *Prunus*, characterized by a naphthoquinone scaffold and a carbohydrate moiety [329]. In the future, an integrated approach, using advanced functional genomic, bioinformatic, chemoinformatic and structural biological tools, could be used to elucidate the functions and structures of RIOKs, whose roles are proposed to be essential and involved intimately in developmental processes.

From a functional perspective, current information on *C. elegans* shows that *riok-1* encodes two isoforms (via alternative splicing) required for viability, fertility, endocytosis, and fat storage. *C. elegans riok-2* also encodes a RIOK required for viability and fertility, and *riok-3* encodes a RIOK expressed in the larval and adult intestine of *C. elegans* [329]. In addition, preliminary experiments have predicted null mutations in *riok-1* and *riok-2*, both of which are lethal, and an uncharacterized predicted null allele of *riok-3* (unpublished). From a structural biology perspective, preliminary comparisons show that the RIOK domain harboring the catalytic site is a conserved fold for nematode RIOKs. However, despite this fold, there are several amino acid substitutions in functionally important, conserved secondary structure elements, whose impact can only be assessed from three-dimensional structures determined experimentally [329]. Thus, structural studies need to assess the particular binding modes of ligands, particularly the phosphate-donating nucleotides, to provide a solid basis for structure-based drug design. Furthermore, the mechanistic aspects of RIOKs are poorly understood, thus requiring detailed structural information. The working model described by Campbell et al. [329] assumes that the two flexible elements in the RIOK domain, the hinge and the flexible loop, serve as docking points for the substrate and might undergo conformational change in the substrate-bound state. Such a process may be further aided by phosphorylation of

Ser165 (in relation to RIOK-1), which is located in the flexible loop and seems to be a conserved residue for RIOKs. Crystal structures of substrate-bound and phosphorylated nematode RIOKs should assist in elucidating the biology of these proteins, providing clues as to how to best design selective and specific inhibitors.

Serine/threonine phosphatases (STPs) are also proposed to be involved in essential biological pathways and, thus, might represent viable anthelmintic targets [99]. In silico structural comparisons between *Hc*-STP-1 and homologues from other parasitic nematodes, including *O. dentatum* and *T. vitrinus*, have revealed conservation of residues and features putatively involved in catalytic activity, whereas phylogenetic analyses of STP sequence data from a range of eukaryotes confirmed the close relationship of nematode STPs, which clustered to the exclusion of homologues from other organisms [99]. In one study, Campbell et al. [311] tested the activity of a series of norcantharidin-derived analogues against *H. contortus*; cf. Subheading 5). Three of these analogues reproducibly displayed 99–100 % lethality against *H. contortus* in a larval development assay [311] and no toxic effects on multiple, independent mammalian (human cancer) cell lines. However, given the difference in structure between these analogues and the original norcantharidin chemotype, it was proposed that these molecules might have targets other than STPs [311]. Further studies are needed to establish the precise mode of action of these effective norcantharidin-derived compounds in nematodes, which show considerable promise as anthelmintics.

7 Challenges and Prospects

Due to the lack of complete genomic sequences for most parasitic nematodes, newly generated transcriptomic and genomic sequence datasets need to be assembled de novo, which means that pooled reads are assembled without a bias towards known sequences [222]. Due to the amount of RNA required for high-throughput sequencing (~5–10 μg; 334, 335), transcriptomes from small nematodes usually originate from multiple individuals, potentially leading to an increased complexity of the sequence data acquired (linked, for instance, to single-nucleotide polymorphisms and other types of sequence variation) and posing some challenges for the assembly. In terms of complexity, and computational and time requirements, de novo assemblies are orders of magnitude slower and much more computationally intensive than knowledge-based (mapping) assemblies, in which reads are aligned and assembled against an existing "backbone" sequence [336]. In addition, reliable de novo assemblies are heavily dependent on the availability of long reads (>100 bases) and of high-coverage, paired-end sequence data [336, 337]. In previous studies, the complementary nature of the 454 and Illumina sequencing platforms has allowed the assembly of raw reads into large scaffolds without need for a reference sequence [338–340]. Thus, clearly, the 454 sequence data assembled in previous studies [203–206] should assist future de novo assemblies of Illumina data (both transcriptomic and genomic) for the species investigated to date.

Some transcriptomic studies have employed 454 sequencing of normalized cDNA libraries [203–206]. Normalization allows transcripts to be studied qualitatively, but this approach does not allow differential gene expression to be investigated quantitatively [203–206]. Exploring differential transcription among stages, sexes and tissues of parasitic nematodes and other helminths provides unique insights into molecular changes occurring, for example, during development and reproduction. Future studies involving the sequencing of non-normalized cDNA libraries by, for instance, Illumina technology [194] will provide an avenue to explore essential biological pathways in parasitic nematodes, such as those linked to the development of neuronal tissue, the formation of cuticle, and the digestion of host hemoglobin in *H. contortus* [204] and in mitochondrial and amino acid metabolism in *N. americanus* [205]. However, the incorporation of gene expression data will inevitably pose new computational challenges for the correct assembly and analysis of sequence datasets and, for instance, for the accurate prediction of alternatively spliced transcripts.

The accurate assembly of ESTs is a crucial step for examining coding genes and, ultimately, addressing biological questions regarding gene and protein function [263]. Knowledge of the function of genes and gene products from organisms is predicted using a process known as "sequence annotation," which has been defined as "the process of gathering available information and relating it to the sequence assembly both by experimental and computational means" [341]. Currently, the annotation of sequence data from parasitic nematodes is primarily based on comparisons with data available in public databases available via multiple portals [203–206] and updated at different rates. The Swiss-Prot database (http://au.expasy.org/sprot), for instance, accepts corrections from its user community, whereas GenBank (www.ncbi.nlm.nih.gov/genbank) only accepts corrections from the author of an entry [342], thus significantly affecting the accuracy and speed with which new sequences are annotated. In addition, some information-management systems evolve to efficiently incorporate data from large-scale projects, but often, the annotation of single records from the literature is slow and cumbersome [343]. Given that, presently, the annotation of sequence data for parasitic nematodes relies heavily on the use of bioinformatic approaches and already annotated/curated sequence data for a wide range of organisms [203–206], these observations are particularly crucial and deserve further consideration. For instance, the analyses and annotation of large-scale transcriptomic sequence datasets for parasitic nematodes could be considerably facilitated through the establishment of a "reference" website, which could provide regular releases of newly developed and validated bioinformatic pipelines for the analyses of sequence datasets as well as links to regularly updated databases. In the future, the establishment of a "centralized" consortium to facilitate the sharing and optimization of bioinformatic pipelines for sequence processing and annotation and, more broadly, to allow access to new sequence data, as well as experimental protocols and relevant literature, would be very useful to the scientific community.

Typically, the annotation of peptides inferred from the transcriptomes of parasitic nematodes is performed by assigning predicted biological function(s) based on comparison with existing information available for *C. elegans* and for other organisms in public databases (e.g., WormBase; InterPro, www.ebi.ac.uk/interpro; Gene Ontology, www.geneontology.org; OrthoMCL, www.orthomcl.org; BRENDA, www.brenda-enzymes.org) [203–206]. Using this approach, predictions for key groups of molecules were made in relation to their function and essential roles in biological processes [203–206]. Such groups included the SCP/TAPS proteins and molecules linked to the physiology of the nervous system, the formation of the cuticle, proteases and protease inhibitors, and protein kinases and phosphatases [203–206]. However, in order to support data inferred from bioinformatic analyses of sequence data, experimental validation is now required. In particular, extensive laboratory experiments need to be conducted to evaluate the functions of molecules in the parasites studied and/or in a suitable surrogate organism. RNAi has been applied to a number of strongylid nematodes of animals, but success has been relatively limited (e.g., 279, 344–351). Current evidence suggests that a number of nematodes of animals, including *H. contortus*, lack critical components of the RNAi machinery [279, 349, 350, 352]. Transgenesis and gene complementation studies have shown considerable promise for evaluating the function of genes from some parasitic nematodes (e.g., 353–355). Indeed, a study demonstrating successful transgenesis in the parasitic nematode *Parastrongyloides trichosuri* (Rhabditida) [356] as well as the use of *C. elegans* as a surrogate system for the analysis of the function of some genes from selected members of the Strongylida and Rhabditida [353–355] provides substantial promise and scope for the application of this methodology to functional genetic studies of selected groups of parasitic nematodes.

In the future, improved bioinformatic prediction and prioritization of potential drug targets in parasitic nematodes will depend on the availability of complete genome sequences. Global repertoires of drug targets could be inferred. For instance, the parasite kinome (the complete set of kinase genes in the genome) could represent a unique opportunity for the design of parasite-selective inhibitors [327]. In addition, the integration of genomic, transcriptomic, and proteomic data will be crucial to identify groups of molecules essential to parasite survival and development, which could represent drug target candidates. Clearly, high-throughput sequencing, such as Illumina, provides the efficiency and depth of coverage required to rapidly define genomes and transcriptomes of eukaryotic pathogens of socioeconomic importance [202, 211, 293]. The combined use of innovative bioinformatic tools will open the door to understanding the molecular biology of parasites and other pathogens on an unprecedented scale. A deep understanding of these pathogens at the molecular level will provide exciting opportunities for the development of novel interventions and diagnostic methods.

8 Update on Next-Generation Sequencing Technologies

In October 2013, Roche announced the closure of its subsidiary 454 Life Sciences and the discontinuation of the 454 sequencer (http://www.bio-itworld.com/2013/10/16/six-years-after-acquisition-roche-quietly-shutters-454.html); this outcome has been attributed largely to major competition by Illumina and Life Technologies, with the release of their respective Personal Genome Machine (PGM), MiSeq, and Ion Torrent sequencing platforms. While, to the best of our knowledge, the latter platform is yet to be utilized for high-throughput sequencing studies of parasites of animals and humans, the high sequencing speed, low cost of sample sequencing, and small instrument size [357] will undoubtedly represent substantial advantages in the quest to fight neglected diseases.

Acknowledgments

Funding from the Australian Research Council, the National Health and Medical Research Council, the Australian Academy of Science, the Alexander von Humboldt Foundation, and Melbourne Water Corporation is gratefully acknowledged (RBG). Our research program was also supported by the Victorian Life Sciences Computation Initiative (grant number VR0007) on its Peak Computing Facility at the University of Melbourne, an initiative of the Victorian Government (RBG).

References

1. de Silva NR, Brooker S, Hotez PJ et al (2003) Soil-transmitted helminth infections: updating the global picture. Trends Parasitol 19:547–551
2. Artis D (2006) New weapons in the war on worms: identification of putative mechanisms of immune-mediated expulsion of gastrointestinal nematodes. Int J Parasitol 36:723–733
3. Bethony J, Brooker S, Albonico M et al (2006) Soil-transmitted helminth infections: ascariasis, trichuriasis, and hookworm. Lancet 367:1521–1532
4. Brooker S, Clements AC, Bundy DA (2006) Global epidemiology, ecology and control of soil-transmitted helminth infections. Adv Parasitol 62:221–261
5. Nikolaou S, Gasser RB (2006) Prospects for exploring molecular developmental processes in *Haemonchus contortus*. Int J Parasitol 36:859–868
6. Hotez PJ, Fenwick A, Savioli L et al (2009) Rescuing the bottom billion through control of neglected tropical diseases. Lancet 373:1570–1575
7. O'Harhay MO, Horton J, Olliaro PL (2010) Epidemiology and control of human gastrointestinal parasites in children. Expert Rev Anti Infect Ther 8:219–234
8. Newton SE, Munn EA (1999) The development of vaccines against gastrointestinal nematode parasites, particularly *Haemonchus contortus*. Parasitol Today 15:116–122
9. Newton SE, Meeusen EN (2003) Progress and new technologies for developing vaccines against gastrointestinal nematode parasites of sheep. Parasite Immunol 25:283–296
10. Roeber F, Jex AR, Gasser RB (2013) Advances in the diagnosis of key gastrointestinal nematode infections of livestock, with an emphasis on small ruminants. Biotechnol Adv 31(8):1135–1152. doi:10.1016/j.biotechadv.2013.01.008, pii: S0734-9750(13)00010-4
11. Wolstenholme AJ, Fairweather I, Prichard R et al (2004) Drug resistance in veterinary helminths. Trends Parasitol 20:469–476
12. Gilleard JS (2006) Understanding anthelmintic resistance: the need for genomics and genetics. Int J Parasitol 36:1227–1239
13. Wolstenholme AJ, Kaplan RM (2012) Resistance to macrocyclic lactones. Curr Pharm Biotechnol 13:873–887
14. Anderson RC (2000) Nematode parasites of vertebrate. Their development and transmission, 2nd edn. CABI Publishing, Wallingford
15. Kennedy MW, Harnett W (2001) Parasitic nematodes: molecular biology, biochemistry and immunology. CABI Publishing, New York
16. Nagaraj SH, Gasser RB, Ranganathan S (2007) A hitchhiker's guide to expressed sequence tag (EST) analysis. Brief Bioinform 8:6–21
17. Parkinson J, Blaxter M (2009) Expressed sequence tags: an overview. Methods Mol Biol 533:1–12
18. Ranganathan S, Menon R, Gasser RB (2009) Advanced *in silico* analysis of expressed sequence tag (EST) data for parasitic nematodes of major socio-economic importance-fundamental insights toward biotechnological outcomes. Biotechnol Adv 27:439–448
19. Cantacessi C, Campbell BE, Gasser RB (2012) Key strongylid nematodes of animals – Impact of next-generation transcriptomics on systems biology and biotechnology. Biotechnol Adv 30:469–488
20. Hugot JP, Baujard P, Morand S (2001) Biodiversity in helminths and nematodes as a field of study: an overview. Nematology 3:199–208
21. Chitwood BG (1950) An outline classification of the Nematoda. In: Chitwood BG, Chitwood MB (eds) Introduction to nematology. University Park Press, Baltimore, MD, pp 12–25
22. Lichtenfels JR (1980) Keys to the genera of the Superfamily Strongyloidea. In: Anderson RC, Chabaud AG, Willmott S (eds) CIH Keys to the nematode parasites of vertebrate. CAB International, Wallingford, pp 1–41
23. Durette-Desset MC, Chabaud AG (1977) Essai de classification des nématodes Trichostrongyloidea. Ann Parasitol Hum Comp 52:539–558
24. Durette-Desset MC, Chabaud AG (1981) Nouvel essai de classification de nematode Trichostrongyloidea. Ann Parasitol Hum Comp 56:297–312
25. Durette-Desset MC (1983) Keys to the genera of the superfamily Trichostrongyloidea. In: Anderson RC, Chabaud AG, Willmott S (eds) CIH Keys to the nematode parasites of vertebrate. CAB International, Wallingford, pp 1–68
26. Skrjabin KI, Sobolev AA, Ivashkin VM (1967) Principles of Nematology. Izdatel'sto Akademii Nauk SSSR. Israel Program for Scientific Translations, Washington
27. Blaxter ML, De Ley P, Garey JR et al (1998) A molecular evolutionary framework for the phylum Nematoda. Nature 392:71–75

28. O'Connor LJ, Walkden-Brown SW, Kahn LP (2006) Ecology of the free-living stages of major trichostrongylid parasites of sheep. Vet Parasitol 142:1–15
29. Anderson N, Dash KM, Donald AD et al (1978) Epidemiology and control of nematode infections. In: Donald AD, Southcott WH, Dineen JK (eds) The epidemiology and control of gastrointestinal parasites of sheep in Australia. CSIRO, Australia, pp 23–51
30. Veglia F (1915) The anatomy and life-history of the *Haemonchus contortus* (Rud.). Rep Dir Vet Res 3–4:347–500
31. Monnig HO (1926) The life histories of *Trichostrongylus instabilis* and *T. rugatus* of sheep in South Africa. 11-12th Annual Report of the Director of Veterinary Education and Research, Union of South Africa, pp. 231–251
32. Olsen OW (1986) Animal parasites. Their life cycles and ecology. The quarterly review of biology. University of Chicago Press, Chicago, IL
33. Sommerville RI (1957) The exsheathing mechanism of nematode infective larva. Exp Parasitol 6:18–30
34. Rogers WP, Sommerville RI (1963) The infective stage of nematode parasites and its significance in parasitism. Adv Parasitol 1:109–177
35. Rogers WP, Sommerville RI (1968) The infectious process, and its relation to the development of early parasitic stages of nematodes. Adv Parasitol 6:327–348
36. Noble ER, Noble GA (1982) Parasitology: the biology of animal parasites, 5th edn. Lea & Febiger, Philadelphia, PA
37. Waller PJ (1997) Anthelmintic resistance. Vet Parasitol 72:391–412
38. Holmes PH (1985) Pathogenesis of trichostrongylosis. Vet Parasitol 18:89–101
39. Barker IK (1973) Scanning electron microscopy of duodenal mucosa of lambs infected with *Trichostrongylus colubriformis*. Parasitology 67:307–314
40. Barker IK (1975) Intestinal pathology associated with *Trichostrongylus colubriformis* infection in sheep – histology. Parasitology 70:165–171
41. Beveridge I, Pullman AL, Phillips PH et al (1989) Comparison on the effects of infection with *Trichostrongylus colubriformis*, *Trichostrongylus vitrinus* and *Trichostrongylus rugatus* in Merino lambs. Vet Parasitol 32:229–245
42. Garside P, Kennedy MW, Wakelin D et al (2000) Immunopathology of intestinal helminth infection. Parasite Immunol 22:605–612
43. Xu LQ, Yu SH, Jiang ZX et al (1995) Soil-transmitted helminthiases: nationwide survey in China. Bull World Health Organ 73:507–513
44. Schneider B, Jariwala AR, Periago MV et al (2011) A history of hookworm vaccine development. Hum Vaccin 7:1234–1244
45. Hotez PJ, Bethony J, Bottazzi ME et al (2006) New technologies for the control of human hookworm infection. Trends Parasitol 22:327–331
46. Schad GA, Warren KS (eds) (1990) Hookworm disease: current status and new directions. Taylor & Francis, London
47. Looss A (1898) Zur Lebensgeschichte des *Ancylostoma duodenale*. Eine Erwiederung an Herrn Prof Dr Leichtenstern. Zentralblatt fur Bakteriologie 24:442–449
48. Bruni A, Passalaqua A (1954) Sulla presenza di una mesomucinasi (jaluronidasi) in *Ancylostoma duodenale*. Boll Soc Ital Biol Sper 30:789–791
49. Lewert RM, Lee CL (1954) Studies on the passage of helminth larvae through host tissues. I Histochemical studies on extracellular changes caused by penetrating larvae II Enzymatic activity of larvae in vitro and in vivo. J Infect Dis 95:13–51
50. Gilman RH (1982) Hookworm disease: host-pathogen biology. Rev Infect Dis 4:824–829
51. Gasser RB, Cantacessi C, Loukas A (2008) DNA technological progress toward advanced diagnostic tools to support human hookworm control. Biotechnol Adv 26:35–45
52. Foster AO, Cross SX (1934) The direct development of hookworms after oral infection. Am J Trop Med 14:565–573
53. Schad GA, Chowdhury AB, Dean CG et al (1973) Arrested development in human hookworm infections: an adaptation to a seasonally unfavourable external environment. Science 180:500–501
54. Gibbs HC (1986) Hypobiosis in parasitic nematodes – an update. Adv Parasitol 25:129–174
55. Arasu P, Kwak D (1999) Developmental arrest and pregnancy-induced transmammary transmission of *Ancylostoma caninum* larvae in the murine model. J Parasitol 85:779–784
56. Hotez PJ, Brooker S, Bethony J et al (2004) Hookworm infection. N Engl J Med 351:799–807
57. Loukas A, Bethony J, Brooker S et al (2006) Hookworm vaccines: past, present, and future. Lancet Infect Dis 6:733–741
58. Gasbarre LC, Nansen P, Monrad J et al (1993) Serum anti-trichostrongyle antibody

responses to first and second season grazing calves. Res Vet Sci 54:340–344
59. Klei TR (1997) Immunological control of gastrointestinal nematode infections. Vet Parasitol 72:507–523
60. Balic A, Bowles VM, Meeusen ELT (2000) The immunobiology of gastrointestinal nematode infections in ruminants. Adv Parasitol 45:181–241
61. Loukas A, Prociv P (2001) Immune responses in hookworm infection. Clin Microbiol Rev 14:689–703
62. Loukas A, Constant SL, Bethony JM (2005) Immunobiology of hookworm infection. FEMS Immunol Med Microbiol 43:115–124
63. Gause WC, Urban JF Jr, Stadecker MJ (2003) The immune response to parasitic helminths: insights from murine models. Trends Immunol 24:269–277
64. Liu Z, Liu Q, Pesce J et al (2004) Requirements for the development of IL-4-producing T cells during intestinal nematode infections: what it takes to make a Th2 cell in vivo. Immunol Rev 201:57–74
65. Maizels RM, Yazdanbakhsh M (2003) Immune regulation by helminth parasites: cellular and molecular mechanisms. Nat Rev Immunol 3:733–744
66. Maizels RM, Balic A, Gomez-Escobar N et al (2004) Helminth parasites—masters of regulation. Immunol Rev 201:89–116
67. Anthony RM, Rutitzky LI, Urban JF Jr et al (2007) Protective immune mechanisms in helminth infection. Nat Rev Immunol 7:975–987
68. Patel N, Kreider T, Urban JF Jr et al (2009) Characterization of effector mechanisms at the host: parasite interface during the immune response to tissue-dwelling intestinal nematode parasites. Int J Parasitol 39:13–21
69. Liu Q, Kreider T, Bowdridge S et al (2010) B cells have distinct roles in host protection against different nematode parasites. J Immunol 184:5213–5223
70. Allen JE, Maizels RM (2011) Diversity and dialogue in immunity to helminths. Nat Rev Immunol 11:375–388
71. White CJ, Maxwell CJ, Gallin JI (1986) Changes in the structural and functional properties of human eosinophils during experimental hookworm infection. J Infect Dis 154:778–783
72. Maxwell C, Hussain R, Nutman TB et al (1987) The clinical and immunological responses of normal human volunteers to low dose hookworm (*Necator americanus*) infection. Am J Trop Med Hyg 37:126–134
73. Miller JE, Horohov DW (2006) Immunological aspects of nematode parasite control in sheep. J Anim Sci 84:E124–E132
74. Larsen RH, Christensen CM, Lind P (1997) Serological assays for the identification of *Oesophagostomum dentatum* infections in pigs. Res Vet Sci 63:5–10
75. Joachim A, Ruttkowski B, Daugschies A (1998) Changes in antigen and glycoprotein patterns during the development of *Oesophagostomum dentatum*. Int J Parasitol 28:1853–1860
76. Joachim A, Ruttkowski B, Christensen CM et al (1999) Identification, isolation and characterisation of a species-specific 30 kDa-antigen of *Oesophagostomum dentatum*. Parasitol Res 85:307–311
77. Stockdale PH (1970) Necrotic enteritis of pigs caused by infection with *Oesophagostomum* spp. Br Vet J 126:526–530
78. Haussler M (1996) Immunhistologische Untersuchungen an der Dickdarmschleimhaut bei der *Oesophagostomum dentatum*-infektion des Schweines zu unterschiedlichen Zeitpunkten nach experimenteller infection. Dr Med. Vet. Thesis, Tierartzliche Hochschule, Hannover, Germany
79. McSorley HJ, Loukas A (2010) The immunology of human hookworm infections. Parasite Immunol 32:549–559
80. Pearson MS, Tribolet L, Cantacessi C et al (2012) Molecular mechanisms of hookworm disease – stealth, virulence, and vaccines. J Allergy Clin Immunol 130:13–21
81. Holden-Dye L, Walker RJ (2007) Anthelmintic drugs. WormBook, ed. The *C. elegans* Research Community, doi:/10.1895/wormbook.1.143.1, http://www.wormbook.org
82. Robertson AP, Clark CL, Martin RJ (2010) Levamisole and ryanodine receptors. I: A contraction study in *Ascaris suum*. Mol Biochem Parasitol 171:1–7
83. Keiser J, Utzinger J (2008) Efficacy of current drugs against soil-transmitted helminth infections: systematic review and meta-analysis. JAMA 299:1937–1948
84. Stepek G, Buttle DJ, Duce IR et al (2006) Human gastrointestinal nematode infections: are new control methods required? Int J Exp Pathol 87:325–341
85. Epe C, Kaminsky R (2013) New advancement in anthelmintic drugs in veterinary medicine. Trends Parasitol 29:129–134
86. Gilleard JS, Beech RN (2007) Population genetics of anthelmintic resistance in parasitic nematodes. Parasitology 134:1133–1147

87. Kwa MS, Veenstra JG, Roos MH (1993) Molecular characterisation of beta-tubulin genes present in benzimidazole-resistant populations of *Haemonchus contortus*. Mol Biochem Parasitol 60:133–143
88. Geerts S, Coles GC, Gryssels B (1997) Anthelmintic resistance in human helminths: learning from problems with worm control in livestock. Parasitol Today 13:149–151
89. Roos MH (1997) The role of drugs in the control of parasitic nematode infections: must we do without? Parasitology 114:S137–S144
90. Geerts S, Gryssels B (2001) Anthelmintic resistance in human helminths: a review. Trop Med Int Health 6:915–921
91. Horton J (2003) Human gastrointestinal helminth infections: are they now neglected diseases? Trends Parasitol 19:527–531
92. Albonico M, Smith PG, Hall A et al (1994) A randomized controlled trial comparing mebendazole and albendazole against *Ascaris*, *Trichuris* and hookworm infections. Trans R Soc Trop Med Hyg 88:585–589
93. Albonico M, Bickle Q, Ramsan M et al (2003) Efficacy of mebendazole and levamisole alone or in combination against intestinal nematode infections after repeated targeted mebendazole treatment in Zanzibar. Bull World Health Org 81:343–352
94. de Clercq D, Sacko M, Behnke J et al (1997) Failure of mebendazole in treatment of human hookworm infections in the southern region of Mali. Am J Trop Med Hyg 57:25–30
95. Reynoldson JA, Behnke JM, Gracey M et al (1997) Failure of pyrantel in treatment of human hookworm infections (*Ancylostoma duodenale*) in the Kimberley region of North West Australia. Acta Trop 68:301–312
96. Sacko M, de Clercq D, Behnke JM et al (1999) Comparison of the efficacy of mebendazole, albendazole and pyrantel in treatment of human hookworm infections in the southern region of Mali, West Africa. Trans R Soc Trop Med Hyg 93:195–203
97. Kotze AC, Kopp SR (2008) The potential impact of density dependent fecundity on the use of the faecal egg count reduction test for detecting drug resistance in human hookworms. PLoS Negl Trop Dis 2:e297
98. Besier B (2007) New anthelmintics for livestock: the time is right. Trends Parasitol 23:21–24
99. Campbell BE, Hofmann A, McCluskey A et al (2010) Serine/threonine phosphatases in socioeconomically important parasitic nematodes—prospects as novel drug targets? Biotechnol Adv 29:28–39
100. Albonico M (2003) Methods to sustain drug efficacy in helminth control programmes. Acta Trop 86:233–242
101. Smits HL (2009) Prospects for the control of neglected tropical diseases by mass drug administration. Expert Rev Anti Infect Ther 7:37–56
102. Morgan ER, Coles GC (2010) Nematode control practices on sheep farms following an information campaign aiming to delay anthelmintic resistance. Vet Rec 166:301–303
103. Knox DP (2000) Development of vaccines against gastrointestinal nematodes. Parasitology 120:S43–S61
104. Dalton JP, Mulcahy G (2001) Parasite-vaccines—a reality? Vet Parasitol 98:149–167
105. Claerebout E, Knox DP, Vercruysse J (2003) Current research and future prospects in the development of vaccines against gastrointestinal nematodes in cattle. Expert Rev Vaccines 2:147–157
106. Bethony JM, Loukas A, Hotez PJ et al (2006) Vaccines against blood-feeding nematodes of humans and livestock. Parasitology 133:S63–S79
107. Diemert DJ, Bethony JM, Hotez PJ (2008) Hookworm vaccines. Clin Infect Dis 46:282–288
108. Hotez PJ, Bethony JM, Oliveira SC et al (2008) Multivalent anthelmintic vaccine to prevent hookworm and schistosomiasis. Expert Rev Vaccines 7:745–752
109. Jarrett WFH, Jennings FW, McIntyre WIM et al (1959) Studies on immunity to *Haemonchus contortus* infection—vaccination of sheep using a single dose of X-irradiated larvae. Am J Vet Res 20:527–531
110. Jarrett WFH, Jennings FW, McIntyre WIM et al (1961) Studies on immunity to *Haemonchus contortus* infection—double vaccination of sheep with irradiated larvae. Am J Vet Res 22:186–188
111. Miller TA (1971) Vaccination against the canine hookworm disease. Adv Parasitol 9:153–183
112. Smith WD, Angus KW (1980) *Haemonchus contortus*: attempts to immunize lambs with irradiated larvae. Res Vet Sci 29:45–50
113. Hotez PJ, Zhan B, Bethony JM et al (2003) Progress in the development of a recombinant vaccine for human hookworm disease: the Human Hookworm Vaccine Initiative. Int J Parasitol 33:1245–1258
114. Munn EA, Smith TS, Graham M et al (1993) Vaccination of merino lambs against haemon-

chosis with membrane-associated proteins from the adult parasite. Parasitology 106:63–66

115. Newton SE (1995) Progress on vaccination against *Haemonchus contortus*. Int J Parasitol 25:1281–1289
116. Newton SE, Morrish LE, Martin PJ et al (1995) Protection against multiply drug-resistant and geographically distant strains of *Haemonchus contortus* by vaccination with H11, a gut membrane-derived protective antigen. Int J Parasitol 25:511–521
117. Smith WD, van Wyk JA, van Strijp MF (2001) Preliminary observations on the potential of gut membrane proteins of *Haemonchus contortus* as candidate vaccine antigens in sheep on naturally infected pasture. Vet Parasitol 98:285–297
118. Knox DP, Smith WD (2001) Vaccination against gastrointestinal nematode parasites of ruminants using gut-expressed antigens. Vet Parasitol 100:21–32
119. Smith TS, Munn EA, Graham M et al (1993) Purification and evaluation of the integral membrane protein H11 as a protective antigen against *Haemonchus contortus*. Int J Parasitol 23:271–277
120. Smith WD, Smith SK, Murray JM (1994) Protection studies with integral membrane fractions of *Haemonchus contortus*. Parasitol Immunol 16:231–241
121. Cachat E, Newlands GF, Ekoja SE et al (2010) Attempts to immunize sheep against *Haemonchus contortus* using a cocktail of recombinant proteases derived from the protective antigen, H-gal-GP. Parasite Immunol 32:414–419
122. Pearson MS, Ranjit N, Loukas A (2010) Blunting the knife: development of vaccines targeting digestive proteases of blood-feeding helminth parasites. Biol Chem 391:901–911
123. Skuce PJ, Redmond DL, Liddell S et al (1999) Molecular cloning and characterization of gut-derived cysteine proteinases associated with a host protective extract from *Haemonchus contortus*. Parasitology 119:405–412
124. Williamson AL, Brindley PJ, Abbenante G et al (2003) Hookworm aspartic protease, *Na*-APR-2, cleaves human hemoglobin and serum proteins in a host-specific fashion. J Infect Dis 187:484–494
125. Smith WD, Newlands GF, Smith SK et al (2003) Metalloendopeptidases from the intestinal brush border of *Haemonchus contortus* as protective antigens for sheep. Parasite Immunol 25:313–323
126. Loukas A, Bethony JM, Williamson AL et al (2004) Vaccination of dogs with a recombinant cysteine protease from the intestine of canine hookworms diminishes the fecundity and growth of worms. J Infect Dis 189:1952–1961
127. Redmond DL, Knox DP (2004) Protection studies in sheep using affinity-purified and recombinant cysteine proteinases of adult *Haemonchus contortus*. Vaccine 22:4252–4261
128. Pearson MS, Bethony JM, Pickering DA et al (2009) An enzymatically inactivated hemoglobinase from *Necator americanus* induces neutralizing antibodies against multiple hookworm species and protects dogs against heterologous hookworm infection. FASEB J 23:3007–3019
129. Knox DP, Smith SK, Redmond DL et al (2005) Protection induced by vaccinating sheep with a thiol-binding extract of *Haemonchus contortus* membranes is associated with its protease components. Parasite Immunol 27:121–126
130. Knox DP, Smith SK, Smith WD (1999) Immunization with an affinity purified protein extract from the adult parasite protects lambs against infection with *Haemonchus contortus*. Parasite Immunol 21:201–210
131. Loukas A, Bethony JM, Mendez S et al (2005) Vaccination with recombinant aspartic hemoglobinase reduced parasite load and blood loss after hookworm infection. PLoS Med 2:e295
132. Xiao S, Zhan B, Xue J et al (2008) The evaluation of recombinant hookworm antigens as vaccine in hamsters (*Mesocricetus auratus*) challenged with human hookworm, *Necator americanus*. Exp Parasitol 118:32–40
133. Pearson MS, Pickering DA, Tribolet L et al (2010) Neutralizing antibodies to the hookworm hemoglobinase *Na*-APR-1: implications for a multivalent vaccine against hookworm infection and schistosomiasis. J Infect Dis 201:1561–1569
134. Hotez P, Haggerty J, Hawdon J et al (1990) Metalloproteases of infective *Ancylostoma* hookworm larvae and their possible functions in tissue invasion and ecdysis. Infect Immun 58:3883–3892
135. Williamson AL, Lustigman S, Oksov Y et al (2006) *Ancylostoma caninum* MTP-1, an astacin-like metalloprotease secreted by infective hookworm larvae, is involved in tissue migration. Infect Immun 74:961–967
136. Hawdon JM, Hotez PJ (1996) Hookworm: developmental biology of the infection process. Curr Opin Genet Dev 6:618–623

137. Hawdon JM, Jones BF, Hoffman DR et al (1996) Cloning and characterization of *Ancylostoma*-secreted protein. A novel protein associated with the transition to parasitism by infective hookworm larvae. J Biol Chem 22:6672–6678
138. Hawdon JM, Narasmihan S, Hotez PJ (1999) *Ancylostoma* secreted protein 2: cloning and characterization of a second member of a family of nematode secreted proteins from *Ancylostoma caninum*. Mol Biochem Parasitol 30:149–165
139. Cantacessi C, Campbell BE, Visser A et al (2009) A portrait of the "SCP/TAPS" proteins of eukaryotes – developing a framework for fundamental research and biotechnological outcomes. Biotechnol Adv 27:376–388
140. Brooker S, Bethony J, Hotez PJ (2004) Human hookworm infection in the 21st century. Adv Parasitol 58:197–288
141. Diemert DJ, Pinto AG, Freire J et al (2012) Generalized urticaria induced by the Na-ASP-2 hookworm vaccine: implications for the development of vaccines against helminths. J Allergy Clin Immunol 130:169–176
142. Zhan B, Santiago H, Keegan B et al (2012) Fusion of Na-ASP-2 with human immunoglobulin Fcγ abrogates histamine release from basophils sensitized with anti-Na-ASP-2 IgE. Parasite Immunol 34:404–411
143. Alwine JC, Kemp DJ, Stark GR (1977) Method for detection of specific RNAs in agarose gels by transfer to diazobenzyloxymethyl-paper and hybridization with DNA probes. Proc Natl Acad Sci U S A 74:5350–5354
144. Higuchi R, Fockler C, Dollinger G et al (1993) Kinetic PCR analysis: real-time monitoring of DNA amplification reactions. Biotechnology 11:1026–1030
145. Liang P, Pardee AB (1992) Differential display of eukaryotic messenger RNA by means of the polymerase chain reaction. Science 257:967–971
146. Pratt D, Cox GN, Milhausen MJ et al (1990) A developmentally regulated cysteine protease gene family in *Haemonchus contortus*. Mol Biochem Parasitol 43:181–191
147. Savin KW, Dopheide TA, Frenkel MJ et al (1990) Characterization, cloning and host-protective activity of a 30-kilodalton glycoprotein secreted by the parasitic stages of *Trichostrongylus colubriformis*. Mol Biochem Parasitol 41:167–176
148. Sangster NC, Bannan SC, Weiss AS et al (1999) *Haemonchus contortus*: sequence heterogeneity of internucleotide binding domains from P-glycoproteins. Exp Parasitol 91:250–257
149. Boag PR, Newton SE, Hansen NP et al (2000) Isolation and characterization of sex-specific transcripts from *Oesophagostomum dentatum* by RNA arbitrarily-primed PCR. Mol Biochem Parasitol 108:217–224
150. Moore J, Tetley L, Devaney E (2000) Identification of abundant mRNAs from the third stage larvae of the parasitic nematode, *Ostertagia ostertagi*. Biochem J 347:763–770
151. Nikolaou S, Hartman D, Presidente PJ et al (2002) HcSTK, a *Caenorhabditis elegans* PAR-1 homologue from the parasitic nematode, *Haemonchus contortus*. Int J Parasitol 32:749–758
152. Hartman D, Cottee PA, Savin KW et al (2003) *Haemonchus contortus*: molecular characterisation of a small heat shock protein. Exp Parasitol 104:96–103
153. Cottee PA, Nisbet AJ, Abs El-Osta YG (2006) Construction of gender-enriched cDNA archives for adult *Oesophagostomum dentatum* by suppressive subtractive hybridization and a microarray analysis of expressed sequence tags. Parasitology 132:691–708
154. Velculescu VE, Zhang L, Vogelstein B et al (1995) Serial analysis of gene expression. Science 270:484–487
155. Velculescu VE, Zhang L, Zhou W et al (1997) Characterization of the yeast transcriptome. Cell 88:243–251
156. Boon K, Osorio EC, Greenhut SF et al (2002) An anatomy of normal and malignant gene expression. Proc Natl Acad Sci U S A 99:11287–11292
157. Liang P (2002) SAGE Genie: a suite with panoramic view of gene expression. Proc Natl Acad Sci U S A 99:11547–11548
158. Datson NA, van der Perk-de Jong J, van der Perk-de Jong MP et al (1999) MicroSAGE: a modified procedure for serial analysis of gene expression in limited amounts of tissue. Nucleic Acids Res 27:1300–1307
159. Skuce PJ, Yaga R, Lainson FA et al (2005) An evaluation of serial analysis of gene expression (SAGE) in the parasitic nematode, *Haemonchus contortus*. Parasitology 130:553–559
160. Adams MD, Kelley JM, Gocayne JD et al (1991) Complementary DNA sequencing: expressed sequence tags and human genome project. Science 252:1651–1656
161. McCombie WR, Adams MD, Kelley JM et al (1992) *Caenorhabditis elegans* expressed sequence tags identify gene families and potential gene homologues. Nat Genet 1:124–131

162. Sanger F, Nicklen S, Coulson AR (1977) DNA sequencing with chain-terminating inhibitors. Proc Natl Acad Sci U S A 74:5463–5467
163. Sanger F, Air GM, Barrell BG et al (1977) Nucleotide sequence of bacteriophage phi X174 DNA. Nature 265:687–695
164. Clifton SW, Mitreva M (2009) Strategies for undertaking expressed sequence tag (EST) projects. Methods Mol Biol 533:13–32
165. Blaxter ML, Raghavan N, Ghosh I et al (1996) Genes expressed in *Brugia malayi* infective third stage larvae. Mol Biochem Parasitol 77:77–96
166. Daub J, Loukas A, Pritchard DI et al (2000) A survey of genes expressed in adults of the human hookworm, *Necator americanus*. Parasitology 120:171–184
167. Hoekstra R, Visser A, Otsen M et al (2000) EST sequencing of the parasitic nematodes *Haemonchus contortus* suggests a shift in gene expression during transition to the parasitic stages. Mol Biochem Parasitol 110:53–68
168. McCarter JP, Abad J, Jones JT et al (2000) Rapid gene discovery in plant parasitic nematodes via gene discovery. Nematology 2:719–731
169. Williams SA, Lizotte-Waniewski MR, Foster J et al (2000) The filarial genome project: analysis of the nuclear, mitochondrial and endosymbiont genomes of *Brugia malayi*. Int J Parasitol 30:411–419
170. Parkinson J, Whitton C, Guiliano D et al (2001) 200,000 nematode ESTs on the net. Trends Parasitol 17:394–396
171. Parkinson J, Mitreva M, Whitton C et al (2004) A transcriptomic analysis of the phylum Nematoda. Nat Genet 36:1259–1267
172. Doyle MA, Gasser RB, Woodcroft BJ et al (2010) Drug target prediction and prioritization: using orthology to predict essentiality in parasite genomes. BMC Genomics 11:222
173. Hartman D, Donald DR, Nikolaou S et al (2001) Analysis of developmentally regulated genes of the parasite *Haemonchus contortus*. Int J Parasitol 31:1236–1245
174. Campbell BE, Nagaraj SH, Hu M et al (2008) Gender-enriched transcripts in *Haemonchus contortus*—predicted functions and genetic interactions based on comparative analyses with *Caenorhabditis elegans*. Int J Parasitol 38:65–83
175. Ranjit N, Jones MK, Stenzel DJ et al (2006) A survey of the intestinal transcriptomes of the hookworms, *Necator americanus* and *Ancylostoma caninum*, using tissues isolated by laser-dissection microscopy. Int J Parasitol 36:701–710
176. Yin Y, Martin J, Abubucker S et al (2008) Intestinal transcriptomes of nematodes: comparison of the parasites *Ascaris suum* and *Haemonchus contortus* with the free-living *Caenorhabditis elegans*. PLoS Negl Trop Dis 2:e269
177. Rabelo EM, Hall RS, Loukas A et al (2009) Improved insights into the transcriptome of the human hookworm *Necator americanus*-fundamental and biotechnological implications. Biotechnol Adv 27:122–132
178. DeRisi J, Penland L, Brown PO et al (1996) Use of a cDNA microarray to analyse gene expression patterns in human cancer. Nat Genet 14:457–460
179. Grant WN, Viney ME (2001) Post-genomic nematode parasitology. Int J Parasitol 31:879–888
180. Gasser RB, Cottee P, Nisbet AJ et al (2007) *Oesophagostomum dentatum*: potential as a model for genomic studies of strongylid nematodes, with biotechnological prospects. Biotechnol Adv 25:281–293
181. Nisbet AJ, Gasser RB (2004) Profiling of gender-specific gene expression for *Trichostrongylus vitrinus* (Nematoda: Strongylida) by microarray analysis of expressed sequence tag libraries constructed by suppressive-subtractive hybridization. Int J Parasitol 34:633–643
182. Moser JM, Freitas T, Arasu P et al (2005) Gene expression profiles associated with the transition to parasitism in *Ancylostoma caninum* larvae. Mol Biochem Parasitol 143:39–48
183. Datu BJ, Gasser RB, Nagaraj SH et al (2008) Transcriptional changes in the hookworm, *Ancylostoma caninum*, during the transition from a free-living to a parasitic larva. PLoS Negl Trop Dis 2:e130
184. Nisbet AJ, Redmond DL, Matthews JB et al (2008) Stage-specific gene expression in *Teladorsagia circumcincta* (Nematoda: Strongylida) infective larvae and early parasitic stages. Int J Parasitol 38:829–838
185. Cantacessi C, Loukas A, Campbell BE et al (2009) Exploring transcriptional conservation between *Ancylostoma caninum* and *Haemonchus contortus* by oligonucleotide microarray and bioinformatic analyses. Mol Cell Probes 23:1–9
186. Yang GP, Kuang WW, Weigel RJ (1999) Combining SSH and cDNA microarrays for rapid identification of differentially expressed genes. Nucleic Acids Res 27:1517–1523

187. Liu MY, Wang XL, Fu BQ et al (2007) Identification of stage-specifically expressed genes of *Trichinella spiralis* by suppression subtractive hybridization. Parasitology 134:1443–1455
188. Huang CQ, Gasser RB, Cantacessi C et al (2008) Genomic-bioinformatic analysis of transcripts enriched in the third-stage larva of the parasitic nematode *Ascaris suum*. PLoS Negl Trop Dis 2:e246
189. Geldhof P, Whitton C, Gregory WF et al (2005) Characterisation of the two most abundant genes in the *Haemonchus contortus* expressed sequence tag dataset. Int J Parasitol 35:513–522
190. Mitreva M, McCarter JP, Arasu P et al (2005) Investigating hookworm genomes by comparative analysis of two *Ancylostoma* species. BMC Genomics 26:58
191. Abubucker S, Martin J, Yin Y et al (2008) The canine hookworm genome: analysis and classification of *Ancylostoma caninum* survey sequences. Mol Biochem Parasitol 157:187–192
192. Wang Z, Abubucker S, Martin J et al (2010) Characterizing *Ancylostoma caninum* transcriptome and exploring nematode parasitic adaptation. BMC Genomics 11:307
193. Margulies M, Egholm M, Altman WE et al (2005) Genome sequencing in microfabricated high-density picolitre reactors. Nature 437:376–380
194. Bentley DR, Balasubramanian S, Swerdlow HP et al (2008) Accurate whole human genome sequencing using reversible terminator chemistry. Nature 456:53–59
195. Harris TD, Buzby PR, Babcock H et al (2008) Single-molecule DNA sequencing of a viral genome. Science 320:106–109
196. Pandey V, Nutter RC, Prediger E (2008) Applied Biosystems SOLiD™ System: Ligation-Based Sequencing. In: Milton JM (ed) Next generation genome sequencing: towards personalized medicine. Wiley, Australia, pp 29–41
197. Mardis ER (2008) The impact of next-generation sequencing technology on genetics. Trends Genet 24:133–141
198. Wang Z, Gerstein M, Snyder M (2009) RNA-seq: a revolutionary tool for transcriptomics. Nat Rev Genet 10:57–63
199. Marguerat S, Bahler J (2010) RNA-seq: from technology to biology. Cell Mol Life Sci 67:569–579
200. Mardis ER (2008) Next-generation DNA sequencing methods. Ann Rev Genom Human Genet 9:387–402
201. Jex AR, Hu M, Littlewood DT et al (2008) Using 454 technology for long-PCR based sequencing of the complete mitochondrial genome from single *Haemonchus contortus* (Nematoda). BMC Genomics 9:11
202. Jex AR, Li B, Young ND et al (2011) *Ascaris suum* draft genome. Nature 479:529–533
203. Cantacessi C, Mitreva M, Campbell BE et al (2010) First transcriptomic analysis of the economically important parasitic nematode, *Trichostrongylus colubriformis*, using a next-generation sequencing approach. Infect Genet Evol 10:1199–1207
204. Cantacessi C, Campbell BE, Young ND et al (2010) Differences in transcription between free-living and CO_2-activated third-stage larvae of *Haemonchus contortus*. BMC Genomics 11:266
205. Cantacessi C, Mitreva M, Jex AR et al (2010) Massively parallel sequencing and analysis of the *Necator americanus* transcriptome. PLoS Negl Trop Dis 4:e684
206. Cantacessi C, Jex AR, Hall RS et al (2010) A practical, bioinformatic workflow system for large data sets generated by next-generation sequencing. Nucleic Acids Res 38:e171
207. Cantacessi C, Gasser RB, Strube C et al (2011) Deep insights into *Dictyocaulus viviparus* transcriptomes provides unique prospects for new drug targets and disease intervention. Biotechnol Adv 29:261–271
208. Young ND, Campbell BE, Hall RS et al (2010) Unlocking the transcriptomes of two carcinogenic parasites, *Clonorchis sinensis* and *Opisthorchis viverrini*. PLoS Negl Trop Dis 4:e719
209. Young ND, Hall RS, Jex AR et al (2010) Elucidating the transcriptome of *Fasciola hepatica*—a key to fundamental and biotechnological discoveries for a neglected parasite. Biotechnol Adv 28:222–231
210. Young ND, Jex AR, Cantacessi C et al (2011) A portrait of the transcriptome of the neglected trematode, *Fasciola gigantica* – biological and biotechnological implications. PLoS Negl Trop Dis 5:e1004
211. Young ND, Jex AR, Li B et al (2012) Whole-genome sequence of *Schistosoma haematobium*. Nat Genet 44:221–225
212. Huang X, Madan A (1999) CAP3: a DNA sequence assembly program. Genome Res 9:868–877
213. Iseli C, Jongeneel CV, Bucher P (1999) ESTScan: a program for detecting, evaluating, and reconstructing potential coding regions in EST sequences. Proc Int Conf Intell Syst Mol Biol 1:138–148

214. Conesa A, Gotz S, Garcia-Gomez JM et al (2005) Blast2GO: a universal tool for annotation, visualization and analysis in functional genomics research. Bioinformatics 21:3674–3676
215. Nagaraj SH, Deshpande N, Gasser RB et al (2007) ESTExplorer: an expressed sequence tag (EST) assembly and annotation platform. Nucleic Acids Res 35:W135–W147
216. Hunter S, Apweiler R, Attwood TK et al (2009) InterPro: the integrative protein signature database. Nucleic Acids Res 37:D211–D215
217. Soderlund C, Johnson E, Bomhoff M et al (2009) PAVE: program for assembling and viewing ESTs. BMC Genomics 10:400
218. Nagasaki H, Michizuki T, Kodama Y et al (2013) DDJB Read Annotation Pipeline: a cloud computing-based pipeline for high-throughput analysis of next-generation sequencing data. DNA Res 20(4):383–390
219. Falgueras J, Lara AJ, Fernandez-Poso N et al (2010) SeqTrim: a high throughput pipeline for pre-processing any type of sequence read. BMC Bioinformatics 11:38
220. Myers EW (1995) Toward simplifying and accurately formulating fragment assembly. J Comput Biol 2:275–290
221. Idury RM, Waterman MS (1995) A new algorithm for DNA sequence assembly. J Comput Biol 2:291–306
222. Zerbino DR, Birney E (2008) Velvet: algorithms for *de novo* short read assembly using de Bruijn graphs. Genome Res 18:821–829
223. Scheibye-Alsing K, Hoffmann S, Frankel A et al (2009) Sequence assembly. Comput Biol Chem 33:121–136
224. Miller JR, Koren S, Sutton G (2010) Assembly algorithms for next-generation sequencing data. Genomics 95:315–327
225. Green P (1996) Documentation for PHRAP. Genome Center, University of Washington, Seattle, http://www.phrap.org/phredphrap/phrap.html, USA
226. Sutton GG, White O, Adams MD et al (1995) TIGR assembler: a new tool for assembling large shotgun sequencing projects. Genome Sci Technol 1:9–19
227. Huang X, Wang J, Aluru S et al (2003) PCAP: a whole genome assembly program. Genome Res 13:2164–2170
228. Chevreux B (2005) MIRA: an automated genome and EST assembler. Ph.D Thesis, German Cancer Research Center Heidelberg, Duisburg, Germany
229. Warren RL, Sutton GC, Jones SJM et al (2007) Assembling millions of short DNA sequences using SSAKE. Bioinformatics 23:500–501
230. Schulz MH, Zerbino DR, Vingron M et al (2012) Oases: robust de novo RNA-seq assembly across the dynamic range of expression levels. Bioinformatics 28:1086–1092
231. Hernandez D, François P, Farinelli L et al (2008) *De novo* bacterial genome sequencing: millions of very short reads assembled on a desktop computer. Genome Res 18:802–809
232. Pevzner PA, Tang H, Waterman MS (2001) An Eulerian path approach to DNA fragment assembly. Proc Natl Acad Sci U S A 98:9748–9753
233. Simpson JT, Wong K, Jackman SD et al (2009) ABySS: a parallel assembler for short read sequence data. Genome Res 19:1117–1123
234. Li R, Li Y, Kristiansen K et al (2008) SOAP: short oligonucleotide alignment program. Bioinformatics 24:713–714
235. Grabherr MG, Haas BJ, Yassour M et al (2011) Full-length transcriptome assembly from RNA-Seq data without a reference genome. Nat Biotechnol 29:644–652
236. Min XJ, Butler G, Storms R et al (2005) OrfPredictor: predicting protein-coding regions in EST-derived sequences. Nucleic Acids Res 33:W677–W680
237. Fukunishi Y, Hayashizaki Y (2001) Amino acid translation program for full-length cDNA sequences with frameshift errors. Physiol Genomics 5:81–87
238. Klassen JL, Currie CR (2013) ORFcor: identifying and accommodating ORF prediction inconsistencies for phylogenetic analysis. PLoS One 8:e58387
239. Hofmann K, Bucher P, Falquet L et al (1999) The Prosite Database, its status in 1999. Nucleic Acids Res 27:215–219
240. Attwood TK, Croning MD, Flower DR et al (2000) Prints-S: the database formerly known as prints. Nucleic Acids Res 28:225–227
241. Bateman A, Birney E, Durbin R et al (2000) The Pfam protein families database. Nucleic Acids Res 28:263–266
242. Corpet F, Gouzy J, Kahn D (1999) Recent improvements of the ProDom database of protein domain families. Nucleic Acids Res 27:263–267
243. Schultz J, Copley RR, Doerks T et al (2000) Smart: a web-based tool for the study of genetically mobile domains. Nucleic Acids Res 28:231–234
244. Ashburner M, Ball CA, Blake JA et al (2000) Gene ontology: tool for the unification of biology. The gene ontology consortium. Nat Genet 25:25–29
245. Krogh A, Larsson B, von Heijne G et al (2001) Predicting transmembrane protein topology with a hidden Markov model: application to complete genomes. J Mol Biol 305:567–580
246. Nielsen H, Engelbrecht J, Brunak S et al (1997) A neural network method for the

identification of prokaryotic and eukaryotic signal peptides and prediction of their cleavage sites. Int J Neural Syst 8:581–599

247. Altschul SF, Gish W, Miller W et al (1990) Basic local alignment search tool. J Mol Biol 215:403–410
248. Benson DA, Karsch-Mizrachi I, Lipman DJ et al (2002) GenBank. Nucleic Acids Res 30:17–20
249. Stoesser G, Baker W, van den Broek A et al (2002) The EMBL nucleotide sequence database. Nucleic Acids Res 30:21–26
250. Tateno Y, Imanishi S, Miyazaki S et al (2002) DNA Data Bank of Japan (DDBJ) for genome scale research in life sciences. Nucleic Acids Res 30:27–30
251. Wheeler DL, Church DM, Lash AE et al (2001) Database resources of the national center for biotechnology information. Nucleic Acids Res 29:11–16
252. Shumway M, Cochrane G, Sugawara H (2010) Archiving next generation sequencing data. Nucleic Acids Res 38:D870–D871
253. Berman HM, Westbrook J, Feng Z et al (2000) The protein data bank. Nucleic Acids Res 28:235–242
254. Bairoch A, Apweiler R (2000) The SWISS-PROT protein sequence database and its supplement TrEMBL in 2000. Nucleic Acids Res 28:45–48
255. Bairoch A, Apweiler R (1996) The SWISS-PROT protein sequence data bank and its new supplement TREMBL. Nucleic Acids Res 24:21–25
256. Cherry JM, Ball C, Weng S et al (1997) Genetic and physical maps of *Saccharomyces cerevisiae*. Nature 387:67–73
257. Tweedie S, Ashburner M, Falls K et al (2009) FlyBase: enhancing *Drosophila* Gene Ontology annotations. Nucleic Acids Res 37:D555–D559
258. Bult CJ, Epping JT, Kadin JA et al (2008) The Mouse Genome Database (MGD): mouse biology and model systems. Nucleic Acids Res 36:D724–D728
259. Harris TW, Antoshechkin I, Bieri T et al (2010) WormBase: a comprehensive resource for nematode research. Nucleic Acids Res 38:D463–D467
260. Bieri T, Blasiar D, Ozersky P et al (2006) WormBase: new content and better access. Nucleic Acids Res 35:D506–D510
261. Schwarz EM, Antoshechkin I, Bastiani C et al (2006) WormBase: better software, richer content. Nucleic Acids Res 34:D475–D478
262. Yook K, Harris TW, Bieri T et al (2012) WormBase 2012: more genomes, more data, new website. Nucleic Acids Res 40:D735–D741
263. Mangiola S, Young ND, Korhonen P et al (2013) Getting the most out of parasitic helminth transcriptomes using HelmDB: implications for biology and biotechnology. Biotechnol Adv 31(8):1109–1119. doi:10.1016/j.biotechadv.2012.12.004, pii: S0734-9750(12)00197-8
264. Brenner S (1974) The genetics of *Caenorhabditis elegans*. Genetics 77:71–94
265. The C. elegans Sequencing Consortium (1998) Genome sequence of the nematode C. elegans: a platform for investigating biology. Science 282:2012–2018
266. Fire A, Xu S, Montgomery MK et al (1998) Potent and specific genetic interference by double-stranded RNA in *Caenorhabditis elegans*. Nature 391:806–811
267. Barstead R (2001) Genome-wide RNAi. Curr Opin Chem Biol 5:63–66
268. Kamath RS, Ahringer J (2003) Genome-wide RNAi screening in *Caenorhabditis elegans*. Methods 30:313–321
269. Simmer F, Moorman C, van der Linden AM et al (2003) Genome-wide RNAi of *C. elegans* using the hypersensitive *rrf-3* strain reveals novel gene functions. PLoS Biol 1:E12
270. Sugimoto A (2004) High-throughput RNAi in *Caenorhabditis elegans*: genome-wide screens and functional genomics. Differentiation 72:81–91
271. Sonnichsen B, Koski LB, Walsh A et al (2005) Full-genome RNAi profiling of early embryogenesis in *Caenorhabditis elegans*. Nature 434:462–469
272. Tabara H, Grishok A, Mello CC (1998) RNAi in *C. elegans*: soaking in the genome sequence. Science 282:430–431
273. Timmons L, Fire A (1998) Specific interference by ingested dsRNA. Nature 395:854
274. Tabara H, Sarkissian M, Kelly WG et al (1999) The *rde-1* gene, RNA interference, and transposon silencing in *C. elegans*. Cell 99:123–132
275. Tavernarakis N, Wang SL, Dorovkov M et al (2000) Heritable and inducible genetic interference by double-stranded RNA encoded by transgenes. Nat Genet 24:180–183
276. Maeda I, Kohara Y, Yamamoto M et al (2001) Large-scale analysis of gene function in *Caenorhabditis elegans* by high-throughput RNAi. Curr Biol 11:171–176
277. Ashrafi K, Chang FY, Watts JL et al (2003) Genome-wide RNAi analysis of *Caenorhabditis elegans* fat regulatory genes. Nature 421:268–272
278. Britton C, Murray L (2006) Using *Caenorhabditis elegans* for functional analysis of genes of parasitic nematodes. Int J Parasitol 36:651–659
279. Geldhof P, Visser A, Clark D et al (2007) RNA interference in parasitic helminths: current situation, potential pitfalls and future prospects. Parasitology 134:609–619

280. Morris KV (2008) RNA-mediated transcriptional gene silencing in human cells. Curr Top Microbiol Immunol 320:211–224
281. Rosso MN, Jones JT, Abad P (2009) RNAi and functional genomics in plant parasitic nematodes. Annu Rev Phytopathol 47:207–232
282. Serkirk ME, Huang SC, Knox DP et al (2012) The development of RNA interference (RNAi) in gastrointestinal nematodes. Parasitology 139:605–612
283. Stinchcomb DT, Shaw JE, Carr SH et al (1985) Extrachromosomal DNA transformation of *Caenorhabditis elegans.* Mol Cell Biol 5:3484–3496
284. Fire A (1986) Integrative transformation of *Caenorhabditis elegans.* EMBO J 5:2673–2680
285. Chalfie M, Tu Y, Euskirchen G et al (1994) Green fluorescent protein as a marker for gene expression. Science 263:802–805
286. Lok JB, Artis D (2008) Transgenesis and neuronal ablation in parasitic nematodes: revolutionary new tools to dissect host-parasite interactions. Parasite Immunol 30:203–214
287. Hobert O, Loria P (2006) Uses of GFP in *Caenorhabditis elegans.* Methods Biochem Anal 47:203–226
288. Reinke V, Smith HE, Nance J et al (2000) A global profile of germline gene expression in *C. elegans.* Mol Cell 6:605–616
289. Kim SK, Lund J, Kiraly M et al (2001) A gene expression map for *Caenorhabditis elegans.* Science 293:2087–2092
290. Jiang M, Ryu J, Kiraly M et al (2001) Genome-wide analysis of developmental and sex-regulated gene expression profiles in *Caenorhabditis elegans.* Proc Natl Acad Sci U S A 98:218–223
291. Chilton NB (2004) The use of nuclear ribosomal DNA markers for the identification of bursate nematodes (order Strongylida) and for the diagnosis of infections. Anim Health Res Rev 5:173–187
292. Bürglin TR, Lobos E, Blaxter ML (1998) *Caenorhabditis elegans* as a model for parasitic nematodes. Int J Parasitol 28:395–411
293. Mitreva M, Jasmer JP, Zarlenga DS et al (2011) The draft genome of the parasitic nematode *Trichinella spiralis.* Nat Genet 43:228–243
294. Williamson AL, Lecchi P, Turk BE et al (2004) A multi-enzyme cascade of hemoglobin proteolysis in the intestine of blood-feeding hookworms. J Biol Chem 279:35950–35957
295. Ranjit N, Zhan B, Hamilton B et al (2009) Proteolytic degradation of hemoglobin in the intestine of the human hookworm *Necator americanus.* J Infect Dis 199:904–912
296. Furmidge BA, Horn LA, Pritchard DI (1996) The anti-haemostatic strategies of the human hookworm *Necator americanus.* Parasitology 112:81–87
297. Milstone AM, Harrison LM, Bungiro RD et al (2000) A broad spectrum kunitz type serine protease inhibitor secreted by the hookworm *Ancylostoma ceylanicum.* J Biol Chem 275:29391–29399
298. Grad LI, Sayles LC, Lemire BD (2007) Isolation and functional analysis of mitochondria from the nematode *Caenorhabditis elegans.* Methods Mol Biol 372:51–66
299. Fetterer RH (1996) Growth and cuticular synthesis in *Ascaris suum* larvae during development from third to fourth stage in vitro. Vet Parasitol 65:275–282
300. Quinn CC, Pfeil DS, Wadsworth WG (2008) CED-10/Rac1 mediates axon guidance by regulating the asymmetric distribution of MIG-10/lamellipodin. Curr Biol 18:808–813
301. Ranjit N, Zhan B, Stenzel DJ et al (2008) A family of cathepsin B cysteine proteases expressed in the gut of the human hookworm, *Necator americanus.* Mol Biochem Parasitol 160:90–99
302. Robinson BW, Venaille TJ, Mendis AH et al (1990) Allergens as proteases: an Aspergillus fumigatus proteinase directly induces human epithelial cell detachment. J Allergy Clin Immunol 86:726–731
303. Björnberg F, Lantz M, Gullberg U (1995) Metalloproteases and serineproteases are involved in the cleavage of the two tumour necrosis factor (TNF) receptors to soluble forms in the myeloid cell lines U-937 and THP-1. Scand J Immunol 42:418–424
304. Hotez PJ, Prichard DI (1995) Hookworm infection. Sci Am 6:42–48
305. Shaw RJ, McNeill MM, Maass DR et al (2003) Identification and characterisation of an aspartyl protease inhibitor homologue as a major allergen of *Trichostrongylus colubriformis.* Int J Parasitol 33:1233–1243
306. Williamson AL, Brindley PJ, Knox DP et al (2003) Digestive proteases of blood-feeding nematodes. Trends Parasitol 19:417–423
307. Cottee PA, Nisbet AJ, Boag PR et al (2004) Characterization of major sperm protein genes and their expression in *Oesophagostomum dentatum* (Nematoda; Strongylida). Parasitology 129:479–490

308. Miller MA, Nguyen VQ, Lee MH et al (2001) A sperm cytoskeletal protein that signals oocyte meiotic maturation and ovulation. Science 291:2144–2147, Erratum in: *Science* **292**, 639
309. Miller MA, Ruest PJ, Kosinski M et al (2003) An Eph receptor sperm-sensing control mechanism for oocyte meiotic maturation in *Caenorhabditis elegans*. Genes Dev 17:187–200
310. Freigofas R, Leibold W, Daugschies A et al (2001) Products of fourth-stage larvae of *Oesophagostomum dentatum* induce proliferation in naïve porcine mononuclear cells. J Vet Med B Infect Dis Vet Public Health 48:603–611
311. Campbell BE, Tarleton M, Gordon CP et al (2011) Norcantharidin analogues with nematocidal activity in *Haemonchus contortus*. Bioorg Med Chem Lett 21:3277–3281
312. McCluskey A, Keane MA, Walkom CC et al (2002) The first two cantharidin analogues displaying PP1 selectivity. Bioorg Med Chem Lett 12:391–393
313. Hill TA, Stewart SG, Sauer B et al (2007) Heterocyclic substituted cantharidin and norcantharidin analogues—synthesis, protein phosphatase (1 and 2A) inhibition, and anticancer activity. Bioorg Med Chem Lett 17:3392–3397
314. Stewart SG, Hill TA, Gilbert J et al (2007) Synthesis and biological evaluation of norcantharidin analogues: towards PP1 selectivity. Bioorg Med Chem 15:7301–7310
315. Olson SK, Bishop JR, Yates JR et al (2006) Identification of novel chondroitin proteoglycans in *Caenorhabditis elegans*: embryonic cell division depends on CPG-1 and CPG-2. J Cell Biol 173:985–994
316. Zhan B, Liu Y, Badamchian M et al (2003) Molecular characterisation of the *Ancylostoma-secreted* protein family from the adult stage of *Ancylostoma caninum*. Int J Parasitol 33:897–907
317. Mulvenna J, Hamilton B, Nagaraj S et al (2009) Proteomic analysis of the excretory/secretory component of the blood-feeding stage of the hookworm, *Ancylostoma caninum*. Mol Cell Proteomics 8:109–121
318. Bethony J, Loukas A, Smout M et al (2005) Antibodies against a secreted protein from hookworm larvae reduce the intensity of hookworm infection in humans and vaccinated laboratory animals. FASEB J 19:1743–1745
319. Bethony JM, Simon G, Diemert DJ et al (2008) Randomized, placebo-controlled, double-blind trial of the *Na*-ASP-2 hookworm vaccine in unexposed adults. Vaccine 26:2408–2417
320. Mendez S, Samuel A D', Antoine AD et al (2008) Use of the air pouch model to investigate immune responses to a hookworm vaccine containing the *Na*-ASP-2 protein in rats. Parasite Immunol 30:53–56
321. Osman A, Wang CK, Winter A et al (2012) Hookworm SCP/TAPS protein structure - a key to understanding host-parasite interactions and developing new interventions. Biotechnol Adv 30:652–657
322. Hopkins AL, Groom CR (2002) The druggable genome. Nature 1:727–730
323. Chang A, Scheer M, Grote A et al (2009) BRENDA, AMENDA and FRENDA the enzyme information system: new content and tools in 2009. Nucleic Acids Res 37:D588–D592
324. Manning G, Whyte DB, Martinez R et al (2002) The protein kinase complement of the human genome. Science 298:1912–1934
325. Manning G, Reiner DS, Lauwaet T et al (2011) The minimal kinome of *Giardia lamblia* illuminates early kinase evolution and unique parasite biology. Genome Biol 12:R66
326. Lucet IS, Tobin A, Drewry D et al (2012) *Plasmodium* kinases as targets for new-generation antimalarials. Future Med Chem 4:2295–2310
327. Liotta F, Siekierka JJ (2010) Apicomplexa, trypanosoma and parasitic nematode protein kinases as antiparasitic therapeutic targets. Curr Opin Invest Drugs 11:147–156
328. Knobloch J, Kunz W, Grevelding CG (2006) Herbimycin A suppresses mitotic activity and egg production of female *Schistosoma mansoni*. Int J Parasitol 36:1261–1272
329. Campbell BE, Boag PR, Hofmann A et al (2011) Atypical (RIO) protein kinases from *Haemonchus contortus* – Promise as new targets for nematocidal drugs. Biotechnol Adv 29:338–350
330. Hu M, Laronde-Leblanc N, Sternberg PW et al (2008) *Tv*-RIO1 – an atypical protein kinase from the parasitic nematode *Trichostrongylus vitrinus*. Parasit Vectors 1:34
331. Ferreira CV, Gusto GZ, Sousa AC et al (2006) Natural compounds as source of protein phosphatase inhibitors: application to the rational design of small-molecule derivatives. Biochemie 88:1859–1873
332. Cho YY, Yao K, Kim HG et al (2007) Ribosomal S6 kinase 2 is a key regulator in tumor promoter induced cell transformation. Cancer Res 67:8104–8112

333. Nöthlings U, Murphy SP, Wilkens LR et al (2007) Flavonoids and pancreatic cancer risk. Am J Epidemiol 166:924–931
334. Meyer M, Briggs AW, Maricic T et al (2007) From micrograms to picograms: quantitative PCR reduces the material demands in high throughput sequencing. Nucleic Acids Res 1:1–6
335. Jarvie T, Harkins T (2008) Transcriptome sequencing with the Genome Sequencer FLX system. Nat Methods 5:6–8
336. Flicek B, Birney E (2009) Sense from sequence reads, methods for alignment and assembly. Nat Methods 6:S6–S12
337. Pepke S, Wold B, Mortazavi A (2009) Computational approaches to the analysis of ChIP-seq and RNA-seq data. Nat Methods 6:S22–S32
338. Reinhardt JA, Baltrus DA, Nishimura MT et al (2009) De novo assembly using low-coverage short read sequence data from the rice pathogen *Pseudomonas syringae* pv. *oryzae*. Genome Res 19:294–305
339. Nagarajan H, Butler JE, Klimes A et al (2010) *De novo* assembly of the complete genome of an enhanced electricity-producing variant of *Geobacter sulfurreducens* using only short reads. PLoS One 5:e10922
340. Tsai IJ, Otto TD, Berriman M (2010) Improving draft assemblies by iterative mapping and assembly of short reads to eliminate gaps. Genome Biol 11:R41
341. Gregory SG, Barlow KF, McLay KE et al (2006) The DNA sequence and biological annotation of human chromosome 1. Nature 441:315–321
342. Karp PD (1998) What we do not know about sequence analysis and sequence databases. Bioinformatics 14:753–754
343. Benitez-Paez A (2009) Considerations to improve functional annotations in biological databases. OMICS 13:527–535
344. Boag PR, Ren P, Newton SE et al (2003) Molecular characterisation of a male-specific serine/threonine phosphatase from *Oesophagostomum dentatum* (Nematoda: Strongylida), and functional analysis of homologues in *Caenorhabditis elegans*. Int J Parasitol 33:313–325
345. Issa Z, Grant WN, Stasiuk S et al (2005) Development of methods for RNA interference in the sheep gastrointestinal parasite, *Trichostrongylus colubriformis*. Int J Parasitol 35:935–940
346. Geldhof P, Murray L, Couthier A et al (2006) Testing the efficacy of RNA interference in *Haemonchus contortus*. Int J Parasitol 36:801–810
347. Kotze AC, Bagnall NH (2006) RNA interference in *Haemonchus contortus*: suppression of beta-tubulin gene expression in L3, L4 and adult worms in vitro. Mol Biochem Parasitol 145:101–110
348. Visser A, Geldhof P, DeMaere V et al (2006) Efficacy and specificity of RNA interference in larval life-stages of *Ostertagia ostertagi*. Parasitology 133:777–783
349. Zawadzki JL, Presidente PJ, Meeusen EN et al (2006) RNAi in *Haemonchus contortus*: a potential method for target validation. Trends Parasitol 22:495–499
350. Knox DP, Geldhof P, Visser A et al (2007) RNA interference in parasitic nematodes of animals: a reality check? Trends Parasitol 23:107–117
351. Samarasinghe B, Knox DP, Britton C (2011) Factors affecting susceptibility to RNA interference in *Haemonchus contortus* and in vivo silencing of an H11 aminopeptidase gene. Int J Parasitol 41:51–59
352. Viney ME, Thompson FJ (2008) Two hypotheses to explain why RNA interference does not work in animal parasitic nematodes. Int J Parasitol 38:43–47
353. Lok JB (2009) Transgenesis in parasitic nematodes: building a better array. Trends Parasitol 25:345–347
354. Hu M, Lok JB, Ranjit N et al (2010) Structural and functional characterisation of the fork head transcription factor-encoding gene, *Hc-daf-16*, from the parasitic nematode *Haemonchus contortus* (Strongylida). Int J Parasitol 40:405–415
355. Stepek G, McCormack G, Page AP (2010) Collagen processing and cuticle formation is catalysed by the astacin metalloprotease DPY-31 in free-living and parasitic nematodes. Int J Parasitol 40:533–542
356. Grant WN, Skinner SJ, Newton-Howes J et al (2006) Heritable transgenesis of *Parastrongyloides trichosuri*: a nematode parasite of mammals. Int J Parasitol 36:475–483
357. Liu L, Li Y, Li S et al (2012) Comparison of next-generation sequencing systems. J Biomed Biotechnol 2012:251364

Chapter 32

Functional Genomics of Tick Vectors Challenged with the Cattle Parasite *Babesia bigemina*

Ana Domingos, Sandra Antunes, Margarita Villar, and José de la Fuente

Abstract

Ticks are obligate hematophagous ectoparasites considered as vectors of animal diseases, having a huge economic impact in cattle industry. *Babesia* spp. are tick-borne pathogens that cause a disease called babesiosis in a wide range of animals and in humans. Control of tick infestations is mainly based on the use of acaricides, which have limited efficacy reducing tick infestations, mostly due to wrong usage, and is often accompanied by the selection of acaricide-resistant ticks, environmental contamination, and contamination of milk and meat products. Vaccines affecting both vector and pathogens constitute new control strategies for tick and tick-borne diseases and are, therefore, a good alternative to chemical control.

In this chapter we describe the identification of *Rhipicephalus (Boophilus) annulatus* genes differentially expressed in response to infection with *B. bigemina* by using suppression-subtractive hybridization (SSH), which allows the identification of differentially expressed genes. The results of the SSH studies are validated by real-time reverse transcription (RT)-PCR. Functional analyses are conducted by RNAi on selected *R. annulatus* genes to determine their putative role in *B. bigemina*–tick interactions. Gathered data may be useful for the future development of improved vaccines and vaccination strategies to control babesiosis.

Key words Tick, Genomics, *Babesia*, *Rhipicephalus*, *Boophilus*, Subtractive hybridization, RNA interference, Vaccines

1 Introduction

Tick-borne pathogens of the genus *Babesia* are *Apicomplexan* parasites responsible for a disease called babesiosis that affects a wide range of animals and, occasionally, humans. The major economic impact of babesiosis is on cattle industry, caused mainly by *Babesia bovis* and *B. bigemina*. *Rhipicephalus (Boophilus)* spp. ticks are their principal vectors, being considered one of the most important cattle ectoparasites due to the direct impact affecting leather quality, meat and milk production and, most importantly, pathogen transmission capacity [1].

In the last decades, new tools have been developed in the molecular biology field, leading to a better knowledge of genes

Mónica V. Cunha and João Inácio (eds.), *Veterinary Infection Biology: Molecular Diagnostics and High-Throughput Strategies*, Methods in Molecular Biology, vol. 1247, DOI 10.1007/978-1-4939-2004-4_32,

involved in the control of biological functions in numerous organisms, such as vector ticks and pathogens transmitted to man and animals. Genomics continues to contribute greatly to this cause by (a) bringing new information about genomes and development of new technologies, (b) allying these new resources to traditional techniques, and (c) enabling the development of new practical interventions in the triangle vector–host–pathogen. Few complete genomes are known for either vector or pathogen but information regarding partial and complete nucleotide sequences from both organisms is being progressively more available. Moreover, sialomes and transcriptomes of different ticks are now accessible. New findings on the genomic field do not replace older strategies developed to study tick and tick-borne pathogens but rather complement them, improving research outputs. As examples, there are techniques such as artificial feeding or cellular lines that remain extremely useful to determine biological effects in cells and organisms.

Within new control strategies for tick and tick-borne diseases, vaccines arise as important alternatives to chemical control since they may affect both vector and pathogen. Molecular interactions at the tick–pathogen interface ensure survival and development of both the pathogen and tick vector. Recent studies demonstrated that tick vaccines reduce tick–pathogen infection when using antigens found to be related with pathogen infection/multiplication, illustrating the complexity of tick–pathogen coevolution [2]. Other experiments have demonstrated that tick gene expression is modified in response to pathogen infection [3–12], but information on the function of differentially expressed genes is limited [7–11, 13–15] mainly because the identification of potential vaccine candidates is not simple, being a crucial step.

In the present example, it is our aim to demonstrate how gene functional analysis can support the identification of genes that are involved in the vector–pathogen interaction using as model the vector *R. annulatus* and the pathogen *B. bigemina*.

To infer about the pressure of infection in the vector, first, two different tick populations had to be produced: a *B. bigemina*-infected population and an uninfected one. Factors like gender, time point in the life cycle, and similar feeding conditions have to be considered and controlled. The only feature that should be different in these samples is the presence of infection that eventually will induce a differential expression of the genes reflecting the effect of the pathogen in the tick organism. Secondly, the differences between these populations have to be identified and measured. The subtractive suppression hybridization (SSH) method allows the detection of transcripts differently expressed in two related mRNA populations with no prior knowledge of these mRNA. This technique relies on the hybridization of equal mRNA present on two different populations, followed by the enrichment of different mRNA (present in only one of the populations) by traditional PCR. When using SSH, the differentially expressed genes need to be quantitatively validated in order to point which are the most relevant transcripts in the picture. Microarrays can appear as a valid option, but due to the costs linked to this technique, the gain must be well weighted. For example, if the objective of the study is to analyze gene expression profiles in different situations, a microarray chip can be a solution, but if the target is the punctual identification of relevant genes, then the real-time PCR technique is a more suitable and simpler way to quantify mRNA.

Another conceptually similar technique to SSH is the direct sequencing of mRNA also known as RNA-Seq. This high-throughput technique offers a complete image of what is happening in the transcriptome in a determined time point, so when comparing an mRNA population corresponding to infected and healthy populations, the transcriptome differences will arise. An extremely important task in the identification of transcripts is the sequence analysis steps. Various tools are accessible online in which a comparison to available datasets is done. The cDNA Annotation System software (dCAS) [16] is a good option for performing an automated sequence clean-up, assembly, and BLAST analysis against the non-redundant (nr) sequence database. Manual curation is imperative after the automated analysis to complete this step. From this step on, it is possible to identify differentially expressed genes that can be further characterized.

The third, and last step, on finding new antigens involved in infection processes, within the example of *B. bigemina*-infected *R. annulatus* ticks, concerns to the functional analysis. These assays allow demonstrating the active role of antigens in a specific process. RNAi or posttranscriptional gene silencing is a conserved and natural process that cells use to turn down, or silence, specific genes [17, 18]. Small interfering RNAs (siRNAs) are the effector molecules of the RNAi pathway that is initiated by double-stranded RNA (dsRNA) and results in a potent sequence-specific degradation of cytoplasmic mRNAs containing the same sequence as the dsRNA trigger [8, 19]. RNAi revealed to be a valuable tool for studying tick gene function, the characterization of the tick–pathogen interface and the screening and characterization of tick-protective antigens [20]. RNAi process in ticks has not yet been revealed but a model has been proposed based in the information available for *Drosophila melanogaster* and *Anopheles gambiae* [21]. This technique has been used to study the function of tick proteins at the tick–pathogen interface in a number of tick species [12, 22–25]. In ticks, depending on the experimental design and targets, four different techniques of dsRNA delivery are known: (a) injection, the most common method; (b) soaking of isolated tissues; (c) the RNAi-inducing capillary feeding; and (d) virus production of dsRNA. Herein, the selected method was the injection of dsRNA directly in the hemolymph in adult female ticks since it was vital that ticks would feed normally after gene silencing. The evaluation of gene knockdown in biological parameters like weight and reproduction success, or even, as in the present case, the infection level, elucidates on the effect gene disruption.

2 Materials

2.1 Organisms

1. *Rhipicephalus annulatus* ticks.
2. *Babesia bigemina* (Moledet strain, provided by Kimron Veterinary Institute, Israel).
3. Holstein–Friesian calves.

2.2 General Laboratory Consumables, Materials, and Equipment

1. Sterile 1 ml syringes and needles with different gauges.
2. Sterile 1.5 ml and 2 ml microcentrifuge tubes.
3. 96 wells plates for PCR.
4. Micropipettes and filter tips.
5. Agar plates (LB Agar, 20 g/L, with appropriate antibiotics and supplements).
6. 1× TAE (Tris-acetate buffer): 40 mM Tris–HCl, 20 mM acetic acid, and 1 mM EDTA.
7. PBS (phosphate buffered saline): 0.027 M potassium chloride, 0.137 M sodium chloride, and 1.76 mM potassium phosphate.
8. 0.5× TBE (Tris-borate-EDTA buffer): 45 mM Tris, 45 mM boric acid, 1 mM EDTA, pH 8.3.
9. Agarose.
10. Nuclease-free water.
11. Refrigerated centrifuge.
12. Thermocycler (e.g., GeneAmp® PCR System 2700, Applied Biosystems Life Technologies, Foster City, CA, USA).
13. Real-time thermal detection system (e.g., IQ5 thermo-cycler, BioRad, Hercules, CA, USA).
14. NanoDrop ND-1000 (Thermo Fischer Scientific, Waltham, MA, USA).
15. Stereo microscope.
16. Humidity chamber.

2.3 Suppression Subtractive Hybridization (SSH) Library Construction

DNA and RNA Extraction

1. RNA*later*™ solution (Ambion Life Technologies, Carlsbad, CA, USA).
2. TRI Reagent® (Sigma-Aldrich, St. Louis, MO, USA). Additional reagents needed: chloroform, isopropanol, absolute ethanol, 75 % ethanol, 1 mM sodium citrate in 10 % ethanol, and 8 mM NaOH.

Detection of Babesia bigemina Infection in Ticks

1. *R. annulatus* DNA.
2. PCR Master Mix (Promega, Fitchburg, WI, USA).
3. Specific primers for *B. bigemina* (e.g., 5′-AGC TTG CTT TCA CAA CTC GCC-3′ and 5′-TTG GTG CTT TGA CCG ACG ACA T-3).

SSH Library Construction

1. Infected and uninfected tick total RNA.
2. FastTrack® 2.0 mRNA Isolation Kit (Invitrogen Life Technologies, Carlsbad, CA, USA).
3. PCR-Select™ cDNA Subtraction Kit (Clontech Laboratories Inc., Mountain View, CA, USA).
4. Advantage® 2 PCR polymerase mix with TITANIUM *Taq* DNA Polymerase (Clontech-Takara, Mountain View, CA, USA).

cDNA Library Cloning

1. TOPO TA Cloning® Kit for sequencing (Invitrogen Life Technologies, Carlsbad, CA, USA).
2. One Shot® TOP10 competent cells (Invitrogen Life Technologies, Carlsbad, CA, USA).
3. PCR Master Mix (Promega, Fitchburg, WI, USA).
4. Universal T3 and T7 primers.
5. Illustra plasmidPrep Mini Spin Kit (GE Healthcare, Buckinghamshire, UK).

2.4 Sequence Analysis and Database Search

1. Sequences from SSH clones.
2. cDNA Annotation System software (dCAS; Bioinformatics and Scientific IT Program (BSIP), Office of Technology Information Systems (OTIS), National Institute of Allergy and Infectious Diseases (NIAID), Bethesda, MD, USA) (http://exon.niaid.nih.gov).
3. AlignX (included in the Vector NTI Suite V 5.5 software, Invitrogen Life technologies, North Bethesda, MD, USA).
4. CLUSTAL 2.1 /W multiple sequence alignment tool (http://www.clustal.org/).

2.5 Validation of SSH Results

1. Infected and uninfected *R. annulatus* RNA.
2. iScript™ cDNA Synthesis Kit (BioRad, Hercules, CA, USA).
3. iQ SYBR Green Supermix (BioRad, Hercules, CA, USA).
4. Specific and housekeeping primers.

2.6 Functional Tick Gene Analysis by RNA Interference

dsRNA Synthesis

1. *R. annulatus* RNA.
2. Specific primers for target genes with T7 extension.
3. Access RT-PCR system (Promega, Madison, USA).
4. PCR products purification kit (e.g., PureLink™ PCR Purification Kit, Life Technologies, Carlsbad, CA, USA).
5. MEGAscript® T7 Kit (Ambion Life Technologies, Carlsbad, CA, USA).

Injection in Ticks

1. Specific dsRNA.
2. Hamilton syringe, with 1 in., 33 G needle.
3. Forceps/tweezers.
4. Double face duck tape.
5. Dental wax plates.
6. Control buffer: 10 mM Tris–HCl, pH 7, 1 mM EDTA.

Tick Feeding

1. Infected *B. bigemina* calf.
2. Freshly molted female *R. annulatus.*
3. Contact glue.
4. Cotton sleeves.
5. Razor blade.

Gene Knockdown Assessment and Infection Assessment

1. *R. annulatus* ticks treated with dsRNA.
2. iScript™ One-Step RT-PCR Kit with SYBR® Green (Biorad, Hercules, CA, USA).
3. Gene-specific and housekeeping primers.

3 Methods

3.1 Ticks Processing

3.1.1 Uninfected and Babesia bigemina-Infected Ticks for SSH Library Construction

Obtain *B. bigemina*-infected and uninfected *R. annulatus* female ticks from experimentally infected and babesiosis-free 3 to 4-month-old male Holstein–Friesian calves, respectively (*see* **Note 1**).

1. Prior to tick infestation, test calves for antibodies against *Babesia* spp. infection, maintained under strict tick-free conditions, using an indirect fluorescent antibody (IFA) assay [26].
2. Inoculate one calf intravenously with 2×10^8 *B. bigemina* cryopreserved parasites (Moledet strain).
3. Monitor calf clinical responses by means of daily examinations of body temperature, packed cell volume (PCV) and of Giemsa-stained blood films.
4. Collect engorged adult female ticks from both infected and uninfected calves after feeding and maintain ticks at controlled conditions (temperature 22–25 °C and relative humidity > 85 %) for blood meal digestion during 4–5 days.

3.1.2 Uninfected R. annulatus for RNA Interference Studies

1. Use a 3–4-month-old male Holstein calf free of babesiosis to obtain uninfected *R. annulatus* freshly molted adult female ticks.
2. Infest the calf with 1 g of tick eggs at day zero (0). Retrieve the freshly molted females from the bovine host at day 21 using fine forceps. Thereafter, observe, clean, and place ticks in a controlled humidity and temperature chamber until dsRNA injection.
3. Glue tick-feeding sleeves (450 mm × 400 mm) (cotton fabric) to calf shaved skin one day prior to infestation with dsRNA-injected ticks.

3.2 SSH Library Construction and Sequencing

3.2.1 Tick Total RNA and DNA Extraction

1. Dissect each tick and place tissues in a tube containing 1 ml of TRI Reagent®. Homogenize using a 21 G × 1½″ (0.8 × 40 mm) needle and 1 ml syringe tube. Isolate total RNA and DNA according to the manufacturer's protocol (*see* **Notes 2** and **3**).
2. Dissolve the RNA and DNA in 30 μl of nuclease-free water and measure the concentration of each sample spectrophotometrically with a NanoDrop ND-1000 (*see* **Note 3**).

3.2.2 Detection of Babesia bigemina in Ticks by PCR

1. Perform a PCR using the following reaction mixture: final volume of 25 μL including 1× PCR Master Mix, 1 μM of forward and reverse primers specific for *B. bigemina*, and 50 ng of tick DNA; and the thermal cycling conditions: initial denaturation step at 95 °C for 10 min followed by 40 cycles of 30 s at 94 °C, 45 s at 64 °C, and 1 min at 72 °C, with a final extension step of 10 min at 72 °C (*see* **Note 4**).
2. Analyze the amplification products in a 1 % TAE agarose gel electrophoresis.

3.2.3 Complementary DNA (cDNA) Library Construction and SSH

1. Check the RNA integrity before proceeding with cDNA synthesis (*see* **Note 5**).
2. Create two pools corresponding to the infected and uninfected tick populations. Seven to ten ticks are enough to obtain sufficient RNA for each pool.

3. Isolate poly A+RNA using the FastTrack® 2.0 mRNA Isolation Kit, according to the manufacturer's instructions. After this isolation, check the integrity of poly A+RNA by electrophoresis.
4. Construct the SSH library using the PCR-Select™ cDNA Subtraction Kit. The procedure is thoroughly explained in the manufacturer instructions. Briefly:
   (a) After the two strands of cDNA are synthesized, digest the molecules into small blunt-ended fragments with the restriction enzyme *Rsa*I.
   (b) Submit the tester sample and part of the control sample to adaptors ligation.
   (c) Perform the first hybridization by mixing the tester samples with different adaptors and each of these with driver cDNA. Denature with heat and allow annealing/hybridization.
   (d) Second hybridization: mix the two samples obtained from the first hybridization and add fresh denatured cDNA driver. The new formed hybrid molecules consist now of differentially expressed cDNA with different adaptors on each end.
   (e) Amplify selectively the differentially expressed cDNAs during two PCR reactions using the Advantage® 2 PCR polymerase mix with TITANIUM *Taq* DNA polymerase.
   (f) Prior to thermal cycling, fill the missing strands of the adaptors by a brief incubation which creates binding sites for the primers used in the PCR. In this first amplification, only double-stranded cDNA with different adaptors sequences on each end is exponentially amplified.
   (g) In the second amplification, nested PCR was used to reduce the background (unwanted PCR products) and improving enrichment of the differentially expressed sequences in the tester sample or infected population (*see* **Note 6**).

3.2.4 cDNA Library Cloning

1. Clone the enriched cDNAs for sequencing with the TOPO TA Cloning® Kit, and transform One Shot® TOP10 competent *Escherichia coli* cells, following the manufacturer's instructions (*see* **Note 7**).
2. Prepare agar plates with the appropriate antibiotic (100 μg/ml of ampicillin) and supplement it with 0.5 mM of Isopropyl β-D-1-thiogalactopyranoside (IPTG). Spread 75 μl and 150 μl of cell culture in each plate.
3. Incubate plates overnight at 37 °C.
4. Perform colony PCR to randomly selected colonies for insertion confirmation analysis.

5. Colonies should be picked from the agar plate with a sterile pipette tip and resuspended in 20 μl of PCR reaction mix, which should include the universal T3/T7 primers at a final concentration of 1 μM.
6. PCR conditions should be: 10 min at 95 °C followed by 30 cycles of 30 s at 94 °C, 45 s at 64 °C, and 1 min at 72 °C and a final extension step of 10 min at 72 °C.
7. Analyze the PCR products on a 1.2 % TAE agarose gel.
8. Prepare the cDNA library for sequencing by inoculating 1 ml of LB medium with plated SSH clones and incubate overnight at 37 °C and 200 rpm to ensure high growth of transformed bacteria.

3.2.5 Plasmid Purification for Sequencing

1. Purify plasmids from the bacterial culture using Illustra plasmidPrep Mini Spin Kit, following the manufacturer's instructions.
2. Randomly select and sequence clones obtained from the SSH library using traditional Sanger sequencing approaches (*see* **Note 8**).

3.3 Sequence Analysis and Database Search

3.3.1 Sequencing and Analysis of SSH Clones

1. Use the available means for automated sequence clean-up, assembly, and BLAST analysis against nonredundant sequence database (nr) and databases of tick-specific sequences (*see* **Note 9**).
2. Analyze protein/gene ontology using a protein reference database (*see* **Note 9**).
3. Align nucleotide and protein sequences using widely available software like CLUSTAL 2.1 multiple sequence alignment tool.

3.3.2 Confirmation of Differential Gene Expression by Real-Time RT-PCR

1. Design appropriate primers manually or using available programs for the selected differentially expressed candidate genes.
2. Use total RNA from uninfected and *B. bigemina*-infected *R. annulatus* female ticks to construct cDNA using the iScript™ cDNA Synthesis Kit following the manufacturer's instructions.
3. Use the previously synthesized cDNA to perform quantitative real-time PCR. iQ SYBR Green Supermix can be used for the real-time PCR following the manufacturer's recommendations, including forward and reverse primers at a final concentration of 500 mM and cDNA at a final concentration of 20–25 ng (500 ng).
4. PCR conditions include an initial denaturation and enzyme activation step at 95 °C for 2 min, followed by 40 cycles of 15 s at 95 °C, 15 s at the primers annealing temperature, and 15 s at 62 °C for extension.

5. The mRNA levels should be normalized against the tick β-actin and 16S rRNA transcripts using the ddCT method [27, 28]. In all cases, the mean of the duplicate values should be used.
6. Compare the data from infected and uninfected ticks using the Student's *t*-test ($P=0.05$).

3.4 Functional Tick Gene Analysis by RNA Interference

3.4.1 dsRNA Synthesis

1. Based in the SSH clone sequences, design specific primers containing T7 promoter sequences (5′-TAA TAC GAC TCA CTA TAG GGT ACT-3′) at the 5′-end. Long fragments are desired.
2. Use RNA as template to amplify the fragments of interest by RT-PCR, using the Access RT-PCR system according to instructions given by the manufacturer, including 1 μM of each primer and 200 ng of template RNA. Conditions of the RT-PCR should be: first-strand synthesis performed at 45 °C for 45 min and AMV reverse transcriptase inactivation performed at 94 °C for 3 min, followed by PCR cycling for 40 cycles of 30 s at 94 °C, 30 s at 55 °C, and 90 s at 68 °C with a final extension step of 7 min at 68 °C.
3. Analyze amplification products on a 0.5× TBE, 1.2 % agarose gel.
4. Purify the PCR products using an appropriated kit like the PureLink™ PCR Purification Kit.
5. Use the MEGAscript® T7 Kit to synthesize dsRNA according to the manufacturer's instructions.
6. Purify and quantify by spectrometry the resulting dsRNA and check it on a 1.2 % TBE agarose gel.

3.4.2 dsRNA Injection in Ticks

1. Obtain freshly molted *R. annulatus* adult female ticks from the bovine host, using fine forceps.
2. Observe, clean, and place the ticks ventral side up on double sticky tape affixed to a 3″ × 6″ sheet of red dental wax. Position them together in groups of 10 leaving the body exposed.
3. Inject the ticks with 0.4 μl of dsRNA (1×10^{11} to 1×10^{12} mol/μl) in the lower right quadrant of the ventral surface of the tick exoskeleton [29] (*see* **Note 10**).
4. Inject at least 30 female ticks per group using a Hamilton syringe with a 1 in., 33 G needle.
5. Inoculate control ticks solely with control buffer (*see* **Note 11**).

3.4.3 Treatment of Ticks After Injection and Tick Feeding

1. Keep injected ticks in a recovery plastic container to wait for tick activation and then place them in a humidity chamber (12 h light/12 h dark photoperiod at 22–25 °C and 95 % relative humidity) for 24 h.
2. Allow the ticks to feed in separated circular patches, for test groups and controls, on a calf experimentally infected with 2×10^{8} *B. bigemina* parasites.

3. Glue patches with inner diameter of 150 mm used for tick feeding to the shaved back of the calf using contact glue.
4. Monitor cattle infection to ensure that feeding occurs at the peak of host parasitemia and perform visual examination of blood smears. Remember to place male ticks together with each group to allow mating.
5. Remove unattached ticks 2 days after infestation and all attached ticks after 7 days of feeding.
6. Keep the ticks in a humidity chamber for 4 days to allow digestion of the blood meal.

3.4.4 Analysis of Ticks After RNA Interference

1. Evaluate the number of ticks that survived as well as tick weighs. Tick mortality is evaluated as the ratio of dead ticks to the total number of fed ticks on the calf. To analyze tick mortality, the Chi-square test ($P = 0.05$) can be used with the null hypothesis that tick mortality was not dependent on gene knockdown.
2. After allowing blood digestion, ticks should be dissected and whole internal organs stored in RNA*later*™ solution for further DNA and RNA extraction.
3. Extract DNA and RNA using the TRI Reagent® as described above.

3.4.5 Gene Knockdown Assessment by Real-Time RT-PCR and Infection Quantification

1. Use the previously extracted RNA to perform real-time RT-PCR.
2. Evaluate gene knockdown of the selected genes by real-time RT-PCR using sequence-specific primers. The iScript One-Step RT-PCR Kit with SYBR® Green can be used to perform mRNA quantification. Manufacturer recommendations should be followed including primers at a final concentration of 500 mM and RNA at a final concentration of at least 25 ng/μl.
3. Incubate the reaction mix in a real-time thermal cycling detection system as follows: 10 min at 50 °C for cDNA synthesis; 5 min at 95 °C for reverse transcriptase inactivation; 40 cycles of 15 s at 95 °C followed by 15 s at primers annealing temperature and 15 s at 62 °C for extension.
4. The mRNA levels should be normalized against tick 16S rRNA transcripts using ddCT method.
5. Compare normalized mRNA levels between dsRNA-injected and control ticks using the Student's *t*-test ($P = 0.05$) (*see* **Note 12**).
6. Determine the *B. bigemina* infection levels by quantitative PCR. The 18S rDNA gene can be used as a genomic target using the specific primers 5′-AAT AAC AAT ACA GGG CTT TCG TCT-3′ and 5′-AAC GCG AGG CTG AAA TAC AAC T-3′.

7. Normalize against the tick 16S rDNA gene using the ddCT method [27, 28].
8. Compare the *B. bigemina* infection levels in ticks between dsRNA and control ticks using *t*-student test ($P = 0.05$).

4 Notes

General note: A project having as target the identification of new vaccine candidates has to be carefully designed and has to surpass different milestones. Experiments have to be properly designed and the obtained biological samples must be in good conditions.

1. Ticks must be reared in a certified laboratory according to animal welfare guidelines. Individual features as tick life cycle must be considered, for instance, if it's a one, two, or three host–tick species. When dealing with cattle ticks like *R. microplus* and *R. annulatus*, some constrains can arise due to their host specificity [30]. Plus, cattle are most of the times a requirement for the conduction of laboratorial experiments. Other species are less selective and smaller vertebrates like rabbits can be used to establish tick colonies. The tick infection can be obtained in different ways such as artificial feeding or even injection of pathogen, but the best way of copying natural infections is to infect the host and promote ordinary feeding.
2. DNA derived from nontarget organisms present on the surface of ticks may yield amplicons with some primers. To overcome this problem, the ticks may be rinsed two times individually in distilled water, once in 75 % ethanol and once more in water.
3. The TRI Reagent® is a mixture of guanidine thiocyanate and phenol that uses a convenient single-step liquid phase separation resulting in the simultaneous isolation of RNA, DNA, and proteins. After adding chloroform or 1-bromo-3-chloropropane and centrifuging, the mixture separates into 3 phases: an aqueous phase containing the RNA, the interphase containing DNA, and an organic phase containing proteins. Each component can then be isolated after separating the three phases. This reagent extracts total RNA, but when poly A+RNA is the target, it is necessary to separate this last type of RNA from the remaining existent RNA in a cell (rRNA and tRNA).
4. A one step PCR can be used to detect the presence of *B. bigemina* in sampled ticks. The example shown here uses primers Bbi400F: 5′-AGC TTG CTT TCA CAA CTC GCC-3′ and Bbi400R: 5′-TTG GTG CTT TGA CCG ACG ACA T-3′ that amplify a 400 bp fragment within the conserved region of the five *rap-1a* paralogous genes [31, 32], but the detection of pathogen infection in ticks can be done using different protocols

and/or using different PCR mixtures. When dealing with low parasitemias, the use of a nested PCR is recommended.

5. RNA quality should be checked by gel electrophoresis to confirm the integrity of RNA preparations since high-quality, pure, and intact total RNA is critical to perform fundamental downstream molecular biology experiments.
6. For SSH library construction, following the manufacturer's protocol usually is sufficient to achieve good results, but small modifications or optimizations can be done that normally are stated in the protocol. It is fundamental to always read the entire protocol before starting any procedure in order to carefully plan the experiments (e.g., the reagents within the PCR-Select™ cDNA Subtraction Kit are limited).
7. The TOPO TA Cloning® Kit uses the pCR™4-TOPO vector which allows the selection of successful transformants by antibiotic and directly by disruption of the lethal *E. coli* gene, *ccd*B [33]. The vector contains the *ccd*B gene fused to the C-terminus of the LacZα fragment. The ligation of a PCR product disrupts expression of the *lac*Zα-*ccd*B gene fusion permitting growth of only positive recombinants upon transformation. Cells that contain nonrecombinant vector are killed upon plating. Therefore, blue/white screening is not required.
8. The number of clones obtained from SSH library varies from assay to assay and might be necessary to make a random selection of clones to sequence, facing the high sequencing costs. As dealing with products of PCR, many clones are expected to be repeated. Sequencing of clones can be done in house or using available outsource academic or commercial sequencing facilities.
9. The cDNA Annotation System software (dCAS) [16] may be used for automated sequence clean-up, assembly, and BLAST analysis against nonredundant sequence database (nr) and databases of tick-specific sequences (http://www.proteinlounge.com, http://www.ncbi.nlm.nih.gov and http://www.vectorbase.org/index.php) and gene ontology (GO) assignments.
10. For visualization of tick gene silencing procedures, please visit: http://www.jove.com/video/2474/rna-interference-in-ticks?ID=2474.
11. Control ticks can be injected with an unrelated dsRNA to control the effect of dsRNA injection in the tick, with a control buffer or even with PBS.
12. In the present study, it was unnecessary to determine the absolute transcript copy number, so the relative change in gene expression suffices. Relative quantification describes the changes in the expression of target genes in the infected tick population relatively to the reference group, the uninfected tick population.

References

1. Bock R, Jackcon L, de Vos A, Jorgensen W (2004) Babesiosis of cattle. Parasitology 129: S247–S269
2. de la Fuente J, Moreno-Cid JA, Canales M et al (2011) Targeting arthropod subolesin/akirin for the development of a universal vaccine for control of vector infestations and pathogen transmission. Vet Parasitol 181: 17–22
3. Macaluso KR, Mulenga A, Simser JA et al (2003) Differential expression of genes in uninfected and rickettsia-infected *Dermacentor variabilis* ticks as assessed by differential-display PCR. Infect Immun 71:6165–6170
4. Mulenga A, Macaluso KR, Simser JA et al (2003) Dynamics of Rickettsia-tick interactions: identification and characterization of differentially expressed mRNAs in uninfected and infected *Dermacentor variabilis*. Insect Mol Biol 12:185–193
5. Nene V, Lee D, Kang'a S, Skilton R et al (2004) Genes transcribed in the salivary glands of female *Rhipicephalus appendiculatus* ticks infected with *Theileria parva*. Insect Biochem Mol Biol 34:1117–1128
6. Rudenko N, Golovchenko M, Edwards MJ et al (2005) Differential expression of *Ixodes ricinus* tick genes induced by blood feeding or *Borrelia burgdorferi* infection. J Med Entomol 42:36–41
7. de la Fuente J, Blouin EF, Manzano-Roman NR et al (2007) Functional genomic studies of tick cells in response to infection with the cattle pathogen, *Anaplasma marginale*. Genomics 90:712–722
8. de la Fuente J, Kocan KM, Almazan C et al (2007) RNA interference for the study and genetic manipulation of ticks. Trends Parasitol 23:427–433
9. Villar M, Torina A, Nunez Y et al (2010) Application of highly sensitive saturation labeling to the analysis of differential protein expression in infected ticks from limited samples. Proteome Sci 8:43
10. Zivkovic Z, Esteves E, Almazan C et al (2010) Differential expression of genes in salivary glands of male *Rhipicephalus* (*Boophilus*) *microplus* in response to infection with *Anaplasma marginale*. BMC Genomics 11:186
11. Mercado-Curiel RF, Palmer GH, Guerrero FD et al (2011) Temporal characterisation of the organ-specific *Rhipicephalus microplus* transcriptional response to *Anaplasma marginale* infection. Int J Parasitol 41:851–860
12. Antunes S, Golovchenko M, Rudenko N et al (2012) Gene silencing of the tick antigens selected after infection with *Babesia bigemina*, in the host tick *Rhipicephalus annulatus* by RNA interference. Int J Parasitol 42:187–195
13. Zivkovic Z, Torina A, Mitra R et al (2010) Subolesin expression in response to pathogen infection in ticks. BMC Immunol 11:7
14. de la Fuente J, Maritz-Olivier C, Naranjo V et al (2008) Evidence of the role of tick subolesin in gene expression. BMC Genomics 9:372
15. Kocan KM, Zivkovic Z, Blouin EF et al (2009) Silencing of genes involved in *Anaplasma marginale*–tick interactions affects the pathogen developmental cycle in *Dermacentor variabilis*. BMC Dev Biol 9:42
16. Guo YJ, Ribeiro JMC, Anderson JM et al (2009) dCAS: a desktop application for cDNA sequence annotation. Bioinformatics 25:1195–1196
17. Fire A, Xu S, Montgomery MK, Kostas SA et al (1998) Potent and specific genetic interference by double-stranded RNA in *Caenorhabditis elegans*. Nature 391:806–811
18. Montgomery MK, Xu SQ, Fire A (1998) RNA as a target of double-stranded RNA-mediated genetic interference in *Caenorhabditis elegans*. Proc Natl Acad Sci U S A 95:15502–15507
19. Mello CC, Conte D (2004) Revealing the world of RNA interference. Nature 431:338–342
20. de la Fuente J, Kocan KM (2006) Strategies for development of vaccines for control of ixodid tick species. Parasite Immunol 28: 275–283
21. Hoa NT, Keene KM, Olson KE et al (2003) Characterization of RNA interference in an *Anopheles gambiae* cell line. Insect Biochem Mol Biol 33:949–957
22. Pal U, Li X, Wang T et al (2004) TROSPA, an *Ixodes scapularis* receptor for *Borrelia burgdorferi*. Cell 119:457–468
23. Ramamoorthi N, Narasimhan S, Pal U et al (2005) The Lyme disease agent exploits a tick protein to infect the mammalian host. Nature 436:573–577
24. Sukumaran B, Narasimhan S, Anderson JF et al (2006) An *Ixodes scapularis* protein required for survival of *Anaplasma phagocytophilum* in tick salivary glands. J Exp Med 203:1507–1517
25. Merino O, Almazan C, Canales M et al (2011) Control of *Rhipicephalus* (*Boophilus*) *microplus* infestations by the combination of subolesin

vaccination and tick autocidal control after subolesin gene knockdown in ticks fed on cattle. Vaccine 29:2248–2254

26. Shkap V, Leibovitz B, Krigel Y et al (2005) Vaccination of older *Bos taurus* bulls against bovine babesiosis. Vet Parasitol 129:235–242
27. Livak KJ, Schmittgen TD (2001) Analysis of relative gene expression data using real-time quantitative PCR and the 2(T)(-Delta Delta C) method. Methods 25:402–408
28. Schefe JH, Lehmann KE, Buschmann IR et al (2006) Quantitative real-time RT-PCR data analysis: current concepts and the novel "gene expression's C-T difference" formula. J Mol Med 84:901–910
29. de la Fuente J, Almazan C, Blouin EF et al (2006) Reduction of tick infections with *Anaplasma marginale* and *A. phagocytophilum* by targeting the tick protective antigen subolesin. Parasitol Res 100:85–91
30. Willadsen P, Kemp DH (1988) Vaccination with concealed antigens for tick control. Parasitol Today 4:196–198
31. Suarez CE, Palmer GH, Florin-Christensen M et al (2003) Organization, transcription, and expression of rhoptry associated protein genes in the *Babesia bigemina* rap-1 locus. Mol Biochem Parasitol 127:101–112
32. Petrigh R, Ruybal P, Thompson C et al (2008) Improved molecular tools for detection of *Babesia bigemina*. Ann N Y Acad Sci 1149: 155–157
33. Bernard P, Gabant P, Bahassi EM, Couturier M (1994) Positive-selection vectors using the F plasmid *ccdB* killer gene. Gene 148: 71–74

Chapter 33

Metagenomic Approaches to Disclose Disease-Associated Pathogens: Detection of Viral Pathogens in Honeybees

Fredrik Granberg, Oskar E. Karlsson, and Sándor Belák

Abstract

Metagenomic approaches have become invaluable for culture-independent and sequence-independent detection and characterization of disease-associated pathogens. Here, the sequential steps from sampling to verification of results are described for a metagenomic-based approach to detect potential pathogens in honeybees. The pre-sequencing steps are given in detail, but due to the rapid development of sequencing technologies, all platform-specific procedures, as well as subsequent bioinformatics analysis, are more generally described. It should also be noted that this approach could, with minor modifications, be adapted for other organisms and sample matrices.

Key words Metagenomics, Sequencing, Unknown viruses, Virus detection, Diagnosis, Unknown etiology

1 Introduction

Metagenomics based on high-throughput sequencing (HTS) allows for cell culture-independent and nucleotide sequence-independent detection of pathogens as well as characterization of the entire microbial flora in a sample. It thus has the potential to detect the full spectrum of emerging new pathogens, including novel viruses and fastidious bacteria, as demonstrated and reviewed [1–4]. Viral metagenomics (or metaviromics) focuses on the viral fraction of a metagenomic sample, and several HTS-based approaches have been developed for unbiased characterization of the viral populations in various organisms and environments. These approaches are usually comprised of several typical steps including sample homogenization, target enrichment, sequence-independent amplification, sequencing library construction, HTS, and bioinformatics analysis [5, 6].

The pre-sequencing steps are similar to the method outlined by Allander et al. [7]. Following homogenization and filtration, nuclease treatment with both DNase and RNase is used to reduce the host

Mónica V. Cunha and João Inácio (eds.), *Veterinary Infection Biology: Molecular Diagnostics and High-Throughput Strategies*, Methods in Molecular Biology, vol. 1247, DOI 10.1007/978-1-4939-2004-4_33, © Springer Science+Business Media New York 2015

background and enrich viral nucleic acid by removing unprotected nucleic acids (i.e., those not in viral capsids), which makes this approach most suitable for detection of actively replicating viruses during the infectious period. The nuclease treatment is efficient and easy to perform, as previously demonstrated [8, 9]. However, the quantities of recovered viral nucleic acid after extraction from nuclease-treated samples are usually insufficient for generation of sequencing libraries. An amplification step is therefore required, and for this purpose, we have incorporated random priming and amplification using the sequence-independent single-primer amplification (SISPA) method. Even though SISPA, or variants thereof, has been extensively used with great success for pre-amplification in viral discovery [10–13], the method has been demonstrated to introduce an amplification bias. This is not necessarily a problem for virus identification, but it makes SISPA an unsuitable choice when whole-genome recovery is of central importance [14, 15].

Most existing HTS platforms have their own protocols to convert extracted and amplified material into a sequencing library suitable for subsequent cluster generation and sequencing. These protocols have differing requirements in terms of the quantity and quality of the starting material, but they are usually comprised of four main steps: (1) fragmentation of DNA; (2) end repair, modification, and ligation of adapters, which enable amplification of the sheared DNA by adapter-specific primers; (3) size selection of DNA molecules with a certain length optimal for the current application or instrument; and (4) enrichment of adapter-ligated DNA by PCR [16]. By also adding specific short sequence tags during the construction of multiple libraries, it is possible to pool them into a single-indexed library for increased throughput and reduced costs. The necessary reagents for preparing a sequencing library can often be purchased as platform-specific commercial kits.

There are currently three major commercial HTS platforms that we have found suitable for metagenomic-based detection of virus: (1) Roche 454; (2) Illumina; and (3) Ion Torrent. The Roche 454 platform has been the high-throughput method of choice for discovery and de novo assembly of novel microorganisms [17–19]. In addition to having the longest read lengths, which simplifies de novo assembly, this was also the first HTS platform on the market. However, Roche recently announced that the 454 platform will be phased out in mid-2016, indicating that it has become outdated and cost ineffective. The field has developed rapidly as a result of continuous improvement of existing systems and release of completely new platforms, and both the Illumina and Ion Torrent platforms have become more attractive alternatives. What they may lack in terms of read length is compensated for by throughput, cost, and accuracy. More specifically, while Illumina currently boasts the industry's most accurate data, Ion Torrent has the shortest run time [20].

Bioinformatics is employed to analyze obtained sequence data. It is important and good practice to first perform a quality control of the dataset, not only to detect deviations but also to aid in the preprocessing of sequencing data, which include removal of adaptor sequences and low-quality reads [21]. The taxonomical content of a metagenomic dataset is usually determined by comparing individual reads against databases of known sequences using a comparison tool such as BLAST. However, for the purpose of pathogen detection, it is often beneficial to first assemble the reads into longer continuous sequences (contigs), thereby substantially decreasing the amount of data to be classified as well as providing longer stretches of nucleotides to match toward the database.

How and when sampling is conducted might greatly affect the outcome of pathogen detection schemes. The presence and prevalence of pathogens in a honeybee colony may vary over time and space and can depend on several factors, such as colony composition regarding age class of bees and brood, physiological status of bees, and/or the presence of brood [22]. For the investigation of colony collapse disorder (CCD), which is recognized by a drastic reduction in adult population despite the presence of abundant food and breeding resources, hives displaying a lack of vitality of adult worker honeybees and unusual depopulation might be suitable for sampling.

We here describe a collection of sequential protocols that outline a metagenomic approach aimed at detection of viral pathogens in honeybees, which successfully has been employed for the detection of viral pathogens in Spanish honeybees [23]. Although variants of the protocols have been described elsewhere, we have combined and augmented them for this specific aim. While the pre-sequencing steps are described in detail, more general recommendations are given regarding sequencing procedures and subsequent bioinformatic analysis. This is mainly due to the rapid development of HTS technologies, which quickly would render detailed and platform-specific descriptions obsolete. Furthermore, the generation of sequencing libraries as well as the actual sequencing is commonly performed by engaging a commercial sequencing provider or an academic sequencing core facility. It should also be noted that the described approach can be adapted for other organism by simply modifying the sample preparation step.

2 Materials

If solutions are not obtained from a commercial supplier, they should be prepared using ultrapure water (prepared by purifying deionized water to attain a sensitivity of 18 MΩ cm at 25 °C) and analytical grade reagents. Prepare and store reagents according to their individual specifications (room temperature if not specified). Special care should be taken to keep enzymes at −20 °C until use. Diligently follow all waste disposal regulations when disposing waste materials.

2.1 Sample Preparation

1. Hand-operated glass homogenizer (or mortar and pestle), 30 ml capacity.
2. Sterile phosphate-buffered saline (1×PBS): 137 mM NaCl, 2.7 mM KCl, 10 mM Na_2HPO_4, and 1.76 mM KH_2PO_4 (pH 7.4).
3. 0.45 μm PVDF syringe filters.
4. 5 ml syringes.
5. 15 ml tubes.
6. 1.5 ml tubes.

2.2 Enrichment by Nuclease Treatment and Nucleic Acid Extraction

1. Desktop mini centrifuge.
2. Refrigerated microcentrifuge.
3. 1.5 ml tubes.
4. DNase I (10 U/μl; e.g., Roche Applied Science).
5. DNase buffer (10×; supplied with DNase I).
6. RNase A (1 μg/μl; e.g., Life Technologies, Sigma-Aldrich, or Thermo Scientific): Dilute to the working concentration using nuclease-free water (not DEPC treated). Gently mix by pipetting or by flicking the tube a few times. Keep on ice until use.
7. Heat block or water bath (with a rack for 1.5 ml tubes).
8. Column-based DNA extraction kit with proteinase K, e.g., QIAamp DNA Mini Kit (Qiagen) or PureLink Genomic DNA Mini Kit (Life Technologies).
9. TRIzol LS Reagent (Life Technologies) or other acid-guanidinium-phenol-based reagents, e.g., TRI Reagent (Sigma-Aldrich), TriPure (Roche Applied Science), or QIAzol (Qiagen).
10. Chloroform.
11. Ethanol (70 %).
12. Column-based RNA extraction kit, e.g., RNeasy Mini Kit (Qiagen) or PureLink RNA Mini Kit (Life Technologies).
13. Fluorescence-based capillary electrophoresis instrument, 2100 Bioanalyzer (Agilent Technologies).

2.3 Sequence-Independent, Single-Primer Amplification (SISPA)

1. Desktop mini centrifuge.
2. Thermocycler.
3. 0.2 or 0.5 ml tubes: Should fit the thermocycler.

4. 1.5 ml tubes.
5. Nuclease-free water (not DEPC treated).
6. Tag labeling primer FR26RV-N (GCCGGAGCTCTGCAG ATATCNNNNNN): Dilute to 10 μM with nuclease-free water.
7. Amplification primer FR20RV (GCCGGAGCTCTGCAGAT ATC): Dilute to 10 μM with nuclease-free water.
8. dNTP mix (10 mM each).
9. dNTP mix (2.5 mM each).
10. Exo(−) Klenow DNA polymerase (5 U/μl; e.g., New England Biolabs or Thermo Fisher Scientific).
11. Exo(−) Klenow Buffer (10×; supplied with Exo(−) Klenow DNA polymerase).
12. DTT (0.1 M).
13. RNase inhibitor (40 U/μl), e.g., RNaseOUT (Life Technologies), RiboLock (Thermo Fisher Scientific), or Protector (Roche Applied Science).
14. Reverse transcriptase (200 U/μl), e.g., SuperScript III (Life Technologies) or Maxima (Thermo Fisher Scientific).
15. Reverse transcriptase (RT) buffer (5×; supplied with reverse transcriptase).
16. $MgCl_2$ (25 mM).
17. DNA polymerase (5 U/μl), e.g., AmpliTaq Gold with Buffer II (Life Technologies).
18. PCR buffer (10×; supplied with DNA polymerase).
19. Column-based PCR purification kit, e.g., QIAquick PCR Purification Kit (Qiagen) or PureLink PCR Purification Kit (Life Technologies).
20. Elution buffer (EB): 10 mM Tris–HCl (pH 8.5).
21. EcoRV (20 U/μl; e.g., New England Biolabs).
22. Restriction enzyme buffer (10×; supplied with EcoRV).
23. Instrument for quantification of nucleic acids, e.g., Qubit 2.0 Fluorometer with Qubit Assay Kits for DNA and RNA (Life Technologies) or NanoDrop ND-1000 spectrophotometer (NanoDrop Technologies).
24. Fluorescence-based capillary electrophoresis instrument, 2100 Bioanalyzer (Agilent Technologies).
25. TBE buffer (0.5×): 45 mM Tris–HCl (pH 8.3), 45 mM boric acid, 1 mM EDTA.

26. Agarose (type LE) gel (1 %): Prepare using your standard protocol in 0.5× TBE buffer. Add GelRed or ethidium bromide for visualization.
27. 1 kb Plus DNA Ladder (e.g., Life Technologies or Thermo Fisher Scientific).

2.4 Library Preparation and Sequencing

See HTS platform-specific protocols, according to manufacturers.

2.5 Data Handling and Bioinformatics

1. Intel-based server: 4× 2 Intel Xeon or similar capacity, 256 GB memory per processor (*see* **Note 1** for bioinformatics and data management considerations).
2. Linux-based operating system.
3. PrinSeq software package (http://sourceforge.net/projects/prinseq/files/).
4. MIRA software package (http://sourceforge.net/projects/mira-assembler).
5. BLAST+ software package (ftp://ftp.ncbi.nlm.nih.gov/blast/executables/blast+).
6. Workstation, Intel i7 or similar, 8 GB of memory.
7. MEGAN 4 software (http://ab.inf.uni-tuebingen.de/software/megan/).
8. Bowtie 2 (http://bowtie-bio.sourceforge.net/bowtie2).
9. Integrative Genomics Viewer (http://www.broadinstitute.org/igv/).

2.6 Confirmation and Retrieval of Near-Full Genome Sequences

1. Thermocycler.
2. 0.2 or 0.5 ml tubes: Should fit the thermocycler.
3. 1.5 ml tubes.
4. Column-based DNA extraction kit with proteinase K, e.g., QIAamp DNA Mini Kit (Qiagen) or PureLink Genomic DNA Mini Kit (Life Technologies).
5. TRIzol LS Reagent (Life Technologies) or other acid-guanidinium-phenol-based reagents, e.g., TRI Reagent (Sigma-Aldrich), TriPure (Roche Applied Science), or QIAzol (Qiagen).
6. Column-based RNA extraction kit, e.g., RNeasy Mini Kit (Qiagen) or PureLink RNA Mini Kit (Life Technologies).
7. First-strand cDNA synthesis kit, e.g., SuperScript III First-Strand Synthesis System (Life Technologies) and RevertAid First-Strand cDNA Synthesis Kit (Thermo Fisher Scientific) or Transcriptor First-Strand cDNA Synthesis Kit (Roche Applied Science).

8. DNA polymerase, e.g., AmpliTaq Gold (Life Technologies), DreamTaq (Thermo Fisher Scientific), or Platinum Taq (Life Technologies).
9. PCR buffer (10×; supplied with DNA polymerase).
10. High-fidelity long-range DNA polymerase, e.g., Phusion Hot Start II High Fidelity (Thermo Fisher Scientific).
11. Agarose (type LE) gel (1 %): Prepare using your standard protocol in 0.5× TBE buffer.
12. UV transilluminator.
13. Scalpel.
14. Column-based gel extraction kit, e.g., QIAquick Gel Extraction Kit (Qiagen) or Purelink Quick Gel Extraction Kit (Life Technologies).

3 Methods

The sequential steps in the metagenomic-based approach outlined below are summarized in Fig. 1. Carry out all laboratory procedures at room temperature unless otherwise specified.

3.1 Sample Preparation

1. For each hive, collect approximately 50 adult worker bees in total, from both inside and outside the hive to ensure the presence of young and adult bees, in sterile containers. Keep frozen during transport at −18 °C or lower.
2. Out of the collected material from a hive, manually homogenize 20 whole bees in a 30 ml glass homogenizer with 6 ml of 1× PBS. If possible, perform the homogenization on ice.
3. Pour the homogenate into a 15 ml tube (or use several 2 ml tubes) and centrifuge at 1,000 × *g* for 10 min at 4 °C to pellet debris.
4. Use a 5 ml syringe and a 0.45 μm PVDF syringe filter to remove any remaining debris. Draw a small amount of air (about 1 ml) into the syringe before filling with the supernatant. Attach the syringe filter and pass the supernatant through the filter into 1.5 ml tubes by applying a steady pressure. Use the air in the syringe to purge the filter. This will minimize fluid retention within the filter device and maximize sample recovery.

3.2 Enrichment by Nuclease Treatment and Nucleic Acid Extraction

1. Aliquot 168 μl of the filtered homogenate into two 1.5 ml tubes and add 20 μl of 10× DNase buffer to each. Mix by vortexing and spin down briefly using a desktop mini centrifuge.
2. To each tube, add 10 μl DNase I (10 U/μl) and 2 μl RNase (1 μg/μl). Mix by pipetting.
3. Incubate at 37 °C for 2 h using a heat block or water bath.

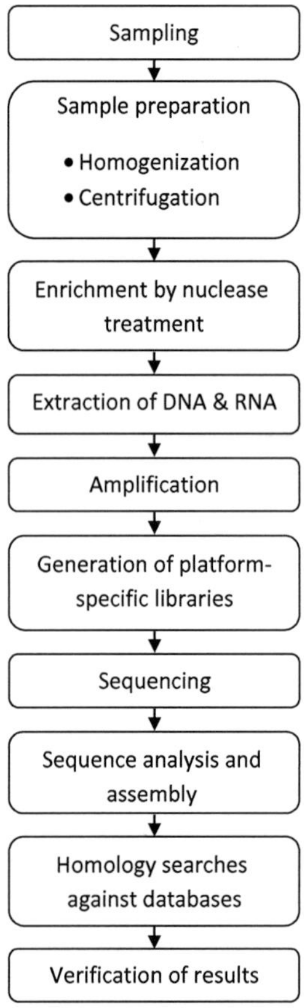

Fig. 1 Flow graph of the described metagenomic-based approach to detect potential pathogens

4. Dry the tubes, if necessary, and put them on ice. Store at –80 °C or proceed directly.

DNA Extraction

1. Use the QIAamp DNA Mini Kit according to the manufacturer's spin protocol for blood and body fluid DNA extraction (*see* **Note 2**).
2. Measure DNA concentration by using a Qubit 2.0 Fluorometer with the dsDNA HS (High Sensitivity) Assay Kit, or use a NanoDrop ND-1000 to make an estimate, according to the manufacturers' instructions. Concentrations are expected to range between 2 and 25 ng/μl.
3. Aliquot the DNA and mark the tubes with the sample ID and date of extraction. Store at –80 °C.

RNA Extraction

The following steps should be carried out under a fume hood due to phenol component.

1. Add 600 μl of TRIzol LS to each nuclease-treated homogenate and pipette the homogenate up and down a couple of times.
2. Incubate the tubes at room temperature for 5 min.
3. Add 160 μl of chloroform.
4. Cap the tube securely and shake and/or vortex it vigorously for 15 s, so the contents of the tube get whitish.
5. Incubate the tube for 2–3 min in room temperature.
6. Centrifuge the tubes at 12,000 × *g* for 15 min at 4 °C. The rest of the centrifugation steps should be carried out at room temperature.
7. Carefully take the tubes to the fume hood. There will be three phases after the centrifugation: an upper, colorless, aqueous phase containing RNA, a white interphase containing DNA, and a lower, red, organic phase.
8. Carefully transfer the aqueous phase to a fresh 1.5 ml tube. Transfer it in small volumes without getting any of the other two phases into the pipette tip.
9. Estimate the volume of the aqueous phase. Add the same volume of 70 % ethanol. Mix thoroughly by vortexing. Do not centrifuge.
10. Pipet up to 700 μl of the sample into an RNeasy Mini Spin Column, or similar, in a 2 ml collection tube. Mark the lid of the column with the sample ID.
11. Centrifuge at ≥8,000 × *g* for 15 s at 15–25 °C. Discard the flow-through. If there is still some of the sample left, transfer it to the Mini Column and centrifuge again.
12. Proceed according to the manufacturer's instructions.
13. Measure the concentration of the extracted RNA by using a Qubit 2.0 Fluorometer with the RNA Assay Kit or control the RNA quality by using a 2100 Bioanalyzer with a RNA Pico Chip (Agilent Technologies) according to the instructions of the manufacturers. Concentrations are expected to range between 2 and 25 ng/μl.
14. Aliquot the RNA and mark the tubes with the sample ID and date of extraction. Store at –80 °C.

3.3 Sequence-Independent, Single-Primer Amplification (SISPA)

Tag Labeling DNA

1. Prepare the reagent mixture described in Table 1 in a 0.2 or 0.5 ml tube.
2. Denature at 94 °C for 2 min in a thermal cycler and chill on ice for 2 min.
3. Add 0.5 μl (2.5 U) of exo(−) Klenow DNA polymerase.

Table 1
Reagent mixture for tag labeling DNA

Component	Volume (μl)
FR26RV-N (10 μM)	2
DNA template	10
dNTP mix (10 mM each)	1.5
Exo(−) Klenow Buffer (10×)	1.5
Total volume	15

Table 2
Reaction mix 1 for tag labeling RNA

Component	Volume (μl)
FR26RV-N (10 mM)	2
RNA template	10
dNTP mix (10 mM each)	1.5
Total volume	13.5

4. Complete a first round of extension by incubating at 37 °C for 1 h. Proceed directly with denaturation at 94 °C for 2 min and chill on ice for 2 min.
5. Add 0.5 μl (2.5 U) of exo(−) Klenow DNA polymerase for a second round of extension.
6. Incubate at 37 °C for 1 h and inactivate the enzyme by incubating at 75 °C for 10 min.
7. Tagged DNA fragments can be stored at −20 °C for several weeks.

Tag Labeling RNA

1. Prepare the reaction mix 1 (Table 2) and 2 (Table 3) in separate 0.2 or 0.5 ml tubes.
2. Keep reaction mix 2 on ice until **step 4**.
3. Incubate reaction mix 1 at 65 °C for 5 min in a thermal cycler to denature the RNA.
4. Chill on ice for 1 min and add reaction mix 2.
5. Perform the reverse transcription by incubating at 25 °C for 5 min, 50 °C for 1 h, and 85 °C for 5 min. Place on ice.
6. Add 0.5 μl (2.5 U) of exo(−) Klenow DNA polymerase for second-strand synthesis and incubate at 37 °C for 1 h. A final incubation at 75 °C for 10 min inactivates the enzyme.

Table 3
Reaction mix 2 for tag labeling RNA

Component	Volume (μl)
Reaction mix 1 (*see* Table 2)	13.5
RT buffer (5×)	4
DTT (0,1 M)	1
RNase inhibitor (40 U/μl)	1
Reverse transcriptase (200 U/μl)	1
Total volume	20.5

Table 4
Reaction mix for PCR amplification

Component	Volume (μl)
PCR buffer (10×)	5
dNTP Mix (2.5 mM each)	4
$MgCl_2$ (25 mM)	5
FR20RV (10 mM)	4
DNA polymerase (5 U/μl)	0.5
Nucleic acid template	2.5
Nuclease-free H_2O	29
Total volume	50

7. Tagged cDNA fragments can be stored at –20 °C for several weeks.

Amplification

1. Perform the PCR amplification by using the complementary primer FR20RV. For each reaction, prepare the reaction mix described in Table 4 in a 0.2 or 0.5 ml tube.
2. Mix gently and, if necessary, spin down briefly using a desktop mini centrifuge.
3. Perform the PCR in a thermal cycler with the conditions described in Table 5.
4. PCR products can be stored at –20 °C for several weeks.

Exonuclease Removal of Amplification Tag Sequences

1. Purify the PCR products with the QIAquick PCR Purification Kit, according to the manufacturer's instructions, or use a similar column-based purification system. Elute in 50 μl of EB buffer or water (pH 7.0–8.5).

Table 5
Thermal cycling conditions

Cycle step	Temperature (°C)	Duration	Number of cycles
Initial denaturation	95	10 min	1
Denaturation	95	60 s	
Annealing	58	60 s	40
Extension	72	60 s	
Final extension	72	10 min	1

Table 6
Restriction reaction mixture

Component	Volume (μl)
Purified PCR product	26
Restriction enzyme buffer (10×)	3
EcoRV (20 U/μl)	0.5
Total volume	29.5

2. Use the restriction enzyme EcoRV to remove the amplification tag. Add purified PCR product, buffer, and restriction enzyme to a 1.5 ml microfuge tube as described in Table 6.
3. Incubate at 37 °C for 1 h using a heat block or water bath.
4. Purify again using the QIAquick PCR Purification Kit or a similar column-based purification system. Elute in 50 μl of EB buffer or water (pH 7.0–8.5).
5. To assess the compositions and concentrations of the final samples, use either a 2100 Bioanalyzer or run the samples on an agarose gel (1 % agarose in 0.5× TBE buffer) and measure the concentration using a Qubit 2.0 Fluorometer. Figure 2a, b illustrates successfully amplified random products when analyzed with the two abovementioned methods, respectively.

3.4 Library Preparation and Sequencing

The generation of sequencing libraries as well as the actual sequencing is commonly performed by engaging a commercial provider or an academic core facility. This paragraph will therefore be kept brief and not outline a detailed protocol.

1. Since the preparation of sequencing libraries are platform specific, it is first necessary to select a sequencing platform. It has been demonstrated that HTS data in the range of 10–50 Mbp is enough to identify viruses with the described approach [24]. Most current platforms have a capacity in this range or higher. There are therefore other factors that might influence the

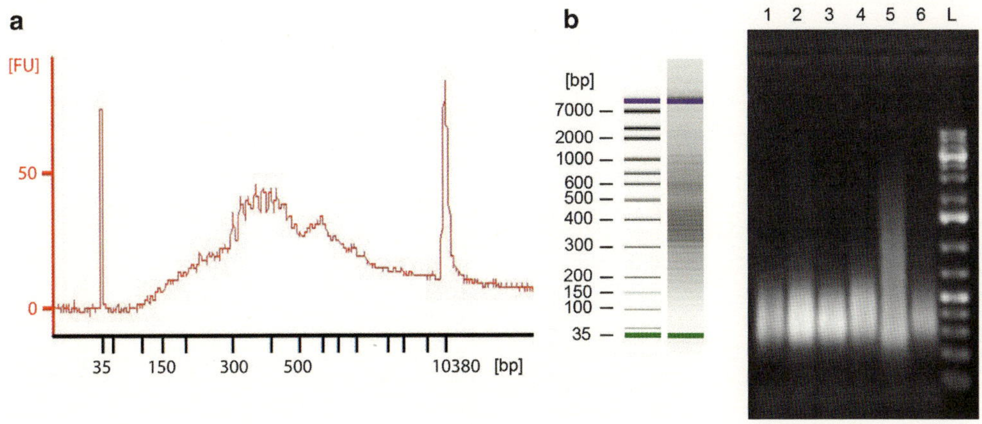

Fig. 2 Successfully amplified random products analyzed using (**a**) the 2100 Bioanalyzer DNA 1000 Assay and (**b**) separation on a 0.8 % agarose gel. The Bioanalyzer produces a graph where the *y*-axis represents fluorescence units [FU] and the *x*-axis is time, which translates to fragment size in base pair (bp). This information is also used to create a gel-like densitometry plot. On the agarose gel, sizes were determined using a 1 kb Plus DNA Ladder. A smear is expected due to the randomness of the amplification procedure and the DNA size typical range from 200 to 1,000 bp, with the mean size ~375 bp

choice, such as read length, cost (both per run and per Mb of DNA sequence), and ease of availability. For comparison, major commercial HTS platforms suitable for metagenomic-based detection and their characteristics are summarized in Table 7. A comprehensive review about HTS platforms has also been made by Glenn et al. [25].

2. The necessary reagents for sequencing library generation can be obtained as platform-specific commercial kits. It should therefore be straightforward to prepare a sequencing library according to the kit manufacturer's protocol. In addition, the use of specific short sequence tags (indexes) is supported by most platforms. They can be added during the construction of multiple libraries to allow multiplexing for increased throughput and reduced costs (for other considerations regarding preparation of sequencing libraries, *see* **Note 3**).
3. Perform sequencing according to the platform manufacturer's protocol.

3.5 Data Handling and Bioinformatics

We here describe a general approach based on publicly available software on a Unix/Linux system.

1. Sequence data is usually received in compressed format, for example, as a .tar.gz file. The software application gzip is preinstalled on most Unix/Linux systems and can be invoked as gunzip from the command line to uncompress files (on the command line type: gunzip –h for help using gunzip).

Table 7
Characteristics and utility grades of HTS platforms suitable for metagenomic-based detection of potential pathogens

Platforms	Library preparation time	Run time[a]	Average read length (bp)	Throughput per run	Reagent cost/run	Reagent cost/Mb	Utility grade[b]
Roche/454[c]							
GS FLX Titanium XL+	2–6 h	23 h	~700	700 Mb	~$6 k	~$8.6	B—average; long read length; high cost per Mb
GS Junior	2–6 h	10 h	~400	35–50 Mb	~$1 k	~$20	B/C—average; suitable for single samples; long read length; low cost per run but high cost per Mb
Illumina							
HiSeq 2500 (rapid)	3–5 h	27 h	2 × 100	180 Gb	~$6 k	~$0.04	B/A—average; limited by short reads (assembly more challenging); highest throughput per run; low cost per Mb
HiSeq 2500 (max)	3–5 h	11 days	2 × 100	600 Gb	~$23 k	~$0.04	
MiSeq	90 min	~24 h	2 × 250	7.5–8.5 Gb	~$1 K	~$0.13	A/B—good; shorter reads than 454 but much greater throughput; low cost per Mb; fastest Illumina run times

Ion Torrent PGM	4–6 h						
314 Chip		2–3 h	~400	10–40 Mb	$350	~$8.5	B/C—average; long read length; lowest experimental cost but high cost per Mb; short run time (but long library prep.)
316 Chip		2–3 h	~400	400 Mb	$550	~$1.38	A/B—good; similar to the 314 chip but higher throughput
318 Chip		2–3 h	~400	~1 Gb	$750	~$0,75	A/B—good; similar to the 316 chip but higher throughput
Ion Proton	4–6 h						
Chip I		2–4 h	~200	~10 Gb	~$1 k	~$0,1	B/A—average; longer reads than HiSeq; low cost per Mb
Chip II		2–4 h	~200	~100 Gb	~$1 k	~$0,01	A/B—good, longer reads than HiSeq; lowest cost per Mb

[a]Instrument time for maximum read length

[b]Initial letter indicates the author's opinion of the overall utility (grade) for a platform for metagenomic-based detection. Utility grades combine data characteristics, cost of data, and ease of assembling the data into the final desired product. Major considerations for utility grades are noted

[c]Roche recently announced that the 454 sequencers will be phased out in mid-2016

2. If necessary, convert the data into a file format, such as FASTQ or FASTA with a corresponding quality file, that is compatible with most sequence analysis software and applications (*see* **Note 4**).
3. Perform a quality control on the data (investigate read length, quality score, and sequence complexity distributions, as well as sequence duplication and number of ambiguous bases) and preprocess the data accordingly. The PrinSeq software can be used both for the quality control and the preprocessing (*see* **Note 5**).
4. Assemble the reads into longer continuous sequences (contigs). The MIRA assembler can be used for data from most available platforms and is publicly available [33] (*see* **Note 6**). There also exist alternative assemblers (*see* **Note 7**).
5. Complete BLASTN, BLASTX, and tBLASTx searches against local copies of NCBI's nucleotide and protein databases using an updated version of NCBI's blast program to enable taxonomic classification (*see* **Note 8**). This can be performed for both reads and contigs. For parsing of blast results, we would recommend using either a custom-made script (*see* **Note 9**) or a ready software solution, such as MEGAN (MEtaGenome ANalyzer) [26].
6. For potential pathogens identified during the evaluation of BLAST results, retrieve candidate reference genomes from GenBank in FASTA format. Map reads and/or contigs against the reference genomes to allow analysis and visualization of similarities and coverage distribution (*see* **Note 10**).

3.6 Verification and Retrieval of Near-Full Genome Sequences

1. Based on the results from the alignments, use the Primer3 program [27] (or similar software) to design PCR primers to confirm the presence of virus in the original material and to close gaps.
2. Extract RNA and DNA from the original material as above, but without nuclease treatment.
3. Generate cDNA by using a first-strand cDNA synthesis kit with random hexamers according to the manufacturer's instructions.
4. PCR products with an expected length shorter than 1,500 bp can be obtained by using a standard DNA polymerase assay. For longer fragments, it is recommended to use a high-fidelity long-range DNA polymerase system, such as the Phusion Hot Start II High-Fidelity system. Optimize reaction conditions, such as annealing temperature, if necessary.
5. Separate the amplified products on an agarose gel and visualize and extract the DNA bands of interest by using a UV transilluminator and a scalpel (for an alternative procedure without potentially damaging UV illumination, *see* **Note 11**).

6. Purify the PCR products by using a column-based gel extraction kit.
7. Perform Sanger sequencing (either in-house or by using a commercial sequencing service). Longer distances can be covered by iterative primer walking and repeated sequencing (*see* **Note 12**).
8. Obtained sequences should be incorporated into the alignment against the reference genome.

4 Notes

1. On the use of bioinformatics, centers, and in-house solutions. One of the major obstacles to using HTS methodologies for detection of viruses is the need for server solutions for bioinformatics analysis as well as for storage of data. Most sequencing centers provide basic bioinformatics as part of their services, but for more in-depth analysis, the baseline service might not be sufficient. The best cost/benefit solution is to attach a bioinformatician to the group and access either a national high-performance center for computing or a local-/university-based solution. The second best alternative is to build the capacity yourself by expanding the group with bioinformaticians and server solutions for handling the data; there, our recommendations are the minimum recommendations. The third option is to outsource the analysis to a commercial partner and/or another group with the needed expertise. This is the least favored option due to the loss of control over a major part of the project.
2. Kits from other manufacturers can be used, but it is preferable to use nucleic acid extraction systems incorporating a spin or vacuum column. This allows for efficient removal of inhibitors since nucleic acid trapped in a silica gel membrane can be very effectively washed before elution [28].
3. For each sample, the SISPA products (from DNA and cDNA, respectively) can be pooled (unless there is a specific reason not to). Additionally, when sequencing SISPA material on HTS platforms that permit longer read lengths (300–600 bp), an alternative to fragmentation is to perform direct size selection since the majority of the SISPA products already are within this size range, as illustrated in Fig. 2. This can be performed by traditional gel electrophoresis or by an automated preparative gel electrophoresis system, such as the Pippin Prep (Sage Science).
4. Most sequencing platforms can deliver the data in a variety of output formats, including FASTQ or FASTA with a corresponding quality (QUAL) file. One noticeable exception is the Roche/454

platform that generates a binary standard flowgram format (SFF) file. However, the Roche/454 software usually comes bundled with "off-instrument" applications that allow conversion from SFF to FASTA and QUAL files. An alternative solution is to use the seq_crumbs package (http://bioinf.comav.upv.es/seq_crumbs/). For the use with certain assemblers, it is also useful to extract the trace.info file in XML format.

5. The PrinSeq software for quality control and preprocessing of metagenomic datasets is a powerful tool for assessing the validity of a dataset [21]. Except for the normal quality measures, such as sequence length and base qualities, PrinSeq also enables the user to overview several statistics valuable for assessing metagenomic datasets. Among these are tag sequence contamination, complexity, and a measurement of possible sequence contamination. PrinSeq can also be used to trim adaptor regions, filter low-quality and low-complexity reads, as well as remove platform-specific duplicates, an artifact of the sequencing technology.
6. The MIRA (Mimicking Intelligent Read Assembly) software is one of the more accomplished stand-alone noncommercial assemblers. For assembly aimed at metagenomes, standard settings for de novo assembly should be sufficient. Consult the MIRA manual for suggested settings and required preprocessing of data.
7. There are several assemblers suitable for assembly of metagenomic datasets. Except for MIRA, the Newbler assembler can be used with good result for 454 and Ion Torrent data. Both MetaVelvet and Ray Meta can produce assemblies taking mixed genomic material into account. For increased quality, several assemblies should be compared, resulting in a master list of verified contigs (sequences that are found in more than one assembly), thereby removing assembly artifacts as an error source.
8. The BLAST software suite released by NCBI can perform a number of different types of homology searches of nucleotide query sequences against databases of nucleotide and amino acid sequences. Updated and preformatted nucleotide and protein databases can be obtained from NCBI as compressed archives (ftp://ftp.ncbi.nih.gov/blast/db/). When performing a BLAST search, it is possible to configure parameters or settings to specify BLAST algorithm, database(s) to be searched, output format, cutoff levels, etc. For example, to compare nucleotide sequence(s) against a nucleotide database with BLASTn and receive the result in XML format, the command would be: blastn –query 'your_query_file'.fasta –db 'your_database' –out 'your_result' –outfmt 5. For more information, see the manual at http://www.ncbi.nlm.nih.gov/books/NBK1763/. In addition to BLASTn, it is preferable to also

perform homology searches with BLASTx, using a nucleotide query toward a protein database, and tBLASTx, querying a translated nucleotide toward a translated nucleotide database. Together, these three search strategies allow an increasingly wider homology search to be performed, enabling direct mapping toward known organisms, indirect mapping toward similar proteins, and finally mapping toward protein families.

9. Tools for computational molecular biology and bioinformatics have been developed using both Perl and Python, two general-purpose scripting languages, and are now being distributed in the modules BioPerl [29] and Biopython [30]. Both have useful tools for parsing BLAST result files in XML format and can be used to create custom-made scripts. More information and installation instructions can be found at http://www.bioperl.org/ and http://biopython.org/.
10. This can be performed by using combinations of sequence aligners and visualization software. The results from aligners such as Bowtie2 [31] and bwa [32] can be inspected using the Integrative Genomics Viewer (IGV) [33]. Another possibility is to use MUMmer and DisplayMUMs [34], or the commercial software CodonCode Aligner (CodonCode Corporation).
11. As an alternative to UV illumination, it is recommended to use SYBR Gold staining and a blue-light transilluminator, such as Safe Imager 2.0 (Invitrogen) or Dark Reader (Clare Chemical).
12. Primer walking can be used to sequence PCR fragments that are too long to be sequenced in a single round of Sanger sequencing. First use the PCR primers that generated the fragment to perform Sanger sequencing from both ends of the fragment. New PCR primers are then designed at the end of the obtained sequences, close to the region not yet covered. Perform another round of Sanger sequencing with the new primers and repeat the procedure if necessary until the whole fragment has been sequenced.

Acknowledgments

The authors would especially like to thank Professor José Manuel Sánchez-Vizcaíno (Animal Health Department, Complutense University of Madrid, Madrid, Spain) and his research group for their contribution to the original paper on which this chapter was based. This work was supported by Epi-SEQ, a research project supported under the 2nd joint call for transnational research projects by EMIDA ERA-NET (FP7 project nr 219235); by the Award of Excellence (Excellensbidrag), provided to SB by the Swedish University of Agricultural Sciences (SLU); and by/executed in the framework of the EU project AniBioThreat (Grant Agreement: Home/2009/ISEC/AG/191) with the financial support from the Prevention of and Fight against Crime Programme of the European Union, European Commission—Directorate General Home Affairs. This publication reflects the views only of the authors, and the European Commission cannot be held responsible for any use, which may be made of the information contained therein. The funders had no role in the study design, data collection and analysis, decision to publish, or preparation of the manuscript.

References

1. Cheval J, Sauvage V, Frangeul L et al (2011) Evaluation of high-throughput sequencing for identifying known and unknown viruses in biological samples. J Clin Microbiol 49:3268–3275
2. Lipkin WI (2010) Microbe hunting. Microbiol Mol Biol Rev 74:363–377
3. Nakamura S, Nakaya T, Iida T (2011) Metagenomic analysis of bacterial infections by means of high-throughput DNA sequencing. Exp Biol Med (Maywood) 236:968–971
4. Tang P, Chiu C (2010) Metagenomics for the discovery of novel human viruses. Future Microbiol 5:177–189
5. Daly GM, Bexfield N, Heaney J et al (2011) A viral discovery methodology for clinical biopsy samples utilising massively parallel next generation sequencing. PLoS One 6:e28879
6. Delwart EL (2007) Viral metagenomics. Rev Med Virol 17:115–131
7. Allander T, Tammi MT, Eriksson M et al (2005) Cloning of a human parvovirus by molecular screening of respiratory tract samples. Proc Natl Acad Sci U S A 102:12891–12896
8. Allander T, Emerson SU, Engle RE, Purcell RH, Bukh J (2001) A virus discovery method incorporating DNase treatment and its application to the identification of two bovine parvovirus species. Proc Natl Acad Sci U S A 98:11609–11614
9. Victoria JG, Kapoor A, Dupuis K, Schnurr DP, Delwart EL (2008) Rapid identification of known and new RNA viruses from animal tissues. PLoS Pathog 4:e1000163
10. Djikeng A, Halpin R, Kuzmickas R et al (2008) Viral genome sequencing by random priming methods. BMC Genomics 9:5
11. Reyes GR, Kim JP (1991) Sequence-independent, single-primer amplification (SISPA) of complex DNA populations. Mol Cell Probes 5:473–481
12. Rosseel T, Scheuch M, Höper D (2012) DNase SISPA-next generation sequencing confirms Schmallenberg virus in Belgian field samples and identifies genetic variation in Europe. PLoS One 7:e41967
13. Ambrose HE, Clewley JP (2006) Virus discovery by sequence-independent genome amplification. Rev Med Virol 16:365–383
14. Karlsson OE, Belák S, Granberg F (2013) The effect of preprocessing by sequence-independent, single-primer amplification (SISPA) on metagenomic detection of viruses. Biosecur Bioterror 11(S1):S227–S234
15. Rosseel T, Van Borm S, Vandenbussche F et al (2013) The origin of biased sequence depth in sequence-independent nucleic acid amplification and optimization for efficient massive parallel sequencing. PLoS One 8:e76144
16. Linnarsson S (2010) Recent advances in DNA sequencing methods—general principles of sample preparation. Exp Cell Res 316:1339–1343
17. Palacios G, Druce J, Du L et al (2008) A new arenavirus in a cluster of fatal transplant-associated diseases. N Engl J Med 358:991–998
18. Briese T, Paweska JT, McMullan LK et al (2009) Genetic detection and characterization of Lujo virus, a new hemorrhagic fever-associated arenavirus from southern Africa. PLoS Pathog 5:e1000455
19. Cox-Foster DL, Conlan S, Holmes EC et al (2007) A metagenomic survey of microbes in honey bee colony collapse disorder. Science 318:283–287
20. Loman NJ, Misra RV, Dallman TJ et al (2012) Performance comparison of benchtop high-throughput sequencing platforms. Nat Biotechnol 30:434–439
21. Schmieder R, Edwards R (2011) Quality control and preprocessing of metagenomic datasets. Bioinformatics 27:863–864

22. Pirk CWW, Miranda JR, Kramer M, et al. (2013) Statistical guidelines for Apis mellifera research. J Apic Res 52 (doi: 10.3896/IBRA.1.52.4.13)
23. Granberg F, Vicente-Rubiano M, Rubio-Guerri C et al (2013) Metagenomic detection of viral pathogens in Spanish honeybees: co-infection by Aphid lethal paralysis, Israel acute paralysis and Lake Sinai viruses. PLoS One 8:e57459
24. Belák S, Karlsson OE, Leijon M, Granberg F (2013) High-throughput sequencing in veterinary infection biology and diagnostics. Rev Sci Tech 32:893–915
25. Glenn TC (2011) Field guide to next-generation DNA sequencers. Mol Ecol Resour 11:759–769
26. Huson DH, Mitra S, Ruscheweyh HJ, Weber N, Schuster SC (2011) Integrative analysis of environmental sequences using MEGAN4. Genome Res 21:1552–1560
27. Rozen S, Skaletsky H (2000) Primer3 on the WWW for general users and for biologist programmers. Methods Mol Biol 132:365–386
28. Ratcliff RM, Chang G, Kok T, Sloots TP (2007) Molecular diagnosis of medical viruses. Curr Issues Mol Biol 9:87–102
29. Cock PJ, Antao T, Chang JT et al (2009) Biopython: freely available Python tools for computational molecular biology and bioinformatics. Bioinformatics 25:1422–1423
30. Stajich JE, Block D, Boulez K et al (2002) The Bioperl toolkit: Perl modules for the life sciences. Genome Res 12:1611–1618
31. Langmead B, Salzberg SL (2012) Fast gapped-read alignment with Bowtie 2. Nat Methods 9:357–359
32. Li H, Durbin R (2009) Fast and accurate short read alignment with Burrows-Wheeler transform. Bioinformatics 25:1754–1760
33. Thorvaldsdottir H, Robinson JT, Mesirov JP (2013) Integrative Genomics Viewer (IGV): high-performance genomics data visualization and exploration. Brief Bioinform 14:178–192
34. Kurtz S, Phillippy A, Delcher AL et al (2004) Versatile and open software for comparing large genomes. Genome Biol 5:R12

Chapter 34

Proteomics Characterization of Tick-Host-Pathogen Interactions

Marina Popara, Margarita Villar, and José de la Fuente

Abstract

Ticks are blood-feeding arthropod ectoparasites of wild and domestic animals that transmit disease-causing pathogens to humans and animals worldwide and a good model for the characterization of tick-host-pathogen interactions. Tick-host-pathogen interactions consist of dynamic processes involving genetic traits of hosts, pathogens, and ticks that mediate their development and survival. Proteomics provides information on the protein content of cells and tissues that may differ from results at the transcriptomics level and may be relevant for basic biological studies and vaccine antigen discovery. In this chapter, we describe various methods for protein extraction and for proteomics analysis in ticks based on one-dimensional gel electrophoresis to characterize tick-host-pathogen interactions. Particularly relevant for this characterization is the use of blood-fed ticks. Therefore, we put special emphasis on working with replete ticks collected after feeding on vertebrate hosts.

Key words Tick-host-pathogen interactions, Proteomics, Protein extraction, Mass spectrometry, LC-MS/MS, Electrophoresis

1 Introduction

Ticks are blood-feeding arthropod ectoparasites of wild and domestic animals that transmit disease-causing pathogens to humans and animals worldwide [1–3]. Tick-host-pathogen interactions consist of dynamic processes involving genetic traits of hosts, pathogens, and ticks that mediate their development and survival [2–4]. In the early 1990s, a cost-effective alternative for tick control became commercially available with the development of vaccines reducing the use of acaricides and the problems associated with them such as selection of acaricide-resistant ticks and the contamination of the environment and animal products with pesticide residues [5]. However, new vaccines are needed for efficient control of vector infestations and pathogen infection and transmission [6].

Mónica V. Cunha and João Inácio (eds.), *Veterinary Infection Biology: Molecular Diagnostics and High-Throughput Strategies*, Methods in Molecular Biology, vol. 1247, DOI 10.1007/978-1-4939-2004-4_34, © Springer Science+Business Media New York 2015

In the post-genomics era, proteomics has emerged as a powerful new tool that includes strategies for the characterization of dynamic interactions that cannot be analyzed by genomics or transcriptomics approaches alone. This technique provides information on the protein content of cells and tissues that may differ from results at the transcriptomics level and may be relevant for basic biological studies and vaccine antigen discovery [2, 3, 6–9]. Regarding proteomics of blood-sucking arthropods, a significant number of studies were done primarily on mosquitoes, sandflies, and tsetse flies [10]. The sequence databases of tick species of agricultural and medical importance are constantly increasing, which enabled the expansion of research into the field of proteomics [11]. However, the application of proteomics research on ticks is still at its infancy [2]. The only tick genome close to completion is that of the black-legged deer tick, *Ixodes scapularis* [12, 13], with 26,066 proteins currently in the UniProt database (data from January 2014). However, for other tick species of medical importance such as *Rhipicephalus*, *Dermacentor*, and *Amblyomma* species, protein information in the databases is very limited, thus making proteomics research in this area very difficult.

Few studies have covered proteomics research in ticks [2, 9–11, 14–17]. Furthermore, some of these studies were done using tick cells lines, but work with ticks is more complex because, in most cases, proteins from the vector, the vector-borne symbionts or pathogenic microorganisms, and the vertebrate hosts are identified [2, 7]. Therefore, proteomics techniques need to be refined to adequately address these challenges. In this chapter, we describe various methods for protein extraction and for proteomics analysis in ticks based on one-dimensional gel electrophoresis to characterize tick-host-pathogen interactions. Particularly relevant for this characterization is the use of blood-fed ticks. Therefore, we put special emphasis on working with replete ticks collected after feeding on vertebrate hosts.

2 Materials

All reagents used for buffer preparations need to be of analytical grade. The solutions are prepared with ultrapure water and stored at 4 °C, except for the solutions containing SDS that are stored at 20 °C to avoid detergent precipitation. Reagents for protein digestions and mass spectrometry analysis need to be of liquid chromatography-mass spectrometry (LC-MS) grade.

2.1 Tick Samples

Ticks are collected after feeding on vertebrate hosts, including both domestic and wild animals. After repletion, ticks are collected and stored in 70 % ethanol at 4 °C until processed (*see* **Note 1**).

2.2 Protein Extraction Buffers

1. Buffer 1: 10 mM phosphate-buffered saline (PBS), pH 7.4 (0.26 g of KH_2PO_4, 2.17 g of $Na_2HPO_4.7H_2O$, 8.71 g of NaCl) supplemented with 1 % sodium dodecyl sulfate (SDS). For preparation of buffer 1, add 1 ml of 10 % stock solution of SDS to 9 ml of 10 mM PBS pH 7.4 and mix (*see* **Note 2**). The buffer is also supplemented with 1 tablet of complete mini protease inhibitor cocktail (Roche, Basel, Switzerland) per 10 ml of solution.
2. Buffer 2: 10 mM PBS, pH 7.4, supplemented with 1 % octyl phenol ethoxylate (Triton X-100). For preparation of buffer 2, add 1 ml of 10 % stock solution of Triton X-100 to 9 ml of 10 mM PBS pH 7.4 and mix (*see* **Note 2**). The buffer is also supplemented with 1 tablet of complete mini protease inhibitor cocktail per 10 ml of solution.
3. Buffer 3: 10 mM PBS, pH 7.4, supplemented with 1 % polyethylene glycol sorbitan monolaurate (Tween 20). For preparation of buffer 3, add 1 ml of 10 % stock solution of Tween 20 to 9 ml of 10 mM PBS pH 7.4 and mix (*see* **Note 2**). The buffer is also supplemented with 1 tablet of complete mini protease inhibitor cocktail per 10 ml of solution.
4. Buffer 4: 7 M urea, 2 M thiourea, 4 % CHAPS, 20 % glycerol, 200 mM KCl and 100 mM sodium hydrogen phosphate dihydrate, pH 7.4. Weigh 4.2 g of urea, 1.52 g of thiourea, 0.4 g of CHAPS, 0.015 g of KCl, and 0.36 g of $Na_2HPO_4.2H_2O$. Add 9 ml of water, m*ix*, and make up to 10 ml with water. The buffer is also supplemented with 1 tablet of complete mini protease inhibitor cocktail per 10 ml of solution.

2.3 Laemmli Sample Buffer

0.125 M Tris–HCl, pH 6.8, 4 % SDS, 20 % glycerol, 0.004 % bromophenol blue, and 10 % β-mercaptoethanol. Mix 1.51 g of Tris–HCl, 4 g of SDS, 20 ml of glycerol, and 0.004 g of bromophenol blue and bring up the volume to 100 ml with water. Make aliquots of 1 ml and store at −20 °C. Supplement the buffer with 10 % final of β-mercaptoethanol before use.

2.4 SDS-PAGE Gel Components

1. Resolving gel buffer: 1.5 M Tris–HCl, pH 8.8. Weigh 181.7 g of Tris, add water to a volume of 900 ml, adjust to pH 8.8 with HCl, and make up to 1 L.
2. Stacking gel buffer: 1.5 M Tris–HCl, pH 6.5. Weigh 181.7 g of Tris, add water to a volume of 900 ml, adjust to pH 6.5 with HCl, and make up to 1 L.
3. Resolving gel: Mix 2.5 ml of resolving gel buffer, 4 ml of 30 % acrylamide/bis-acrylamide solution (Bio-Rad, Hercules, CA, USA), 100 μl of 10 % SDS, and 4 ml of water and mix well. Add 100 μl of 10 % ammonium persulfate and 5 μl of TEMED and cast gel.

4. Stacking gel: Mix 0.84 ml of stacking gel buffer, 0.84 ml of 30 % acrylamide/bis-acrylamide solution, 50 μl of 10 % SDS, and 3 ml of water and mix well. Add 50 μl of 10 % ammonium persulfate and 5 μl of TEMED and cast gel.
5. Make 1.5 mm-thick gels with wells of 5 mm wide for conventional one-dimensional gels and 1.2 cm wide for proteome band concentration.

2.5 SDS-PAGE Running Buffer

Tris-glycine SDS-PAGE buffer (10×): 0.25 M Tris–HCl, pH 8.3, 1.92 M glycine, and 1 % SDS. This buffer is diluted 10 times with water before use.

2.6 Protein In-Gel Digestion Buffers

1. 50 mM ammonium bicarbonate, pH 8.8: Add 0.04 g of ammonium bicarbonate to 9 ml of LC-MS grade water, mix, and adjust pH to 8.8 with 5 N ammonium hydroxide. Complete to 10 ml with water to obtain a 50 mM final solution.
2. 10 mM dithiothreitol (DTT): Add 1.54 mg of DTT to 1 ml of 50 mM ammonium bicarbonate, pH 8.8.
3. 55 mM iodoacetamide: Add 10.2 mg to 1 ml of 50 mM ammonium bicarbonate, pH 8.8.
4. Sequencing grade trypsin (Promega, Madison, WI, USA) is dissolved in 50 mM ammonium bicarbonate, pH 8.8, to a final concentration of 60 ng/μl.

2.7 Other Reagents, Consumables, Equipments, and Software

1. Ice-cold acetone.
2. Trifluoroacetic acid.
3. 0.1 % formic acid.
4. 10 % (v/v) acetonitrile.
5. Methanol.
6. Chloroform.
7. GelCode Blue Stain Reagent (Thermo Scientific, San Jose, CA, USA).
8. BCA Protein Assay (Thermo Scientific, San Jose, CA, USA).
9. Liquid nitrogen.
10. Sterilized mortar and pestle.
11. Syringe equipped with a 21 gauge needle.
12. OMIX pipette tips C18 (Agilent Technologies, Santa Clara, CA, USA).
13. Ultrasonic cooled bath.
14. SDS-PAGE apparatus.
15. Centrifuge.
16. Freezer (−20 °C).
17. Vertical rotating shaker.
18. Confocal microscope.

19. Reverse-phase liquid chromatography-mass spectrometer (we use Easy-nLC II system coupled to an ion trap LCQ Fleet mass spectrometer, Thermo Scientific, San Jose, CA, USA).
20. SEQUEST algorithm (Proteome Discoverer 1.3, Thermo Scientific, San Jose, CA, USA).
21. PEAKS Studio v 6.0 software (Bioinformatics Solutions Inc., Waterloo, Ontario, Canada).

3 Methods

3.1 General Considerations

Up to date, tick proteome characterization has not been widely developed, and the methodologies used are based on the analysis of either unfed ticks or the specific tick tissue of interest. Herein, we focus on establishing standardized conditions to work with replete ticks after feeding on vertebrate hosts and with one-dimensional gel electrophoresis. One important consideration, especially for quantitative proteomics analysis, is to perform protein extraction as simple as possible reducing the number of steps to minimum in order to avoid protein losses during the extraction procedure. The application of detergents for protein solubilization in a sample is widely used for routine protein extraction as for the enrichment of membrane proteins that are involved in the first contact between pathogen, vector, and the host. However, to date, there is no universal detergent or detergent mixtures that allow the complete solubilization of all proteins in the sample. For proteomics analysis, buffers based on the use of chaotropic reagents such as urea and thiourea, combined with detergents and salts are also widely used for protein solubilization in one single step. Therefore, the optimal method always needs to be determined empirically depending on the sample type.

3.2 Tick Protein Extraction

Carry out all the procedures at 4 °C until the SDS-containing buffer is used, requiring 20 °C to avoid detergent precipitation:

1. Remove the ticks from the ethanol storage and leave for 1–2 min in a fume hood to evaporate excess of ethanol.
2. Remove the cuticle by dissecting the ticks using a confocal microscope and add 10 mM PBS for constant hydration of the tissues during dissection (*see* **Note 3**).
3. Homogenize the tick internal organs by quick-freezing in liquid nitrogen and pulverizing with a sterilized mortar and pestle.
4. Add at least 2 ml of protein extraction buffer 1, 2, 3, or 4 per 100 μg of tissue. Homogenize in a glass homogenizer with a minimum of 10 strokes of a glass rod.
5. Sonicate the sample for 1 min in an ultrasonic cooled bath followed by 10 s vortex and leave to rest on ice for 1 min. Repeat these cycles 2–3 times or until the sample becomes

completely solubilized. Moderately shake the crude extracts for 20 min at 4 °C and then additionally pass the extract through a syringe equipped with a 21 gauge needle to assist breakdown of remaining nucleic acids.

6. Centrifuge the samples for 5 min at 200 × *g* at 20 °C to remove the cell debris.
7. Collect the supernatant, quantify the protein content of the crude extracts with the BCA Protein Assay (Table 1), and analyze by SDS-PAGE (Fig. 1), according to standard procedures.

Table 1

Identification of proteins extracted using different extraction buffers[a]

Database search	Buffer 1	Buffer 2	Buffer 3	Buffer 4
Ixodida	62.9 %	48.2 %	44.4 %	82.0 %
Pecora	72.4 %	44.2 %	40.2 %	72.7 %

[a]The efficacy of different detergents on tick protein extraction is compared by using protein extraction buffers 1–4. We have observed that extraction with buffer 4 gives the highest yield for both tick and host proteins identification, compared to the detergent-based buffers 1–3. Of the three detergent-based buffers, SDS-containing buffer 1 shows the best efficiency in proteins extraction, whereas the nonionic detergents in buffers 2 and 3, Triton X-100 and Tween 20, show similar values for protein extraction. Proteins are expressed as percentages of the total proteins identified

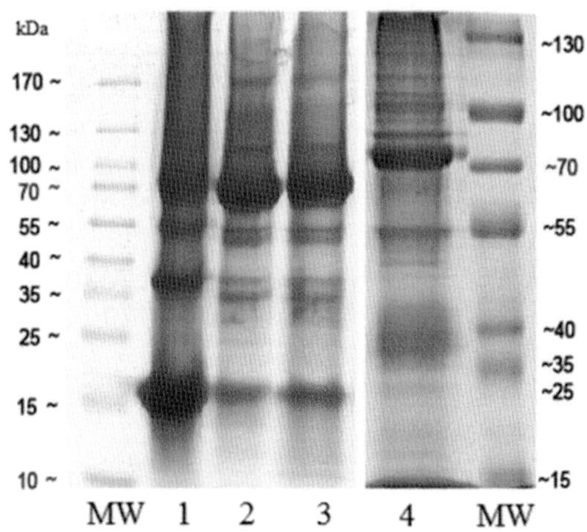

Fig. 1 Representative one-dimensional SDS-PAGE gel showing protein band patterns in extracts prepared using different protein extraction buffers. (1) Proteins extracted with buffer 1. (2) Proteins extracted with buffer 2. (3) Proteins extracted with buffer 3. (4) Proteins extracted with buffer 4. MW: molecular weight markers (PageRuler Plus Prestained Protein Ladder, Scientific, San Jose, CA, USA). Twenty micrograms of soluble fractions are run on a 5 mm wide conventional 12 % SDS-PAGE gel performing electrophoresis at 180 V of constant voltage. Bands are visualized by staining with GelCode Blue Stain Reagent by manufacturer's protocol

3.3 Protein Fractionation Method

In this extraction method, an additional step is introduced for sample processing, thus resulting in the fractionation of the crude extract into cytosolic (supernatant) and plasma membrane-associated (pellet) protein fractions:

1. Extract the tick proteins following the same steps as in the previous method (Subheading 3.2, **steps 1–6**).
2. After the centrifugation at 200×*g*, additionally centrifuge the obtained supernatant at 12,000×*g* for 20 min obtaining two fractions: cytosolic-enriched protein supernatant and crude plasma membrane-enriched protein pellet.
3. Collect the supernatant and quantify the protein content with the BCA Protein Assay (Fig. 2a) (*see* **Note 4**).
4. Resuspend the pellet containing the crude plasma membrane fraction directly in 100 μl of Laemmli sample buffer and leave on a vertical rotating shaker for 30 min to 1 h at 20 °C with vigorous shaking to enable solubilization.
5. Centrifuge the sample for 30 s on a benchtop centrifuge to remove insoluble fragments and collect the supernatant (Fig. 2b) (*see* **Note 5**).

3.4 Proteome In-Gel Digestion

1. Precipitate 200 μg of protein extracts to be analyzed by adding four volumes of ice-cold acetone to one volume of sample. Vortex the mixture, incubate at −20 °C for at least 4 h, and centrifuge at 12,000×*g* for 15 min at 4 °C. Discard the supernatant, air-dry the pellet, and resuspend in 100 μl of Laemmli sample buffer supplemented with 5 % β-mercaptoethanol.
2. Apply the samples onto 1.2 cm wide wells in a 12 % SDS-PAGE gel.
3. Stop the electrophoretic run as soon as the front enters 3 mm into the resolving gel, so that the whole proteome becomes concentrated in the stacking/resolving gel interface (*see* **Note 6**).
4. Stain with GelCode Blue Stain Reagent for visualization of the unseparated protein bands, excise the gel-containing bands, cut into 2×2 mm cubes, and transfer into a microcentrifuge tube.
5. Destain gel pieces, alternating 50 mM ammonium bicarbonate/acetonitrile (1:1, v/v) with neat acetonitrile, incubating for 10 min at room temperature with occasional vortexing until the gel pieces become white and shrink; remove acetonitrile; and dry gel pieces.
6. Cover gel pieces with 60 ng/μl of sequencing grade trypsin at 5:1 protein/trypsin (w/w) ratio in 50 mM ammonium bicarbonate, pH 8.8, containing 10 % (v/v) acetonitrile and leave it in an ice bucket for 2 h to saturate them with trypsin. If all solution was absorbed, add 20–30 μl of 50 mM ammonium bicarbonate and digest overnight at 37 °C.

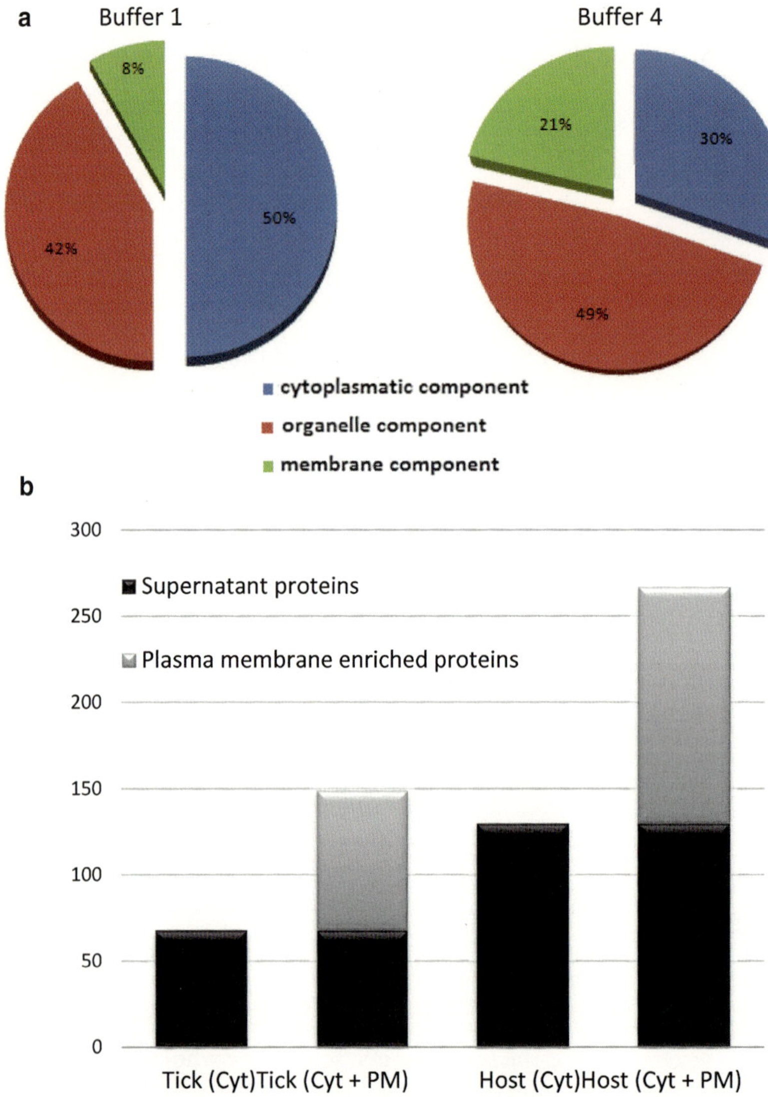

Fig. 2 The subcellular distribution of the extracted proteins depends on the buffer used. (**a**) Subcellular distribution of identified tick proteins after extraction with buffer 1 and buffer 4. We observed that buffer 4, a more astringent buffer, allows the extraction of a greater number of internal organelle and membrane proteins. (**b**) Number of identified tick and host proteins in the different fractions obtained using the buffer 1. An average of 41 % increase in the number of tick proteins and up to 72 % for host proteins is detected when crude plasma membrane fraction is included in the analysis compared to the supernatant fraction only. Therefore, it is necessary to process both fractions, cytoplasmatic soluble, and plasma membrane pellet, obtained after detergent extraction and separated by ultracentrifugation, in order to characterize the entire proteome. Identification is performed using the SEQUEST algorithm of Proteome Discoverer 1.3 against Ixodida and Ruminantia databases for tick and host proteins identification, respectively. An FDR<0.05 for tick and an FDR<0.01 for host proteins identification are considered as cutoff. Abbreviations: Cyt, cytoplasmic soluble protein fraction; PM, plasma membrane protein fraction

7. Add trifluoroacetic acid to a final concentration of 1 % to stop the digestion.
8. Desalt the samples using OMIX pipette tips C18 following the manufacturer instructions, vacuum dry, and store at −20 °C until the mass spectrometry analysis.

3.5 Reverse-Phase Liquid Chromatography (RP-LC)-MS/MS Analysis

1. Resuspend the protein digests in 0.1 % formic acid and analyze by RP-LC-MS/MS in an Easy-nLC II system coupled to an ion trap LCQ Fleet mass spectrometer (Thermo Scientific, San Jose, CA, USA).
2. The peptides are concentrated (online) by reverse-phase chromatography using a 0.1 mm × 20 mm C18 RP precolumn (Thermo Scientific) and then separated using a 0.075 mm × 100 mm C18 RP column (Thermo Scientific) operating at 0.3 μl/min.
3. Elution of peptides is done using a 180 min gradient from 5 to 35 % solvent B (solvent A, 0.1 % formic acid in water; solvent B, 0.1 % formic acid in acetonitrile). ESI ionization is done with nano-bore emitters stainless steel ID 30 μm (Thermo Scientific) interface (*see* **Note 7**).
4. Peptides are detected in survey scans from 400 to 1,600 amu (1 μscan), followed by three data-dependent MS/MS scans (Top 3), using an isolation width of 2 in mass-to-charge ratio units, normalized collision energy of 35 %, and dynamic exclusion applied during 30 s periods (*see* **Note 8**).

3.6 Proteomics Data Analysis

Peptide identification from raw data is carried out using the SEQUEST algorithm (Proteome Discoverer 1.3, Thermo Scientific):

1. Database search is performed against Uniprot-Ixodida.fasta (57,021 entries in January 2014), Uniprot-Pecora.fasta (67,200 entries in January 2014), and Uniprot-Alphaproteobacteria.fasta (2,480,730 entries in January 2014) (http://www.uniprot.org) for tick, host, and pathogen proteins identification, respectively.
2. The following constraints may be used for the searches: tryptic cleavage after Arg and Lys, up to two missed cleavage sites, and tolerances of 1 Da for precursor ions and 0.8 Da for MS/MS fragment ions and the searches were performed allowing optional Met oxidation and Cys carbamidomethylation. Search against decoy database (integrated decoy approach) is done using false discovery rate (FDR) <0.01.

3.7 Hemoglobin Removal

In ticks collected after feeding on a host, the major constrain for the successful protein identification is the large amount of the host proteins, predominantly blood. These proteins, such as hemoglobin, serum albumin, and immunoglobulins, are very abundant and mask the detection of vector and pathogen proteins. In engorged tick samples, a high abundance of host hemoglobin is detected

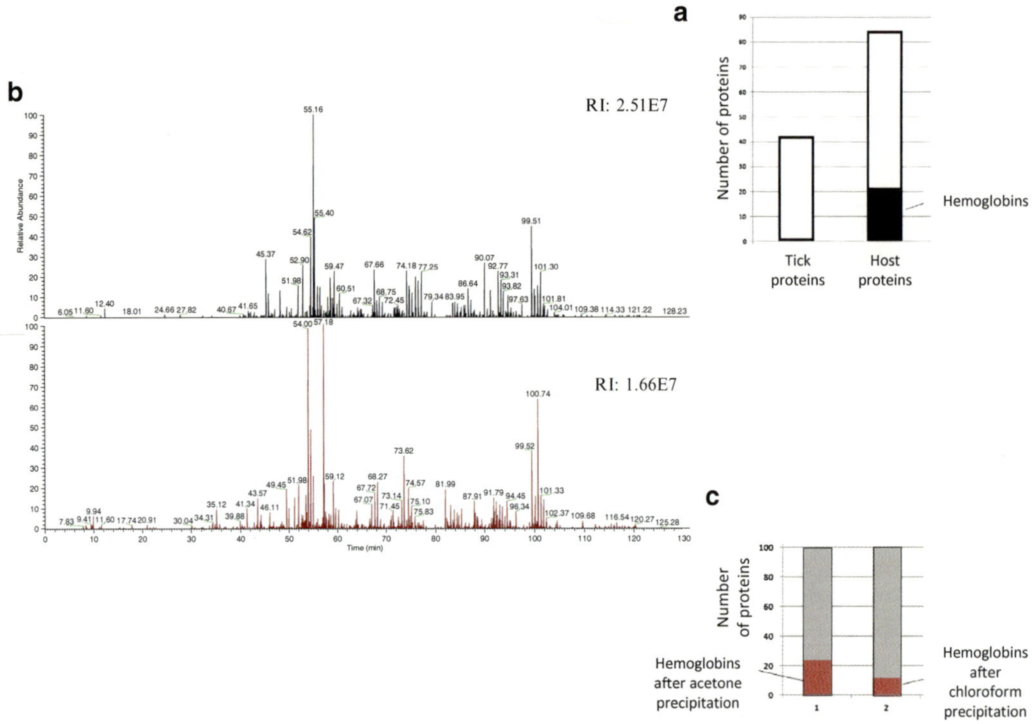

Fig. 3 Removal of host hemoglobin from tick protein samples. (**a**) Representative protein distribution in engorged tick samples. (**b**) Mass spectra comparing the MS/MS fragment peptides of two precipitation methods: acetone- (above) and chloroform-based method (below). The same profile is observed with a slight increase in the intensity of the spectra using the acetone precipitation method. (**c**) Presence of hemoglobins in the sample before and after treatment. Chloroform-methanol precipitation decreases the number of detected hemoglobins in a total sample where hemoglobins represented 14 % of total of proteins identified compared to 23 % of hemoglobins present after acetone precipitation. Additionally, the hemoglobins that remain in the sample are identified with a lower number of peptides. This method is therefore very helpful in treating the engorged tick samples, but it does not completely eliminate host hemoglobins

within an average of 20 % of the total number of identified proteins (Fig. 3a) (*see* **Note 9**). We next describe the comparison of the efficacy of two methods for removal of these hosts proteins from tick samples: a method reported to remove hemoglobin from blood samples [18] with minor modifications and a conventional precipitation method with ice-cold acetone that was used as a control:

1. Process two samples of 200 μg each of a tick protein extract.
2. One sample is directly precipitated following a conventional acetone precipitation method.
3. To the other sample, slowly add a mixture of methanol and chloroform under homogenization to a final concentration of 19 % of methanol and 0.6 % chloroform. Keep the mixture at 4 °C and homogenize for an additional 20 min to obtain

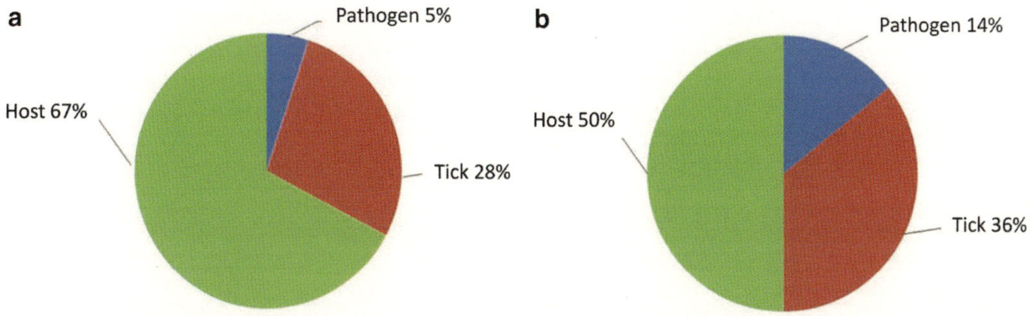

Fig. 4 Identification of tick, host, and pathogen proteins in a single sample with a high level of confidence. Protein extract of engorged ticks was obtained by total protein extraction method with buffer 4. (**a**) Database search is performed against a database composed of Uniprot-Ruminantia.fasta, Uniprot-Ixodida.fasta, and Uniprot-Alphaproteobacteria.fasta. Data is analyzed using the SEQUEST algorithm of Proteome Discoverer 1.3 software applying a 1 % FDR as criteria for assignations. (**b**) The application of de novo sequencing software PEAKS Studio 6.0 significantly increases the number of identified proteins, primarily tick and pathogen proteins that are usually masked by host proteins in engorged ticks

hemoglobin elimination. Centrifuge the sample at 2,500 × *g* for 10 min at 4 °C and discard the resulting hemoglobin containing precipitate.

4. Precipitate the resulting supernatant with acetone (*see* **Note 10**).
5. Both pellets resulting from the two methods may be dissolved in Laemmli buffer, concentrated on conventional SDS-PAGE gel and compared by LC-MS/MS analysis (Fig. 3b, c).

3.8 Pathogen Identification

Proteomics is one of the most powerful technologies that allow simultaneous detection of proteins originating from different organisms in the same sample. Pathogen proteins present in ticks can be successfully detected with a high level of confidence in the same protein extract where tick and host proteins are identified if the search is performed against a database containing pathogen proteins built by combination of Ixodida and Alphaproteobacteria UniProt databases (www.uniprot.org) (Fig. 4a).

3.9 De Novo Sequencing and Homology Analyses

PEAKS Studio v 6.0 software (Bioinformatics Solutions Inc.) permit protein identification by generating de novo peptide sequences, which is especially useful when working with organisms such as ticks with limited sequence information available. These analyses may be done with the same general parameters as for the routinely applied software Proteome Discoverer 1.3 (as described in Subheading 3.6). Additionally, in PEAKS a special algorithm is used to generate de novo sequences of the input spectrum, and the SPIDER module is used to identify variations from sequences using a homology match query. The filtering of the scores for all identified peptides is done by assigning a −10lg P value of 30 that was established after manual analyses of the obtained peptide matches to assure quality of the identifications. The application of PEAKS software using the above listed parameters gives 10 % to 20 % average increase in the number of detected proteins by applying homology search and generating de novo peptide sequences (Fig. 4b). This approach enables the identification of every peptide in the dataset, whether it is in a database or not, modified or mutated.

3.10 Quantitative Proteomics Analyses

Proteomics analyses are intended not only to obtain the identification of as many proteins as possible in a given sample but also to allow focusing on the differences between several samples of interest, which is possible through the application of quantitative proteomics techniques. Quantitative proteomics approaches can be divided into label-based or label-free methodologies depending on the use or not of stable isotopic or isobaric labeling reagents to "mark" the proteins or peptides under comparison before mass spectrometry analysis. Additionally, gel-based and gel-free approaches using multidimensional chromatography can be developed for quantitative proteomics analyses (a good review of these quantitative methodologies can be found in [19]). The combination of more than one technique is the best way to obtain greater proteome coverage and to identify a bigger number of differentially represented proteins between samples due to the complementarity of the quantitative approaches. The application of quantitative proteomics to the characterization of the tick-pathogen interface is still in its infancy [2], but its development is crucial for the identification of proteins involved in pathogen infection, multiplication, and transmission, as well as possible antigens for vaccine development.

4 Notes

1. When working in field experiments such as epidemiology studies or vaccine trials, collected ticks are generally stored in ethanol and not deep-frozen because it is easier under field conditions and makes their shipment from one lab to another cheaper. Therefore, this work focused on optimizations on this kind of samples.
2. Triton X-100 and Tween 20 detergents are diluted to a 10 % stock solution to reduce their viscosity and facilitate pipetting. SDS is also prepared in a 10 % stock solution in order to work in a similar manner.
3. Removing the cuticle from a tick enables a better detection of low-abundance tick proteins. Our previous studies showed that processing the entire tick results in the detection of over

50 % of abundant cuticle proteins masking other minority tick proteins that might be a key for understanding ticks metabolical processes. The removal of the cuticle of completely engorged ticks is relatively easy to perform. Care should be taken to completely remove the tissues around the mouthparts. However, if not working with freshly collected ticks, differentiating tick tissues is very difficult due to a large presence of coagulated host blood.

4. When using a urea-containing buffer such as buffer 4, the obtained pellet containing the protein fraction is less abundant than when using buffers 1–3 in which the solubility of the proteins is higher. However, it has to be taken into consideration that the obtained pellet protein fraction cannot be processed further since a dense and insoluble viscous pellet is formed, probably due to the accumulation of nucleic acids or coagulation of abundant host blood proteins. However, the obtained protein extracts in the soluble fraction remain stable through time and do not show signs of degradation after long-term storage. Samples of the soluble fraction, if very diluted, can be successfully concentrated using columns for protein concentration. Millipore (Billerica, MA, USA) columns give a good result, and four times concentration is accomplished by centrifuging a 1 ml sample for 10 min at 4,800 × *g*.
5. Due to the impossibility of direct quantification of insoluble pellet fraction, equal amount of micrograms of dried pellet is measured, and the protein concentration is determined by running the same amount of the sample on a one-dimensional gel and comparing to an albumin standard. Pellet is very difficult to dissolve and needs to be left on a shaker for at least 30 min. It is best to store dry pellets at −20 °C and directly solubilize them in Laemmli buffer prior to the analysis.
6. The concentration of proteins in one single band is the only gel-based approach that allows quantitative comparisons between samples without using protein-labeling approaches because all proteins from the samples under comparison are located in the same band avoiding the gel-cutting effect [20].
7. The development of long gradients promotes peptide separation and increases the number of identified proteins. When a HPLC working on microliters instead of nanoliters is used, it is recommended to increase the duration of the gradient time.
8. In the case of using a mass spectrometer with scan speed and mass resolution higher than LCQ Fleet (e.g., a LTQ), it is recommended to increase the numbers of dependent MS/MS scans to 15 or more, allowing the detection of low-abundant proteins.

9. Even in unfed ticks, host blood proteins can persist months after feeding and molting. Vertebrate actins are found in *Ixodes ricinus* nymphs and *Rhipicephalus microplus* larvae even weeks after molting [14, 16, 17].
10. When precipitating with acetone, a special care needs to be taken to allow it to evaporate from the obtained pellet before further processing. Otherwise, the efficiency of protein detection after this method decreases significantly [21, 22].

Acknowledgments

We thank the CMBSO proteomics facility (Centro de Biología Molecular Severo Ochoa, Madrid, Spain) for technical assistance. This research was supported by grants BFU2011-23896 and the EU FP7 ANTIGONE project number 278976. M. Popara is an early-stage researcher supported by the POSTICK ITN (postgraduate training network for capacity building to control ticks and tick-borne diseases) within the FP7-PEOPLE—ITN program (EU Grant No. 238511).

References

1. de la Fuente J, Estrada-Peña A, Venzal JM et al (2008) Overview: Ticks as vectors of pathogens that cause disease in humans and animals. Front Biosci 13:6938–6946
2. Villar M, Popara M, Bonzón-Kulichenko E et al (2012) Characterization of the tick-pathogen interface by quantitative proteomics. Ticks Tick Borne Dis 3:154–158
3. de la Fuente J, Kocan KM, Blouin EF et al (2010) Functional genomics and evolution of tick-Anaplasma interactions and vaccine development. Vet Parasitol 167:175–186
4. Galindo RC, de la Fuente J (2012) Transcriptomics Data integration reveals Jak-STAT as a common pathway affected by pathogenic intracellular bacteria in natural reservoir hosts. J Proteomics Bioinform 5:108–115
5. de la Fuente J, Almazán C, Canales M et al (2007) A ten-year review of commercial vaccine performance for control of tick infestations on cattle. Anim Health Res Rev 8: 23–28
6. de la Fuente J (2012) Vaccines for vector control: exciting possibilities for the future. Vet J 194:139–140
7. Villar M, Torina A, Nuñez Y et al (2010) Application of highly sensitive saturation labeling to the analysis of differential protein expression in infected ticks from limited samples. Proteome Sci 8:43
8. Sebatjane SI, Pretorius A, Liebenberg J et al (2010) In vitro and in vivo evaluation of five low molecular weight proteins of *Ehrlichia ruminantium* as potential vaccine components. Vet Immunol Immunopathol 137: 217–225
9. Marcelino I, de Almeida AM, Ventosa M et al (2012) Tick-borne diseases in cattle: applications of proteomics to develop new generation vaccines. J Proteomics 75:4232–4250
10. Patramool S, Choumet V, Surasombatpattana P et al (2012) Update on the proteomics of major arthropod vectors of human and animal pathogens. Proteomics 12:3510–3523
11. Rachinsky A, Guerrero FD, Scoles G et al (2007) Differential protein expression in ovaries of uninfected and *Babesia*-infected southern cattle ticks, *Rhipicephalus (Boophilus) microplus.* Insect Biochem Mol Biol 37: 1291–1308
12. Hill CA, Wikel SK (2005) The *Ixodes scapularis* genome project: an opportunity for advancing tick research. Trends Parasitol 21: 151–153
13. Meyer JM, Kurtti TJ, Van Zee JP, Hill CA (2010) Genome organization of major tandem

repeats in the hard tick, *Ixodes scapularis*. Chromosome Res 18:357–370
14. Villar M, Ayllón N, Busby AT et al (2010) Expression of heat shock and other stress response proteins in ticks and cultured tick cells in response to Anaplasma spp infection and heat shock. Int J Proteomics 2010:657261
15. Untalan PM, Guerrero FD, Haines LR, Pearson TW (2005) Proteome analysis of abundantly expressed proteins from unfed larvae of the cattle tick, *Boophilus microplus*. Insect Biochem Mol Biol 35:141–151
16. Vennestrøm J, Jensen PM (2007) *Ixodes ricinus*: the potential of two-dimensional gel electrophoresis as a tool for studying host-vector-pathogen interactions. Exp Parasitol 115: 53–58
17. Wickramasekara S, Bunikis J, Wysocki V, Barbour AG (2008) Identification of residual blood proteins in ticks by mass spectrometry proteomics. Emerg Infect Dis 14:1273–1275
18. Tanaka K, Sawatani E, Shigueoka EM et al (2001) Isolation of bovine plasma albumin by liquid chromatography and its polymerization for use in immunohematology. Braz J Med Biol Res 34:977–983
19. Megger DA, Bracht T, Meyer HE, Sitek B (2013) Label-free quantification in clinical proteomics. Biochim Biophys Acta 1834:1581–1590
20. Bonzon-Kulichenko E, Pérez-Hernández D, Núñez E et al. (2011) A robust method for quantitative high-throughput analysis of proteomes by 18O labeling. Mol Cell Proteomics 10(1):M110.003335
21. Fic E, Kedracka-Krok S, Jankowska U et al (2010) Comparison of protein precipitation methods for various rat brain structures prior to proteomic analysis. Electrophoresis 31:3573–3579
22. Simpson DM, Beynon RJ (2010) Acetone precipitation of proteins and the modification of peptides. J Proteome Res 9:444–450

Index

Mónica V. Cunha and João Inácio (eds.), *Veterinary Infection Biology: Molecular Diagnostics and High-Throughput Strategies*, Methods in Molecular Biology, vol. 1247, DOI 10.1007/978-1-4939-2004-4, © Springer Science+Business Media New York 2015

N

O

P

Q

R

S

T

U

V

W

X

Y

Z

Printed by Printforce, the Netherlands